Issues and Trends in Nursing: Essential Knowledge for Today and Tomorrow

Welcome to *Issues and Trends in Nursing: Essential Knowledge for Today and Tomorrow!*

Along with useful tables and figures, each chapter includes:

LEARNING OUTCOMES

These objectives provide instructors and students with a snapshot of the key information they will encounter in each chapter. They can serve as a checklist to help guide and focus study.

chapter

1

History of Nursing

Karen J. Egenes

LEARNING OUTCOMES

After reading this chapter you will be able to:

- Discuss the importance to a profession's understanding of its own history.
- Identify the contributions of selected leaders in the development of U.S. nursing.
- Trace the origins and purposes of major professional nursing organizations.
- Describe the influences of war on the development of nursing.
- Discuss the influences of faith traditions on the development of nursing.
- Analyze the impact of government on the growth of health care and the development of nursing.
- Explore the development of advanced practice roles in nursing.

History can be defined as a study of events from the past leading up to the present time. However, the study of history focuses on not just the chronology of events, but also the impact and influence those events continued to have throughout time. Over the passage of time, events unfold and trends emerge. These historical trends, in turn, influence or shape the destiny of an

1

KEY TERMS

Found in the margins throughout each chapter, these terms will create an expanded vocabulary in nursing. Visit **http://nursing.jbpub.com** to see these terms in an interactive glossary and use flashcards and word puzzles to master the definitions!

Nursing Education: Past, Present, Future

The quality of nursing programs is measured through nationally established standards or criteria. Standards can include such things as how the school is fulfilling its mission and philosophy, how its curriculum is preparing students for nursing practice, and to what extent the qualifications of nursing faculty facilitate preparing future nurses.

The NLNAC and CCNE accredit schools for a period of time, usually 8–10 years, depending upon the agency and the review findings. Throughout the accreditation period, schools continue to use professional standards as benchmarks to evaluate their program, making necessary changes to ensure they maintain quality. Contemporary Practice Highlight 2-3 addresses the essential qualities and competencies that one of nursing's professional organizations, AACN, has deemed necessary for contemporary nursing practice; this document is used as a framework by many baccalaureate schools to ensure quality curricula.

KEY TERM

Curriculum: The overall structure of learning experiences within nursing education programs that reflects a school of nursing's mission and philosophy, program outcomes, course of study, and program evaluation methods.

Curriculum and Instruction in Nursing Education

Central to nursing education is curriculum and instruction. **Curriculum** is the overall structure of nursing education programs that reflects schools' mission and philosophy, course of

CONTEMPORARY PRACTICE HIGHLIGHT 2–3

THE AACN BSN ESSENTIALS OF BACCALAUREATE EDUCATION

In 1986 the AACN developed a document titled *The Essentials of Baccalaureate Education for Professional Nursing Practice*. The purpose of the document was to provide faculty in schools of nursing with an understanding of the competencies nursing students needed to function in contemporary health-care systems. Many schools of nursing use the "essentials" to structure the curriculum of their nursing education programs. Due to social, political, and economic trends and issues this document was updated in 1998. In 2007, the AACN determined it was necessary to update the document once again. Changes in the

document will likely mean revisions are on the horizon for many nursing curricula in order to remain current and up-to-date with contemporary practice. For instance, it is anticipated that the revised document will address the need to prepare students for evidence-based practice, information management, and expertise in evaluating patient outcomes (Martin, 2007).

Similar AACN documents for master's degree and DNP programs also exist, entitled the *Essentials of Master's Education for Advanced Practice Nursing* and the *Essentials of Doctoral Education for Advanced Nursing Practice*.

CONTEMPORARY PRACTICE HIGHLIGHTS

A close look at a nursing issue and its implication for professional practice.

Visit **http://nursing.jbpub.com**

KEY TERM REVIEW
Key terms are listed and defined here for quick and easy reference.

REFLECTIVE PRACTICE QUESTIONS
Critical thinking questions highlighting relevant research or demographic findings that inform the issue and guide nursing practice.

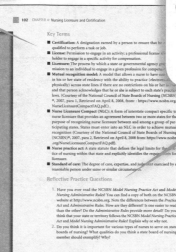

FEATURED BOXES
These colorful boxes call your attention to strategic information to help synthesize and reinforce concepts.

Other key features include:

SIDEBARS
These notes emphasize pertinent pieces of data, trends, or perspectives.

SUMMARY
A concise summary that serves as a checkpoint for you to be sure you have a firm grasp of all topics discussed in that particular chapter.

or interactive exercises and additional review.

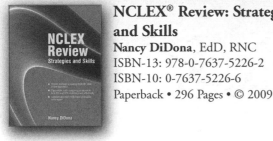
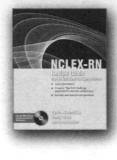
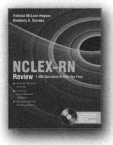
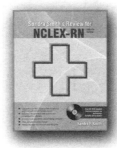
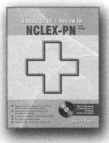
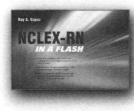

Issues and Trends in Nursing: Essential Knowledge for Today and Tomorrow

EDITED BY

Gayle Roux, PhD, RN, CNS, NP-C

Associate Professor
Associate Dean for Faculty
Loyola University Chicago
Marcella Niehoff School of Nursing
Chicago, Illinois

Judith A. Halstead, DNS, RN, ANEF

Professor and Executive Associate Dean for Academic Affairs
Indiana University School of Nursing
Indianapolis, Indiana

JONES AND BARTLETT PUBLISHERS

Sudbury, Massachusetts

BOSTON   TORONTO   LONDON   SINGAPORE

World Headquarters

Jones and Bartlett Publishers	Jones and Bartlett Publishers Canada	Jones and Bartlett Publishers International
40 Tall Pine Drive	6339 Ormindale Way	Barb House, Barb Mews
Sudbury, MA 01776	Mississauga, Ontario L5V 1J2	London W6 7PA
978-443-5000	Canada	United Kingdom
info@jbpub.com		
www.jbpub.com		

Jones and Bartlett's books and products are available through most bookstores and online booksellers. To contact Jones and Bartlett Publishers directly, call 800-832-0034, fax 978-443-8000, or visit our website www.jbpub.com.

Substantial discounts on bulk quantities of Jones and Bartlett's publications are available to corporations, professional associations, and other qualified organizations. For details and specific discount information, contact the special sales department at Jones and Bartlett via the above contact information or send an email to specialsales@jbpub.com.

The authors, editor, and publisher have made every effort to provide accurate information. However, they are not responsible for errors, omissions, or for any outcomes related to the use of the contents of this book and take no responsibility for the use of the products and procedures described. Treatments and side effects described in this book may not be applicable to all people; likewise, some people may require a dose or experience a side effect that is not described herein. Drugs and medical devices are discussed that may have limited availability controlled by the Food and Drug Administration (FDA) for use only in a research study or clinical trial. Research, clinical practice, and government regulations often change the accepted standard in this field. When consideration is being given to use of any drug in the clinical setting, the health care provider or reader is responsible for determining FDA status of the drug, reading the package insert, and reviewing prescribing information for the most up-to-date recommendations on dose, precautions, and contraindications, and determining the appropriate usage for the product. This is especially important in the case of drugs that are new or seldom used.

Production Credits
Publisher: Kevin Sullivan
Aquisitions Editor: Emily Ekle
Aquisitions Editor: Amy Sibley
Associate Editor: Patricia Donnelly
Editorial Assistant: Rachel Shuster
Associate Production Editor: Amanda Clerkin
Associate Marketing Manager: Ilana Goddess
Manufacturing and Inventory Control Supervisor: Amy Bacus
Composition: Shawn Girsberger
Cover Design: Kristin E. Ohlin
Cover Image Credit: © sgame/ShutterStock, Inc.
Printing and Binding: Malloy, Inc.
Cover Printing: Malloy, Inc.

Library of Congress Cataloging-in-Publication Data
Roux, Gayle M.
  Issues and trends in nursing : essential knowledge for today and tomorrow / [edited by] Gayle Roux, Judith A. Halstead.
     p. ; cm.
  Includes bibliographical references and index.
  ISBN-13: 978-0-7637-5225-5 (pbk.)
  ISBN-10: 0-7637-5225-8 (pbk.)
  1. Nursing--United States. I. Halstead, Judith A. II. Title.
  [DNLM: 1. Nursing--trends. 2. Nursing Care--trends. WY 16 R871i 2009]
  RT4.R69 2009
  610.73068--dc22
                            2008027304
6048

Printed in the United States of America
12 11 10 09 08   10 9 8 7 6 5 4 3 2 1

Contents

Preface

From its origins, nursing was described by Florence Nightingale as a distinct discipline concerned with the relationship between the patient, nurse, and environment. Nightingale defined nursing as having "charge of the personal health of somebody…and what nursing has to do….is to put the patient in the best condition for nature to act upon him" (1859/1992, p. 75). Nursing has advanced as a scientific discipline, with a wide scope of responsibility for nursing as a goal-directed and evidence-based practice. The goal of health and "putting the patient in the best condition for nature to act" requires the nurse to address a constantly expanding body of knowledge, technology, and sociocultural change. It is with this challenge in mind that this textbook was created. The graduating nurse must understand the complicated context of the issues that impact the nurse–patient relationship including political policy, professional organizations, performance outcomes, emergency preparedness, and global health issues.

While many different viewpoints of nursing theory have been debated, there is general agreement on the domains of nursing. Fawcett concluded there is a consensus about the central concepts of the discipline—person, environment, health, and nursing. These concepts constitute its metaparadigm (Fawcett, 1989). Therefore, the concepts of nursing, environment, person, and health were selected to form the organizational units of this textbook. The chapter topics do indeed aggregate into these four concepts, lending validity to the umbrella of the metaparadigm to describe the essence of nursing.

Unit I addresses *The **Nursing** Profession*. The unit begins with a discussion of the historical origins of nursing with emphasis on the history and development of the nursing profession in the United States. Nursing education is also addressed with a description of the various educational nursing programs that exist within the profession and a focused discussion on contemporary issues impacting nursing education curricula. Other chapter topics in Unit I identify the essential information a graduating nurse needs to know to be socialized into the profession, including preparing for the NCLEX examination and professional licensure and regulation, developing professionally through membership in professional nursing organizations, and engaging in interprofessional practice and research.

Unit II focuses on *The **Environment** and Nursing Practice.* To be safe and effective practitioners, nurses must fully understand and appreciate the complexity of the healthcare environment within which they practice. Systematized knowledge about safety, research, and the regulatory mechanisms in health care are essential in nursing to produce cost-effective, evidence-based patient health outcomes. The chapters within Unit II address current trends and issues existing within the healthcare environment including the movement towards a culture of safety, quality management and performance outcomes in the workplace, healthcare delivery systems, and evidence-based practice. Global nursing workforce issues and the role of the nurse in disaster preparedness are also addressed.

In Unit III, *The **Person** in Health Care*, the patient becomes the focus of our discussion. Maintaining a caring relationship with the patient that facilitates health and healing requires the nurse to be socially conscious. Sociocultural changes in the United States, increasing numbers of clients without insurance, legal directives, and federal and state policy embody an infrastructure for the person seeking health care. The increasing cultural diversity of the United States population and rising numbers of vulnerable patients requiring access to health care has multiple implications for nurses in their role as patient advocates. The legal and ethical issues related to nursing care are discussed with an emphasis on the nurse's role in ensuring attention to the legal and ethical rights of patients.

Unit IV addresses ***Health** and Nursing Issues*. Risk factors and health issues related to care of individuals in rural and urban settings are important considerations for nurses who practice in these settings. Informatics and health technology are increasingly influential in delivering effective, high quality health care and nurses are personally accountable for increasing their understanding of the use of technology in their practice. The unit ends with a discussion of transitioning into nursing practice and the future of nursing profession.

The essentials of information given in each chapter are intended to provide the undergraduate nursing student with the necessary details to think critically about issues and trends in nursing, engage in relationships with clients within an informed context of the issues and their environment, and create therapeutic plans to improve health outcomes. The editors and authors are sensitive to the fact that this text is one of a multitude of resources that is needed to achieve excellence in nursing. Internet sites are provided for the reader to obtain further information. As organizations frequently change Internet addresses, we regret if any sites listed are not current.

The editors, authors, and Jones and Bartlett staff have shared their expertise as a commitment to nursing education. We hope the contributions of this textbook are a component of your knowledge development and this knowledge makes a significant difference in how you think about and practice nursing.

Gayle Roux
Judith A. Halstead

References

Fawcett, J. (1989). *Analysis and evaluation of conceptual models of nursing* (2nd ed.). Philadelphia, PA: Davis.
Nightingale, F. (1859/1992). *Notes on nursing.* Philadelphia, PA: J.B. Lippincott.

Contributors

Amanda Alonzo, RN, MSN
Nursing Instructor
Mary Grimes School of Nursing
Neosho County Community College
Chanute, Kansas

Lisa S. Anderson, MPH
Instructor
Department of Epidemiology &
    Community Health, School of Medicine
Virginia Commonwealth University
Richmond, Virginia

Wanda Bonnel, RN, PhD, ARNP
Associate Professor
University of Kansas
School of Nursing
Kansas City, Kansas

**Patricia Gail Colo Braun, RN, MS,
    DNSc**
Loyola University Medical Center
Loyola University
Maywood, Illinois

Patricia E. Conejo, RN, MSN, WHNP
Assistant Professor of Nursing
Avila University
School of Nursing
Kansas City, Missouri

Karen L. Courtney, PhD, RN
Assistant Professor
Department of Health and Community
    Systems
Nursing Informatics
School of Nursing
University of Pittsburgh
Pittsburgh, Pennsylvania

Patricia Ebright, DNS, CNS, RN
Associate Professor
Indiana University School of Nursing
Indiana University-Purdue University
    Indianapolis
Indianapolis, Indiana

Karen J. Egenes, RN, EdD
Associate Professor
Marcella Niehoff School of Nursing
Loyola University Chicago
Chicago, Illinois

Gilan EL Saadawi, MD, PhD, MS
Assistant Professor
Department of Health and Community
    Systems
Nursing Informatics
School of Nursing
University of Pittsburgh
Pittsburgh, Pennsylvania

Joan C. Engebretson, DrPH, RN, AHN-BC
Professor
Department of Integrative Nursing Care
University of Texas Health Science Center at Houston School of Nursing
Houston, Texas

Beverly S. Farmer, RN, MSN, CCRN
Patient Safety Officer and Accreditation Coordinator
Deaconess Hospital
Evansville, Indiana

Eileen K. Fry-Bowers, JD, MS, RN, CPNP
Assistant Professor
Loma Linda University School of Nursing
Loma Linda, California

Nena R. Harris, MSN, CNM, FNP-BC
Faculty
Frontier School of Midwifery and Family Nursing
Hyden, Kentucky

Judith A. Headley, PhD, RN, AOCN, CCRP
Associate Professor, Division of Oncology
Director, Clinical Research Management, School of Nursing
University of Texas Health Sciences Center – Houston
Houston, Texas

Sylvia Heinze, MS, RN, APN, ACNS-BC, AOCN
Nurse Manager
Tunnell Cancer Center
Becbe Medical Center
Lewes, Delaware

Sharon Kimball, MS, RN, CNL, CRRN
Clinical Nurse Leader
Providence Portland Medical Center
Portland, Oregon

Pamela B. Koob, PhD, APRN, BC, FNP
Private Practice
Internal Medicine Associates
Hopkinsville, Kentucky

Elizabeth M. LaRue, PhD, MLS, AHIP
Assistant Professor
Department of Health and Community Systems
Nursing Informatics
School of Nursing
University of Pittsburgh
Pittsburgh, Pennsylvania

Kristi L. Lewis, PhD, MPH
Assistant Professor
Department of Health Sciences
College of Integrated Sciences and Technology
James Madison University
Harrisonburg, Virginia

Lillia Loriz, PhD, ARNP, BC
Associate Professor and Director of School of Nursing
University of North Florida
Brooks College of Health
Jacksonville, Florida

Beverly A. Mendes, APRN, MS, DNS-C
Hartford Hospital
Cardiac Catheterization Lab APRN
Hartford, Connecticut

Susan K. Newbold, PhD, RN-BC, FAAN, FHIMSS
Associate Professor, Nursing Informatics
Vanderbilt University School of Nursing
Nashville, Tennessee

Mary R. Nichols, PhD, APRN, BC, FNP
Faculty and Course Coordinator
Family Nursing Department
Frontier School of Midwifery and Family Nursing
Hyden, Kentucky

Karen Peddicord, RNc, PhD
Director of Research, Education, and Publications
Association of Women's Health, Obstetric and Neonatal Nurses (AWHONN)
Washington, DC

Monique Ridosh, MSN, RN
Faculty and Clinical Placement Coordinator
Marcella Niehoff School of Nursing
Loyola University Chicago
Chicago, Illinois

Mary E. Riner, DNS, RN
Associate Professor and Director
World Health Organization Collaborating Center in Healthy Cities
Indiana University School of Nursing
Indianapolis, Indiana

Martha Scheckel, PhD, RN
Assistant Professor
Department of Nursing
Winona State University
Winona, Minnesota

Wendy Stoelting-Gettelfinger, FNP, DNS, JD
Assistant Professor
Indiana University School of Nursing
Bloomington, Indiana

Lucy B. Trice, PhD, ARNP, BC
Brooks College of Health, School of Nursing
University of North Florida
Jacksonville, Florida

Kevin Valadares, PhD
Associate Professor of Health Services Administration
University of Southern Indiana
Evansville, Indiana

Joanne R. Warner, DNS, RN
Dean and Professor
University of Portland
School of Nursing
Portland, Oregon

Ellen Wathen, PhD, RN, BC
Staff Development Specialist
Deaconess Hospital
Evansville, Indiana

Diane Baer Wilson, EdD, MS, RD
Associate Professor
Department of Internal Medicine and Massey Cancer Center
School of Medicine
Virginia Commonwealth University
Richmond, Virginia

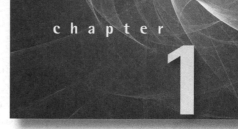

History of Nursing

Karen J. Egenes

LEARNING OUTCOMES

After reading this chapter you will be able to:

- Discuss the importance to a profession's understanding of its own history.
- Identify the contributions of selected leaders in the development of U.S. nursing.
- Trace the origins and purposes of major professional nursing organizations.
- Describe the influences of war on the development of nursing.
- Discuss the influences of faith traditions on the development of nursing.
- Analyze the impact of government on the growth of health care and the development of nursing.
- Explore the development of advanced practice roles in nursing.

History can be defined as a study of events from the past leading up to the present time. However, the study of history focuses on not just the chronology of events, but also the impact and influence those events continued to have throughout time. Over the passage of time, events unfold and trends emerge. These historical trends, in turn, influence or shape the destiny of an individual or a group. The development and evolution of the nursing profession is intricately connected to historical influences throughout the ages, beginning in antiquity. The study of the history of nursing helps us to better understand the societal forces and issues that continue to confront the profession. Understanding the history of nursing also allows nurses to gain an appreciation of the role the profession has played in the healthcare system of the United States (Donahue, 1991). The purpose of this chapter is to provide an overview of the history of nursing with an emphasis on nursing in the United States, describe the influence of societal trends on the development of nursing as a profession, and identify the contributions of selected leaders in U.S. nursing.

Nursing in Antiquity

In primitive societies, the decision to be a caregiver was often made for a person long before he or she had the ability to make such a choice. For example, among the members of the Zuni tribe, if an infant was born with a part of the placenta covering the face, it was taken as a sign that he or she had been marked as one who was destined to be a caregiver (Henly & Moss, 2007). In many societies, the provision of nursing care was a role that was assigned to female members. Because women traditionally provided nurturance to their own infants, it was assumed these same caring approaches could be extended to sick and injured community members as well. Yet in other societies, care of the sick was a role assigned to medicine men, shamans, or other male tribesmen.

Because no formal education in the care of the sick was available, the earliest nurses learned their art through oral traditions passed from generation to generation, from observations of others caring for the sick, and many times, through a process of trial and error. Those who acquired a reputation for expert care of the sick with a succession of positive outcomes were often sought after to provide care to friends and relatives. In this way, they established themselves in a practice of nursing care.

Available evidence indicates that nurses first formed themselves into organized groups during the early Christian era. The nursing ideals of charity, service to others, and self-sacrifice were in harmony with the teachings of the early Christian church. The role of **deaconess** gave women a meaningful way of participating in the work of the church. Deaconesses were often Roman matrons or widows with some educational background who were selected by the church's bishops to visit and care for the sick in their homes. Fabiola was a deaconess who is credited with the establishment and operation of the first Christian hospital in Rome. The deaconess Phoebe is often cited as the first "visiting nurse" because of the expert home nursing care she provided (Nutting & Dock, 1907).

KEY TERM

Deaconesses: Women with some educational background who were selected by the church to provide care to the sick.

Throughout antiquity, the preferable, and often safest, nursing care was provided in one's own home, where one was cared for by family members, clansmen, or friends. Care in a hospital was sought only by those who had no family members nearby, such as persons whose work took them away from their homes, or persons who had been ostracized or who were destitute. Early hospitals were begun by members of religious communities—nuns and monks who devoted their lives to the care of the sick. One example is the convent hospital at Beaune in France, where the sick were cared for in beds that lined the walls surrounding the main altar of the convent's church. Another example was the Hôtel-Dieu in Paris, a hospital operated by the Augustinian sisters, which was founded by the bishop of Paris in 651 A.D. Since its founding, the hospital has had an unbroken record of care "for all who suffer." The detailed records that survive from this hospital provide many interesting insights into the state of medical and nursing care during the Middle Ages. More than one patient was placed in each bed, with the feet of one patient opposite the face of another. Because patients received no diagnosis upon admission, a patient with a leg fracture might be placed in the same bed with a patient with smallpox and another with tuberculosis (Robinson, 1946).

Nursing in Early Modern Europe

In England, in the wake of the Protestant Reformation, monasteries and convents were closed and their lands were seized. Care of the sick fell to "common" women, often those of the lower classes who were too old or too ill to find any other type of work. Hospital records of the day report that nurses were often sanctioned for fighting, use of foul language, petty theft, and extortion of money from patients (Pavey, 1953). The sick who lacked families to tend to their needs were warehoused in almshouses and municipal hospitals, overseen by attendants who lacked any knowledge of nursing care. Charles Dickens, a Victorian-era author who championed social reform, described the poor conditions of nursing care through his characters Sairey Gamp and Betsey in his novel *Martin Chuzzlewit*. Dickens's nurses were often drunk while on duty, engaged in intimate relationships with their patients, and took delight in their patients' deaths (Dolan, 1968).

During the first half of the 19th century, a variety of British social reformers advocated for the formation of groups of religious women to staff the existing hospitals. To answer this need, in 1840, Elizabeth Fry, a Quaker who had earlier fought for prison reform in England, founded the Protestant Sisters of Charity. Members of this sisterhood received only a rudimentary education in nursing; their only practical nursing experiences consisted of observing patients at two London hospitals.

The nurses of St. John's House, an English Protestant sisterhood founded in 1848, lived together as a community under the direction of a clergyman and a lady superintendent. Pupils paid 15 pounds sterling for a training program that was 2 years in length, but were then required to work for St. John's House for 5 years in return for room and board, and a small salary. Although they received instruction in nursing in the Middlesex, Westminster, and King's College hospitals in London, they nursed for only a few hours each day, spending the remainder of their time engaged in religious instruction and prayer (Pavey, 1953).

On the European continent, Theodor Fliedner, a German Lutheran pastor, in an attempt to create a role for women in the church, established a Deaconess Home and Hospital at Kaiserswerth, a city in Germany on the Rhine River. Pastor Fliedner had traveled to England, where he was impressed with the work of Elizabeth Fry. Together with his wife, Frederike, Pastor Fliedner founded a deaconess training program. Although the deaconesses' primary instruction was in nursing, they also received education in religious instruction and in the provision of social services. According to the plan of Pastor Fliedner, deaconesses took no vows, but instead promised to continue to carry out their work as long as they felt called to this role. In return, the deaconesses were cared for by their mother house, which provided them with a permanent home. Although they were sent on assignments, they remained under the protection of their home organization (Gallison, 1954).

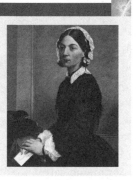

Florence Nightingale and the Origin of Professional Nursing

Into this setting entered **Florence Nightingale**, the woman who would not only reform nursing as it existed at that time, but also lay the foundation for nursing as a profession. Florence Nightingale was born into a wealthy British family. For their honeymoon, her parents embarked on an extensive tour of Europe. Their first child, Parthenope (the Greek name for Naples), was born while they visited Naples, and their second child, Florence, was born in the Italian city of that name. When the family returned to England, Mr. Nightingale took charge of the education of his daughters. Florence was educated in Greek and Latin, mathematics, natural science, ancient and modern literature, German, French, and Italian (Nutting & Dock, 1907).

It was assumed that Florence would follow the traditional path dictated for women of the upper class during the Victorian era, which included marriage and the rearing of a family. Although Florence was courted by various wealthy suitors, she rebuffed their approaches, stating she instead believed she had been called to dedicate her life to the service of humanity. Nightingale's parents at first were appalled by her desire to care for the sick, because such work was considered improper for a woman of her class. As steadfast members of the Church of England, they were even more shocked at her suggestion that she might seek admission to a convent of Irish Catholic nursing sisters. With time they consented to her attendance for a 2-week period at Pastor Fliedner's Deaconess Home and Hospital in Germany. In July 1851, she was able to return to Kaiserswerth for 3 months, during which time she worked with the deaconesses, learned basic information about patient care, and observed the Fliedners' methods of instruction in nursing.

When Nightingale returned to England, she was appointed superintendent of the Upper Harley Street Hospital, a small hospital for sick and elderly women of the upper class who had experienced financial difficulties. During her time in this position, she also made a journey to Paris to observe the hospital work of the Catholic Sisters of Charity, and volunteered as a nurse at the Middlesex Hospital during a cholera epidemic there.

In 1854, the Crimean War broke out, in which Russia waged war against the combined armies of England, France, and Turkey. Nightingale was appalled to learn that the mortality rate for British troops was 41 percent. More disturbing was the fact that whereas the French had nursing nuns to care for their troops, the British army lacked any kind of nurses. In fact, most British soldiers were dying from disease rather than from injuries incurred on the battlefield. From her travels, observations of nursing care provided in hospitals abroad, and practical experiences in nursing, she had a far greater knowledge of the elements of skilled nursing care than the majority of medical workers of her time (Pavey, 1953).

Using her political influence, Nightingale sought permission for her and a band of ladies drawn from the upper class to travel to the Crimea and to care for the sick and wounded. Because Nightingale believed that dirt, rather than microscopic pathogens, were the cause of disease, she embarked on a campaign to thoroughly scrub the soldiers' barracks and hospital wards, and to let in sunshine and fresh air. Within months, the number of deaths decreased dramatically. Nightingale, who had learned the principles of statistics from her father's tutelage, carefully documented the results of her care and used these as the basis for further interventions (Woodham-Smith, 1951). Through her work, she laid the foundation for modern evidence-based practice.

When Nightingale returned to England, she was hailed as a heroine. The British people, in recognition for her work, established a trust fund to be used at her discretion. Through this Nightingale Fund, she established the Nightingale School of Nursing at **St. Thomas' Hospital** in London for the education of professional nurses. The school differed from earlier forms of nursing education because student nurses received classes in theory coupled with clinical experiences on hospital wards. In addition, a set curriculum guided the students' experiences, so that during their program, they received training in various aspects of nursing care for patients in many of the hospital's specialty areas. Because the Nightingale School had the Nightingale

KEY TERM

St. Thomas' Hospital: A hospital in London where Florence Nightingale established the Nightingale School of Nursing.

Fund as its financial base, students' experiences were planned by Nightingale and her instructors (Baly, 1997; Seymer, 1960). Emphasis was placed on the proper education of the nurse, rather than on the needs of the hospital.

Origins of Professional Nursing in the United States

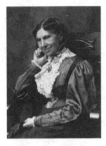

Clara Barton

Within a decade of Nightingale's return from the Crimea, the United States experienced the outbreak of civil war. When the war began, there was no provision for military nurses in either the Union or the Confederacy. At the time, there were no nursing schools, no "trained" nurses, and no nursing credentials. The title "nurse" was also rather vague, and could refer to an officer's wife who accompanied her husband to the battlefield, a woman who came to care for a wounded son or husband and remained to care for others, a member of a Catholic religious community in a hospital that cared for military personnel, or a volunteer. It is estimated that more than 3,000 women served as nurses during the Civil War, caring for sick or wounded soldiers on the battlefields, in field hospitals, in hospitals removed from battle sites, or even in their own homes. These female volunteer nurses went to the war with only the most basic knowledge of nursing care derived from their personal experiences caring for loved ones. They learned about the care of battle-related injuries and illnesses through their own wartime experiences (Livermore, 1888). Table 1-1 identifies some of the nurses who provided care to soldiers during the Civil War.

Influences of the U.S. Civil War

The Civil War nurses listed in Table 1-1 laid the foundation for professional nursing in the United States. The work they performed changed the public's perception of work by women outside of their homes. Many Civil War nurses had left their husbands and/or families to serve in situations that had not previously been considered a proper "place" for ladies. The work of the Civil War nurses also changed public opinion about women's work in health care. Women, who had volunteered as nurses during the Civil War, had come to realize the value of formal education in the care of the sick. Some of them became instrumental in the establishment of the first nurse training schools (schools of nursing) in the United States. In 1868, just 3 years after the end of the war, Samuel Gross, MD, president of the American Medical Association, strongly endorsed the formation of training schools for nurses (Larson, 1997).

The Effects of Social Change in the United States

Following the Civil War, cities in the United States experienced a rapid growth. Fueled by the rise of industries, many persons from rural areas flocked to cities to find work in factories. Hordes of immigrants from Eastern and Southern Europe

TABLE 1.1 CIVIL WAR NURSES

DOROTHEA DIX (1802–1887), superintendent of Union Army nurses during the war. She was a teacher and reformer of mental hospitals who, at the outbreak of the war, was charged with recruitment of nurses and supervision of nursing activities.

KATE CUMMINGS (1836–1909), a nurse for the Confederate Army. During the war, she kept a diary that she later published. Her book presents a realistic record of Confederate hospitals and nursing.

JANE WOOLSEY (1830–1900), a volunteer nurse for the Union Army, she became a superintendent of a Union hospital in Virginia. She later published her memoirs, which describe medical practices, the work of nurses, and the lives of wounded soldiers. Following the war, she helped to found the nurse training school at Presbyterian Hospital in New York City.

CLARA BARTON (1821–1912), a volunteer nurse who served in battlefield hospitals and prisoner of war camps. Following the war, she founded and became the first president of the American Red Cross.

WALT WHITMAN (1819–1892), a poet who worked as a volunteer nurse in a Union military hospital in Washington, D.C. He later memorialized in his poetry the work of wartime nurses in the care of wounded and dying soldiers.

HARRIET TUBMAN (1820–1913), born into slavery, escaped to Philadelphia. During the war she nursed soldiers using herbs and other home remedies.

MARY LIVERMORE (1820–1905), a teacher and abolitionist who served as a volunteer nurse. As director of the Northwestern branch of the U.S. Sanitary Commission, she directed the solicitation and distribution of food and medical supplies to military hospitals.

LOUISA MAY ALCOTT (1832–1888), an author and volunteer nurse for the Union Army. Her book *Hospital Sketches*, which was based on letters she had written home from an army hospital, aroused public awareness of the work of nurses in the grim environments of military hospitals.

MARY ANN "MOTHER" BICKERDYKE (1817–1901), a nurse for the Union Army. Before the war she had studied botanic medicine. She is renowned for her work in founding, cleaning, and sanitizing Union military hospitals in the face of opposition from Union officers. She also collected food and medical supplies for Union military hospitals.

came to the cities to meet the factories' insatiable appetite for manpower. In fact, the population of many U.S. cities nearly doubled during each decade from 1880 until 1920. Crowded living conditions in the burgeoning cities often fostered the spread of disease. Because these new arrivals to cities often lacked family members with sufficient resources to care for them in time of illness and need, their only option was to seek care in municipal almshouses.

In many large cities in the United States, the sick wards of the almshouses evolved into public hospitals. Conditions in these municipal institutions in the United States were equal to the horrors in England that were described by Dickens.

A group of reform-minded citizens who visited public charitable facilities in New York City during the 1870s reported that much of the nursing care was provided by drunkards and former convicts. It was reported that prostitutes sentenced in the city's courts were given the choice of going to prison or going into hospital service. No nurses were on duty at night; instead, the patients were supervised by night watchmen (Pavey, 1953).

Establishment of the First Nurse Training Schools

The success of the Nightingale School of Nursing became known around the world. Social activists in many countries wrote to Nightingale with requests for her to send one of her graduates to found a nurse training school and hospital in their city. It was not long before social reformers and some physicians in the United States espoused the idea that provision of safe nursing care was important and could best be delivered by persons who had received a formal education in nursing. Small groups of public-minded women grew increasingly concerned about the welfare of the patients housed in the massive hospitals and almshouses, and worked to establish nurse training schools to sanitize the institutions and to give patients care far better than that rendered by the untrained and politically chosen attendants then employed (Schryver, 1930).

The first permanent school of nursing in the United States is reputed to be the **nurse training school of Women's Hospital of Philadelphia**, which was established in 1872. The staff of the hospital was predominantly female physicians, who sought to open the field of nursing to a better-quality type of woman. Following the Nightingale model, the school had a set curriculum, paid instructors, equipment for the practice of nursing skills, provision for student experiences in other Philadelphia hospitals, and a nurses' library.

In the same year, a training school for nurses was founded at the New England Hospital for Women and Children, another hospital with a staff composed of female physicians. Located in Boston, the school was founded and administered by two physicians, Dr. Susan Dimrock, who had been educated in Switzerland and was familiar with the educational methods of Kaiserswerth, and Dr. Marie Zakrzewska, who taught bedside nursing. **Linda Richards**, who is purported to be the first educated nurse in the United States, was a graduate of this program. Another notable graduate was **Mary Mahoney**, the first African American graduate nurse (Dolan, 1968). Table 1-2 describes some of the early leaders in nursing from this era.

Unfortunately, physicians' support for the formal education of nurses was absent in the establishment of other

KEY TERM

Nurse training school of Women's Hospital of Philadelphia: Established in 1872, reputed to be the first permanent school of nursing in the United States.

KEY TERM

Richards, Linda: Purported to be the first educated nurse in the United States, a graduate of the New England Hospital for Women and Children in Boston.

KEY TERM

Mahoney, Mary: The first African American graduate nurse.

TABLE 1.2 EARLY LEADERS IN NURSING

LINDA RICHARDS (1841–1930), awarded the title "America's first trained nurse." She was the first graduate of the year-long nurse-training program at the New England Hospital for Women and Children. She established the first nurse-training program in Japan, and then returned to the United States to found nurse-training programs in Michigan, Massachusetts, and Pennsylvania.

ISABEL HAMPTON ROBB (1860–1910), superintendent of nurses at the Illinois Training School and the Johns Hopkins School for Nurses. She became the first president of the Society of Superintendents of Training Schools for Nurses (forerunner of the National League for Nursing) and the Associated Alumnae Association (forerunner of the American Nurses Association).

SOPHIA PALMER (1853–1920), a founder of the New York State Nurses Association and campaigner for nurse licensure in New York. She became the first editor of the *American Journal of Nursing*. She authored a history of nursing, as well as other nursing textbooks and journal articles.

LAVINIA DOCK (1858–1956), a lecturer, author, and activist. Her campaign for women's suffrage and participation in anti-war protests sometimes led to her arrest. She authored many nursing textbooks and, because of her leadership in the International Council of Nurses, served as editor for the *American Journal of Nursing*'s Foreign Department.

MARY ADELAIDE NUTTING (1858–1948), the appointed head of the Department of Nursing and Health at Teachers College of Columbia University. She became the world's first professor of nursing.

ISABEL MAITLAND STEWART (1878–1947), a professor of nursing at Teachers College of Columbia University. She worked tirelessly for the establishment of a standardized nursing curriculum. She insisted on the need for nursing research to give the profession a solid scientific base.

LILLIAN WALD (1867–1940), from her work providing home nursing care and teaching home nursing to immigrant women on New York City's Lower East Side, she went on to found the Henry Street Settlement and the first Visiting Nurse Association.

MARY BRECKENRIDGE (1881–1965), a nurse midwife. She founded the Frontier Nursing Service to provide maternity services to women in the Appalachian mountains of eastern Kentucky. Nurses visited families on horseback. This service significantly lowered the maternal mortality rate of the region served.

early nurse training schools. Indeed, for many years a number of eminent physicians were opposed to any education for nurses other than the most basic training (Goodnow, 1953). Despite this, in 1873, three notable nurse training schools were established: the Bellevue Hospital Training School in New York City, the Connecticut Training School in New Haven Hospital, and the Boston Training School in Massachusetts General Hospital. It is significant that these schools were founded through the efforts of committees of laywomen, rather than physicians.

Conditions in Nurse Training Schools

In 1883, 10 years after the first training schools were founded, the number of training schools across the country had grown to 35. The majority of these schools were located on the east and west coasts, with isolated schools located in large cities across the nation's heartland. However, unlike the Nightingale School, training schools in the United States were economically dependent upon the hospitals in which they were located. Because of this, the needs of the hospital took precedence over the students' educational needs.

Hospital boards and physicians soon realized the economic advantages of the use of student labor, under the aegis of "clinical training," in the delivery of care to hospitalized patients. Because students tended to be compliant and obedient, the care they provided was cheap, efficient, and more cost effective than if graduate nurses had been hired by hospitals. The student nurses in effect traded their labor for the opportunity to be educated in a profession. Students worked 12-hour shifts with little or no clinical supervision. Some were required to sleep on hospital wards in beds that adjoined those of their patients. Classes were irregularly scheduled and were often cancelled when students were needed to staff the wards. Some hospitals earned additional funds by sending students to care for patients in private homes, a setting in which students were typically overworked and lacked both supervision and access to instruction (Kalisch & Kalisch, 1995).

By 1900, the number of schools had increased to 432. Many of these schools had been founded in state mental hospitals, tuberculosis sanatoria, and other "specialty" hospitals that provided very limited experiences. Still other schools were founded in hospitals with fewer than 25 beds, which because of their size, provided less than adequate clinical experiences (Baer, 1990).

Following the completion of their training, only a select handful of graduates were offered hospital positions as supervisors and clinical faculty. The majority of graduates found employment in the homes of clients who could afford their services. The need for these private duty nurses was great because the majority of infants were delivered in the home, and some surgical procedures were performed there. In addition, many medical conditions, such as typhoid fever and pneumonia, were treated in the home setting. Often a private duty nurse slept in the same room as her patient, and was also responsible for laundry chores and meal preparation. Despite these harsh work conditions, nursing offered women a socially acceptable means of self-support and economic independence.

Advances in Science and Medicine

The 19th century was marked by vigorous intellectual activity and the expansion of knowledge in the sciences. These advances profoundly influenced both medicine and the burgeoning profession of nursing. By the beginning of the 20th

century, the symptoms and natural life histories of many diseases had been identified. Because of advances in the development of microscopes, in some cases,
the causative organisms of disease had been identified as well. Newly developed
instruments aided in the assessment of bodily function. Through the development of antiseptic agents and anesthesia, complicated surgical procedures were
possible. Increasingly the practice of medicine was based on scientific knowledge
and aimed to both control and cure disease.

The expansion of scientific knowledge and the increased used of complex technological procedures were linked to the growth of schools of nursing. The work
of curing patients was best carried out in hospitals where physicians and surgeons
had access to modern technology. With the expansion of medical care, educated
nurses were needed to aid in the care and treatment of patients with increasingly
more complex conditions and needs.

The Origins of Public Health Nursing

At the end of the 19th century, the field of public health nursing was instituted,
which provided a third area in which nurse graduates could find employment.
District nursing originated in England during the 1860s. Through funding from
wealthy philanthropists, nurses provided care to "sick poor"
persons in their homes, and also provided food and medical
supplies. In 1886, the idea spread to the United States, and
two district nurse associations were established in Boston and
Philadelphia. In 1893, **Lillian Wald** originated settlement
house nursing, an offshoot of district nursing, among the
immigrant populations on the lower east side of New York.

KEY TERM

Wald, Lillian: A public health nurse
who founded Henry Street Settlement
House to provide home nursing care to
the immigrant populations on the lower
east side of New York.

Following her graduation from the New York Hospital Training School, Wald
taught a home nursing class in a neighborhood populated by recent immigrants.
One day a young child came to her, asking for her aid in the care of his mother who
had given birth only 2 days before. He escorted her to a dreary apartment where she
found the young mother lying on a bed in a pool of blood. Wald was so moved by
this scene that she made the commitment to care for the destitute immigrant population of her city. With funding provided by women of the upper class, she and
a classmate, Mary Brewster, moved into a small apartment in the neighborhood,
offering nursing care to recent immigrants who sought their help. They were soon
joined by other nurses and by social workers. Within 2 years, they helped to found
the Henry Street Settlement House to provide both home nursing care and a variety
of social services to New York's immigrant population (Wald, 1934).

In an attempt to demonstrate the positive outcomes that could be realized by
a public health nurse in a school setting, in October 1902 Wald sent one of her
Henry Street nurses, Lina Ravanche Rogers, to work for a month in the New York
public schools. At that time, any child could be barred from school if the teacher

believed there was reason for the exclusion. However, no attempt was made to determine whether there was a medical cause for the exclusion, nor was any attempt made to secure treatment for the child if this were necessary. The school nurse experiment was so successful in reducing the number of absences among schoolchildren that by December 1902, Lina Rogers was appointed to the Board of Health and 12 additional nurses were employed to aid her provision of school health services.

Wald was the first person to use the term *public health nursing* to describe the work of nurses in patients' homes as well as in other community settings. This field of nursing gained such prominence that in 1912 the National Organization for Public Health Nursing (NOPHN) was founded to set standards and to plan for the expansion of community-based nursing services (Randall, 1937).

The Origins of Nursing Associations

The World's Fair and Colombian Exposition was held in Chicago from May until October 1893 to celebrate the 400th anniversary of Columbus' arrival in the New World. Various conventions and conferences were held at the exposition, including the International Congress of Charities, Correction and Philanthropy. A section of this conference was chaired by Isabel Hampton. Prominent nurses presented papers on topics related to nursing. Of concern to the nurses gathered was the fact that at that time, only one-tenth of the persons who practiced nursing in the United States were graduates of hospital nurse training schools. The other 90 percent, who received equal pay for their care of the sick, had little or no formal education in nursing. Nurse licensure was considered vital to the protection of the public by providing a distinction between educated nurses and uneducated nurses. Nurse leaders voiced their concerns about the need for licensure, called for nurses to unite to advance their new profession, and proposed strategies to unite nurses.

KEY TERM

Nurses' Associated Alumnae of the United States and Canada: Originally founded in 1896 with the intent of achieving licensure for nurses; became the American Nurses Association (ANA).

In 1896, the **Nurses' Associated Alumnae of the United States and Canada**, which later became the American Nurses Association (ANA), was founded with the intent of achieving licensure for nurses. This escalating concern for nurse licensure led to the formation of state nurses' associations that were committed to the attainment of nurse registration through the passage of a nurse practice act in each state of the union. Other goals of the association included the establishment of a code of ethics, promotion of the image of nursing, and provision of attention to the financial and professional interests of nursing (American Nurses Association & National League of Nursing Education, 1940).

Another concern voiced was the lack of educational standards in nursing. The programs offered in nurse training schools varied in length from a few months to 3 years, and curricula and entrance requirements varied greatly. This issue was of particular concern to the 18 superintendents of nurse training schools who attended the Congress. As a result of their conversations, they joined together in 1893 to form the **American Society of Superintendents of Training Schools of Nursing**, a national nursing organization focused on elevating the standards of nursing education. This association later became the National League for Nursing Education, and still later, the National League for Nursing (NLN).

> **KEY TERM**
>
> **American Society of Superintendents of Training Schools of Nursing:** A national nursing organization founded in 1893 to elevate the standards of nursing education; later became the National League for Nursing Education, and ultimately, the National League for Nursing (NLN).

Licensure for Nurses

In 1901, New York, New Jersey, Illinois, and Virginia were the first states that organized state nurses' associations with the goal of enacting a nurse practice act for their states. In 1903, North Carolina passed the first nurse licensure act in the United States. By 1921, 48 states, as well as the District of Columbia and the territory of Hawaii, had enacted laws that regulated the practice of professional nursing. These early versions of nurse practice acts provided for licensure as a "registered nurse" (Birnbach, in Schorr & Kennedy, 1999).

Although the passage of these acts marked a tremendous milestone in the professionalization of nursing, a serious weakness of the early nurse practice acts was that they were permissive laws, rather than mandatory. They were "permissive" in that only nurses who were licensed were permitted to use the title "registered nurse." Thus, untrained persons were not prohibited from practice as nurses as long as they did not use the title "registered nurse."

This deficiency caused hardships for registered nurses during the Great Depression of the 1930s. Because the states lacked mandatory nurse licensure, any person was legally able to work as a "nurse" for pay. Thus licensed graduate nurses competed with uneducated "nurses" for the few available positions. The American Nurses Association argued that if only licensed nurses were allowed to practice, there would be enough work for each of them. Mandatory licensure laws, which made it unlawful for any person to practice nursing without a valid nursing license, were not passed by states until the late 1940s.

Effects of the Great Depression on Nursing

The stock market crash of 1929 plunged the United States into the throes of the Great Depression. Although every group of workers was devastated by the collapse of the nation's economy, nurses were particularly affected. Most nurses were independent practitioners, self-employed in private duty work in patients' homes. However, the patients who once employed private duty nurses were now unable to pay for this service.

Nurses who attempted to move from private duty work in patients' homes to hospital settings encountered problems in this venture. The depression years saw reductions in the number of hospital beds occupied. Patients who were forced to seek medical care were often without financial resources. Most hospitalized patients were in hospitals with training schools that used their students for bedside care. Hospitals without training schools were usually staffed with uneducated attendants. It is estimated that of the hospitals with training schools, 73 percent had no graduate nurse employees, and of these, only 15 percent had four or more graduate nurse employees. Graduate nurses who engaged in bedside patient care were looked down on as nurses not able to succeed in private duty work. After much debate, some hospital administrators decided to accept the services of unemployed registered nurses in exchange for a room, meals, and laundry, but offered the nurses no salary (Kalisch & Kalisch, 1995).

The National Recovery Act, passed by the U.S. Congress in 1933 in an effort to find employment for those without work, did not apply to unemployed nurses. The law stated, "The Agreement . . . shall not apply to professional persons employed in their profession" (President's Re-employment Agreement, 1933). In response to the implications of the National Recovery Act for the nursing profession, the Board of Directors of the American Nurses Association issued the following position statements:

1. Any plan for economic recovery must consider the thousands of unemployed graduate registered nurses.
2. In all cases, the most effective type of nursing service should be made available to patients.
3. Wherever possible, the nurse should be employed on the basis of an 8-hour day or 48-hour week.
4. The salaries of nurses should be kept above sustenance levels.
5. Nurses caring for acutely ill patients should not be expected to work more than 8 hours out of 24.

By 1933, the 8-hour day for hospital nurses was gaining ground. This schedule for nurses gained support because it helped to alleviate the problem of unemployment of nurses. When nurses were on duty for 8 hours instead of 12 hours, three nurses, rather than two, could work during each 24-hour period.

A milestone was reached in 1933 when the federal government announced that a program offered through the Civil Works Service would provide funds for bedside nursing care in the homes of recipients of unemployment relief. The care would be paid for from Federal Emergency Relief Administration funds at a set rate per visit, not to exceed the established rate charged by accredited visiting nurse associations in the local district. The program also included the use of graduate nurses for instruction to home workers, health education programs, instruction in hygiene, preventative measures, care of infants and children, first aid, and nutrition. This program served to interest many nurses in the specialty area of public health nursing (The NRA and Nursing, 1933).

Nursing and Times of War

Times of war have increased both the nation's need for nurses and the public's recognition of nurses' work in saving lives. Educated nurses first served as army nurses in 1898, in the Spanish-American War. At the outbreak of the war, nurse training schools had been educating nurses for nearly 20 years. Congress authorized the Surgeon General to hire as many nurses as would be needed. At first, the educated nurses had difficulty winning acceptance from medical officers, but because they had been approved by the Surgeon General, their presence was tolerated. However, as the war progressed, their skills in caring for ill and wounded soldiers won recognition, and army doctors came to depend on them. More than 1,500 nurses entered the army during the war. Table 1-3 presents information about some of the early military nurses in our country's history.

TABLE 1.3 MILITARY NURSES

CLARA MAAS (1876–1901), following service in the Spanish-American War, participated in a study to determine the cause of yellow fever. She allowed herself to be bitten by a mosquito known to have bitten infected patients, contracted the disease, and died a few days later.

JANE DELANO (1862–1919), credited with the creation of American Red Cross Nursing. She recruited nurses for army service in World War I through the American Red Cross. While touring Red Cross hospitals in France following the Armistice, she contracted an ear infection and died a few days later.

ANNIE GOODRICH (1866–1954), a professor at Teachers College of Columbia University. During World War I, she organized and served as dean of the Army School of Nursing. Following the war, she served as the first dean of the Yale University School of Nursing.

JULIA STIMSON (1881–1948), during World War I, served as chief nurse of the American Expeditionary Forces. Following the war, she served as dean of the Army School of Nursing and was appointed the first superintendent of the Army Nurse Corps. During World War II she recruited nurses for military service.

FLORENCE BLANCHFIELD (1882–1971), superintendent for the Army Nurse Corps during World War II. She was one of a few women to reach the rank of colonel. Following the war, she worked for passage of the bill that granted army and navy nurses the pay, benefits, and privileges prescribed for commissioned officers.

LUCILE PETRY (1902–1999), served as head of the Cadet Nurse Corps during World War II. This program provided a free nursing education to women who agreed to provide military service until the end of the war.

In 1901, an Act of Congress established a permanent Army Nurse Corps, followed in 1908 by the establishment of the Navy Nurse Corps. However, military nursing did not achieve prominence until 1917, when the United States entered World War I. At the beginning of the war there were fewer than 500 nurses in the Army Nurse Corps. However, by the war's end, aided by reserve nurses from the American Red Cross National Nursing Service, the number had increased to over 21,000 army nurses and 1,386 navy nurses. During the war, over 10,000 U.S. nurses served overseas.

In 1914, when war first broke out in Europe, Jane Delano was appointed Director of Nursing Services for the American Red Cross Department of Nursing. Because the American Red Cross was regarded as the unofficial reserve for the military in times of national emergency, it became Delano's responsibility to recruit nurses for the Army Nurse Corps, Navy Nurse Corps, and U.S. Public Health Service, as well as to equip nurses for duty overseas. Traditionally, only graduates of nurse training school were eligible for military service. However, as the war progressed and the supply of nurses became depleted, society women, filled with a spirit of patriotism but unwilling to commit to a formal educational program in nursing, increasingly pressured the government for the right to serve as volunteer nurses. Although various schemes were developed to conserve the supply of nurses through the uses of volunteer nurses' aides, nurse leaders remained resolute that only educated nurses could serve as military nurses.

In an effort to recruit college-educated women into military nursing, in 1918 Vassar College offered its campus as a training camp to provide a 12-week preclinical program in basic science and basic nursing skills as part of a nursing program for college women. Upon successful completion of the Vassar Training Camp program, the college women were assigned to select nurse training schools as regular students for the completion of their education in nursing. During that summer, 432 women from 115 colleges and representing 41 states participated in the Vassar program. Their enthusiasm spread interest in nursing across U.S. college campuses. Many graduates of the Vassar Training Camp became leaders in nursing education during the following decades.

In a related effort, the Army School of Nursing was founded in 1918, with Annie Goodrich, a former faculty member from Teachers College of Columbia University, as its dean. Following the model used by the best civilian hospitals of the time, Goodrich's goal in founding the school was to provide patients in military hospitals with quality care provided by student nurses supervised by educated faculty. The school's curriculum was 3 years in length, with 9 months credit awarded to college graduates. Most clinical experiences were provided in army hospitals, with affiliations in civilian hospitals for pediatrics and other experiences. There were 500 students in the class of 1921, the first class to graduate from the Army School of Nursing. Although the school had been planned to be a permanent institution, it was closed in 1933 because of financial constraints imposed by the Great Depression. However, the Army School of Nursing was well organized and offered a high standard of nursing education that served as a model for nurse training schools in the civilian sector (Jensen, 1950).

In 1940, as a second world war threatened, the American Nurses Association and other nursing organizations established the Nursing Council of National Defense to recruit more student nurses as well as to assess the number of graduate nurses who might be available for military service. The council worked closely with the American Red Cross in attempts to recruit registered nurses for military service. When a national inventory of nursing personnel conducted by the National Nursing Council revealed an acute shortage of nurses, the council joined with U.S. Representative Frances Payne Bolton of Ohio in the sponsorship of the first bill passed by Congress that provided government funding for the education of nurses for national defense. This bill was followed closely by the **Bolton Act of 1942**, which created the U.S. Cadet Nurse Corps, a program to prepare nurses as quickly as possible to meet the needs of the armed forces, civilian and government hospitals, and war industries. The entire nursing education of students enrolled in this program, including tuition, housing, uniforms, books, and monthly stipends, was subsidized by the federal government. Students were required to promise to work in either civilian or military nursing roles that were deemed essential to the national defense for the duration of the war. The Bolton Act further stipulated that the length of study for members of the Cadet Nurse Corps be reduced from 36 months to 30 or fewer months. By the beginning of 1944, students in the Cadet Nurse Corps began reporting to military hospitals for the clinical experiences that composed their senior year. The Bolton Act had a widespread influence on nursing education, mandating standards for nursing education programs and the removal of school policies that discriminated against students' gender, marital status, ethnicity, or race.

> **KEY TERM**
>
> **Bolton Act of 1942:** Legislation that created the U.S. Cadet Nurse Corps, a program subsidized by the federal government and designed to quickly prepare nurses to meet the needs of the armed forces, civilian and government hospitals, and war industries.

During the war, over 77,000 nurses, more that two-fifths of the active nurses at the time, served in the armed forces. Despite these valiant efforts, the number of nurses in military service remained inadequate. In his address to Congress in January 1945, President Roosevelt requested a national draft of nurses. Although the leading nursing organizations were supportive of a national service act for all men and women, they opposed a law aimed specifically at nurses. Discussion about the bill ended with the Allies' victory in Europe.

During times of war, the profession of nursing has attained a positive image and has enjoyed the highest level of respect from members of the lay public (Kalisch & Kalisch, 1981). During World War II, the great need for nurses caused the U.S. government to provide the resources that were needed to both increase the supply of nurses and improve the quality of nursing education. Nurse leaders seized on this opportunity to advance not only military nursing, but also the profession in general.

Collective Bargaining in Nursing

Following World War II, the United States experienced one of its most drastic shortages of nurses. Many nurses who returned from the war sought the idealized role of wife and mother. Until the 1960s, nurses who worked in hospitals were expected to resign from their positions when they married. In addition, returning military nurses who had experienced such profoundly autonomous roles during the war were now reluctant to return to the subservient role of staff nurse in a hospital.

During the years that immediately followed the end of the war, despite the acute nursing shortage, nurses were paid far less than elementary school teachers, the professional group to whom nurses were most often compared. In fact, a study conducted in 1946 by the California Nurses Association found that the majority of staff nurses were paid only slightly more than hotel maids and seamstresses.

During the 1940s, Shirley Titus, Executive Director of the California Nurses Association, lobbied for economic empowerment for nurses. At the American Nurses Association convention of 1946 she successfully argued for nurses' rights to economic security through collective bargaining, insurance plans, benefit packages, and access to consultation from state nurses associations. In 1949, the American Nurses Association approved state nurses associations as collective bargaining agencies for nurses. However, a 1947 revision of the Taft-Hartley Labor Act exempted not-for-profit institutions such as hospitals from the requirement to enter into labor negotiations with their employees to address workplace grievances. Because the American Nurses Association had adopted a "no-strike" policy, and hospitals were not required to enter into labor negotiations with nurse employees, nurses often had no means to improve their work conditions other than by threats of mass resignation. Although hospitals were not required to enter into collective bargaining agreements with nurses, many times nurses working collectively were able to pressure their employers into voluntary labor agreements.

In 1966, the American Nurses Association rescinded its no-strike clause, opening the way for nurses' strikes for improvements in work conditions and salaries. Although relatively few strikes by nurses have occurred, when they have, nurses have ensured that care for those in need continued to be provided. Both nurses and members of the general public are often opposed to the idea of nurses entering into labor negotiations with employers, which they view as "unprofessional." However, collective bargaining has provided nurses with both increased economic security and a greater voice in decisions that affect patient care (Stafford, Taylor, Zimmerman, et al 2000).

Advances in Nursing Education

The apprentice system used in nursing education was often criticized by academicians and external review agencies because of its lack of intellectual rigor and its exploitation of student labor. In 1919, a Committee for the Study of Nursing Education, supported by the Rockefeller Foundation, was established to examine the state of both public health nursing and nursing education. The committee's published report, the **Goldmark Report** (1923), recommended that nursing education should have educational standards, and that schools of nursing should have a primary focus on education, rather than on patients. The report further recommended that nursing education be moved to universities, and that nurse educators receive the advanced education that was required for their roles. Although some changes in nursing education were implemented after the publication of the Goldmark Report, the changes were neither far-reaching nor permanent. Hospital administrators resisted change in nursing education that would eliminate the "free" labor provided by nursing students.

> **KEY TERM**
>
> **Goldmark Report:** Published in 1923, this report recommended that nursing education develop educational standards, schools of nursing adopt a primary focus on education and be moved to universities, and nurse educators receive advanced education.

In 1926, the Committee on the Grading of Nursing Schools was organized to analyze the work of nurses and to study the educational preparation of student nurses. The committee's published report, *Nurses, Patients, and Pocketbooks*, became known as the Burgess Report (1928). The committee recommended that admission criteria be adopted for applicants to schools of nursing, and that hospital nursing schools focus on education rather than provision of patient care. The report further decried a hospital's use of funds collected for care of the sick to finance its nurse training school. Unfortunately, the recommendations of the Burgess Report were also largely ignored.

A third evaluation of nursing education, *The Future of Nursing*, authored by Esther Brown (1948), was funded by the Carnegie Foundation. Like the two previous reviews, Brown recommended that schools of nursing strive for autonomy from hospital administration, improve the quality of their programs, recruit faculty with baccalaureate or graduate degrees, and use discretion in the selection of sites to be used for students' clinical experiences. To relieve the acute shortage of nurses that followed World War II, Brown strongly advocated the employment of married nurses and the recruitment of men into nursing. Brown further recommended that nursing practice be based on principles from the physical and social sciences.

The years that followed World War II saw a significant increase in the number of students who sought college degrees. This trend was coupled with dramatic changes in health care as technological advances increasingly led to specialized practice in medicine and nursing (Kalisch & Kalisch, 1995). However, during the 1950s and 1960s, the number of baccalaureate programs in nursing grew at a very slow rate. The vast majority of schools of nursing continued to be hospital-based diploma programs. Many of the diploma nursing programs had improved in quality as a result of the Brown Report, as well as measures instituted by the National League for Nursing, such as the publication of a standardized curriculum and the establishment of a process of voluntary accreditation. However, the diploma programs continued to be dependent on hospitals for financial support, and continued to give higher priority to the service needs of the hospitals rather than to their students' educational needs.

In response to the acute nursing shortage that followed World War II, an associate degree in nursing (ADN) was initiated. The ADN program was conceived by **Mildred Montag** as the topic of her doctoral dissertation. It was initiated on an experimental basis in 1951 to provide a large number of nurses in a relatively short time period. It was intended that the ADN nurse would practice solely at the bedside and would have a significantly narrower scope of practice than the traditional registered nurse. The ADN programs were tested for 5 years (1952–1957) and successfully produced nurses who were proficient in technical skills and could successfully function as registered nurses despite the fact that their program was only 2 years in length (Haase, 1990). The number of ADN programs increased as the number of community colleges increased. The ADN programs provided a pathway to the nursing profession for men, married women, mature students, and other groups who had traditionally been excluded from admission to nursing programs. By the end of the 1970s, the number of graduates from ADN programs exceeded the number of graduates from baccalaureate programs and diploma programs. As the number of ADN programs increased, the number of diploma programs rapidly declined.

In 1965, the American Nurses Association published the document *Educational Preparation for Nurse Practitioners and Assistants to Nurses*, which became known as the ANA position paper. This document reaffirmed the stand that nursing education should occur in institutions of higher education, rather than in hospitals. In addition, the position paper stated that the minimum preparation for beginning professional nurses should be a baccalaureate degree, the minimum preparation for beginning technical nurses should be an associate degree, and the educational preparation of nursing assistants should be a short, intensive pre-service program in an institution that offered vocational education (ANA, 1965). Although the ANA position paper arose from the association's concern that societal changes and advances in technology required significant changes in nursing education, publication of this document led to an enduring rift in the profession and has discouraged movement toward the baccalaureate degree as the requirement for entry level into practice for professional nursing.

During the first half of the 20th century, the number of baccalaureate and graduate programs in nursing increased slowly. The slow rate of growth of

KEY TERM

Montag, Mildred: Developed the concept for associate degree in nursing programs.

collegiate programs can be partly attributed to the nursing profession's uncertainty about the curriculum these programs should follow and the ways in which they should differ from diploma programs. At the beginning of the 1960s, only 14 percent of all basic students in nursing were enrolled in baccalaureate programs. In addition, there were only 14 higher degree programs in nursing to prepare the faculty needed to staff schools of nursing. A study commissioned in 1963 by the Surgeon General of the U.S. Public Health Service revealed that faculty in all schools of nursing, including baccalaureate programs, lacked the minimal educational preparation required for teaching. The published report of the study, *Toward Quality in Nursing, Needs and Goals*, recommended increased federal funding for nursing programs, and led to the passage of the Nurse Training Act of 1964 (Kalisch & Kalisch, 1995). This federal assistance was particularly important in the development of graduate programs in nursing. Prior to this time, nurses were often required to seek graduate degrees in education or in related disciplines. The 1970s saw a rapid increase in graduate programs focused on clinical specialties and laid the basis for an expansion in advanced practice roles in nursing.

Advances in Nursing Practice

The growth of master's degree programs in nursing opened many new advanced practice roles for nurses, including the roles of clinical specialist, nurse practitioner, researcher, and nurse administrator. Clinical nurse specialists have expertise in a defined clinical area. They are educated to provide expert care to patients who have complex health problems that require specialized care, to serve as role models for staff nurses, to provide consultation to nurses from other clinical areas, and to identify and research clinical problems associated with patient care. By the 1970s, clinical specialist roles had been developed in a variety of nursing practice areas including psychiatric/mental health nursing, cardiac nursing, oncology nursing, and community health nursing.

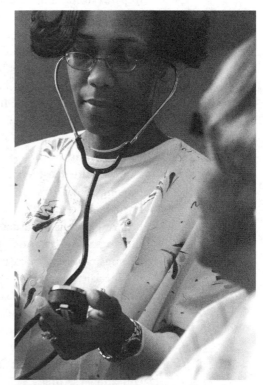

During the 1960s, concern for extending access to primary care services to traditionally underserved populations led to the evolution of the nurse practitioner role. It was long believed that the role of the nurse could be expanded and that nurses with specialized education could perform many of the primary care functions traditionally performed by physicians, but at a substantially lower cost. The title *nurse*

A nurse takes the blood pressure of a patient.
Source: © Liquid Library

practitioner was first used in a demonstration project at the University of Colorado, which was designed to prepare nurses to deliver well child care in ambulatory care settings. By the 1970s nurse practitioner preparation increasingly occurred in graduate programs in nursing. Provision of primary care by nurse practitioners became widely accepted by the general public.

The expansion of nurses' roles necessitated changes in the extant state nurse practice laws. At times, the extended roles for nurses, especially prescriptive authority for nurses, were met with criticism and opposition by medical associations. Nurses in advanced practice roles honed their skills in political activism as they fought for the changes in legislation that were required for roles for which they had been educated.

Advances were also made in nursing research. Over time, nurse leaders had struggled to establish nursing as a discipline that was separate and unique from medicine. However, this could be accomplished only when nursing developed its own unique theory base and body of knowledge. In addition, technological advances in medicine called for concurrent advances in clinical nursing practice, which could best be developed and validated through research. The journal *Nursing Research*, which was first published during the 1950s, provided a great impetus to nursing scholarship. The National Institutes of Health, Division of Nursing Research, was initiated in 1956. This body provided extramural grants for nursing research projects, and primarily funded proposals focused on applied research aimed to improve nursing practice. Nursing research further spawned the development of nursing theory by nurse scholars such as Martha Rogers, Hildegarde Peplau, Imogene King, Myra Levine, and Dorothy Orem. Prior to the work by these nurse theorists, frameworks for nursing research had often been "borrowed" from other disciplines. The new emphasis on the development and refinement of nursing theories allowed nursing to be established as a distinct discipline.

As early as the mid-1930's hospital and public health nursing administration were identified as areas of graduate study for nurses. It was acknowledged that nursing administration required a specialized set of knowledge and skills, and as such, in the 1950's the W. K. Kellogg Foundation funded 13 universities in order to establish graduate nursing programs that prepared nurses for hospital nursing administration. This emphasis continued into the 1970's as nursing administration was increasingly recognized as a practice area and certification for the specialty of nursing administration was established. However, the increasing emphasis on clinical specialization in nursing during the 70's and early '80's eventually resulted in decreased numbers of nurses enrolling in educational programs that were focused on nursing administration (Simms, 1989). Today nursing administration is recognized as an advanced practice role requiring graduate education to adequately prepare nurses to lead in complex health care practice and educational settings.

Summary

From the beginnings of mankind, persons have been designated, called, or educated to perform the functions we now refer to as nursing care. The history of nursing has been distinctly linked to a tradition of caring. Nurses have felt a true responsibility to reach out to those in need and to advocate on their behalf. See Contemporary Practice Highlight 1-1 for a further illustration of this call to caring.

The history of nursing reveals a pattern of recurrent issues that the profession has been required to confront over time. Some of these issues have included maintenance of standards for the profession, autonomy for nurses, and maintenance of control of professional nursing practice. Over time, the profession has also addressed phenomena such as nursing shortages, new categories of health-care providers, and ethical dilemmas. Each decade has brought new insight into ways the profession can better meet these challenges.

Nurses of the future must continue to monitor changes in technology, advances in scientific knowledge, and changes in society and in the health care delivery system. Perhaps through study of the challenges of the past we will have the insights to best meet our future.

CONTEMPORARY PRACTICE HIGHLIGHT 1-1

Susan Reverby. (1987). A caring dilemma: Womanhood and nursing in historical perspective. *Nursing Research*, 36(1), 5–11.

Susan Reverby, a noted historian, argues that "caring" is the central dilemma of U.S. nursing. She asserts that the history of nursing is intimately entwined with the history of U.S. womanhood. She believes that throughout history, nurses have viewed caring as the basis of their practice. Indeed, nurses believe it their "order," or mandate, to care if they are to fulfill the proper role of a professional nurse. However, nurses have difficulty fulfilling this mandate in a society that refuses to value caring.

In her historical research article, she traces the history of the "mandate" to care from Florence Nightingale, through the origins of U.S. nurse training schools, to the present day. In her analysis, she suggests that nursing continues to be plagued by the dilemma of "altruism versus autonomy" and offers implications of this dilemma for modern professional nursing practice. Too often nurses have equated the "order" to care and empower others with the need for self-immolation. She suggested that nurses need "to create a new political understanding for the basis of caring and to find ways to gain the power to implement it (p.10)" and in the process gain an understanding of how to practice altruism *with* autonomy.

Key Terms

■ **American Society of Superintendents of Training Schools of Nursing:** A national nursing organization founded in 1893 to elevate the standards of nursing education; later became the National League for Nursing Education, and ultimately, the National League for Nursing (NLN).

■ **Bolton Act of 1942:** Legislation that created the U.S. Cadet Nurse Corps, a program subsidized by the federal government and designed to quickly prepare nurses to meet the needs of the armed forces, civilian and government hospitals, and war industries.

■ **Deaconesses:** Women with some educational background who were selected by the church to provide care to the sick.

■ **Goldmark Report:** Published in 1923, this report recommended that nursing education develop educational standards, schools of nursing adopt a primary focus on education and be moved to universities, and nurse educators receive advanced education.

■ **Mahoney, Mary:** The first African American graduate nurse.

■ **Montag, Mildred:** Developed the concept for associate degree in nursing programs.

■ **Nightingale, Florence:** The founder of professional nursing in England.

■ **Nurse training school of Women's Hospital of Philadelphia:** Established in 1872, reputed to be the first permanent school of nursing in the United States.

■ **Nurses' Associated Alumnae of the United States and Canada:** Originally founded in 1896 with the intent of achieving licensure for nurses; became the American Nurses Association (ANA).

■ **Richards, Linda:** Purported to be the first educated nurse in the United States, a graduate of the New England Hospital for Women and Children in Boston.

■ **St. Thomas' Hospital:** A hospital in London where Florence Nightingale established the Nightingale School of Nursing.

■ **Wald, Lillian:** A public health nurse who founded Henry Street Settlement House to provide home nursing care to the immigrant populations on the lower east side of New York.

Reflective Practice Questions

1. What are some of the issues that the profession of nursing has confronted in the past? What solutions were proposed or implemented? What can we learn from these successful (or unsuccessful) efforts?

2. What contributions has military nursing made to the entire profession? What current nursing practices are the legacy of military nursing?

3. Although advanced practice nursing roles were formally introduced to the profession during the latter half of the 20th century, it has been argued that nurses began to function in expanded roles long before that time. Give examples of expanded roles assumed by nurses (community health nurses, military nurses) early in the 20th century.

4. What do you envision for the profession of nursing 50 years from now? What current trends in nursing practice do you believe will be the basis for future practice?

References

American Nurses Association. (1965). American Nurses Association's first position paper on education for nursing. *American Journal of Nursing, 65*(12), 106–111.

American Nurses Association & National League of Nursing Education. (1940). *Nurse practice acts and board rules: A digest*. New York: Authors.

Baer, E. (1990). *Editor's notes for nursing in America: A history of social reform*. New York: National League for Nursing.

Baly, M. (1997). *Florence Nightingale and the nursing legacy* (2nd ed.). London: Whurr.

Birnbach, N. (1999). Registration. In Schorr, T. and Kennedy, M. (Eds.) *100 years in American nursing: Celebrating a century of caring*. Hagertown, MD: Lippincott Williams and Wilkins, p. 17–22.

Brown, E. L. (1948). *Nursing for the future*. New York: Russell Sage Foundation.

Burgess, M. A. (1928). *Nurses, patients, and pocketbooks*. New York: Committee on the Grading of Nursing Schools.

Dolan, J. A. (1968). *History of nursing* (12th ed.). Philadelphia: W.B. Saunders.

Donahue, P. (1991). Why nursing history? *Journal of Professional Nursing, 7*, 77.

Gallison, M. (1954). The *ministry of women: One hundred years of women's work at Kaiserswerth, 1836–1936*. London: Butterworth.

Goldmark, J. (1923). *Nursing and nursing education in the United States*. New York: MacMillan.

Goodnow, M. (1953). *Nursing history* (9th ed.). Philadelphia: W.B. Saunders.

Haase, P. (1990). *The origins and rise of associate degree education*. Durham, NC: Duke University Press.

Henly, S. J., & Moss, M. (2007). American Indian health issues. In S. Boslaugh (Ed.), *Encyclopedia of epidemiology*. Thousand Oaks, CA: Sage.

Jensen, D. (1950). *History and trends of professional nursing* (2nd ed.). St. Louis: Mosby.

Kalisch, P., & Kalisch, B. (1981). When nurses were national heroines: Images of nursing in American film, 1942-1943. *Nursing Forum, 20*(1), 14–61.

Kalisch, P., & Kalisch, B. (1995). *The advance of American nursing* (3rd ed.). Philadelphia: Lippincott.

Larson, R. D. (1997). *White roses: Stories of Civil War nurses*. Gettysburg, PA: Thomas.

Livermore, M. (1888). *My story of the war, a woman's narrative of four years' experience as a nurse in the Union Army*. Hartford, CT: A.D. Worthington.

The NRA and Nursing. (1933). *Illinois State Nurses' Association Bulletin, 30*, 6.

Nutting, M. A., & Dock, L. (1907). *A history of nursing: The evolution of nursing systems from the earliest times to the foundation of the first English and American training schools for nurses*. New York: G.P. Putnam's Sons.

Pavey, A. E. (1953). *The story of the growth of nursing as an art, a vocation, and a profession* (4th ed.). Philadelphia: J.B. Lippincott.

President's Re-employment Agreement. (Blanket Code), July 22, 1933.

Randall, M. G. (1937). *Personnel policies in public health nursing.* New York: Macmillan.

Robinson, V. (1946). *White caps: The story of nursing.* Philadelphia: J.B. Lippincott.

Schryver, G. F. (1930). *A history of the Illinois Training School for Nurses, 1880–1929.* Chicago: Board of Directors of the Illinois Training School for Nurses.

Seymer, L. (1960). *Florence Nightingale's nurses: The Nightingale Training School, 1860–1960.* London: Pitman Medical.

Simms, L. (1989). The evolution of education for nursing administration. In Henry, Arndt, Di Vincenti, and Marriner-Tomey (Eds.), *Dimensions of nursing administration.* Cambridge, MA: Blackwell Scientific Publications

Stafford, M., Taylor, J., Zimmerman, A., Henrick, A., Perry, K., and Lambke, M. (2000). Letters to the editor: "A new vision for collective bargaining," *Nursing Outlook, 48*(2), 92.

Wald, L. (1934). *Windows on Henry Street.* Boston: Little, Brown.

Woodham-Smith, C. (1951). *Florence Nightingale.* New York: McGraw-Hill.

Nursing Education: Past, Present, Future

Martha Scheckel

LEARNING OUTCOMES

After reading this chapter you will be able to:

- Develop an understanding of the historical evolutions, contributions, and differences of various nursing education programs.
- Critique contemporary options for nursing education in the context of social, political, and economic trends and issues.
- Explain the process of accreditation in nursing education.
- Analyze curriculum and instruction in relation to learning nursing practice.
- Develop a personal philosophy of nursing education that reflects trends and issues in nursing education and practice.

Introduction

This chapter provides a descriptive account of nursing education including how its past has shaped its present and how current times are influencing and delineating its future. Understanding the continuum of development in nursing education promotes an awareness of the diversity that exists within nursing education and the common purposes that bind it together, encourages shared understandings of the various pathways that exist within nursing education, and promotes community among nursing students, nurse educators, and nurses regarding the complexities surrounding educational preparation for nursing practice.

This chapter begins with a discussion of the levels of nursing education prevalent since the turn of the 20th century and the issues associated with each program (see Table 2-1). The discussion begins with practical nursing, the most basic level of nursing education, and progresses to describing more advanced nursing education programs. The second half of the chapter focuses on curriculum and instruction in nursing education, beginning with a description of curriculum and instruction and including exemplars that describe what students learn and how they learn it in today's nursing schools. One might wonder why it is important for nursing students to understand curriculum and instruction. In the past, what and how students learned was the specialty of faculty. However, recent evidence suggests that student-centered curriculum and instruction can improve learning outcomes (Candela, Dalley, & Benzel-Lindley, 2006). As faculty respond to this trend, they seek approaches that overcome learning environments where teaching and learning as well as the teacher and the learner are separate, discrete, polarizing entities, each with his or her own predetermined roles, functions, and expected responsibilities. This means that students play an increasingly active role in their own learning. Therefore, a goal of the latter part of this chapter is to promote dialogue between teachers and students to encourage mutual trust, respect, and understanding for the content and processes involved in the preparation of nursing students for contemporary nursing practice.

TABLE 2.1 THE HISTORICAL EVOLUTION OF NURSING EDUCATION PROGRAMS

Early 1900s	1920s–1930s	1940s–1950s	1960s–present
Practical nursing	Practical nursing	Practical nursing	Practical nursing
Nightingale Schools	Diploma schools	Diploma schools	Diploma schools
Diploma schools	BSN	BSN	BSN
		ADN	ADN
Postgraduate education	Postgraduate education	Master's degree	Master's degree and CNL
	EdD for nurses	Doctorates for nurses	PhD, DNSc, ND, DNP

Abbreviations key for Table 2-1: ADN – associate degree in nursing; BSN – bachelor's of science in nursing; CNL – clinical nurse leader; DNP – doctorate of nursing practice; DNSc – doctorate of nursing science; EdD – doctorate of education; ND – nursing doctorate; PhD – doctorate of philosophy

As with any chapter in a nursing textbook, it is important to remember that this chapter provides an extensive synopsis of nursing education, particularly important aspects of the topics at hand. Students and teachers are encouraged to use this chapter as a platform for discussion, which can be further enriched by exploring the reference list provided at the end of the chapter. In this way, this chapter provides an excellent gateway to engage readers in the study of nursing education and to pursue ways of integrating its content with other sources of knowledge.

Understanding Nursing Education Programs

To gain an understanding of the various nursing education programs and the context within which they were developed, the discussion for each program includes a historical account of the program's development, the unique and significant issues and challenges associated with the program, and information on contemporary trends related to the program. This approach provides a comprehensive overview that captures the essence of available avenues to achieving a nursing degree. A description of mobility programs and a discussion of the educational accreditation process and its important role in ensuring high quality nursing education programs are also included.

Practical Nursing Education

"Unlike the historically untrained or poorly trained practical nurse, who had unlimited and unsupervised freedom to practice, the present practical nurse is often a hybrid. Today's practical/vocational nursing student is being taught basic skills during the educational program. After licensing, the LPN/LVN [practical nurse] is permitted to perform complex nursing, as delegated by the registered nurse and allowed by the nurse practice act" (Hill & Howlett, 2005, p. 80).

Responding to a Need: A Historical Overview of Practical Nursing Education

Practical nursing, the most basic level of nursing practice, began with the industrial revolution of the late 1800s. To meet labor workforce demands during this time, many people moved from rural areas to urban areas. Women needing employment often provided domestic services, including those associated with caring for the sick (Kurzen, 2005). To support the skills of this new healthcare provider, in 1892 the Young Women's Christian Association (YWCA) located in Brooklyn, New York, offered the first formal practical nursing course. Over time, landmark reports about the state of nursing education contributed to the development of practical nursing programs. For example, in 1923 Josephine Goldmark compiled a report (see Table 2-2) titled *Nursing and Nursing Education in the United States.* In it she recommended higher education standards for practical nurses, laws

TABLE 2.2 DOCUMENTS INFLUENCING TRENDS AND ISSUES IN NURSING EDUCATION		
Name of Document	Year Published	Contribution to Nursing Education
Goldmark Report	1923	Studied the field of nursing education and recommended minimal education standards
Burgess Report	1928	Studied nursing practice and education and addressed the need for major changes in the profession and for the development of a more comprehensive educational philosophy
Brown Report	1948	Recommended vocational education for practical nurses and recommended that education for registered nurses be in an institution of higher learning
Ginzberg Report	1949	Suggested it would be more economical for hospitals to eliminate diploma nursing programs and begin a 2-year course of study for student nurses in colleges
Nursing Schools at Mid-Century (West & Hawkins)	1950	Identified that many schools of nursing were not meeting standards, which provided evidence for reforming diploma nursing education

regulating their practice, and improved environments for their training. In 1948 Lucille Brown compiled another report, *Nursing for the Future*, which hastened the growth of practical nursing programs by emphasizing vocational schools as good environments for practical nursing programs. Today most practical nursing programs are in vocational schools.

Working as a Practical Nurse: Scope and Function

Since the first half of the 20th century, the scope and function of practical nurses have become increasingly sophisticated. They are licensed to practice either as licensed practical nurses (LPNs) or as licensed vocational nurses (LVNs), and they work under the supervision of registered nurses. Nurse practice acts for the practical nurse vary from state to state, but generally, the practical nurse is responsible for stable patients and patients with common health conditions. They also are responsible for collecting and reporting abnormal data, offering suggestions for developing and changing nursing care, providing bedside care, teaching health

TABLE 2.2 DOCUMENTS INFLUENCING TRENDS AND ISSUES IN NURSING EDUCATION *(continued)*

Name of Document	Year Published	Contribution to Nursing Education
Community College Education for Nursing (Montag)	1959	Established the validity of the ADN (2-year nursing) program as adequate preparation for nursing practice
American Nurses' Association Position Statement (ANA)	1965	Stated that those licensed to practice nursing should be educationally prepared in institutions of higher education
Toward Quality in Nursing (U.S. Public Health Service)	1963	Cautioned against preparing all nurses at the baccalaureate level
National Commission for the Study of Nursing and Nursing Education	1970	Cautioned against preparing all nurses at the baccalaureate level
Pew Health Professions Report	1998	Identified competencies nurses would need to prepare for nursing practice in the 21st century

maintenance, and participating with the healthcare team in evaluating nursing care (Kurzen, 2005).

Understanding Practical Nursing Education Today

The scope and function of practical nurses reflect the need for appropriate knowledge and capabilities to fulfill this supportive healthcare role (Mahan, 2005). Practical nursing education programs are often offered in community colleges. Most programs are 12 to 18 months in length, and graduates of these programs complete a state practical nursing exam (National Council Licensure Examination for

A nurse checks the heart rate of a patient. *Source:* © Andrew Gentry/ Shutterstock, Inc.

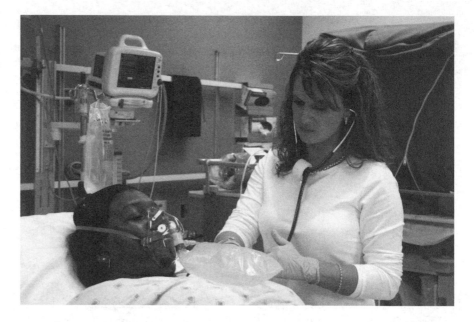

Practical Nurses [NCLEX-PN]; see Chapter 4) prior to being employed. For some individuals, this short course of study is a stepping stone to pursuing advanced nursing education. It also allows them to work as a practical nurse while obtaining further education. For others, practical nursing becomes a long-term career option. In either case, employment possibilities for practical nurses vary and are more plentiful in some states than in others. Long-term care facilities, clinics, hospitals, and home health care are the largest employers of practical nurses, with home health care leading the way in employment options. According to the Bureau of Labor Statistics (2006a), rising elderly populations, in-home medical technologies, and patient preference for home health care will increase the number of practical nurses needed in this area. As a result, one can expect that practical nursing will continue to be an integral part of the fabric of nursing education and nursing practice.

Diploma Nursing Education

"Your own first steps toward a nurse's skill—and toward the coveted nurse's cap," Miss Reamer said, "Will be classes. But not for long." They [student nurses] would learn the hospital routine gradually on the wards, then more and more, until each student would be responsible for her own patients" (Wells, 1943, p. 29).

Training vs. Educating: The History of Diploma Nursing Education

The quote above is from *Cherry Ames*, a fictional series of books about nurses that enamored many, encouraged the pursuit of nursing careers, and indeed reflected diploma nursing programs of that time in nursing education's history. Diploma nursing (originally known as "hospital nursing") began during the latter part of the 19th century with a growth in hospitals. Knowledge of asepsis partially spurred hospitals' growth and precipitated a demand for more nurses. Training of hospital nurses at this time was based on an **apprenticeship model** where nursing students provided service (direct patient care) in exchange for a few educational lectures, room and board, and a monthly allowance (King, 1987). The apprenticeship model flourished because it offered women an opportunity for a vocation, it improved care of the sick, and decreased the cost of nursing service in hospitals while student nurses provided patient care services for a minimal allowance (Bullough & Bullough, 1978).

> **KEY TERM**
>
> **Apprenticeship model:** A model of nursing education that was prevalent during the first half of the 20th century, where student nurses learned nursing practice by providing service to hospitals.

Despite the benefits of the apprenticeship model, it underwent criticism from nursing education leaders. Goldmark (1923) in particular emphasized that the training needs of students and the service needs of hospitals were incongruent. She wrote that when "the needs of the sick must predominate; the needs of education must yield" (Goldmark, p. 195). In other words, Goldmark argued that the hospital training of nurses was unbalanced. Training in the care of children, for example, was relinquished if students were needed to care for patients on the surgical ward. Similarly, May Ayres Burgess published a report in 1928 titled *Nurses, Patients, and Pocketbooks* (later known as the Burgess Report) that argued that within the apprenticeship model, students' patient assignments were based on the hospital's needs rather than on the educational needs of the students.

To balance the academic needs of nursing students with their need for clinical experiences, Dr. Richard Olding Beard advocated for university education for nursing students. He contended that university education would eliminate the incongruence between the hospital's service needs and the educational needs of students. In 1909 Beard began a nursing program at the University of Minnesota. This program is often heralded as the first baccalaureate nursing program. However, it closely resembled diploma education because, even though nursing students met university standards for admission and coursework, they were required to work 56 hours a week on the hospital ward (Bullough & Bullough, 1984).

> **KEY TERM**
>
> **National League for Nursing Education (NLNE):** A professional organization in nursing that fostered excellence in nursing education by supporting nursing education research, engaging in policy making and advocacy efforts related to nursing education, and promoting faculty development. It was the precursor to the National League for Nursing.

Shifting to a New Era in Diploma Nursing Education

Following Dr. Beard's efforts, the **National League for Nursing Education (NLNE)** made numerous attempts to redesign diploma nursing education programs. In 1917, 1919, 1927, and 1937 the NLNE published *Standard Curriculum for*

Schools of Nursing. This report encouraged diploma programs to decrease students' time working on the ward and to increase their education by offering 3 years of course work in the sciences and clinical experiences caring for diverse populations (e.g., medical surgical, pediatric, and obstetric patients). The work of Beard, the NLNE, and other reports on the state of nursing education did contribute to restructuring diploma nursing education. Stewart (1943), in fact, related that these efforts better informed the public about the state of nursing education, promoted experiments with new models of nursing education, and encouraged reform in schools of nursing (pp. 182–183).

During the middle of the 20th century, diploma nursing programs continued to thrive, and other reports such as *Nursing Schools at the Mid-Century*, compiled by West and Hawkins and published in 1950, promoted high standards in diploma nursing programs. Nonetheless, changes in health care such as rapid advances in medical technology and the expansion of knowledge in treatments for diseases required nurses to have sound theoretical preparation (Melosh, 1982). These changes signified a decline in hospital-based diploma programs and the beginning of a new era in nursing education where education would occur predominantly in colleges and universities.

Understanding Diploma Nursing Education Today

As of 2006 there were only about 60 diploma programs in the United States, with most of them located in the northeast (National League for Nursing [NLN], 2006). Hospitals that continue to support diploma programs maintain this educational option because these programs supply the nurses needed in their hospitals, they provide a geographically accessible program for some students, they offer a nursing degree in a short length of time, and they often offer tuition remission. To meet the educational needs of diploma students, many of these programs collaborate with colleges and universities to offer students options to obtain associate and baccalaureate degrees. Additionally, it is important to note that despite the reasons for the decline of diploma programs mentioned earlier, some studies suggest that diploma nurses are as competent in research, leadership, and critical thinking as graduates from other undergraduate nursing programs (Clinton, Murrells, & Robinson, 2005). Thus, for now it seems that diploma programs, though having experienced a turbulent history, are persisting and will continue to be a valuable asset to the nursing profession.

Associate Degree Nursing Education

"Every story in the mosaic of history has a beginning, a cast of characters, a set of social circumstances, and its own momentum. The development of a new, two year program for educating professional nurses during the years just after World War II is no exception" (Haase, 1990, p. 1).

Creating New Models of Nursing Education: The History of Associate Degree Nursing Education

As noted previously, in 1943 Isabel Stewart remarked that efforts to redesign diploma nursing education included experimenting with new nursing education models. One model was associate degree nursing education. It began in response to the post–World War II nursing shortage and it gained momentum following the Ginzberg Report (1949), which suggested that in comparison to a 4-year nursing program it would be more efficient and economical for colleges to offer a 2-year course of study in nursing. Ginzberg believed that not all nurses needed baccalaureate education to provide patient care. Nurses could be prepared to provide safe and competent patient care in less time than baccalaureate education, which would provide a feasible solution to the nursing shortage.

It was at this time that Mildred Montag (1951) described how 2-year associate degree nursing programs, housed in community colleges, could prepare registered nurses (RNs) as semi-professionals. This group of RNs would meet the demand for nurses by acquiring enough nursing skill and judgment to provide nursing care, but not the expert skill and judgment of baccalaureate-prepared nurses. Further study by Montag (1959) suggested that nurses prepared with an associate degree were performing similarly to staff nurses prepared with baccalaureate degrees. Moreover, those within the nursing profession believed that, with the exception of preparation in leadership and public health, nurses with an associate degree provided outstanding bedside nursing care (Smith, 1960). Others contended the associate degree program's focus on learning rather than on service to hospitals provided educationally sound preparation for nursing practice (Lewis, 1964). Still others believed that its accessibility and affordability through community colleges made this degree inclusive. For the first time in the history of nursing education, the associate degree in nursing offered those with little access to baccalaureate nursing programs the opportunity to become registered nurses (Hassenplug, 1965).

Emerging Controversies in Associate Degree Nursing Education

Indeed there were many advantages to associate degree nursing education, and these advantages remain present in today's associate degree nursing programs. Nevertheless, at the height of this program's success, in 1965, the **American Nurses Association (ANA)** published a position paper stating that those licensed to practice nursing should be prepared in institutions of higher education (universities). It also stated that the minimum preparation for the professional nurse should be a baccalaureate degree. In other words, the position paper equated

KEY TERM

American Nurses Association (ANA): A professional organization for nurses that develops various standards of nursing practice and promotes change through policy development.

professional nursing with baccalaureate education. This potentially meant that associate degree–prepared nurses could not practice as registered nurses unless they had licensure requirements that were different from baccalaureate-prepared nurses.

Despite these challenging circumstances, studies conducted since the ANA's position paper through the 1990s showed that, especially in hospital settings, there were unclear differentiations between nurses prepared in associate degree nursing programs and those prepared in baccalaureate degree programs (Bullough, Bullough, & Soukup, 1983; Bullough & Sparks, 1975; Haase, 1990). In fact, many studies showed registered nurses performed essentially the same in practice regardless of academic preparation. Studies occurring in the 2000s, however, are beginning to present a different picture. Current research suggests that baccalaureate-prepared nurses are associated with improved patient outcomes, that hospitals prefer to hire baccalaureate-prepared nurses, and that "magnet" hospitals have a higher percentage of baccalaureate-prepared nurses (Graf, 2006). This is not to say that associate degree nursing programs (like many diploma programs) will disappear. However, these studies do indicate mobility programs (discussed later in this chapter), through which associate degree–prepared nurses obtain baccalaureate and higher degrees in nursing, will take on even greater significance than they have in the past.

Understanding Associate Degree Nursing Education Today

According to the U.S. Department of Health and Human Services Health Resources and Services Administration, National Center for Health Workforce Analysis (2006), 52.8 percent of those wishing to become nurses enter associate degree nursing (ADN) or associate degree in science (ASN) programs. As a result, these programs remain one of the most feasible options of becoming an RN, and they address the nursing shortage by preparing nurses who are safe practitioners. Moreover, faculty members of ADN/ASN programs take responsibility for ensuring graduates are prepared for registered nurse roles in advocacy, leadership, professional involvement, lifelong learning, and evidence-based practice (National Organization for Associate Degree Nursing [N-OADN], 2006). Clearly, the nursing profession must support such nurses in practice and the educational programs that prepare them. However, it is important to note that only 20.7 percent of associate degree nurses return to school for baccalaureate and higher degrees (U.S. Department of Health and Human Services, 2006). Because the associate degree in nursing is considered an initial entry degree into practice as a registered nurse, it is important to investigate why so few associate degree–prepared nurses return to school. Advocates of nursing education need to provide opportunities and incentives for associate degree–prepared nurses to pursue further education.

Baccalaureate Nursing Education

"Very many private schools [hospital schools] of nursing still exist, but like the private schools of medicine that remain, there is a handwriting upon the walls of their future. . . . It says that their days are numbered, that "the old order changeth, giving place to the new," that the day of the university education of the nurse has come" (Beard, 1920, p. 955).

Advocating for University Education: The History of Baccalaureate Nursing Education

Dr. Richard Olding Beard (quoted above), a great supporter of baccalaureate nursing education, followed the thinking of Florence Nightingale and the **Nightingale Schools**. Nightingale believed that nursing education should occur outside of hospitals and the medical model (Stewart, 1943). This model of nursing education would avoid apprenticeships where nursing students received less education in the principles of nursing care because they were providing long hours of service to hospitals. Nightingale advocated for nursing students to learn sound theory in anatomy and physiology, surgery, chemistry, nutrition, sanitation, and professionalism; to train under the guidance of ward sisters who were nurses with experience and dedication to the profession; and to be part of a system that was financially independent from hospitals (Stewart).

> **KEY TERM**
>
> **Nightingale Schools:** Schools of nursing developed by Florence Nightingale that promoted student nurses learning the theory and practice of nursing outside of hospital control.

The Nightingale philosophy initially succeeded in the United States when Bellevue School of Nursing in New York adopted it in 1873. However, opposition to it, which included arguments that nurses do not need to be overeducated, that hospitals needed nurses for service, and that independent funding for nursing schools was unrealistic, maintained diploma nursing education. Despite the overwhelming support for diploma schools, several nursing education leaders during the early 1900s continued to believe in university education for nurses and subsequently persisted in advocating for baccalaureate nursing education.

For example, in 1901, Ethel Gordon Bedford Fenwick, founder of the International Council of Nurses, asserted it was time for nurses to be educated in universities where they could become skilled practitioners able to address local, national, and international health issues (Fenwick, 1901). Additionally, Dr. Beard supported leaders in nursing education who wanted higher educational standards for nurses. He convinced the University of Minnesota to begin moving nursing education into higher education. In 1909 this university began its first nursing program. Though, as referred to previously, it resembled diploma programs, it did represent the beginning of a slow movement in nursing education toward baccalaureate education for nurses.

Struggling to Develop Baccalaureate Nursing Education

Many schools followed the University of Minnesota's lead to offer students courses that supplemented diploma education. The most progressive of these programs was started at Teachers College, Columbia University, in 1917. Here students received 2 years of science at the university, 2 years of nursing at Presbyterian Hospital in New York, and 1 year of specialization in either public health or education (Bullough & Bullough, 1978). By the 1930s the number of students completing this "collegiate curricula" doubled, but these emerging baccalaureate programs remained chaotic and often resembled today's graduate education with an emphasis on specialization in public health, teaching, administration, and clinical specialties (Stewart, 1943, p. 276).

In the 1940s the development of baccalaureate nursing education continued, but the struggle to define it, develop curricula for it, and understand nursing roles from within it remained problematic. The Brown Report was especially helpful in making bold statements about baccalaureate nursing education. Brown (1948) wrote that nursing education belonged in institutions of higher education and that curricula in higher education for nursing education be integrated (including liberal and technical training for professional practice). She also wrote that the degree granted from integrated curriculum should be the Bachelor of Science in Nursing and that these nurses be prepared for complex clinical situations requiring high levels of education and skill.

By the 1960s baccalaureate education was taking shape. In particular, preparation in liberal education, intellectual skills, and content in leadership, management, community health, and teaching differentiated it from diploma or associate degree education (Kelly & Joel, 2002). The struggle for baccalaureate education seemed to be resolving, and the American Nurses Association position paper (1965) calling for the baccalaureate to be the entry-level degree for nursing certainly strengthened the argument for baccalaureate education. Nonetheless, other groups, including the Surgeon General's Consultant Group's document *Toward Quality in Nursing* (U.S. Public Health Service, 1963) and the National Commission for the Study of Nursing and Nursing Education (1970) were cautious in firmly stating that all licensed nurses needed baccalaureate preparation. These groups advocated for additional research to understand the skills and responsibilities required for high quality patient care. But this specific research (described in the next section) would not occur until nearly 40 years later.

Understanding Baccalaureate Nursing Education Today

Since the 1960s, baccalaureate nursing education programs have doubled. Today there are approximately 674 baccalaureate programs (Amos, 2005). Although there was a decline in enrollments in these programs during the 1990s, since 2001 enrollments have increased, with an 18 percent increase in baccalaureate-prepared nursing graduates (AACN, 2006b). Until recently, little research existed that responded to calls put forth in the 1960s to understand the relationship between educational preparation and quality patient care. As described previously, studies showed registered nurses, regardless of academic preparation, perform similarly in practice. A series of recent studies is changing this understanding because each of these studies has shown that hospitals with more baccalaureate-prepared nurses have lower patient mortality rates (Aiken, Clarke, Cheung, Sloane, & Silber, 2003; Estabrooks, Midodzi, Cummings, Ricker, & Giovannetti, 2005; Tourangeau, 2007).

As evidence mounts showing the relationship between higher education for nurses and improved patient outcomes, one could expect the momentum for the baccalaureate degree as the degree needed for entry-level practice as a registered nurse to increase. See Contemporary Practice Highlight 2-1 for an example of one state's proposal to address baccalaureate registered nurse preparation. What matters here is that support for baccalaureate nursing education does not mean opposing practical, associate, or diploma nursing education. Rather, it means striving to encourage nursing peers without baccalaureate degrees to pursue this degree, becoming active in making baccalaureate education accessible and affordable, and working as a team regardless of the academic preparation of a nurse.

CONTEMPORARY PRACTICE HIGHLIGHT 2-1

BACCALAUREATE EDUCATION IN THE STATE OF NEW YORK

In 2007 the New York State Nurses Association introduced a bill (A2480/S294) that would require registered professional nurses to attain a baccalaureate degree in nursing within 10 years of their initial licensure. The bill is modeled after an existing requirement in the state of New York that requires public school teachers to obtain a master's degree within 5 years of their initial teaching certification. If this bill to advance nursing education within the state of New York succeeds and becomes a law, it may mean that other states follow suit, thus increasing the number of baccalaureate-prepared nurses nationwide. A coalition entitled Coalition for Advancement of Nursing Education (CANE) has been formed to generate support within the state of New York for this bill (http://www.rneducationadvanceny.org). As of February 2008, bill A2480/S294 had been referred to the higher education committees of the New York State Assembly and State Senate. The status of this bill can be tracked on the New York State Nurses Association website (Retrieved 4/10/08 from http://www.nysna.org/advocacy/acti).

Graduate Education

"When one turns to the other . . . he [sic] finds a distinct possibility that a fresh and conspicuously enlarged contribution may soon come from many more nurses who find places of great social and professional usefulness in consultation, planning, research, writing, and the promotion of health services. . ." (Brown, 1948, p. 98).

Advancing Nursing Education: The History of Master's Preparation in Nursing Education

The quote above by Esther Lucille Brown was a prelude to the formation of nursing education programs that granted nurses master's degrees. At the time of her statement few nurses had master's degrees (known at that time as "specialties"), and many who had preparation beyond basic nursing education had postgraduate education. Postgraduate education was training nurses received through internships in areas such as pediatrics and infection control, practicum experiences in midwifery and anesthesia, or theoretical preparation in public health and nursing education (Bullough, Bullough, & Soukup, 1983). It also included additional training for nursing supervision and administration (Brown, 1948). Prior to the 1950s, if nurses wanted to obtain a master's degree rather than postgraduate education, they had to seek an advanced degree in another field such as sociology or psychology (Bullough & Bullough, 1984).

During the 1950s nurses first had the opportunity to obtain a master's degree in nursing when Rutgers University in New Jersey offered a master's degree in psychiatric nursing. This first master's degree prompted additional programs, which interestingly reflected specializations of the early postgraduate education in nursing (e.g., teaching, pediatrics, administration). As masters in nursing programs grew, support for them also increased. In 1969 and 1978 the ANA advocated for nurses' advanced preparation in theory to improve practice and in specialty nursing roles to offer high levels of competence in particular areas of nursing practice. By the 1970s societal trends encouraged an even greater demand for masters in nursing programs (Murphy, 1981). For instance, healthcare environments needed nurses with advanced preparation in areas such as research, teaching, administration, and clinical areas of nursing practice. The Council of Baccalaureate and Higher Degree Programs (1985) provided further support for master's preparation by stating that the nation needed nurses prepared with master's degrees in nursing to meet society's nursing needs.

Reforming Master's Preparation in Nursing Education

Despite support for master's education for nurses, Starck (1987) argued that by the 1980s there were far too many master's preparation programs, which served only to confuse the public. She pointed out that by the later 1980s there were 257 titles of masters in nursing programs. She provided recommendations for reforming master's degree programs whereby all master's-prepared nurses would receive core preparation in leadership, management, teaching, intellectual curiosity, creative inquiry, collaborative and consultative skills, and professionalism (p. 20). This preparation would provide the public with a clear understanding of a master's-prepared nurse. It would also prepare nurses to work in settings where autonomy and fiscal management were needed. For instance, she projected trends in healthcare costs would lead to the need for master's-prepared nurses to manage community-based nursing centers and to oversee companies providing services to hospitals.

Understanding Master's Preparation in Nursing Education Today

Starck (1987) was correct in projecting the need for master's-prepared nurses to function within a greater scope (e.g., there are now community-based clinics managed by nurse practitioners). Today there are a variety of master's degree programs, and according to the Bureau of Labor Statistics (2006b) there will continue to be a great demand for clinical nurse specialists, nurse practitioners, midwives, and anesthetists, especially in medically underserved areas. For a nurse wishing to seek graduate preparation, the continued variety of specializations from which to choose is appealing and personally satisfying. Nonetheless, in today's healthcare environment, it has become important to "think outside the box." Will the master's-prepared nurse of today be able to meet the needs of society in the future?

Recent trends include a movement toward a new model of graduate education called the Clinical Nurse Leader (CNL). The CNL focuses on generalist preparation, rather than specialist preparation (AACN, 2007b). The reason for developing such a role comes from evidence suggesting a need for nurses with master's education to develop methods for improving patient outcomes, coordinate evidence-based practice, and promote client self-care and client decision making. The AACN does not suggest that the CNL replace other master's-

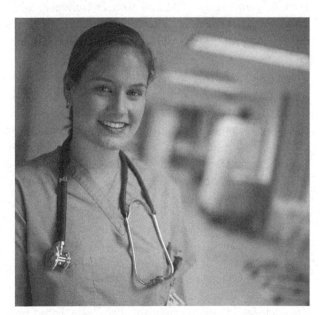

An emergency room nurse.
Source: © Ryan McVay/ Photodisc/Getty Images

prepared nurses; however, it contends this role will provide the public with nurses who have a comprehensive understanding of the broader healthcare system.

Despite the movement to develop the CNL, it is controversial. There are those who contend that the CNL only adds confusion to the multiple existing graduate education pathways, that its development undermines the roles of other nursing specialists (e.g., nurse practitioners and clinical nurse specialists), and that it minimizes the leadership role of every professional nurse (Erickson & Ditomassi, 2005). The AACN has attempted to address such concerns by describing the differences between these roles and the importance of the CNL (AACN, 2005). These conflicts highlight the need for continued dialogue about the CNL, the need for research on its efficacy, and the overall impact of this role in nursing practice specifically, and in healthcare systems generally.

It is clear, however, that there is an ever-increasing need in the United States for nurses prepared at the master's-degree level. The complexity of the healthcare system, the critical shortage of nurse educators, and the need for advanced practice nurses to deliver cost-effective, evidence-based patient care are just three of the driving forces that require nurses be prepared beyond the baccalaureate level to provide leadership in nursing administration, education, and practice.

Developing the Discipline of Nursing: The History of Doctoral Education

Doctoral education for nurses has existed since the 1920s. Doctoral programs originally prepared nurses for administrative and teaching roles. The first program was offered in 1924 at Teachers College, Columbia University, where nurses received an educational doctorate (EdD). Nurses received EdDs because the nursing profession had not developed its own doctoral programs, these doctorates were accessible through programs that offered part-time study, and the programs discriminated less against women as compared to programs in other fields (Bullough & Bullough, 1984). It was not until the latter part of the 20th century that doctoral programs in nursing developed. They developed out of recognition that the nursing profession needed its own research and theoretical base. As a result, doctoral programs in nursing dramatically increased, and offered nurses the opportunity to conduct research and develop theory within their own discipline.

Evolving Doctoral Programs in Nursing Education

The PhD (doctorate of philosophy) in nursing is often referred to as the "gold standard" for adequate doctoral preparation because it ensures nurses are competent to conduct research, which develops nursing knowledge and theory (Kirkman, Thompson, Watson, & Stewart, 2007). Despite the merit of the PhD, in the 1960s Boston University challenged it by beginning the DNSc, or the clinical doctorate. Many thought this doctorate would prepare nurses for doctoral level work in clinical practice, rather than research and theory (Loomis, Willard, & Cohen, 2007). Regardless of its original intent, over time, studies indicated that the DNSc (also known as the DNS or DSN), in many respects, is equivalent to the PhD (Loomis et al., 2007). Another challenge to the PhD occurred in the 1970s when Margaret Newman of New York University advocated for the ND (Nursing Doctorate) program. Similar to the DNSc, with the noted exception that the ND also prepares individuals for basic licensure as a registered nurse, she believed an ND would prepare nurses just as medical schools prepare physicians—for application of advanced knowledge in clinical practice. The first ND program began in 1979 at Case Western Reserve University in Cleveland, Ohio. This evolution of doctoral programs has essentially created two pathways for doctoral education in nursing, one that is research oriented and another that is practice oriented.

Understanding Doctoral Preparation in Nursing Education Today

Doctoral programs are entering a new and progressive era. The DNP (doctorate of nursing practice), proposed by the **American Association of Colleges of Nursing** (AACN, 2007a) to become the terminal degree for advanced practice nursing by 2015, is the newest doctorate focusing on advanced preparation in clinical practice. It is comparable to practice doctorates in fields such as pharmacy and physical therapy. The DNP provides advanced preparation in scientific foundations of nursing practice, leadership, evidence-based practice, healthcare technologies, healthcare policy, interprofessional collaboration, clinical prevention and population-based health care, and advanced nursing practice in specialty areas (AACN, 2006c).

> **KEY TERM**
>
> **American Association of Colleges of Nursing (AACN):** A professional organization in nursing that serves baccalaureate nursing and higher degree nursing education programs by influencing the quality of nursing education and practice through research, advocacy efforts, policy making, development of quality educational standards and indicators, and faculty development.

A great deal of controversy has surrounded the development of the DNP. Those supporting it suggest it offers improved formal preparation for advanced practice nursing roles not obtained by a master's degree in nursing (Hathaway, Jacob, Stegbauer, Thompson, & Graff, 2006). Nurses who have completed the DNP degree report that it provides them with improvement in their clinical expertise and the ability to shape healthcare policy (Loomis et al., 2007). Opponents of the DNP believe that it only serves to confuse the public about various nursing roles and functions. Additionally, its development precludes preparation for the role of nurse educator, creates possible shortages of advanced practice nurses who cannot afford to take the additional coursework needed to complete the DNP, and excludes schools of nursing that may not have the resources to develop a DNP program (Chase & Pruitt, 2006).

Despite these debates, today there are 46 DNP programs, with 140 more nursing schools considering starting this program (AACN, 2007c). As the DNP gains momentum and nurses prepared with the DNP begin to enter the workforce, it will be important for all in the nursing profession to understand how the DNP-prepared advanced practice nurse can potentially contribute to the nursing profession. For example, outcome studies that demonstrate how nurses with a DNP influence the health of individuals, groups, and populations will be necessary to document their contributions to health care. Although not necessarily receiving academic preparation as educators, in response to the nurse faculty shortage many DNP-prepared nurses will likely find roles as nurse educators in schools of nursing—will they be adequately prepared to assume these roles? (See Contemporary Practice Highlight 2-2.) Another important consideration will be what resources are needed to assist in the development of DNP programs in significant enough numbers in schools of nursing with diverse educational missions to produce the number of advanced practice nurses needed in the United States.

It will also be essential to help the public and other healthcare providers understand the DNP role. Nurses who are considering the pursuit of doctoral education will need to carefully consider which doctoral degree is the best fit for their professional career goals—the PhD, DNS, or DNSc degree with a research focus or a practice doctorate such as the DNP.

Mobility Programs in Nursing Education

"There is more depth to my practice now. I see nursing theory behind everything I do." (Delaney & Piscopo, 2007, p. 170)

CONTEMPORARY PRACTICE HIGHLIGHT 2-2

PREPARATION FOR TEACHING NURSING

The AACN has supported the development of the Doctorate in Nursing Practice (DNP) role. Yet, until recently, the NLN had not taken a position on the creation of the DNP role. In April 2007 the NLN released a statement that emphasized its support of all nursing programs. In this statement, the NLN stressed the need to ensure that nurses with advanced degrees be prepared in nursing education as much as they are prepared for advanced clinical practice, research, and theory development. It recommended a minimum of a certificate in teaching and learning principles to ensure a qualified pool of nursing faculty prepared to teach nursing students.

Source: National League for Nursing. (2007). *Doctorate of nursing practice—reflection and dialogue.* Retrieved February 19, 2008, from http://www.nln.org/aboutnln/reflection_dialogue/refl_dial_l.htm

Creating Options: Advancing Nursing Careers

Deepening one's knowledge base and understanding of nursing as well as advancing one's nursing career often occur through mobility programs. **Mobility programs** (also known as educational mobility or career ladder programs) enable individuals to enter the nursing profession from different educational points or pursue professional career development through additional academic preparation without losing credits from previous degree work. This additional academic preparation often involves articulating or making a transition from one nursing degree to another, more advanced nursing degree.

> **KEY TERM**
>
> **Mobility programs:** Nursing programs that facilitate the seamless articulation or transition from one degree in nursing to another degree (e.g., LPN to RN, ASN to BSN, ASN to MSN, BSN to PhD).

For example, there are LPN to RN, RN to BSN, RN to MSN, and even BSN to PhD mobility programs to name a few of the educational mobility options that are available in nursing. The RN to BSN or RN to MSN degree programs enable RNs who hold a diploma in nursing or an ADN (ASN) degree to return to school to pursue either a BSN or an MSN degree and receive credit for their previous coursework and possibly their work experience. There are also programs for those individuals who hold previous non-nursing baccalaureate degrees that enable them to complete a BSN in an accelerated time frame, usually within 12–18 months. These are commonly referred to as second-degree, fast track, or accelerated nursing programs. Accelerated programs for those individuals with previous non-nursing baccalaureate degrees who wish to receive a generic master's degree in nursing also exist. The commonality in all of these mobility options is that they enable the learner to achieve the advanced degree in a timely manner by recognizing and giving credit for previous academic accomplishments and frequently allowing the learner to prepare a portfolio documenting work experiences that can also be evaluated for potential academic credit.

Advancing one's nursing practice can also occur through continuing education programs that result in specialized credentials, certifications, or continuing education credits. For example, nurses can obtain additional education to become certified in diabetes education, critical care, or wound and ostomy care. They can also obtain continuing education by attending conferences or completing online courses or independent studies on particular topics relevant to their area of practice. Given this chapter's focus on academic nursing education programs, what follows is a description of issues and trends related to formal academic mobility options.

Supporting Mobility Programs

Mobility programs have a long history in nursing education and, in recent years, many of these programs have grown due to progress in distance education technologies, making the acquisition of advanced education more accessible. These programs have also flourished under pressure from various nursing organizations to promote baccalaureate and higher degrees in nursing. For example, in 1991 the National League for Nursing issued a position statement urging schools of nursing to coordinate articulation from one degree to another. They promoted the idea that schools should develop fair and equitable policies that allow students who have received credits for prior learning to transfer credits from one school of nursing to another. The American Association of Colleges of Nursing issued a similar position statement in 1998. The feasibility of these statements has increased in part because of governmental support, specifically Title II of the Nurse Reinvestment Act of 2002. This legislation funded mobility programs in a variety of ways to retain qualified nurses and to combat the nursing shortage.

Efforts to support mobility programs have resulted in many different degree articulation models. Some of these models are state mandated whereas others are voluntary. For example, some states have legislation in place mandating academic credit transfer from associate degree nursing programs to baccalaureate degree programs (AACN, 2006a). This model prevents graduates of associate degree nursing programs from encountering barriers to degree advancement, which can occur if baccalaureate programs do not accept academic credits from associate degree nursing programs. Voluntary programs, on the other hand, also exist to streamline the process of advancing from one degree to another. Some of these articulation programs are statewide initiatives (AACN), whereas others are agreements that exist between schools or within healthcare institutions (Eckhardt & Froehlich, 2004).

Reflecting on the Options: Advantages and Disadvantages of Mobility Programs

Regardless of the mobility options available, those considering a nursing career must weigh the advantages and disadvantages of mobility programs. On one hand they offer students flexible and dynamic options for advancing nursing careers. They are also often affordable and accessible and can expedite particular nursing degrees. For instance, students who wish to start their nursing career as an associate degree–prepared registered nurse can attend a community college. Once they decide to pursue a baccalaureate degree, they can continue working as an RN and complete an online baccalaureate completion program or a program at a nearby college or university. Or they may decide to pursue a master's degree in nursing and opt to enroll in an RN-MSN program.

Possible disadvantages of mobility options can include, but are not limited to, increased time commitments to complete coursework, problems with transferring credits from school to school and gaining credit for prior learning, and risks associated with returning to school when one is faced with competing demands. For example, students who complete an associate degree program in 2 years and then return to school for a baccalaureate degree may return to school and struggle through completing this degree on a part-time basis. Career and family commitments and demands may mean it takes longer to complete a baccalaureate degree than if pursuing the baccalaureate degree to begin with. These students may also encounter barriers in transferring credits and may need to show evidence of prior learning that can count toward their baccalaureate degree.

Regardless of the mobility program a student chooses, the likelihood of his or her success within it depends on the school's willingness to develop flexible and creative curricula (Boland & Finke, 2005). In response to the need for nurses prepared with baccalaureate and higher degrees, many schools of nursing are indeed designing flexible curricula and delivery methods that can accommodate learners returning to school to pursue nursing degrees.

Accreditation in Nursing Education

Accreditation is a process by which an institution's (e.g., school of nursing's) programs, policies, and practices are reviewed by an external accrediting body to determine whether professional standards are being met. Accreditation can also be considered to be a means of fostering continuous quality improvement in programs as the faculty also participate in the process to review and reflect upon all aspects of their program, with the goal of maintaining and improving quality.

Schools of nursing are accredited by the **National League for Nursing Accrediting Commission (NLNAC)** and/or the American Association of Colleges of Nursing **Commission on Collegiate Nursing Education (CCNE)**. Both NLNAC and CCNE are approved by the U.S. Department of Education. The NLNAC accredits all programs of nursing, whereas the CCNE limits it accreditation to BSN and MSN programs, and will eventually accredit DNP programs. Participation in the accreditation process of either NLNAC or CCNE is essentially a voluntary activity that schools undertake for the professional and public acknowledgment of the quality of their programs. Although accreditation by NLNAC or CCNE is a voluntary activity, it is an extremely meaningful one to the school and its students, because in some cases students can be denied access to scholarships/grants or admission to graduate programs if they are not enrolled in or graduates of a professionally accredited school. In addition to nursing's professional accrediting bodies, all schools of nursing are required to be accredited by the appropriate state board of nursing. Rules and regulations governing the operation and curricula of schools of nursing can be found in state board of nursing practice acts.

KEY TERM

Accreditation: A process by which an institution's (e.g., school of nursing's) programs, policies, and practices are reviewed by an external accrediting body to determine whether professional standards are being met.

KEY TERM

National League for Nursing Accrediting Commission: Affiliated with the National League for Nursing, this commission is an accrediting body for all types of nursing education programs.

KEY TERM

Commission on Collegiate Nursing Education: Affiliated with the American Association of Colleges of Nursing, this commission is an accrediting body for baccalaureate and higher degree nursing education programs.

The quality of nursing programs is measured through nationally established standards or criteria. Standards can include such things as how the school is fulfilling its mission and philosophy, how its curriculum is preparing students for nursing practice, and to what extent the qualifications of nursing faculty facilitate preparing future nurses.

The NLNAC and CCNE accredit schools for a period of time, usually 8–10 years, depending upon the agency and the review findings. Throughout the accreditation period, schools continue to use professional standards as benchmarks to evaluate their program, making necessary changes to ensure they maintain quality. Contemporary Practice Highlight 2-3 addresses the essential qualities and competencies that one of nursing's professional organizations, AACN, has deemed necessary for contemporary nursing practice; this document is used as a framework by many baccalaureate schools to ensure quality curricula.

Curriculum and Instruction in Nursing Education

Central to nursing education is curriculum and instruction. **Curriculum** is the overall structure of nursing education programs that reflects schools' mission and philosophy, course of

> **KEY TERM**
>
> **Curriculum:** The overall structure of learning experiences within nursing education programs that reflects a school of nursing's mission and philosophy, program outcomes, course of study, and program evaluation methods.

CONTEMPORARY PRACTICE HIGHLIGHT 2-3

THE AACN BSN ESSENTIALS OF BACCALAUREATE EDUCATION

In 1986 the AACN developed a document titled *The Essentials of Baccalaureate Education for Professional Nursing Practice*. The purpose of the document was to provide faculty in schools of nursing with an understanding of the competencies nursing students needed to function in contemporary healthcare systems. Many schools of nursing use the "essentials" to structure the curriculum of their nursing education programs. Due to social, political, and economic trends and issues this document was updated in 1998. In 2007, the AACN determined it was necessary to update the document once again. Changes in the document will likely mean revisions are on the horizon for many nursing curricula in order to remain current and up-to-date with contemporary practice. For instance, it is anticipated that the revised document will address the need to prepare students for evidence-based practice, information management, and expertise in evaluating patient outcomes (Martin, 2007).

Similar AACN documents for master's degree and DNP programs also exist, entitled the *Essentials of Master's Education for Advanced Practice Nursing* and the *Essentials of Doctoral Education for Advanced Nursing Practice*.

study, outcomes of learning, and methods of program evaluation. **Instruction** is the teaching and learning strategies and
experiences faculty and students engage in to achieve the elements of the curriculum. Throughout the history of nursing
education various trends and issues have influenced curriculum

and instruction. For example, advances in germ theory added to
what students learned about aseptic technique, progress in pharmacology changed
what students learned about drug therapies, and research in educational theory
changed how teachers taught as well as understandings of how students learn.

What follows are examples of some of the most prevalent trends and issues
influencing curriculum and instruction today. The areas listed are not all inclusive nor do they signify a certain level of importance. The purpose of the overview
is to provide you with an understanding of why you are learning what you are
learning in your curriculum (i.e., important topics) as well as why teachers use
particular methods of teaching and learning (i.e., important methods).

Learning Nursing: Important Topics in Nursing Education

Patient Safety

Patient safety has always been a priority in nursing education. In recent years, due
to widely publicized medical errors, patient safety has taken on even greater importance. The book *To Err Is Human: Building a Safer Health System* (Kohn, Corrigan,
& Donaldson, 1999) brought national attention to the issue of patient safety by discussing the number of people who die each year from medical errors. This, in turn,
sharpened the focus of patient safety in nursing education. Gregory, Guse, Dick, and
Russell (2007) urged nursing educators to begin the process of improving patient
safety by examining how curriculum and instruction are contributing to students
making errors and taking action to change teaching systems to reduce errors. Thus,
nursing students today and in the future may experience a system of nursing education that prepares them differently than in the past to understand the practices and
principles of reducing medical errors. Chapter 8 provides a further discussion of
patient safety and creating a culture of safety in healthcare systems.

Cultural Competence

Cultural competence is the extent to which a nurse understands and has the skills
required to effectively address the healthcare needs of individuals who hold cultural beliefs and values that are different from his or her own. As society continues
to become increasingly diverse and global in nature, there is an increased emphasis
on teaching concepts related to cultural competence in nursing curricula. For
example, the U.S. Census Bureau (2004) reported that Hispanic and Asian populations are growing faster than the population as a whole. Therefore, all nurses are
likely to work with healthcare providers and provide care to patients who have

A nurse giving medication to an elderly patient. *Source:* © Andrew Gentry/Shutterstock, Inc.

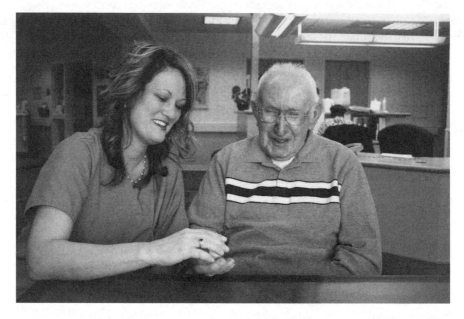

cultural backgrounds with which they are not familiar. Nursing programs are integrating coursework and clinical experiences related to cultural diversity and global health care into the curriculum. These experiences can include, but are not limited to, clinical experiences in other countries and learning with nursing students who live in other countries (Fitzpatrick, 2007). Chapter 14 provides a comprehensive discussion of cultural issues that impact nursing practice.

Gerontology

According to the Centers for Disease Control and Prevention (2007), by 2030 the number of people over the age of 65 will have doubled to 71 million, which will comprise 20 percent of the American population. In a response to this trend, Thornow, Latimer, Kingsborough, and Arietti (2006) have developed a guide for nursing faculty to assist them in preparing nursing students to care for the elderly population. The importance of having a critical mass of nurses prepared to care for the growing population of elderly in the United States cannot be overstated. It is important for gerontology concepts and experiences to be integrated throughout nursing curricula to provide students with the skills required to care for both the well and ill elderly. The elderly as a vulnerable population is addressed in Chapter 13.

Evidence-Based Practice

Evidence-based practice is an approach to nursing care where nurses draw on the best available evidence to make clinical decisions. In nursing, evidence-based practice includes nurses' use of research studies and theory from within nursing and outside of nursing (e.g., medicine, psychology, sociology) to make clinical decisions. For example, a nurse caring for a child with asthma draws on many sources of evidence to develop a therapeutic care plan for this child. Today's nursing students can expect to learn evidence-based practice through various activities where teachers provide instruction in best practices for gathering, analyzing, and synthesizing evidence. See Chapter 11 for a further discussion of evidence-based practice.

Technology and Informatics

Regardless of the practice setting in which students learn nursing care, it will include using various technologies and knowledge of informatics to assist with patient care. These technologies can include, but are not limited to, medical devices patients will use to provide self-care, as well as information retrieval, clinical information management, and documentation technologies. For example, students may have clinical experiences where they need to understand the use of various insulin pumps or pain management technologies that patients use at home, and that have patient teaching implications. Many schools of nursing are incorporating the use of personal digital assistants (PDAs) into the curriculum to help students immediately access information on medical terminology, laboratory values, and evidence-based information. Students' use of this device has important implications for improving their clinical judgment (Newman & Howse, 2007). Students are also being exposed to the use of a variety of clinical management systems. For instance, there are computerized physician order entry systems, telemedicine systems, and patient surveillance systems (Maffei, 2006), many of which have implications for ensuring patient quality and safety. Chapter 20 further addresses informatics and healthcare technology and their implications for nursing practice.

Interprofessional Education

A major movement in healthcare education is that of interprofessional education. It is defined as occasions when professionals learn with, from, and about each other to improve collaboration and quality of care (Barr, Freeth, Hammick, Koppel, & Reeves, 2006). The need for such education originates from concerns about patient care quality and safety and the overall importance of innovative ways to ensure good patient care outcomes. Preliminary research on interprofessional education indicated that it assists students in overcoming stereotypes about disciplines other than their own, promotes understandings across disciplinary boundaries, and improves students' ability to engage in teamwork (Freeth et al., 2001). Research on interprofessional education continues. For instance, current studies are investigating it as an approach to improving psychosocial care of oncology patients (see, for example, the Interprofessional Psychosocial Oncology Distance Education (IPODE) project at http://www.ipode.ca). Nursing students today will benefit from being open to and actively participating in emerging models of interprofessional education. Chapter 6 further explores the topic of interprofessional research and practice.

Learning Nursing: Important Methods in Nursing Education

New Pedagogies

Pedagogy is a term used in nursing education that means the processes of teaching and learning. In the 1980s, nursing education experienced what was known as the curriculum revolution. It began when the National League for Nursing called for nursing schools to examine what students learn and how they learn (Tanner, 2007). In other words, teachers were urged to critically assess the pedagogies they were using and to use new pedagogies to better prepare students for nursing practice. This movement, along with educational research providing evidence for best teaching practices, has led teachers to avoid passive learning strategies (e.g., lectures). For instance, problem-based learning, cooperative learning, and service learning promote student-centered, active learning. Nursing students today can expect to be much more engaged and involved in the teaching and learning process as compared to nursing students of the past.

Critical Thinking

A significant movement that accompanied the curriculum revolution involved using pedagogies to ensure students could think critically in clinical practice. Critical thinking is variously defined, but put simply, it is the ability of nursing students to make sound clinical judgments and to provide safe patient care. Traditionally, students who learned the nursing process were thought to be learning critical thinking. During the past few decades the nursing process has been challenged as the best approach to developing students' critical thinking. It is still the case that the nursing process does assist students in thinking through assessment of patients' health status, devising nursing diagnoses, planning care, deciding on nursing interventions to support that care, and evaluating patients' responses to care. However, current research in nursing education suggests that students also need to engage in thinking processes that promote reflective thinking, where they build practical knowledge (knowledge from experience); embodied thinking, where they learn the importance of intuition; and pluralistic thinking, where they consider a clinical situation using many perspectives (Scheckel & Ironside, 2006). Today's nursing student can expect learning experiences where teachers use the nursing process, but also use other strategies to develop students' critical thinking practices.

Distance Education

With the advent of new learning technologies there has been tremendous growth in distance education. Distance education is instruction students receive in a location other than that of the faculty providing the instruction (Clark & Ramsey,

2005). Nursing students today can expect that many of the degree options covered previously in this chapter will be offered in distance education formats. For example, some students may choose a distance education format to obtain a master's or doctoral degree. There are even distance education programs for undergraduate education. What is important to understand is how a distance education program will serve the learning needs of the nursing student and whether enrollment in a distance education program is the best choice for the individual student.

Simulation

Simulation is a clinical situation that allows student nurses to function in an environment that is as close as possible to a real-life situation (Scheckel, 2008). It traditionally includes the use of live actors, written scenarios, games, virtual reality, and simple mannequins (Bearnson & Wiker, 2005). Teachers use these forms of simulation to foster critical thinking, an understanding of patients' values and needs, decision making, and hands-on skills. In recent years simulation has become more sophisticated, through the use of high-fidelity human patient simulators (HPSs). HPSs are computerized mannequins that include preprogrammed but modifiable patient scenarios, allowing a teacher to direct the simulator's actions so the simulator reacts in real time in response to actions taken by the student nurse (McCartney, 2005). For example, a teacher can program a simulator so that the student uses both critical thinking and psychomotor skills to provide care in an emerging complex patient situation such as an acute myocardial infarction. One significant advantage to the use of HPSs is that it allows students to experience clinical scenarios that they may not get exposed to in real clinical settings. There is emerging research supporting the effectiveness of HPSs in nursing education.

The Future of Nursing Education

In 1998 the Pew Health Professions Commission, a group of healthcare leaders charged with assisting health policy makers and educators teaching health professionals to meet the changing needs of healthcare systems, completed a report listing competencies healthcare providers of the future would need. The competencies listed in this *Fourth Report of the Pew Health Professions Commission* (O'Neal & Pew Health Professions Commission, 1998) included many of the issues discussed in this chapter. For example, the list included the need for healthcare professionals to be competent in evidence-based practice and critical thinking and to take responsibility for patient outcomes. Now 10 years later it is important to reflect on how the commission's projections were so accurate. How will nursing education need to prepare nurses in these competencies and future competencies as changes in the healthcare needs of society occur? Reflecting current initiatives in professional education, Contemporary Practice Highlight 2-4 addresses the Carnegie Foundation for the Advancement of Teaching's Preparation for the Professions Program, a multiyear, multidisciplinary study that is investigating learning and effective teaching for nursing and other professions. The results of this study will undoubtedly influence future trends in nursing education.

Summary

This chapter provided insight into how nursing education will match the healthcare needs of society with the educational preparation of nurses. In particular, practical nursing will continue to have a place in nursing practice, especially in home health care. Diploma and associate degree nursing programs will remain, but evidence linking baccalaureate education with improved patient outcomes suggests there will be a continued movement to prepare a workforce of registered nurses who will need a baccalaureate degree in nursing to be licensed as a registered nurse. Master's education in nursing will continue, but it may be accompanied by Clinical Nurse Leaders (CNL) who will provide oversight and coordination of many of the competencies the Pew Health Professions Commission projected. For example, one important role of the CNL may be to coordinate evidence-based practice in a hospital. Doctoral education can be expected to grow, especially with the development and implementation of the DNP. This newly formed role will prepare nurses for a high level of competency in direct service roles for a variety of clients with complex healthcare needs. Accompanying

CONTEMPORARY PRACTICE HIGHLIGHT 2-4

PREPARATION FOR THE PROFESSIONS PROGRAM

In 2004 and 2005 the Carnegie Foundation for the Advancement of Teaching, an organization committed to the improvement of teaching and learning, began a study to examine teaching and learning in schools of nursing. The Preparation for the Professions Program is a study where investigators are comparing nursing with other professions such as clergy, engineering, legal education, and medicine to determine what is common and different among these professions (Benner & Sutphen, 2007). The hope is that such a study will show how these disciplines can inform one another about ways of changing and improving higher education for professional preparation. For example, are there caring practices of clergy that nurses can learn? This study has implications for shaping curriculum and instruction in nursing programs. Additional information can be found at the Carnegie Foundation for the Advancement of Teaching website: http://www.carnegie foundation.org/general/index.asp?key=30.

the progression in nursing education will be changes in accreditation standards. As nurse educators keep pace with changes in health care, so too will the standards by which schools are accredited need to change. Changes in standards will subsequently mean ongoing but important changes in curriculum and instruction.

Nursing education is dynamic. This chapter explored the landscape of nursing education, including moments of celebration and times of turbulence and instability. Throughout the history of nursing education the nursing programs offered have been a direct reflection of social, political, and economic trends and issues. Nursing leaders and nurses have responded to changing needs by offering a variety of nursing programs. For example, during the 20th century, diploma programs were thought necessary to meet the needs of hospitals, which, with advances in medicine and technology, were multiplying rapidly.

A consistent theme throughout all of the changes in nursing education has been the presence of nursing leaders who diligently investigated the state of nursing education and advocated for reforms to improve the delivery of health care through quality nursing education. Amid the reforms, nursing education leaders and nurses educated within its systems have not wavered in keeping the patient at the center of care. The accreditation standards that arose from leadership in nursing education and the flexibility of nursing educators and nursing students in changing curriculum and instruction are evidence of the patient-centered care the nursing profession strives to provide. Nursing students of today are beneficiaries of a long history in nursing education that has been characterized by a sustained emphasis on advocacy for ensuring they are prepared for nursing practice.

Key Terms

■ **Accreditation:** A process by which an institution's (e.g., school of nursing's) programs, policies, and practices are reviewed by an external accrediting body to determine whether professional standards are being met.

■ **American Association of Colleges of Nursing (AACN):** A professional organization in nursing that serves baccalaureate nursing and higher degree nursing education programs by influencing the quality of nursing education and practice through research, advocacy efforts, policy making, development of quality educational standards and indicators, and faculty development.

■ **American Nurses Association (ANA):** A professional organization for nurses that develops various standards of nursing practice and promotes change through policy development.

■ **Apprenticeship model:** A model of nursing education that was prevalent during the first half of the 20th century where student nurses learned nursing practice by providing service to hospitals.

■ **Commission on Collegiate Nursing Education:** Affiliated with the American Association of Colleges of Nursing, this commission is an accrediting body for baccalaureate and higher degree nursing education programs.

■ **Curriculum:** The overall structure of learning experiences within nursing education programs that reflects a school of nursing's mission and philosophy, program outcomes, course of study, and program evaluation methods.

■ **Instruction:** Teaching and learning strategies and experiences faculty and students engage in to achieve the elements of a curriculum.

■ **Mobility programs:** Nursing programs that facilitate the seamless articulation or transition from one degree in nursing to another degree (e.g., LPN to RN, ASN to BSN, ASN to MSN, BSN to PhD).

■ **National League for Nursing Accrediting Commission:** Affiliated with the National League for Nursing, this commission is an accrediting body for all types of nursing education programs.

■ **National League for Nursing Education (NLNE):** A professional organization in nursing that fostered excellence in nursing education by supporting nursing education research, engaging in policy making and advocacy efforts related to nursing education, and promoting faculty development. It was the precursor to the National League for Nursing.

■ **Nightingale schools:** Schools of nursing developed by Florence Nightingale that promoted student nurses learning the theory and practice of nursing outside of hospital control.

Reflective Practice Questions

1. As you reflect on this chapter, what are the advantages and disadvantages of the various degree options in nursing education today?

2. Nursing educators have often made changes in nursing education based on society's needs. How important is it to examine who decides what these needs are and who decides what changes are made in nursing education in response to these needs?

3. Nursing education has had many leaders who have ushered in important changes in the education of nursing students. What kind of leadership are you demonstrating that develops your ability to participate in leading nursing education in the future?

4. As knowledge in health care continues to proliferate, reflect on how you are learning nursing practice. Is it possible to know "all there is to know" about nursing practice? Is learning to think like a nurse more important than memorizing information?

5. A critique of nursing education is that its methods of curriculum and instruction have not changed—that is, teachers are still teaching using models of nursing education from the past. After reflecting on this chapter do you agree or disagree with this statement, and why?

6. After reading this chapter, in a few sentences can you describe what it means to be a nursing student today? How does the meaning you describe highlight areas of nursing education that will be important in preparing you for nursing practice?

References

Aiken, L. H., Clarke, S. P., Cheung, R. B., Sloane, D. M., & Silber, J. H. (2003). Educational levels of hospital nurses and surgical patient mortality. *Journal of the American Medical Association, 290,* 1617–1623.

American Association of Colleges of Nursing. (1997). *The essentials for baccalaureate education for professional nursing practice.* Washington, DC: Author.

American Association of Colleges of Nursing. (1998). *AACN position statement: Educational mobility.* Washington, DC: Author.

American Association of Colleges of Nursing. (2005). *CNL toolkit table of contents.* Retrieved November 23, 2007, from http://www.aacn.nche.edu/CNL/tkmats.htm

American Association of Colleges of Nursing. (2006a). *Articulation agreements among nursing education programs.* Washington, DC: Author.

American Association of Colleges of Nursing. (2006b). *Press release. Student enrollment rises in U.S. nursing colleges and universities for the 6th consecutive year.* Retrieved July 15, 2007, from http://www.aacn.nche.edu/06Survey.htm

American Association of Colleges of Nursing. (2006c). *The essentials of doctoral education for advanced practice.* Washington, DC: Author.

American Association of Colleges of Nursing. (2007a). *Doctor of nursing practice (DNP) programs.* Retrieved July 15, 2007, from http://www.aacn.nche.edu/DNP/DNPProgramList.htm

American Association of Colleges of Nursing. (2007b). *White paper on the education and role of the clinical nurse leader.* Washington, DC: Author. Retrieved July 15, 2007, from http://www.aacn.nche.edu/Publications/pdf/2-07CNLWhitePaperf.pdf

American Nurses Association. (1969). *Statement on graduate education in nursing.* Kansas City, MO: Author.

American Nurses Association. (1978). *Statement on graduate education in nursing.* Kansas City, MO: Author.

American Nurses Association. (1965). American Nurses Association first position on education for nurses. *American Journal of Nursing, 65*(120), 106–111.

Amos, L. K. (2005). *Baccalaureate nursing programs.* Retrieved July 15, 2007, from http://www.aacn.nche.edu/Education/nurse_ed/BSNArticle.htm

Barr, H., Freeth, D., Hammick, M., Koppel, I., & Reeves, S. (2006). The evidence base and recommendations for interprofessional education in health and social care. *Journal of Interprofessional Care, 20*(1), 75–78.

Beard, R. O. (1920). The social, economic and educational status of the nurse. *The American Journal of Nursing, 12*(20), 955–962.

Bearnson, C. S., & Wiker, K. M. (2005). Human patient simulators: A new face in baccalaureate nursing education at Brigham Young University. *Journal of Nursing Education, 44*(9), 421–425.

Benner, P., & Sutphen, M. (2007). Learning across the professions: The clergy, a case and point. *Journal of Nursing Education, 46*(3), 103–108.

Boland, D. L., & Finke, L. M. (2005). Teaching and learning at a distance. In D. M. Billings & J. A. Halstead (Eds.), *Teaching in nursing: A guide for faculty* (2nd ed., pp. 145–166). St. Louis, MO: Elsevier Saunders.

Brown, E. L. (1948). *Nursing for the future: A report prepared for the National Nursing Council.* New York: Russell Sage Foundation.

Bullough, V. L., & Bullough, B. (1978). *The care of the sick: The emergence of modern nursing.* New York: Prodist.

Bullough, V. L., & Bullough, B. (1984). *History, trends, and politics of nursing.* Norwalk, CT: Appleton-Century-Crofts.

Bullough, B., Bullough, V., & Soukup, M. C. (1983). *Nursing issues and nursing strategies for the eighties.* New York: Springer.

Bullough, B., & Sparks, C. (1975). Baccalaureate vs. associate degree nurses: The care–cure dichotomy. *Nursing Outlook, 23*(11), 688–992.

Bureau of Labor Statistics. (2006a). *Occupational outlook handbook: Licensed practical and licensed vocational nurses.* Retrieved June 4, 2007, from http://www.bls.gov/oco/ocos102.htm

Bureau of Labor Statistics. (2006b). *Registered nurses.* Retrieved July 13, 2007, from http://www.bls.gov/oco/ocos083.htm#training

Burgess, M. A. (1928). *Nurses, patients and pocketbooks: Report of a study of the economics of nursing conducted by the Committee on the Grading of Nursing Schools.* New York: Committee on the Grading of Nursing Schools.

Candela, L., Dalley, K., & Benzel-Lindley, J. (2006). A case for learning-centered curricula. *Journal of Nursing Education, 45*, 59–66.

Centers for Disease Control and Prevention & The Merck Company Foundation. (2007). *The state of aging and health in America 2007.* Whitehouse Station, NJ: The Merck Company Foundation. Retrieved July 12, 2007, from http://www.cdc.gov/aging/saha.htm

Chase, S. K., & Pruitt, R. H. (2006). The practice doctorate: Innovation or disruption? *Journal of Nursing Education, 45*(5), 155–161.

Clark, C. E., & Ramsey, R. W. (2005). Teaching and learning at a distance. In D. M. Billings & J. A. Halstead (Eds.), *Teaching in nursing: A guide for faculty* (2nd ed., pp. 397–439). St. Louis, MO: Elsevier Saunders.

Clinton, M., Murrells, T., & Robinson, S. (2005). Assessing competency in nursing: A comparison of nurses prepared through degree and diploma programmes. *Journal of Clinical Nursing, 14*(1), 82–94.

Council of Baccalaureate and Higher Degree Programs. (1985). *Master's education in nursing. Route to opportunities in contemporary nursing: 1984–1985.* New York: National League for Nursing.

Delaney, C., & Piscopo, B. (2007). There really is a difference: Nurses' experiences with transitioning from RNs to BSNs. *Journal of Professional Nursing, 23*(3), 167–173.

Eckhardt, J., & Froehlich, H. (2004). An education-service partnership: Helping RNs obtain baccalaureate degrees in nursing at their practice sites. *Journal of Nursing Education, 43*(12), 558–561.

Erickson, J. I., & Ditomassi, M. (2005). The clinical nurse leader: New in name only. *Journal of Nursing Education, 44*(3), 99–100.

Estabrooks, C. A., Midodzi, W. K., Cummings, G. G., Ricker, K. L., & Giovannetti, P. (2005). The impact of hospital nursing characteristics on 30-day mortality. *Nursing Research, 54*(2), 74–84.

Fenwick, E. B. (1901). A plea for the higher education of trained nurses. *The American Journal of Nursing, 2*(1), 4–8.

Fitzpatrick, J. (2007). From the editor: Cultural competence in nursing revisited. *Nursing Education Perspectives, 28*(1), 5.

Freeth, D., Reeves, S., Goreham, C., Parker, P., Haynes S., & Pearson, S. (2001). "Real life" clinical learning on an interprofessional training ward. *Nursing Education Today, 21,* 366–372.

Ginzberg, E. (1949). *A pattern for hospital care: Final report of the New York State hospital study.* New York: Columbia University Press.

Goldmark, J. (1923). *Nursing and nursing education in the United States: The Committee for Study of Nursing Education.* New York: Macmillan.

Graf, C. M. (2006). ADN to BSN: Lessons from human capital theory. *Nursing Economics, 24*(3), 135–141.

Gregory, D. M., Guse, L. W., Dick, D. D., & Russell, C. K. (2007). Research briefs: Patient safety: Where is nursing education? *Journal of Nursing Education, 46*(2), 79–82.

Haase, P. T. (1990). *The origins and rise of associate degree nursing education.* Durham, NC: Duke University Press.

Hassenplug, L. W. (1965). Preparation of the nurse practitioner. *The Journal of Nursing Education, 1,* 29–33.

Hathaway, D., Jacob, S., Stegbauer, C., Thompson, C., & Graff, C. (2006). The practice doctorate: Perspectives of early adopters. *Journal of Nursing Education, 45*(12), 487–496.

Hill, S. S., & Howlett, H. S. (2005). *Success in practical/vocational nursing: From student to leader.* St. Louis, MO: Elsevier Saunders.

Kelly, L. Y., & Joel, L. A. (2002). *The nursing experience: Trends, challenges, and transitions* (4th ed.). New York: McGraw-Hill.

King, M. G. (1987). *Conflicting interests: Professionalization and apprenticeship in nursing education. A case study of the Peter Bent Brigham Hospital.* Unpublished doctoral dissertation, Boston University.

Kirkman, S., Thompson, D. R., Watson, R., & Stewart, S. (2007). Are all doctorates equal or are some more "equal than others?" An examination of which ones should be offered by schools of nursing. *Nursing Education in Practice, 7,* 61–66.

Kohn, L. T., Corrigan, J. M., & Donaldson, M. S. (Eds.). (1999). *To err is human.* Washington, DC: Institute of Medicine.

Kurzen, C. R. (2005). *Contemporary practical/vocational nursing* (5th ed.). Philadelphia: Lippincott Williams & Wilkens.

Lewis, E. P. (1964). The associate degree program. *American Journal of Nursing, 64*(5), 78–81.

Loomis, J. A., Willard, B., & Cohen, J. (2007). Difficult professional choices: Deciding between the PhD and the DNP in nursing. *Online Journal of Issues in Nursing, 12*(1).

Maffei, R. (2006). Pros and cons of healthcare information technology implementation: The pros win. *JONA's Healthcare Law, Ethics, and Regulation, 8*(4), 116–122.

Mahan, P. (2005). It's time to unite. *Journal of Practical Nursing, 55*(4), 25–26.

Martin, P. (2007). 10 questions . . . with Patricia A. Martin Ph.D., RN. *Syllabus, 33*(2), 6.

McCartney, P. (2005). The new networking. Human patient simulators in maternal-child nursing. *MCN: The American Journal of Maternal/Child Nursing, 30*(3), 215.

Melosh, B. (1982). *"The physician's hand." Work culture and conflict in American nursing.* Philadelphia: Temple University Press.

Montag, M. (1951). *The education of nursing technicians.* New York: G.P. Putnam's Sons.

Montag, M. (1959). *Community college education for nurses.* New York: McGraw-Hill.

Murphy, M. I. (1981). *Master's programs in nursing in the eighties: Trends and issues.* Washington, DC: American Association of Colleges of Nursing.

National Commission for the Study of Nursing and Nursing Education. (1970). Summary report and recommendations. *American Journal of Nursing, 70*(2), 279–294.

National League for Nursing. (1991). *Position statement: Educational mobility.* New York: Author.

National League for Nursing. (2006). *A guide to state approved schools of nursing 2006 RN.* New York: Author.

National League for Nursing. (2007). *Doctorate of nursing practice—reflection and dialogue.* Retrieved February 19, 2008, from www.nln.org/aboutnln/reflection_dialogue/refl_dial_1.htm

National League for Nursing Education. (1917). *Standard curriculum for schools of nursing.* Baltimore: Waverly Press.

National League for Nursing Education. (1919). *Standard curriculum for schools of nursing.* New York: Author.

National League for Nursing Education. (1927). *Standard curriculum for schools of nursing.* New York: Author.

National League for Nursing Education. (1937). A *curriculum for schools of nursing.* New York: Author.

National Organization for Associate Degree Nursing. (2006). *Position statement of associate degree nursing.* Pensacola, FL: Author.

Newman, K., & Howse, E. (2007). The impact of a PDA-assisted documentation tutorial on nurses' students attitudes. *Computer Informatics Nursing, 25*(2), 76–83.

O'Neal, E. H., & the Pew Health Professions Commission. (1998). *Recreating health professional practice for a new century: The fourth report of the Pew Health Professions Commission.* San Francisco, CA: Pew Health Professions Commission.

Scheckel, M. (2008). Selecting learning experiences to achieve curriculum outcomes. In D. M. Billings & J. A. Halstead (Eds.), *Teaching in nursing: A guide for faculty* (3rd ed.). St. Louis, MO: Elsevier Saunders, pp. 154–172.

Scheckel, M. M., & Ironside, P. M. (2006). Cultivating interpretive thinking through enacting narrative pedagogy. *Nursing Outlook, 54,* 159–165.

Smith, D. W. (1960). Different programs; different objectives. *Nursing Outlook, 8*(12), 688–689.

Starck, P. L. (1987). The master's-prepared nurse in the marketplace: What do master's-prepared nurses do? What should they do? In S. E. Hart (Ed.), *Issues in graduate nursing education* (pp. 3–23). New York: National League for Nursing.

Stewart, I. M. (1943). *The education of nurses: Historical foundations and modern trends.* New York: Macmillan.

Tanner, C. A. (2007). Editorial. The curriculum revolution revisited. *Journal of Nursing Education, 46*(2), 51–52.

Thornow, D., Latimer, D., Kingsborough, J., & Arietti, L. (2006). *Caring for an aging America: A guide for nursing faculty.* Washington, DC: American Association of Colleges of Nursing and the John A. Hartford Foundation. Retrieved July 12, 2007, from http://www.aacn.nche.edu/Education/Hartford/pdf/monograph.pdf

Tourangeau, A. Press releases. Hospital death rate study reveals wide variations and stresses importance of registered nurses. *Journal of Advanced Nursing.* Retrieved July 12, 2007, from http://www.journalofadvancednursing.com/default.asp?File=pressdetail&id=195

U.S. Census Bureau. (2004). *People: Race and ethnicity.* Retrieved July 11, 2007, from http://factfinder.census.gov/jsp/saff/SAFFInfo.jsp?_pageId=tp9_race_ethnicity

U.S. Congress. (2001). *Nurse reinvestment act. Public law.* Report No. PL-107-205. (ERIC Document Reproduction Service No. ED 468 471). Retrieved December 10, 2007, from www.eric.ed.gov/ERICWebPortal/recordDetail?accno=ED468471

U.S. Department of Health and Human Services Health Resources and Services Administration, National Center for Health Workforce Analysis. (2006). *The registered nurse population: Findings from the 2004 national sample survey of registered nurses.* Retrieved July 7, 2007, from http://bhpr.hrsa.gov/healthworkforce/rnsurvey04/

U.S. Public Health Service. (1963). *Toward quality in nursing.* Report of the Surgeon General's Consultant Group on Nursing (Pub No. 992). Washington, DC: U.S. Government Printing Office.

Wells, H. (1943). *Cherry Ames student nurse.* New York: Grosset & Dunlap.

West, M. D., & Hawkins, C. (1950). *Nursing schools at the mid-century.* New York: National Committee for the Improvement of Nursing Services.

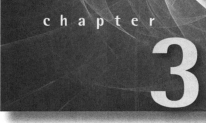

Understanding the NCLEX-RN

Lillia Loriz and Lucy B. Trice

LEARNING OUTCOMES

After reading this chapter you will be able to:

- Explain the purpose of the NCLEX-RN.
- Describe how the NCLEX-RN was developed.
- Analyze the components of the NCLEX-RN test plan.
- Discuss the CAT testing format, including the benefits of this form of testing.
- Explore the various types of questions on the NCLEX-RN.
- Develop strategies to assist in preparing for the NCLEX-RN.

Introduction

As students near the end of their nursing program and prepare to graduate, their thoughts turn naturally to two major events in their professional lives—acquiring their first position as a registered nurse and passing the registered nurse licensure examination. For many students, taking the licensure examination can be a stressful event; after all, one cannot practice as a registered nurse without passing the examination. However, with proper preparation, much can be done to raise self-confidence levels and decrease the normal feelings of anxiety and stress associated with taking the examination.

63

National Council Licensing Examination for Registered Nurses (NCLEX- RN): This examination must be taken by all graduates of diploma, associate degree, and baccalaureate degree nursing programs prior to a license being issued. Successful completion of the NCLEX-RN is a requirement for practice as a registered nurse.

National Council of State Boards of Nursing (NCSBN): The body given the task of providing a means to ensure that those who are licensed to practice as nurses are "safe" in terms of their knowledge base.

The purpose of this chapter is to provide you with an overview of the **National Council Licensure Examination for Registered Nurses (NCLEX-RN)** examination and with suggestions on how to best prepare yourself to take the examination. A brief overview of the purpose of the examination and how it was developed will help introduce to you to the NCLEX-RN. This will be followed by a discussion of the examination, content areas, and test question formatting. Finally, suggestions on how to prepare and take the examination are included.

Purpose of the NCLEX-RN

The **National Council of State Boards of Nursing (NCSBN)** is the body given the task of providing a means to ensure that those who are licensed to practice as registered nurses are "safe" in terms of their knowledge base. The NCSBN performs this function by providing an examination that those educated as registered nurses through diploma, associate degree, and baccalaureate degree programs must successfully complete in order to receive a license to practice nursing. This test is the National Council Licensure Examination for Registered Nurses, more commonly known as the NCLEX-RN. The NCSBN performs the same function for those educated as practical nurses, through the National Council Licensure Examination for Practical Nurses or NCLEX-PN.

The need for a means of ensuring that all nurses who have graduated from a nursing program have a minimal level of competency was recognized as early as 1867 in England; however, this notion did not take root in the United States until 1896 (Kelly & Joel, 1996). As discussed in Chapters 1 and 2, in the early days of nursing education in this country, nursing schools were designed to meet the individual needs of the hospitals housing the programs. Some schools of nursing existed in full-spectrum hospitals, which offered a wide variety of services including medical, surgical, obstetric, and pediatric care, as well as in hospitals offering specialized care only, such as psychiatric and children's hospitals. Nurses graduating from schools associated with full-spectrum hospitals had a different skill set from those educated in single specialty hospitals. Additionally, many of those practicing as nurses had no formal training at all, but could call themselves nurses because there were no legal restrictions on their representing themselves as such (Kalisch & Kalisch, 2004).

This wide disparity in the skills of those calling themselves nurses was the impetus for the movement to license nurses. The movement began in this country in the early part of the 20th century, and by 1923, every state had instituted a form of licensure known as permissive licensure. Licensure was not required, hence the term *permissive*. The rules were voluntary and basically provided a means for licensure to be permitted but not required. In each state, requirements for licensure included educational requirements, rules for examinations, as well as provision for revocation of the license (Kalisch & Kalisch, 1995). Although this type of licensure was not mandatory, it was required in order to use the title "registered nurse." Licensure did not become universally mandatory in all 50 states until the middle of the 20th century.

The purpose of all activities associated with nursing licensure is to address safety for the public who are the recipients of nursing care. Licensing examinations for entry-level nurses and practical nurses are measures of minimal safety. They do not indicate that the individual who has passed these examinations and obtained a license has an exceptional amount of knowledge, but rather that he or she has the minimal amount believed necessary for "safe" practice. The nursing profession has a duty to protect the public from unsafe care, and the NCLEX-RN is one measure designed to accomplish this task (Wall, Miller, & Widerquist, 1993). Nursing programs must have the approval of their state board of nursing in order for their graduates to be granted permission by the NCSBN to take the NCLEX-RN. Part of the evaluation process of nursing programs by the constituent state boards of nursing is reviewing the performance of the school's graduates on the examination. The success of first-time test takers in particular is tracked, and it is possible for schools to be put on probation or have their state board of nursing approval revoked if their success rate falls below the accepted range stipulated by the particular state's board of nursing.

Development of the NCLEX-RN

Initial Development

During the early 1940s, nursing schools recognized that the current method of testing for licensure, tailored to individual states, was inadequate. The National League of Nursing Education (NLNE) recommended that a standardized licensing examination be used by all of the states. Following World War II, the American Nurses Association created the Council of State Boards of Nursing. The council was made up of representatives from each of the states in existence at that time, as well as from each of the other jurisdictions of the United States. The council joined forces with the NLNE in advocating for this standardized licensing examination, and further recommended that the NLNE assist in the development of this test. Each state board was asked to submit sample test questions, and the NLNE's Committee on Nursing Tests selected the ones they believed to be most suitable. The examinations were set up so that each could be graded by machine, rather than by hand, and the examination became known as the State Board Test Pool Examination (Kalisch & Kalisch, 2004; Scherubel, 2005).

By the end of the first year of operation, 15 states had administered the examination. Initially, the examination was made up of 13 separate tests dealing with anatomy and physiology, chemistry, biology, and other areas of the sciences, as well as nutrition and diet therapy, pharmacology, and the various nursing specialties. Within 5 years, this number was reduced to six: medical nursing, surgical nursing, obstetrical nursing, nursing of children, communicable disease, and psychiatric nursing. The tests were designed to assess understanding of scientific principles as well as nursing skills and abilities in specific clinical areas (Kalisch & Kalisch, 2004). Questions were developed to test application of knowledge rather than concentrating on factual knowledge, which had been a criticism of the earlier tests. By 1950, the test was being given in all 48 of the contiguous states, as well as Hawaii (not yet a state) and the District of Columbia. This action made nursing the first profession to have the same licensing examination used throughout the nation (Kalisch & Kalisch, 2004).

During this period, each state or territory set its own standard for what constituted a passing score. This practice tended to hamper nurses' geographic mobility, because a passing score in one state might not be high enough for licensure to be granted in another state. For this reason, in 1951, the council recommended that a minimum score of 350 on each test be adopted as the standard passing score. Most states, but not all, chose to adopt this recommendation.

An advantage of the individual tests was that it was possible for a candidate to pass some portions of the exam and fail others. In this event, only the tests failed needed to be retaken, depending on the number failed. California, for example, allowed no more than two portions to be failed and retaken without needing to retake the entire test. All tests had to be successfully passed before the individual would be issued a license and be entitled to use the designation of registered nurse.

Pencil and paper tests were given at set times during the year, generally in large centrally located cities in each state. At that time, candidates were required to take the test in the state in which they wished to be licensed. In order to be licensed in another state, they applied to that state for reciprocity. Reciprocity refers to the practice of providing licensure in one state based on licensure in another state. This means the registered nurse does not have to retake the NCLEX-RN in each state in order to be licensed in that state. Once the initial licensure has been obtained, registered nurses can apply for licensure by reciprocity in other states. Contemporary Practice Highlight 3-1 addresses the nursing licensure compact, which is currently changing the concept of reciprocity as the profession has historically known it.

In 1952 the NLNE joined forces with several other organizations to become the National League for Nursing (NLN). This body functioned as the accrediting body for schools of nursing as well as the testing service for the national licensing

CONTEMPORARY PRACTICE HIGHLIGHT 3-1

NURSE LICENSURE COMPACT

Recognizing the increased mobility of nurses, over a decade ago the NCSBN proposed a nurse licensure compact to allow nurses to be licensed in their state of residence, but practice in other states participating in the compact without having to obtain specific licensure in those states. As of October 2007 there were 22 compact. member states, with more states considering this option. More recently, the NCSBN has also approved a similar model for advanced practice nurses; however, this model has not yet been implemented. Further information on the nurse licensure compact model can be found at https://www.ncsbn.org/156.htm

examination, which continued to be developed and revised by the council until 1978. At that time, the National Council of State Boards of Nursing was established, which continued the work of the ANA's Council of State Boards of Nursing (Chitty & Black, 2007).

Changes in the NCLEX-RN

Since the early days of the national licensing examination, its purpose has been to protect the public by providing a means of establishing minimal competency for entry into practice. That same desire has been the driving force behind continued efforts to revise and refine the current test. The term *NCLEX-RN* was first used in 1982. The NCLEX-RN format was revised from separate tests for the various nursing specialties to one test addressing all of the specialties. Additionally, the format for question presentation was changed to reflect the use of the nursing process. Questions addressed the various specialties and were presented within the context of each component of the nursing process (Scherubel, 2005). The content of the test was also redesigned to integrate the various components related to client needs considered to be at the heart of nursing practice. These needs include: 1) a safe and effective care environment, 2) health promotion and maintenance, 3) psychosocial integrity, and 4) physiologic integrity. These areas will be discussed at length later in the chapter.

Initially, the minimal passing score was determined by the NCSBN. Each candidate taking the test was given a score as well as the pass or fail designation. However, within a few years, the decision was made to simply score the tests as pass or fail, without the disclosure of actual scores. Until 1994, the NCLEX-RN continued to be administered via paper and pencil. Tests were given twice yearly in large metropolitan areas throughout the country. Each testing round took the better part of two full days. At this time, as previously, the candidate for licensure was required to take the test in the state in which initial licensure was desired.

The last major change in the NCLEX-RN testing format occurred in 1994. At this time the NCLEX-RN was converted to a **computerized adaptive testing (CAT)** format, and the test was administered by computer. Although the content was the same as in the paper and pencil format, the CAT format brought a number of changes. Although one did not need sophisticated computer skills to take the test, having the test appear on a screen rather than on a piece of paper represented a significant change. Perhaps the greatest change in terms of the format, however, was that one could no longer go back and forth from a current question to an earlier question. Each question had to be answered before another question would appear. This particular change effectively eliminated any ability for one question to inadvertently provide a clue to a previously answered question. The CAT format will be discussed in more detail later in this chapter.

The advent of the computerized NCLEX-RN brought about several other changes in the overall process. The test can now be taken as soon as permission is granted for the individual by the appropriate state board of nursing and an appointment is made at any of the many sites administering the test throughout the country. New graduates may sit for the examination within a month after completing requirements for their nursing degree. Additionally, new graduates can take the examination at any authorized testing site, regardless of where they wish to be licensed initially. The amount of time for testing has also changed dramatically. Instead of two full days of testing, the maximum allowable time is now 6 hours or 265 questions, whichever comes first. The test results are mailed to the candidate from the respective state board of nursing approximately 1 month from the date of testing. Finally, should the need to retest arise, the waiting time is 45–90 days (depending on the state) rather than 6 months. The actual amount of time between retesting is set by the individual state boards of nursing. The candidate bulletin explaining the test plan, how to register for the examination, and other pertinent details about the examination are available online at https://www.ncsbn.org.

Initially, the structure of the test questions themselves did not change from the paper and pencil test; they retained the multiple choice format. However, this has evolved so the examination currently has a number of other testing formats in addition to the standard multiple choice testing option. These formats include multiple response, fill-in-the-blank/calculations, hot spots, exhibits, and drag

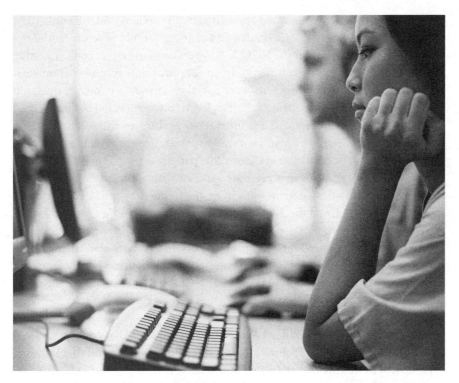

A nurse uses a computer. *Source:* © Photos.com

and drop/ordered response items. Each of these testing formats will be discussed in detail later in this chapter.

Forces Driving the NCLEX-RN Changes

Just as the knowledge explosion in health care continues to drive changes in nursing practice, it will also necessitate changes in NCLEX-RN test content as well as methods of testing in order to verify minimal competence to practice. Every 3 years, the NCSBN explores the entry-level skills and knowledge needed by beginning nurses. The NCSBN is responsible for preparing a licensing examination that is psychometrically sound as well as legally defensible. The triannual job analysis studies assist the NCSBN in doing this (Wendt & Brown, 2000; Wendt & O'Neill, 2006).

As an example, for the 2005 job analysis study, a panel of subject matter experts (SME) representing all geographic areas of the country and all major nursing specialties and practice settings was brought together to develop the job analysis survey. All members of the panel worked with and/or supervised newly licensed registered nurses. The panel reviewed summaries of activity logs completed by a group of newly licensed registered nurses who worked in various practice settings across the United States. Following this review, the panel developed a survey instrument containing a list of nursing activities performed by new nurses.

The instrument was then reviewed and edited by the 2005 NCSBN Examination Committee. The survey was distributed to a random sample of 6,000 candidates who had been successful on the NCLEX-RN between January 1, 2005, and May 31, 2005. The sample was stratified to include appropriate numbers from each NCSBN jurisdiction. Respondents were asked to answer a two-part question in relation to each of the nursing activities listed in the survey. The first part of the question asked whether and how often they performed the activity in their work setting. The second part of the question asked them to rank the activity in terms of priority for patient safety. The SME panel was asked to independently estimate the percentage of new registered nurses with whom they worked who performed the activities listed on the survey, the frequency with which they performed the activities, and the average priority of the activities in terms of patient safety. When the ratings of the SME were compared to the results of the survey analysis, there were only four ratings out of the 150 activity statements in the survey in which there was more than a one-point difference. The results of the analysis were considered valid, and the 2007 NCLEX-RN test plan was modified accordingly (Wendt & O'Neill, 2006). The test plan is kept as is, or revisions are made, based on these triennial analyses.

Further, the growth in minority populations mandates that concepts related to cultural competence be included in the educational process and that minimal competence in this area be addressed in the licensing examination (Fitzpatrick, 2007; Joel, 2003; Wessling, 2006). Additionally, Joel (2006) maintained that in the administration of the test itself, cultural and gender factors on the part of the test taker should be taken into consideration. Changes on the horizon for the 21st century include the possibility of skill demonstration requirements, as well as possible testing of some sort for relicensure (Huston, 2006). Another issue that continues to be debated within the profession is the question of differentiated practice and whether separate licensure examinations should exist for graduates of different educational programs. Contemporary Practice Highlight 3-2 addresses this issue and current studies being conducted by the NCSBN.

Components of the NCLEX-RN Test Plan

The National Council of State Boards of Nursing is responsible for the development of the NCLEX-RN exam (Wendt, Kenny, & Anderson, 2007). As previously discussed, the examination is developed from an analysis of the job functions performed by selected entry-level nurses in the first year of employment. The 2007 NCLEX-RN **test plan** was developed from the 2005 job analysis study described in the preceding section (Wendt et al.). The current test plan can be obtained at http://www.ncsbn.org. Students are encouraged to go to the NCSBN website and obtain a copy of the test

KEY TERM

Test plan: A blueprint for the licensing examination that outlines the examination's content areas and the percentage of questions devoted to each content area.

CONTEMPORARY PRACTICE HIGHLIGHT 3-2

STUDY ON THE 5-YEAR POST-ENTRY COMPETENCE OF RNs

The debate over which educational program—associate degree or baccalaureate degree—best prepares nurses for entry-level practice has been on-going in the profession for decades. Current data from NCSBN retrospective studies indicates that nurses from all types of programs function at approximately the same level during the first 6 months following graduation. The NCSBN is currently doing a prospective, post-entry competence study to explore the characteristics of registered nurses during the first 5 years of practice. Among the areas looked at will be how the characteristics of practice change over time. A potentially interesting outcome of this study will be whether the characteristics differ over time among graduates of the various types of nursing programs. Further information on the purpose and design of this study can be found at https://www.ncsbn.org/986.htm.

plan because it provides a framework for the development of test items and can be used by students as they organize their study materials and begin their preparation for taking the examination.

The test plan is organized around a client needs framework, providing a structure within which nursing actions and competencies can be defined. The term *client* is used interchangeably with *patient* because this provides a broader population for nursing care. This framework also focuses on clients in all care settings (Wendt et al., 2007).

It is important to remember that four main processes are considered fundamental to nursing practice and integrated throughout the test; these processes can be tested in relation to any client or any setting. These four fundamental processes are the Nursing Process, Caring, Communication and Documentation, and Teaching/Learning (NCSBN, 2006, p. 3). Definitions for each of these processes can be found in the most current NCLEX test plan. The implications this has for you, as the learner, are that it is essential that you be competent in understanding and applying the principles and concepts related to using the nursing process; developing mutually collaborative, respectful, and trusting relationships with clients; communicating, verbally and nonverbally, with clients, families, and other healthcare providers and accurately documenting these interactions; and teaching clients and their families/significant others in the care of all clients in any setting.

Framework of Client Needs

The client needs framework is divided into four categories: Safe and Effective Care Environment, Health Promotion and Maintenance, Psychosocial Integrity, and Physiological Integrity. Two of these categories, Safe and Effective Care

Environment and Physiological Integrity, have additional subcategories. The Safe and Effective Care Environment category is further subdivided into Management of Care and Safety and Infection Control. The Physiological Integrity category is further divided into the following four subcategories: Basic Care and Comfort, Pharmacological and Parenteral Therapies, Reduction of Risk Potential, and Physiological Adaptation (NCSBN, 2006, p. 4). Each of these categories is described in the following sections; for a complete and detailed description of each category, please see the most current NCLEX-RN test plan available at the NCSBN website.

Safe and Effective Care Environment

The nurse is responsible for promoting the achievement of client outcomes by directing and providing nursing care in a care setting in a manner that protects clients, family/significant others, and other healthcare providers (Wendt et al., 2007). This category is further divided into Management of Care and Safety and Infection Control. Management of Care addresses concepts related to providing and directing nursing care in a healthcare delivery setting that is designed to protect patients, family, and other healthcare personnel; this subcategory accounts for approximately 13–19 percent of the test plan (NCSBN, 2006, pp. 5–6). Management of care can include, but is not limited to, such nursing responsibilities as prioritizing client care, delegating and supervising care, making appropriate referrals to community resources, maintaining client confidentiality, and providing and participating in staff education.

Safety and Infection Control is focused on health and environmental hazards (NCSBN, 2006, p. 7) in the care setting and constitutes approximately 8–14 percent of the test plan (p. 5). Safety issues, for both the patient and the nurse, have gained increasing importance, and the NCLEX-RN test plan is reflective of this change in emphasis. Examples of content areas that may be addressed in this subcategory include medical and surgical asepsis, safe use of medical devices and restraints, and disaster planning, to name just a few topics.

Health Promotion and Maintenance

This category addresses incorporating concepts from growth and development, and the prevention and early detection of health problems into the provision of nursing care, as well as nursing strategies designed to promote the achievement of optimal client health (Wendt et al., 2007). Approximately 6–12 percent of the test plan is devoted to health promotion and maintenance activities (NCSBN, 2006, p. 5). Throughout this content area, the candidate is expected to demonstrate knowledge related to providing care to individuals across the life span (e.g., care of the pregnant client and newborn, elder care); providing adequate education to meet the needs of the client, family, or significant other (e.g., lifestyle choices, sexually transmitted diseases, self-care activities); and anticipating and preventing potential future health problems (e.g., immunizations).

Psychosocial Integrity

This category addresses content areas related to promoting and supporting the "emotional, mental and social well-being of the client and family/significant others experiencing stressful events, as well as clients with acute or chronic mental illness" (NCSBN, 2006, p. 7). Throughout this content area, the candidate should be able to demonstrate the ability to assess clients and families at risk of mental health problems, provide care to clients in a variety of situations, lead group therapy sessions, incorporate client management techniques, and use therapeutic communication. This category accounts for approximately 6–12 percent of the test plan (NCSBN, 2006, p. 5).

Physiological Integrity

As a single category, physiological integrity accounts for the largest percentage of the total test plan, ranging anywhere from 43 to 67 percent (NCSBN, 2006, p. 5). The category topics are focused on nursing care that is related to safely meeting the client's activities of daily living; providing safe administration of medications; decreasing the potential for client complications; and managing the nursing care of clients with acute, chronic, and/or life-threatening health problems (Wendt et al., 2007).

This category is further subdivided into four subcategories: Basic Care and Comfort, Pharmacological and Parenteral Therapies, Reduction of Risk Potential, and Physiological Adaptation. The subcategory of Basic Care and Comfort, consisting of 6–12 percent, of the test plan (NCSBN, 2006, p. 5), addresses knowledge and competencies related to performing basic nursing skills, including, but not limited to, monitoring vital signs, height and weight, hydration status, and application and removal of orthopedic devices.

The subcategory of Pharmacological and Parenteral Therapies includes all aspects of nursing care related to safe medication administration such as basic dosage calculations; medication administration via all routes, including parenteral; monitoring client responses and outcomes related to medication administration; administration of blood products; total parenteral nutrition; and client and family education regarding medications. In addition, the basic information regarding common medications, their mechanism of action, uses and contraindications, and drug interactions is also part of this subcategory. This subcategory accounts for approximately 13–19 percent of the total test plan (NCSBN, 2006, p. 5).

The subcategory of Reduction of Risk Potential, accounting for 13–19 percent of the test plan (NCSBN, 2006, p. 5) is related to decreasing the likelihood of the client developing complications from existing health problems or care received.

Monitoring the patient for complications is an important nursing responsibility that is addressed in this category, as is the nursing care related to preparing the client for diagnostic tests and surgical procedures, monitoring the patient following the procedures, and understanding the implications of laboratory values to client care.

The final subcategory for this section is Physiological Adaptation, which is related to providing nursing care to clients who are acutely or chronically ill, or experiencing life-threatening health problems (Wendt et al., 2007). This category constitutes 11–17 percent of the test plan (NCSBN, 2006, p. 5). Such health problems as fluid and electrolyte imbalances, hemodynamic instabilities, and medical emergencies, as well as other physiological alterations, are addressed in this category.

As you prepare to study for the NCLEX, using the content area information that is provided to you in the NCLEX test plan framework can help you determine how to most effectively plan and use your study time. You can also use this information to actively seek out learning experiences in the final semesters of your program to ensure that you are developing the necessary knowledge and competencies in all areas of nursing practice to be successful on the examination.

Computer Adaptive Testing (CAT)

Computer adaptive testing (CAT) is a method of computerized testing that adapts to the test taker's responses on test items and alters the level of complexity of subsequent test items based upon previous item responses. As the test taker answers each question, the CAT will adjust subsequent test items to the level of the test taker's knowledge and abilities (as demonstrated by answers on previous items) until, ultimately, the test taker either demonstrates satisfactory performance at the level designated for passing the examination or demonstrates unsatisfactory performance on the examination, as evidenced by the inability to consistently reach and accurately respond to items at a preset level of complexity, thus failing the examination. This is the format in which all candidates for the NCLEX take the examination.

Taking an examination that is administered via the CAT format requires that test candidates understand certain concepts about the administration of the test. First, it is important to understand that all questions must be answered in the order they appear on the computer screen; candidates cannot go back and forth between test items. The candidate can take as long as needed to read and respond to each question; however, the question must be answered before progressing to the next test item. Second, candidates should plan their time spent on each test item, so as to allow enough time to answer the maximum number of questions (265) in the maximum allowed time (6 hours), should that be necessary. It is estimated that most candidates average about 1 minute per multiple choice test item (NCSBN, 2006). If uncertain of an answer, the candidate should make a best guess based on critical reasoning skills and then move on to the next item.

Third, as previously indicated, CAT testing does not allow the candidate to return to an item once an answer has been submitted. The difficulty of the test items is adjusted as the candidate answers the items and demonstrates proficiency in various areas. Essentially, the candidate will be tested at a certain level of difficulty, and if he or she correctly responds to that specific item, the next test item generated by the CAT program is again at that level. After the candidate is again successful at this level, the next item generated will then be at a higher level of difficulty; if unsuccessful at answering that item correctly, the level of difficulty for the next item will be lower. The goal is to determine when the candidate remains at a consistent level of ability. The ability estimate is based on the percentage of test items answered correctly and the difficulty of the items that were administered. The test will automatically stop when either the test bank is exhausted (the candidate took 265 questions), the test length is reached (6 hours for the NCLEX-RN), or the ability level is estimated with sufficient accuracy (Wendt et al., 2007).

The Passing Standard

The passing standard is the minimum level of ability required for safe and effective entry-level nursing practice (Wendt et al., 2007). In order to pass the NCLEX-RN exam, the candidate must perform above the passing standard.

The passing standard is evaluated once every 3 years and adjusted accordingly. The NCSBN Board of Directors makes this determination based on information gathered during that period of time. The information used by the board includes results of surveys, performance of past graduates, and past passing standards. Standard-setting surveys and exercises are conducted to determine the passing standard and what that standard would mean. In addition, the Board of Directors reviews the historical record of the passing standard and correlates these findings with summaries of candidate performance. Information regarding the current educational readiness of high school graduates wanting to study nursing is also reviewed. All these factors are considered as decisions are made in order to determine the passing standard. Once this passing standard is set, all candidates must perform above this standard in order to pass the NCLEX-RN examination (Wendt et al., 2007).

Types of Questions on the NCLEX-RN Examination

As mentioned earlier, the NCLEX-RN examination uses a variety of test item formats. Many of the questions are multiple choice; however, other test item formats used include multiple answer/multiple response, fill-in-the blank/calculations, hot spots, exhibits, and drag and drop/ordered response.

Multiple choice items are the most common test items on the examination. For these items, the candidate will be presented with a question or clinical situation in the question's stem and then asked to select the one best answer from a list of four possible options. Box 3-1 provides an example of a traditional multiple choice item.

Multiple answer/multiple response questions present the candidate with a question, followed by a list of possible answers/responses. The candidate is asked to select all options that apply, allowing for more than one correct response. The candidate must select *all* of the appropriate responses for the item to be answered correctly. Box 3-2 provides an example of a multiple answer/multiple response test item.

Fill-in-the-blank items present a question and then ask the candidate to type in a response. Frequently, fill-in-the-blank items represent drug dosage calculation problems or situations in which the candidate is required to calculate the client's intake/output record. The candidate is expected to calculate the response without the benefit of potential answers. A drop-down calculator is provided to assist with calculations; it can be found by clicking on the calculator button located at the bottom right side of the computer screen. Box 3-3 provides an example of a fill-in-the-blank test item.

BOX 3-1   MULTIPLE CHOICE TEST ITEM

Which of the following assessments would the nurse conduct to evaluate the patient's cerebellar function as part of a neurological assessment?

1. Abdominal reflex
2. Romberg test
3. Glasgow coma scale
4. Babinski test

Answer: 2

BOX 3-2   MULTIPLE ANSWER/MULTIPLE RESPONSE ITEMS

The nurse is providing post-mortem care for a client. Which of the following interventions would be appropriate for the nurse to complete prior to allowing the family to see the client? Select all that apply:

1. Clean and reposition the client's body.
2. Call the physician to verify the time of death.
3. Provide sterile gloves to family members.
4. Freshen the bed linens and pull covers to the client's shoulders.

Answer: 1, 4

BOX 3-3   FILL-IN-THE BLANK ITEMS

A patient has an order for sodium phenobarbital 60 milligrams intramuscularly every 8 hours. You have a vial that reads sodium phenobarbital 100 milligrams/2 milliliters. How many milliliters will you need to administer?

Provide a numeric answer.

_____ milliliters

Answer: 1.2

Hot spots present candidates with a question and a diagram or figure. The candidate needs to use the mouse to identify and select an area on the diagram/figure, then click on the left mouse button in order to indicate an answer. As an example, these types of questions can be used to ask candidates to select appropriate areas to auscultate heart, lung, and abdominal sounds. Box 3-4 provides an example of a "hot spot" test item.

BOX 3-4   HOT SPOT TEST ITEM

Place an X over the anatomical location that the nurse would hear bronchial breath sounds.

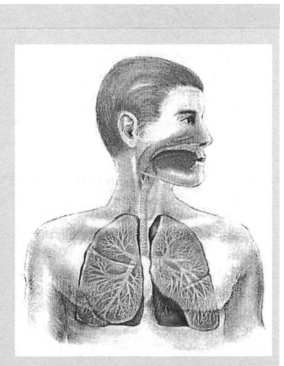

Exhibit items present the candidate with a scenario and an exhibit that contain information required to answer the question. The exhibit may be in the form of a table, graph, or diagram. For example, an exhibit may provide the candidate with a listing of a client's arterial blood gas values, to enable the candidate to respond to a question about the client's physiological status. Box 3-5 provides an example of an "exhibit" question asking the test taker to identify a cardiac rhythm.

Sequencing/prioritizing (drag and drop) test items present the candidate with a question and a list of options that the candidate is required to sequence, prioritize, or rank order to answer the question. In this type of test format, the unordered options appear on the left side of the computer screen. The candidate must use the mouse to click and drag the options to the right side of the screen, place them in the appropriate order, and then confirm completion of that test item to record the answer. Box 3-6 provides an example of a sequencing test item.

BOX 3-5   EXHIBIT TEST ITEM

How would the nurse interpret this cardiac rhythm?

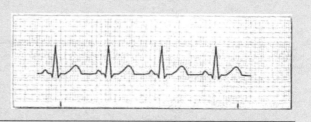

Answer: Sinus bradycardia

Source: Image from Arrhythmia Recognition: The Art of Interpretation, courtesy of Tomas B. Garcia, MD.

BOX 3-6   SEQUENCING/PRIORITIZING TEST ITEM

This question will require you to use the mouse to place the responses in a correct sequence of actions based on the situation.

A patient has just been admitted to the hospital to receive treatment for an exacerbation of his COPD. In which order should the nurse complete the following sequence of events?

1. Place allergy band on patient arm.
2. Order patient meals and procedures.
3. Complete the patient assessment.
4. Call the healthcare provider to obtain admission orders.

Answer: 3, 1, 4, 2

Preparing for the NCLEX-RN

There are multiple ways to prepare for taking the NCLEX-RN. The most important point is actually having a plan for preparation and implementing it prior to graduation from your program. It is also important that candidates select a method of review and preparation that will work best for them. Learning styles differ from individual to individual; some learn best visually, others prefer an auditory approach. Some prefer to study in isolation, whereas group study work is most effective for others. The only constant in preparing for the NCLEX is that preparation must be done. All students can benefit by reviewing and preparing for the NCLEX, even those students who have performed consistently well in school.

How to go about reviewing for the NCLEX is up to the individual. There are many well-written NCLEX review books on the market; most of these books use the NCLEX test plan as a framework for organizing the content and also have an accompanying CD with computerized test questions. Candidates should review and select the book that they find most helpful; it is especially helpful to select a book that provides rationales for right and wrong answers, and offers questions in all of the testing formats utilized on the NCLEX. In addition, there are a variety of computerized and online test review products; these products can help candidates get a sense of what it is like to take a test with the CAT format. There are also formal review programs that are offered over various lengths of time. These review programs may be offered by the school of nursing or potential employers.

Faculty may be helpful in assisting candidates to evaluate the worthiness of any given review product. A good rule of thumb is that what has worked for a candidate in the past in terms of preparing for a test will probably work best when preparing for the NCLEX-RN, so don't abandon or change previously proven methods of helpful study. Although how to structure and plan your review is an individual preference, the following guidelines may be helpful when preparing to take the NCLEX-RN. Box 3-7 summarizes these preparation tips.

- *Conduct a self-assessment:* To begin, review the NCLEX test plan and assess your own knowledge base; identify the content areas you know well, and the areas you know less well. Identify content areas that you may not have

---

BOX 3-7   TIPS ON PREPARING FOR THE NCLEX-RN

- Conduct a self-assessment.
- Develop a timetable.
- Become familiar with the NCLEX-RN test plan.
- Know the item formats used on the NCLEX-RN.
- Practice answering test questions.
- Enroll in review courses.
- Hone test-taking skills.

reviewed for a while. It is normal to have a tendency to want to stay in your comfort zone, which in this case means studying the things you know well. However, in preparing for the NCLEX-RN, you want to spend more time reviewing areas that you are not comfortable with or that you have not reviewed recently.

- *Develop a timetable for your review:* After completing the self-assessment of your own knowledge, look at the volume of material that must be reviewed and how much time you have before you take the test, and then plan how much time you need to spend each day in review. Depending on the volume of material that must be reviewed and other events occurring in your life, a better plan may be to look at how much time you know you can realistically spend each day in review, and then decide when you will request an appointment to take the NCLEX-RN. However, do not unduly delay taking the examination; evidence suggests that those first-time takers who delay taking the examination are more likely to do poorly. The important thing to remember is that a timetable must be set that provides the opportunity for a thorough review and fosters the self-discipline to actually do the review. Don't wait until you graduate to begin your review; beginning the review while you are still in school can help you identify areas where additional learning experiences, especially in the clinical setting, will help increase your knowledge of the content. If you feel you lack the self-discipline to adhere to a review schedule, it may be helpful to find and commit to a study partner who will help keep you on your review schedule.

- *Become familiar with the NCLEX-RN test plan:* As mentioned previously, familiarize yourself with the NCLEX-RN test plan before you begin your review. When you are reviewing, consider the material in light of how the test plan is organized—remember to focus on concepts and fundamental processes, not factual information. A complete and up-to-date description of the test plan is always available for downloading from the NCSBN website at https://www.ncsbn.org.

- *Know the item formats used on the NCLEX-RN:* Just as knowing the test plan around which the NCLEX-RN is organized is important, knowing what type of questions to expect is also important. The format of the question often drives how to study. For example, in a typical, one answer only, multiple choice question, the correct answer must be recognized and selected from among the options provided. However, in fill-in-the-blank and hot spot questions, you will need to be able to critically reason and supply the answer without prompting or validation from a list of options. Being aware of the types of questions you will be asked will assist you in developing your review plan. The various types of question formats are described earlier in this chapter.

■ *Practice answering test questions:* Just as knowing the types of questions to expect is important, practice in answering various types of questions is equally valuable. As discussed previously, there are many sources of practice questions similar to those on the NCLEX-RN. An important part of taking the practice questions is developing an understanding of the rationale of why the correct answer is correct and why the wrong answers are wrong. Examining the rationale will help you develop insight into the context in which the questions are posed, as well as what words in the stem of the question are important to note before choosing an answer. Words or phrases such as *first, first step, next step, best represents, priority action,* or *primary reason* often indicate which of the answer options is the "best" choice, even though all of the answers might actually represent correct actions that could be taken in the situation posed in the question.

■ *Enroll in review courses:* There are many review courses available, ranging from a few days to as long as 2 weeks in length. The advantage to review courses is that they organize the content and provide a structured approach by which to conduct your review. These courses are designed to cover content that is common to all types of nursing programs. They are not meant to teach content, but rather to review it. A good way to approach these reviews is if a topic comes up that is new to you, make note of the topic and plan to study it in detail later. Pay particular attention to content that you experienced more difficulty understanding when initially introduced to you in your nursing program curriculum.

The downside to review courses is that they can be expensive, and are usually offered at specific times that may not be convenient, depending on your own personal schedule. However, if you have any concern that you may not have the self-discipline to do your own review, a review course is well worth the price. Also, some employers will pay the registration costs associated with review courses. Characteristics of a good review course include competent and current faculty, comprehensiveness, opportunities to answer test questions throughout the review, a comprehensive computerized examination to assist with self-assessment prior to the course and/or provide a measure of how prepared you are for the NCLEX-RN exam following completion of the course, and a guarantee that you may repeat the course at least once free of charge, should you be unsuccessful on the NCLEX-RN.

■ *Hone test-taking skills:* It is important to spend time honing test-taking skills, especially if you feel you are not a good test taker. There are books that can help with this, and most colleges and universities housing nursing programs have academic support services to assist in test-taking skills. These kinds of support are often available to alumni as well as current students. It is best to investigate the availability of these services prior to graduation to ensure being able to take advantage of them.

Another area to consider is test anxiety. If you have experienced this in the past, it is something you will want to prepare for now as well. Again, most colleges and universities offer support for students in this area. Just as in test-taking skills, you will want to investigate the availability of this support prior to graduation from your nursing program, in order to ensure that you can take advantage of the assistance.

Finally, if you have any kind of disability for which you could benefit from an accommodation, you will want to investigate obtaining the accommodation as you are applying to take the NCLEX-RN. In general, if you need accommodation for a disability during your nursing educational program, particularly if it dealt with testing, you will want to make that known when you apply to the state board of nursing. A good rule of the thumb is that if you are going to need accommodation, apply for the examination early, at least 60 days in advance of when you expect to take it, because it will take longer for your application to be processed.

Taking the NCLEX-RN

We all understand there are significant consequences to the NCLEX-RN. If you pass, you will receive your license to practice as a registered nurse and will be on your way to a wonderful career filled with new and fulfilling experiences. However, if you do not pass the examination, the consequences are also significant. You will not be able to practice as a registered nurse until you are able to pass the examination. In addition, you are taking this examination in an unfamiliar environment sitting next to people you likely do not know. For these reasons, for many candidates the anxiety level associated with this examination can be very high. It is important to feel confident you are prepared for the examination. Following the preparation tips already provided can help increase your feeling of self-confidence and decrease any feelings of anxiety.

As you prepare for your examination, prepare yourself mentally to take the maximum number of questions (265). You will want to be comfortable at pacing yourself through the test, allotting about 1–2 minutes per test question, with 1 minute being the average amount of time spent on a question. This way you will not become frustrated or anxious if you are required to answer more than the minimum allotment of 75 questions. You also want to know that you will not become excessively fatigued after answering 100 questions. It is also important to remember that you cannot tell how well you are doing on the examination based on the length of time that your test is administered; you may pass the test within either a short or long testing time period.

Once you feel you are prepared for the exam and you have scheduled your testing date, conduct a practice run to the testing facility. Know where you will be testing and what route to take to get there. Become familiar with traffic patterns on the specific day of the week you will be testing. Allow yourself plenty of time to arrive at the testing site on the day of the examination, on time and unrushed.

During the final few days before the examination you should be focusing on obtaining plenty of rest and only engaging in brief periods of review time. Schedule some time for relaxation, such as going to the movies or your favorite restaurant the day before the examination. Make sure you get plenty of rest the night before. Wear comfortable clothes. Have a nutritious breakfast with plenty of "brain food" including protein, and avoid excessive amounts of caffeine. Remember, you will not be allowed to bring anything into the testing site with you. You can bring snacks and leave them in the locker provided; two brief optional break periods are automatically provided during the examination when you may opt to eat a snack. The first optional break is offered 2 hours into the testing time, and the second optionally scheduled break is offered 3 1/2 hours into the testing time (NCSBN, 2008). Unscheduled breaks may also be taken. Take breaks as needed, because not taking them can affect your concentration if you become uncomfortable. Remember, any and all breaks will be counted as part of your total testing time.

Summary

This chapter has presented some basic information regarding the NCLEX-RN examination. The purpose of the NCLEX-RN and how it was developed were discussed. This chapter also provided you with the components of the NCLEX-RN test plan. Using the test plan will help you as you organize preparation for the examination. Finally, a section on the types of questions found on the NCLEX-RN and how to prepare for the examination was included. The information provided in this chapter and your educational preparation should help set you well on your way to a successful NCLEX-RN examination.

Key Terms

- **Computer adaptive testing (CAT):** An interactive testing format used on the NCLEX-RN to adjust the type of question and level of testing difficulty based on the test taker's previous response. In the NCLEX-RN examination, the testing continues until the student either achieves a consistent level of test item difficulty that indicates a satisfactory performance level and passing of the examination, does not achieve a consistent level of testing difficulty required to indicate a satisfactory performance level and thus fails the examination, or completes all of the test items on the examination or time expires on the test.
- **National Council Licensing Examination for Registered Nurses (NCLEX-RN):** This examination must be taken by all graduates of diploma, associate degree, and baccalaureate degree nursing programs prior to a license being issued. Successful completion of the NCLEX-RN is a requirement for practice as a registered nurse.
- **National Council of State Boards of Nursing (NCSBN):** The body given the task of providing a means to ensure that those who are licensed to practice as nurses are "safe" in terms of their knowledge base.
- **Test plan:** A blueprint for the licensing examination that outlines the examination's content areas and the percentage of questions devoted to each content area.

Reflective Practice Questions

1. Consider your own plans for preparing to take the NCLEX-RN. Are you satisfied with the steps that you have taken to date? What else can you do to develop and implement a plan that will support your success on the examination?

2. Conduct a self-assessment of your areas of strengths and areas that need improvement related to taking the NCLEX-RN. What learning experiences can you capitalize on in your remaining time in your educational program to assist you in your preparation for the examination?

3. Do you think the job analysis process as it is currently conducted is a satisfactory method of determining the content that should be on the NCLEX-RN? What are the benefits of this methodology? Are there any inherent limitations?

References

Chitty, K. K., & Black B. P. (2007). *Professional nursing concepts and challenges* (5th ed.). St. Louis, MO: Elsevier Saunders.

Fitzpatrick, J. (2007). Cultural competence in nursing education revisited. *Nursing Education Perspectives, 28*(1), 5.

Huston, C. J. (2006). Assuring provider competence through licensure, continuing education, and certification. In C. J. Huston (Ed.), *Professional issues in nursing challenges & opportunities* (pp. 348–367). New York: Lippincott Williams & Wilkins.

Joel, L. A. (2003). *Kelly's dimensions of professional nursing* (9th ed.). New York: McGraw-Hill.

Joel, L. A. (2006). *The nursing experience: Trends, challenges, and transitions* (5th ed.). New York: McGraw-Hill.

Kalisch, P. A., & Kalisch, B. J. (1995). *American nursing: A history* (3rd ed.). Philadelphia: Lippincott Williams & Wilkins.

Kalisch, P. A., & Kalisch, B. J. (2004). *American nursing: A history* (4th ed.). Philadelphia: Lippincott Williams & Wilkins.

Kelly, L., & Joel, L. (1996). *The nursing experience: Trends, challenges, and transitions* (3rd ed.) New York: McGraw-Hill.

National Council of State Boards of Nursing. (n.d.). *Nurse licensure compact administrators.* Retrieved July 31, 2007, from https://www.ncsbn.org/156.htm

National Council of State Boards of Nursing. (2006). *Test plan for the National Council Licensure Examination for registered nurses.* Retrieved February 20, 2008, from https://www.ncsbn.org/RN_Test_Plan_2007_Web.pdf

National Council of State Boards of Nursing. (2008). *2008 NCLEX examination candidate bulletin.* Retrieved February 20, 2008, from https://www.ncsbn.org/2008_NCLEX_Candidate_Bulletin.pdf

Scherubel, J. C. (2005). Nursing licensure and certification. In B. Cherry & S. Jacob (Eds.), *Contemporary nursing issues, trends, & management* (3rd ed., pp. 91–106). St. Louis, MO: Elsevier Mosby.

Wall, B. M., Miller, D. E., & Widerquist, J. G. (1993). Predictors of success on the newest NCLEX-RN. *Western Journal of Nursing Research, 15*(5), 628–643.

Wendt, A., & Brown, P. (2000). The NCLEX examination preparing for future nursing practice. *Nurse Educator, 25*(6), 297–300.

Wendt, A., Kenny, L., & Anderson, J. (2007). *2007 NCLEX-RN detailed test plan.* Chicago: NCSBN.

Wendt, A., & O'Neill, T. (2006). 2005 RN practice analysis: Linking the NCLEX-RN examination to practice. *NCSBN Research Brief, 21*, 1–97. Retrieved September 28, 2007, from http://www.ncsbn.org/vol_21_web.pdf

Wessling, S. (2006). Does the NCLEX-RN pass the test for cultural sensitivity? Retrieved February 20, 2007, from http://www.minoritynurse.com/features/undergraduate/06-02-03.html

Nursing Licensure and Certification

Wendy Stoelting-Gettelfinger

LEARNING OUTCOMES

After reading this chapter you will be able to:

- Explain the purpose of nursing practice regulation.
- Describe the function of state boards of nursing.
- Understand the historical context of state boards of nursing and their regulatory functions.
- Describe the mutual recognition model.
- Define licensure.
- Explain the history of nursing licensure.
- Differentiate between licensure and certification.

As healthcare consumers, we often take it for granted that the nurse, dentist, physician, or other healthcare provider who we seek services from is competent and qualified to provide those services. Regulation of healthcare providers exists to protect the public. Healthcare outcomes are directly impacted by nursing practice, how it is defined, and ultimately how it is regulated. Nursing regulation is designed to protect public safety; therefore, effective regulation can promote better patient safety and improved health outcomes. Nursing practice is governed by state nurse practice acts and regulatory procedures. This chapter discusses the regulation of nursing practice, licensure, and certification.

The Regulation of Nursing Practice

Nursing, like most other health professions, is regulated because individuals can be harmed by the actions of an incompetent or unqualified practitioner. The public relies upon this regulatory oversight of healthcare providers because they themselves may not be able to identify whether specific healthcare providers are competent or incompetent. In order to regulate the practice of nursing, governmental oversight is provided on a state level by a regulatory authority known as a state board of nursing. Nursing practice is carefully defined within the profession's scope of practice through the nurse practice acts of individual states.

The American Nurses Association (ANA) defines nursing as "the protection, promotion, and optimization of health and abilities; prevention of illness and injury; alleviation of suffering through the diagnosis and treatment of human response; and advocacy in health care for individuals, families, communities, and populations"(ANA, 2007; p. 6; ANA, 2004, p. 7). The American Nurses Association maintains a website (http://www.nursingworld.org) that contains resources and policy updates concerning the practice of nursing. In addition, the practice of nursing is further defined in each state by a piece of regulatory state legislation called a nurse practice act. The nurse practice act defines the scope of nursing practice, creates regulatory entities for nursing practice such as state boards of nursing, empowers delegated entities with regulatory authority, and ensures accountability for nurses. In summary, the nurse practice act is the most authoritative and controlling piece of governing law that regulates nursing practice within a state's borders.

The National Council of State Boards of Nursing (NCSBN) published a position statement entitled *Nursing Regulation and the Interpretation of Nursing Scopes of Practice* that summarizes why and how the practice of nursing is regulated (NCSBN, 2005). NCSBN holds that state/territory nurse practice acts provide the legal basis for the regulation of nursing activities and that the responsibility for interpreting the legal scope of nursing practice rests solely with the individual boards of nursing (Courtesy of: NCSBN ®, 2007).

Nurse practice acts vary among states; however, many of them are based on the model act that was originally published by the American Nurses Association in 1988. The NCSBN also maintains a model nurse practice act and model rules entitled *NCSBN Model Nursing Practice Act* and *Model Nursing Administrative Rules.* The model act and administrative rules provide recommended or model language that individual states or territories may utilize in the development of their state/territory specific nurse practice acts (Courtesy of: NCSBN ®, 2007).

KEY TERM

Nurse practice act: A state statute that defines the legal limits for the practice of nursing within that state and explicitly identifies the requirements for licensure.

The *NCSBN Model Nursing Practice Act* and *Model Nursing Administrative Rules* provide a resource that state legislators and members of individual state/territory boards of nursing can use to compare their existing nurse practice act against. This comparison can identify language that may be missing in a state/territory's existing nurse practice act or provide language that can be utilized for new regulation. Because each state/territory has its own unique version of a nurse practice act, models provide examples and guidance for the use of standardized or uniform language that helps to facilitate a shared knowledge or understanding of what constitutes the practice of nursing (Courtesy of: NCSBN®, 2007). The challenge for many individual practicing nurses can be how to locate their own state or jurisdiction's current nurse practice act.

Accessing Your State's Nurse Practice Act and Administrative Rules

Many states and jurisdictions now post the most current version of their nurse practice act on the Internet. The NCSBN, whose mission is to promote regulatory excellence, maintains a database that contains electronic contact information for state boards of nursing for all 50 states, the District of Columbia, and four U.S. territories (Guam, the Northern Mariana Islands, Puerto Rico, and the Virgin Islands). Simply go to http://www.ncsbn. org and click on the desired home state or territory (or use a pull-down menu) to obtain the current contact information for that state. A sample contact map from the NCSBN website is included in Figure 4-1 to familiarize you with how to contact your home state or territory's nursing board. In addition, contact information for all state boards of nursing can be found in Appendix C.

Many of the state nursing board websites include links to the current state nurse practice act. For those states that do not

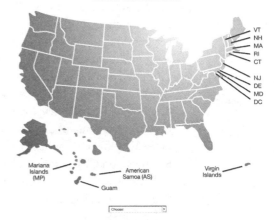

Click on a jurisdiction in the map below or choose a jurisdiction from the drop-down menu to obtain specific member board information:

Choose a jurisdiction from the map or the list of states below to obtain specific member board information:

Alabama Alaska American Samoa Arizona Arkansas California - RN California - VN Colorado Connecticut Delaware District of Columbia Florida Georgia - PN Georgia - RN Guam Hawaii Idaho Illinois - Chicago Office Illinois - Springfield Office Indiana Iowa Kansas Kentucky Louisiana - PN Louisiana - RN Maine Maryland Massachusetts Michigan Minnesota Mississippi Missouri Montana Nebraska Nevada New Hampshire New Jersey New Mexico New York North Carolina North Dakota Northern Mariana Islands Ohio Oklahoma Oregon Pennsylvania Rhode Island South Carolina South Dakota Tennessee Texas Utah Vermont Virgin Islands Virginia Washington West Virginia - PN West Virginia - RN Wisconsin Wyoming

"Weblink" Online: http://www.nysed.gov/prof/nurse.htm

Contact Person: Barbara Zittel, PhD, RN, Executive Secretary

(Permission: National Council for State Boards of Nursing (NCSBN ®)

Figure 4-1 Contacts Map Graphic from NCSBN. *Source:* National Council for State Boards of Nursing (NCSBN®).

include links, there is contact information. Your state or territory's state nursing board or designated regulatory agency also can help answer many of your questions concerning the practice of nursing within your jurisdiction.

If you are not certain whether a website is official or up-to-date, call your state or territory's state board of nursing, and they can direct you to the most current version of their jurisdiction's nurse practice act. Because nurse practice acts can be written in a legal format that may be difficult to interpret, you may also want to consult the accompanying administrative rules for the nurse practice act. Administrative rules help to further define the nurse practice act, providing additional details. Administrative rules are very helpful in answering specific questions that you might have about your nurse practice act.

As a licensed registered nurse it is imperative that you also become familiar with your employer's practice policies and guidelines. For example, some employers will utilize more stringent guidelines concerning delegation than are dictated by the jurisdiction's nurse practice act. The concept of delegation is specifically addressed in each state's nurse practice act. Therefore, it is important for registered nurses to be familiar with the concept of delegation as many states' nurse practice acts define parameters that authorize registered nurses to delegate certain tasks under specific conditions. "All decisions related to delegation and assignment are based on the fundamental principles of protection of the health, safety and welfare of the public" (Courtesy of NCSBN, 2007®, para 6, Retrieved April 8, 2008, from: https://www.ncsbn.org/Joint_statement.pdf). The Joint Statement on Delegation developed by the American Nurses Association (ANA) and the National Council of State Boards of Nursing (NCSBN) lists the five rights of delegation that are applicable to each state's nurse practice act. A copy of the Joint Statement on Delegation can be found at https://www.ncsbn.org/Joint_statement .pdf. A registered nurse must apply professional judgment when following the five rights of delegation within his or her state's nurse practice act to ensure the following: the right task, under the right circumstances, to the right person, with the right directions and communication, and under the right supervision and evaluation (Courtesy of NCSBN, 2007®, para 6, Retrieved April 8, 2008, from: https://www.ncsbn.org/Joint_statement.pdf). The topic of delegation should be covered during your employment orientation. If the topic of delegation and your employer's policies are not discussed in your orientation, you should request copies of these policies for your review and use.

The History of State Boards of Nursing and Their Regulatory Functions

In the early 1900s, states initiated the development of government-established boards of nursing to protect the public's health by overseeing and ensuring the safe practice of nursing (NCSBN, 2007). In 1903, New York, North Carolina, New Jersey, and Virginia developed some of the first nurse practice acts (Roberts, 1954). In addition to establishing standards for safe nursing care, boards of nursing issue licenses to practice nursing. However, once a license is issued to a nurse, a nursing board's job is not complete. State nursing boards continue to monitor each nurse's adherence to governing laws. If a nurse engages in an unsafe or unlawful practice of nursing, a state board of nursing can revoke a license (Courtesy of: NCSBN®, 2007). Box 4-1 provides a further description of the functions of the state boards of nursing.

Individuals who serve on a board of nursing are appointed to their position, in many states by the governor. State law often determines the membership or composition of a state board of nursing, which is usually a mix of different types of nurses with various educational backgrounds as well as healthcare consumers. Generally, boards of nursing consist of licensed practical nurses, registered nurses, advanced practice registered nurses, and healthcare consumers. The members of a state board of nursing convene to oversee nursing activities, including nursing education within a state, and also to take regulatory actions including discipline on nurse licenses when the state nurse practice act is violated (Courtesy of : NCSBN ®, 2007). In some states, state boards of nursing also regulate certified nursing assistants (CNAs) and other healthcare professionals. Individual state nurse practice acts dictate the scope of regulatory authority and powers for individual state and territory boards of nursing.

The membership for the NCSBN is composed of members from the boards of nursing in the 50 states, the District of Columbia, and four U.S. territories— Guam, the Virgin Islands, American Samoa, and the Northern Mariana Islands. Four states currently maintain two separate boards of nursing for registered nurses and licensed practical nurses—California, Georgia, Louisiana, and West Virginia (Courtesy of : NCSBN®, 2007).

BOX 4-1   FUNCTIONS OF THE STATE BOARDS OF NURSING

- Issue licenses; manage the renewal process
- Establish nursing practice standards
- Regulate advanced practice nursing
- Approve and accredit nursing education programs

- Investigate complaints against licensed practitioners
- Hold disciplinary hearings, suspending or revoking licensure if deemed necessary
- Promulgate all rules related to the regulation of nursing practice

Nurse Licensure Compact (NLC): A form of interstate compact specific to nurse licensure that provides an agreement between two or more states for the purpose of recognizing nurse licensure between and among a group of participating states. States must enter into an NLC in order to achieve mutual recognition (Courtesy of the National Council of State Boards of Nursing (NCSBN) ®, 2007, para 2, Retrieved on April 8, 2008, from: https://www.ncsbn.org/NurseLicensureCompactFAQ.pdf.)

The Nurse Licensure Compact

The **Nurse Licensure Compact** (**NLC**) is an agreement that allows a nurse to be licensed in his or her state of primary residency and to practice in other states that agree to mutually recognize that nurse's license from the primary resident state. Essentially, the NLC authorizes licensed nurses who reside in a compact-participating state to practice in another compact-participating state without obtaining additional practice licenses. Participating states acknowledge another state's licensure through a NLC. Multistate licensure privilege means that a nurse has the privilege of practicing in any participating compact state that is not his/her state of residency (Courtesy of NCSBN®, 2007). The NLC allows nurses to practice in other states both physically and electronically through multi-state licensure privilege. However, it is important to note that nurses who reside in states that participate in the NLC who want to practice across state lines in other participating states are subject to the laws and regulations of each state they practice within. Although nursing licensure is tied to the nurse's state of primary residence, accountability for nursing practice is tied to the laws and regulations of the state where a patient is located at the time nursing care and services are rendered. This type of accountability is not unique to nursing licenses; it also applies to other licenses such as a driver's license. For example, a person driving in Wyoming must obey the speeding laws of Wyoming even if his or her driver's license was issued in California. Similarly, nurses must abide by the nursing practice laws in the states where they are practicing (Courtesy of: NCSBN®, 2007). For example, a nurse whose primary residence is in the state of Kentucky, but who is providing case management services through telehealth, Internet, or telephone connections to a patient who resides in South Carolina, would be governed by the South Carolina nurse practice act for care provided to that patient. Nursing practice is no longer limited to the provision of physical patient care, but also includes nursing care such as counseling, education, and prior authorization of services through the use of technology.

A nurse's primary state of residence is defined by the mutual recognition model as "the state of a person's declared fixed permanent and principal home or domicile for legal purposes" (Courtesy of NCSBN®, 2008, p. 1, Retrieved March 23, 2008, from: https://www.ncsbn.org/358.htm). The state of primary residency is used to determine jurisdiction for nursing licensure. Licensure is not based on the state

Mutual recognition model: A model that allows a nurse to have one license in his or her state of residency with the ability to practice (electronically or physically) across state lines if there are no restrictions on his or her license and that person acknowledges that he or she is subject to each state's practice laws. (Courtesy of the National Council of State Boards of Nursing (NCSBN)®, 2007, para 1, Retrieved on April 8, 2008, from: https://www.ncsbn.org/NurseLicensureCompactFAQ.pdf.)

of practice because with the implementation of telenursing and other forms of nursing such as case management through managed care, it is sometimes difficult to determine the state of practice for the specific purpose of licensure. In addition, nurses who are not currently in the workforce or who are working temporarily could be subject to difficulties with state licensure. Tracing complaints and investigations is also facilitated by linking licensure to the state of primary residence rather than employment (NCSBN, 2004).

For states not participating in the mutual recognition model, nurses must apply for separate licensure within the state where they are going to practice either physically or electronically, regardless of residence. Even though there is a national licensure examination, individual state licensure in non–compact participating states is required. The number of states in which a nurse can be licensed is unlimited.

There are very few potential negatives associated with the mutual recognition model. One potential negative is the need for increased vigilance on the part of nurses who practice across state lines to understand the particular standards of care, scope of practice, and state laws that apply within the state where care is rendered. Without separate application for licensure, it may be less apparent to nurses that they must fully understand each state's nurse practice act and governing laws where they render care.

History of the Nurse Licensure Compact

The NCSBN Delegate Assembly began the creation of the Nurse Licensure Compact in 1996. At that time, NCSBN delegates voted to begin the process of studying and inspecting various mutual recognition models and report their findings. By 1997, the NCSBN Delegate Assembly unanimously agreed to endorse a mutual recognition model. In 1998, the NCSBN Board of Directors endorsed the goal of "removing regulatory barriers to increase access to safe nursing care." (Courtesy of NCSBN® (2008), Nurse licensure compact, p. 1, Retrieved on March 23, 2008, from: https://www.ncsbn.org/156.htm). The registered nurses (RN) and licensed practical nurses and vocational nurses (LPN/VN) compact was initiated on January 1, 2000. The first states to pass the RN and LPN/VN Nurse Licensure Compact into law were Maryland, Texas, Utah, and Wisconsin. In 2000 the Nurse Licensure Compact Administrators (NLCA) was organized to protect the public's health and safety. The mission of the NLCA is to promote compliance with laws governing the practice of nursing in each party state through the mutual recognition of party state licenses (Philipsen & Haynes, 2007). For detailed information on frequently asked questions concerning the Nurse Licensure Compact, visit the NCSBN website at https://www.ncsbn.org/NurseLicensureCompactFAQ.pdf. The NCSBN website also has the most up-to-date listing of all states participating in the NLC.

Nursing Licensure

Nursing **licensure** is a form of credentialing or regulatory method that is used when the activities being regulated are complex and require specialized knowledge coupled with the ability to make independent decisions. At the very heart of licensure are public safety and the need to ensure minimal competency in a set of nursing skills that a licensed nurse must possess in order to competently provide consistent quality nursing care for a defined level of nursing practice. Nursing licensure is defined by the NCSBN as "the process by which an agency of state government grants permission to an individual to engage in a given profession upon finding that the applicant has attained the essential degree of competency necessary to perform a unique scope of practice" (Courtesy of: NCSBN® (2008), Practice and discipline. p. 1, Retrieved on March 23, 2008, from: https://www.ncsbn.org/168.htm). The requirements for licensure define what is necessary for individuals to be able to practice the profession of nursing safely and ensure that each person meets those minimal requirements.

> **KEY TERM**
>
> **Licensure:** The process by which a state or governmental agency grants permission to an individual to engage in a given profession for compensation.

The licensure process addresses both qualification and disciplinary activities. First, licensure encompasses predetermination of the qualifications that are required to perform a defined scope of practice (e.g., LPN vs. RN) safely and an objective evaluation process to determine that the qualifications for the defined scope of practice are met. Generally speaking, the objective evaluation is accomplished through an examination (NCLEX-RN; NCLEX-PN) that must be passed before the individual can practice. In addition, licensure provides title protection for the roles and functions that registered nurses perform, and it gives authority to take disciplinary action against a licensee if he or she violates the nurse practice act and governing laws, thus ensuring that the public health, safety, and welfare are protected (NCSBN, 2007). In the United States, nursing licensure is a regulatory function of each state. Currently, each state's board of nursing or a designated entity grants licensure to registered nurses within that jurisdiction. Each state has the ability through enforcement powers to designate an entity with licensing authority to ensure that each individual who claims to be a nurse can function at a minimal level of competency. Many states' nurse practice acts also contain language that provides protection for the title of "registered nurse" to persons who hold a valid license and prevents other persons from using the title or credentials. One example of this type of title protection can be found in Arizona's Nurse Practice Act (see Box 4-2).

The History of Nursing Licensure

Nursing licensure originally came about to protect the public from unsafe nursing practice. During the 1900s nurse practice acts consisted mainly of lists of the names of trained nurses. The state of North Carolina was the first state to

BOX 4-2   ARIZONA'S NURSE PRACTICE ACT

NURSE PRACTICE ACT: SECTION 32-1636: A person who holds a valid and current license to practice professional nursing in this state may use the title "registered nurse" "graduate nurse" or "professional nurse" and the abbreviation "R.N." No other person shall assume or claim any such titles or use such abbreviation or any other words, letters, signs or figures to indicate that the person using it is a registered, graduate or professional nurse.

enact a nurse practice act, in 1903. By 1923, all states had enacted nurse practice acts. From the 1930s through the 1950s, nurse licensure laws were enacted to help define the practice of nursing and to prevent unlicensed individuals from practicing nursing. In 1955, the American Nurses Association issued a model definition of nursing that affirmed that not all nursing duties required physician supervision and that some duties were independent nursing functions. However, the definition did forbid nurses from diagnosing conditions or prescribing medications. Over time, the practice of nursing has expanded, with regulatory focus on professional accountability (Damgaard, Hohman, & Karpiuk, 2000).

Historically, when a registered nurse wanted to work in a state other than his or her home state he/she had to apply for licensure in that other state. In the past, there was no national licensure examination. That meant there was no consistency between states' nurse licensure exams. The NCSBN was instrumental in developing the national licensure exam for registered nurses, which changed in 1982 to the National Council Licensure Examination for Registered Nurses (NCLEX-RN). Thanks to the elimination of state-specific licensure exams, nurses can be more mobile and more easily pursue career opportunities in multiple states.

Requirements for Nursing Licensure

To ensure public protection, each state or territory in the United States through its state board of nursing or designated licensure body requires a candidate for nursing licensure to pass the National Council Licensure Examination for Registered Nurses (NCLEX-RN) or the NCLEX for Practical Nurses (NCLEX-PN) computerized adaptive testing (CAT) exam and meet other requirements before granting a nursing license. The passing level for the exam is set to ensure that at a minimum, a sufficient skill set is demonstrated to protect the public. The NCLEX examination measures the competencies needed to perform safely and effectively as a newly licensed, entry-level nurse (NCSBN, 2007). The requirements for nursing licensure for applicants who wish to become licensed registered nurses include successful graduation from high school or completion of a

GED, successful graduation from an approved nursing school, application to the appropriate state agency for licensure, and payment of required fees. In addition, applicants must not have a criminal history such as a felony conviction that prohibits them from taking the NCLEX-RN. If an applicant successfully meets all these requirements, then a state nursing board or licensure body may grant the applicant a nursing license. Simply passing the NCLEX-RN is no guarantee that an applicant will automatically be granted a nursing license. Only after all state requirements have been satisfied will a candidate be considered for licensure. Although these requirements may seem extensive, the responsibility associated with nursing licensure and safely caring for patients demands such consideration. See Chapter 3 for more information on the NCLEX-RN.

Certification

Certification is a form of credentialing that demonstrates attainment of increased knowledge, but does not address a legal scope of practice like licensure does. Individual certification is the most common type of certification and is awarded when a nurse demonstrates a level of competency above the licensure level for a specific area of nursing practice. Individual certification is granted through a professional organization that offers an examination that demonstrates a higher level of competency or skill set than licensure (American Board of Nursing Specialties, 2005). Numerous state boards of nursing use professional certification as a requirement toward granting authority for advanced practice registered nurses (APRNs).

Organizations, like individuals, also can be certified. However, the certification process for organizations is very different from individual or personal certification. Organizations such as hospitals or healthcare institutions can be certified by external/reviewing entities (ANA, 2007a). Organizational certification is referred to as *accreditation*. The Joint Commission (TJC) is one example of an external entity that accredits hospitals. Hospitals go through an accreditation process to ensure that they are achieving a defined set of performance measures. In essence, hospital accreditation provides a "seal of approval" for hospitals achieving those standards. This approval rating allows consumers to make choices based upon standardized measures that reflect the quality of care provided at that hospital (The Joint Commission, 2008, para 1, Retrieved April 8, 2008, from: http://www.jointcommission.org/AccreditationPrograms/Hospitals). Another type of organizational recognition that has particular meaning for nurses is "magnet status." Magnet status is an award given by the American Nurses Credentialing Center (ANCC), an affiliate of the American Nurses Association, to hospitals that satisfy specific criteria based on the strength and quality of nursing in that facility (American Nurses Credentialing Center, 2007). A magnet hospital is an organization or facility that exhibits nursing excellence through patient outcomes, communication, and delivery of care. Other entities provide voluntary accrediting services for community-based facilities. An example of such a voluntary accrediting agency is the Commission on Accreditation of Rehabilitation Facilities. Potential for confusion exists because regulatory agencies and professional associations in different contexts may use the term *certification* differently (NCSBN, 2007).

As technology advances and the number of nursing specialty areas continue to grow, nurses are pursuing certification to increase their knowledge and skill beyond what they learned in their basic nursing programs. For example, the American Nurses Credentialing Center (ANCC) offers certifications in over 35 areas of nursing practice. However, certification is a concept that is frequently misunderstood by employers, the public, and even other nurses. Examining the current certification process for APRNs provides a unique opportunity for understanding nursing certification in general, because it mirrors the previous development of nursing licensure. APRN certification is in an earlier phase of evolution than is RN licensure. Therefore, APRNs today find that both the uniformity of standards and recognition of their advanced practice expertise lag behind those of their RN status. For example, APRNs' ability to prescribe medications, professional titles, and the ability to bill third party payors vary from state to state. Therefore, APRNs still face many of the challenges and barriers to practicing in different states that registered nurses faced in the recent past. Patients in remote and medically underserved areas who have the greatest need continue to face the greatest difficulties in accessing quality nursing care by APRNs because of some of these barriers (Philipsen & Haynes, 2007).

However, numerous studies have demonstrated that nurses experience positive benefits if they obtain certification. In 2000, the Nursing Credentialing Research Coalition studied the relationship between certified nurses and patient care quality. In 2002, an American Board of Nursing Specialties survey of nurse managers demonstrated that nearly 90 percent of respondents clearly preferred hiring certified nurses over non-certified nurses. Furthermore, 58 percent stated that they saw a positive performance difference in certified nurses. Additionally, a 2002 AACN study demonstrated that certification has a significant positive impact on patient care and patient safety (American Board of Nursing Specialties, 2005).

Requirements for Certification

The requirements for certification are diverse and depend on the organization granting certification. Requirements usually address the candidate's RN licensure status, educational preparation, and number of clinical practice hours in the chosen specialty. Historically, large numbers of professional and specialty groups have offered certification exams. Therefore, the requirements are extremely varied. For example, the American Association of Critical-Care Nurses (AACN) has different certification requirements than the American Association of Operating Room Nurses (AAORN). To determine the exact requirements for certification, nurses should check with the specialty organization through which they wish to become certified.

Differences between Licensure and Certification

Certification, on its face, appears to be very similar to licensure. Licensure and certification are two different terms that carry different meanings both professionally and legally. Certification is the granting of credentials that indicate a person has achieved a level of specialization higher than the minimal level of competency indicated by licensure (American Board of Nursing Specialties, 2005). Licensure is actually a form of legal certification. Although some very specific forms of certification carry a legal status, most certifications only imply a specific professional status. Licensure, on the other hand, always implies a legal status (Mills & McSweeny, 2002).

The Regulation of Advanced Practice Registered Nurses

The regulation of advanced practice registered nurses (APRNs) differs significantly from state to state among boards of nursing. Currently, the NCSBN recommends the use of APRN certification examinations as a basis for determining APRN credentialing. However, the scope of practice and prescriptive privileges that APRNs have depend on each state's nurse practice act. Currently, APRNs must still seek and receive recognition from each state in which they practice, regardless of whether their state of residency participates in the mutual recognition model. The model applies only to basic nursing licensure and currently does not apply to APRN certifications (Philipsen & Haynes, 2007). Generally, an APRN would need to contact the state in which he or she anticipates practicing as an APRN and meet the requirements for certification as an APRN and prescribing privileges (as permitted) in that state. The APRN who resides in a state that is part of the mutual recognition model may go to another compact state and practice as an RN because he or she has a compact RN license, but may *not* practice as an APRN *until* he or she receives advanced practice certification from that state (Philipsen & Haynes).

In April 2000, the NCSBN Board of Directors appointed a special Advanced Practice Task Force to continue to examine the issue of regulatory sufficiency of advanced practice certification examinations. The task force conducted a retrospective evaluation of the current certification review process and made recommendations to ensure consistency in certification to support the nursing boards in protecting the public.

In January 2002, the Board of Directors approved standardized criteria both for the certification programs and for the accrediting agencies that were developed by the Advanced Practice Task Force. For more information concerning APRN certification, you can review *Requirements for Accrediting Agencies and the Criteria for Certification Programs* (available at https://www.ncsbn.org/Requirements_for_ Accrediting_Agencies_and_the_Criteria_for_Certification_Programs.pdf). This document provides the required elements of certification programs that provide examinations suitable for the regulation of advanced practice nurses (Courtesy of: NCSBN®, 2007).

Standard of Care

A **standard of care** is a legal concept that all nurses should become familiar with and understand. This concept is used to depict a standard or measure of behavior that describes how a nurse is expected to act or professionally conduct him- or herself according to an accepted reasonable practice of nursing care. Standards of care can be published within a state's administrative code, and are generally defined within each state's jurisdiction. For example, in the state of Indiana, nurses have a defined responsibility to apply the nursing process and to act in a specific manner as a member of the registered nursing profession. Nursing behaviors including acts, knowledge, and practices that fail to meet defined minimal standards of acceptable current practice that could endanger the health, safety, and welfare of the public, represent unprofessional nursing conduct in Indiana (Indiana Administrative Code, n.d.: Retrieved April 8, 2008, from: http://www.in.gov/legislative/iac/T08480/A00020. PDF).

> **KEY TERM**
>
> **Standard of care:** The degree of care, expertise, and judgment exercised by a reasonable person under same or similar circumstances.

Nurses should conduct themselves with the degree of care, skill, and knowledge that reasonably competent nurses would exhibit in comparable situations. It is important to note that the standard of care represents a minimum level of practice that a nurse must stay within to avoid being found negligent or guilty of malpractice. Nurses must exercise good judgment using their nursing education to the best of their ability under the circumstances. In addition, a standard of care can be used to compare the performance of a nurse with another in the same specialty.

Standards of Care for Particular Areas of Nursing Practice

In malpractice actions, the adequacy of a nurse's performance is based on a professional standard that is then compared with the performance of other nurses in the same specialty area. This type of comparison allows nurses to be compared more accurately with the performance of their peers. For example, neonatal intensive care nurses determine the standard of care for other neonatal intensive care nurses. The conduct of a surgical nurse would not be compared with the conduct of a public health nurse. Standards of care apply to specific areas of nursing practice (American Nurses Association, 2007).

Malpractice actions are premised on allegations of failure to comply with a professional standard of care or performance. If a nurse's actions fall below the accepted professional standard of care, he or she may be found guilty of malpractice. It is extremely important for nurses to be familiar with and understand the professional standard of care that applies to their practice area. There are various layers of accountability for nursing practice ranging from broad national/general practice guidelines to narrow specialty- and state-specific guidelines. Nurses can go to their professional organization's website to determine appropriate standards of care for particular practice settings. For example, nurses can visit the American Nurses Association (ANA) website at http://www.nursingworld.org/ MainMenuCategories/ThePracticeofProfessionalNursing/Regulation.aspx to access information concerning appropriate standards of care. The ANA states that a registered nurse's practice "flows through several levels of accountability in order to ensure safe, competent practice" (ANA, 2007c, para 1). The ANA states that the *Scope and Standards of Nursing Practice* developed by the ANA on behalf of the profession provides the keystone for practice and accountability. The *Scope and Standards* "create the foundation for nursing specialty practice standards" and provide new information that can be incorporated into state nurse practice acts, which provide another layer of accountability. Rules and regulations promulgated by states that are specific to that state's nurse practice act, may further restrict the RN's practice. Additional restrictions upon nursing practice can be enforced by institutions or agencies of employment through policies and procedures (ANA, 2007c, para 1).

See Contemporary Practice Highlight 4-1 for additional discussion of patient safety and standards of care.

Official Resources for Determining Standards of Care

A variety of resources for nursng practice standards exist. Nurses may wish to utilize different resources depending on the states in which they decide to practice. In addition, standards are interpreted and applied differently depending on the state of jurisdiction. In malpractice actions, courts rely on some or all of these resources to help determine the applicable standard of care in each individual case. Some of these resources include:

- State statutes and administrative codes
- Nurse practice acts (a complete listing of resources and contact information concerning nurse practice acts can be found at http://www.ncsbn.org)

CONTEMPORARY PRACTICE HIGHLIGHT 4-1

EMPHASIS ON PATIENT SAFETY

Since the Institute of Medicine (IOM) released its report *To Err Is Human: Building a Safer Healthcare System* (IOM, 2000), which revealed only 55 percent of patients received recommended care, there has been a renewed interest in patient safety and standards of care. Medication errors, in particular, provide an example of high-risk situations that can result in a breach of standards of care and patient safety while exposing nurses to potential liability. Another excellent resource that nurses can access regarding patient safety and standards of care is *Patient Safety: Achieving a New Standard of Care* by Phillip Aspden, published by the Institute of Medicine.

- American Nurses Association (a complete listing of specialty care nursing standards and scopes of practice can be found at http://nursingworld.org/books/)
- The Joint Commission (information concerning the Joint Commission can be found at http://www.jointcommission.org/)
- State and federal case law and published opinions by judges
- Hospital policies

Summary

It is important for registered nurses to understand how and why nursing practice is regulated. By understanding the basic concepts of nursing regulation, licensure, certification, and standards of care, registered nurses are empowered with the necessary skills to provide safe nursing care. State nurse practice acts vary from state to state, and nurses must be aware of their governing nurse practice act when delivering and/or delegating care. As nursing continues to advance, and with the emergence of the field of telehealth, it is becoming increasingly important for nurses to understand that the care they deliver across state lines is impacted by varying state laws and the regulatory process.

Key Terms

- **Certification:** A designation earned by a person to ensure that he or she is qualified to perform a task or job.
- **License:** Permission to engage in an activity; a professional license allows the holder to engage in a specific activity for compensation.
- **Licensure:** The process by which a state or governmental agency grants permission to an individual to engage in a given profession for compensation.
- **Mutual recognition model:** A model that allows a nurse to have one license in his or her state of residency with the ability to practice (electronically or physically) across state lines if there are no restrictions on his or her license and that person acknowledges that he or she is subject to each state's practice laws. (Courtesy of the National Council of State Boards of Nursing (NCSBN) ®, 2007, para 1, Retrieved on April 8, 2008, from: : https://www.ncsbn.org/NurseLicensureCompactFAQ.pdf.) .
- **Nurse Licensure Compact (NLC):** A form of interstate compact specific to nurse licensure that provides an agreement between two or more states for the purpose of recognizing nurse licensure between and among a group of participating states. States must enter into an NLC in order to achieve mutual recognition (Courtesy of the National Council of State Boards of Nursing (NCSBN)®, 2007, para 2, Retrieved on April 8, 2008 from: https://www.ncsbn.org/NurseLicensureCompactFAQ.pdf).
- **Nurse practice act:** A state statute that defines the legal limits for the practice of nursing within that state and explicitly identifies the requirements for licensure.
- **Standard of care:** The degree of care, expertise, and judgment exercised by a reasonable person under same or similar circumstances.

Reflective Practice Questions

1. Have you ever read the NCSBN *Model Nursing Practice Act* and *Model Nursing Administrative Rules*? You can find a copy of both on the NCSBN website at http://www.ncsbn.org. Note the differences between the *Practice Act* and *Administrative Rules*. How are they different? Is one easier to read than the other? Do the *Administrative Rules* provide more detail? Do you think that your state or territory follows the NCSBN *Model Nursing Practice Act* and *Model Nursing Administrative Rules*? Explain why or why not.

2. Do you think it is important for various types of nurses to serve on state boards of nursing? What qualities do you think a state board of nursing member should exemplify? Why?

3. What state do you want to obtain nursing licensure from after graduating from nursing school? Can you list your state's nursing licensure requirements? Is it a Nursing Licensure Compact participating state? Do you plan to practice outside your state of residency? What entity should you contact to find out the exact requirements for nursing licensure?

4. How does certification affect an individual's nursing practice? What are some of the benefits associated with certification?

References

American Nurses Association (2007a). Home page. Retrieved August 21, 2007, from http://www.nursingworld.org.

American Nurses Association. (2007b). *Certification.* Retrieved August 21, 2007, from http://www.nursingworld.org/MainMenuCategories/CertificationandAccreditation/Certification.aspx

American Nurses Association. (2007c). *Regulation and accountability for practice.* Retrieved August 11, 2007, from http://www.nursingworld.org/MainMenuCategories/ThePractice ofProfessionalNursing/Regulation.aspx

ANA: Nursing: scope and standards of practice. (2004), p. 7, Retrieved April 8, 2008, from: http://www.nursingworld.org/MainMenuCategories/CertificationandAccreditation/AboutNursing.aspx).

ANA: Nursing's social policy statement, second edition. (2003), p. 6, Retrieved April 8, 2008, from: http://www.nursingworld.org/MainMenuCategories/CertificationandAccreditation/AboutNursing.aspx).

American Nurses Credentialing Center. (2007). *What is the magnet recognition program?* Retrieved December 26, 2007, from http://nursecredentialing.org/magnet/

Arizona Nurse Practice Act. Section 32-1636. Retrieved December 26, 2007, from http://www.needlestick.org/gova/titlepro.htm

Damgaard, G., Hohman, M., & Karpiuk, K. (2000). *History of nursing regulation.* Colleagues in Caring Project. Retrieved August 17, 2007, from http://doh.sd.gov/boards/nursing/White%20Paper%20History%20of%20Nursing%20Reg%202000.pdf

Henson, S., Burke, D., Crow, S. M., & Hartman, S. (2005). Legal and regulatory education and training needs in the healthcare industry. *JONAS Healthcare, Law, Ethics, and Regulation, 7*(4), 114–118.

Indiana Administrative Code. (n.d.). Article 2. Standards for the competent practice of registered and licensed practical nursing. Retrieved August 11, 2007, from http://www.in.gov/legislative/iac/T08480/A00020.PDF

Joint Commission. (2006). *Sentinel event glossary of terms.* Retrieved August 20, 2007, from http://www.jointcommission.org/SentinelEvents/se_glossary.htm

Joint Commission. (2007). *Facts about patient safety.* Retrieved August 20, 2007, from http://www.jointcommission.org

Joint Commission. (2008). *Hospitals.* Retrieved April 8, 2008, from: http://www.jointcommission.org/AccreditationPrograms/Hospitals/

Kleinman, C. S., & Saccomano, S. J. (2006). Registered nurses and unlicensed assistive personnel: An uneasy alliance. *Journal of Continuing Nursing Education, 37*(4), 162–170.

Mills, A. C., & McSweeny, M. (2002). Nurse practitioners and physician assistants revisited. *Journal of Professional Nursing, 18*(1), 36–46.

National Council of State Boards of Nursing. (2002). *Requirements for accrediting agencies and criteria for APRN certification programs.* Retrieved August 19, 2007, from https://www.ncsbn.org/Requirements_for_Accrediting_Agencies_and_the_Criteria_for_Certification_Programs.pdf

National Council of State Boards of Nursing. (2005). *Nursing regulation and the interpretation of nursing scopes of practice.* Retrieved August 19, 2007, from https://www.ncsbn.org/NursingRegandInterpretationofSoP.pdf

National Council of State Boards of Nursing. (2007a). The joint statement on delegation developed by the American Nurses Association and the National Council of State Boards of Nursing. Retrieved April 8, 2008, from: https://www.ncsbn.org/Joint_statement.pdf.

National Council of State Boards of Nursing. (2007b). *Nurse licensure compact.* Retrieved March 23, 2008 from: https://www.ncsbn.org/156.htm

National Council of State Boards of Nursing. (2007c). *Practice and discipline.*, Retrieved March 23, 2008, from: https://www.ncsbn.org/168.htm.

Nevidjon, B., & Erickson, J. I. (2001). The nursing shortage: Solutions for the short and long term. *The Online Journal of Issues in Nursing, 6.* Retrieved August 10, 2007, from http://www.nursingworld.org/MainMenuCategories/ANAMarketplace/ANAPeriodicals/OJIN/TableofContents/Volume62001/Number1January2001/NursingShortageSolutions.aspx

New York State Education Department, Office of the Professions. (2007). *Professional misconduct and discipline.* Retrieved August 21, 2007, from http://www.op.nysed.gov/opd.htm

News Blaze. (2007). *NCSBN welcomes Kentucky as the 22nd state to join the Nurse Licensure Compact.* Retrieved August 17, 2007, from http://newsblaze.com/story/2006040312000200002.mwir/topstory.html

Nurse Licensure Compact Administrators. (2004). *Frequently asked questions regarding the National Council of State Boards of Nursing (NCSBN) Nurse Licensure Compact (NLC).* Retrieved August 17, 2007, from https://www.ncsbn.org/NurseLicensureCompactFAQ.pdf

Perovich, S. (2004). *Malpractice: Will you be sued?* Retrieved August 21, 2007, from http://www.rd411.com/ce_modules/MAL05.pdf

Philipsen, N. C., & Haynes, D. (2007). The Multi-State Nursing Licensure Compact. Making nurses mobile. *Journal for Nurse Practitioners, 3*(1), 36–40.

Roberts, M. M. (1954). *American nursing, History and interpretation.* New York: MacMillan Company.

Studdert D. M., Mello, M. M., & Brennan, T. A. (2004). Medical malpractice. *New England Journal of Medicine, 350*(3), 283–292.

U.S. Department of Labor. (2007). *Federal vs. state family medical leave laws.* Retrieved August 20, 2007, from http://www.dol.gov/esa/programs/whd/state/fmla/index_PF.htm

Virginia Board of Nursing. (2007). *Nurse Licensure Compact.* Retrieved August 11, 2007, from http://www.dhp.state.va.us/nursing/nursing_compact.htm

Professional Nursing Organizations

Karen Peddicord

LEARNING OUTCOMES

After reading this chapter you will be able to:

- Describe what a professional nursing organization is and what purposes it can serve.
- Analyze the importance of matching the mission of the organization with the member's expectations.
- Describe at least three different nursing organizations and what their missions are.
- List three member benefits associated with professional nursing organizations.
- Explain how nursing organizations provide a voice for nursing in the political arena.
- List two potential deterrents to nurses joining professional nursing organizations.
- Consider individual career plans and the function of professional organizations in advancing career development.

Giving a Voice to Nursing

For a particular job to be described as a profession, several critical elements must exist. These criteria include a distinct body of knowledge, a role within the larger society, and **standards of practice** or some form of gudieline for behavior. There are approximately 2.9 million nurses in this country, but few of this number belong to a **professional nursing organization**. Only about 10 percent of nurses hold **membership** in the American Nurses Association (ANA, 2007). There is also a disturbing trend of either stagnant or declining membership in the professional nursing organizations (White & Olson, 2004). Clearly, the nursing voice could be amplified if more nurses joined professional nursing associations.

There are approximately 74 nursing organizations in the United States, each with a varying type, purpose, and size (Nursing Organizations Alliance, 2007). Membership may vary from a few thousand to as many as 250,000 (Wakefield, 1999). Helping nurses to understand the purpose of professional nursing organizations and the benefits of participation in these groups may help to increase membership.

This chapter provides an overview of what nursing organizations are and a description of the various types of nursing organizations. Within this discussion, a variety of significant functions of these types of organizations, including clinical, political, and regulatory, are presented. The purpose of this chapter is to provide information about the variations in professional nursing organizations as well as the benefits of membership for individual nurses, the profession, and the public. The chapter will provide information for the nurse to examine how professional organizations can be a vehicle for his or her career development. The information is provided within the context of what motivates nurses to join nursing associations and what some of the barriers are based on membership research to date. Membership benefits and opportunities are described, as well as some specific information about individual organizations.

What Are Professional Nursing Organizations?

Professional nursing organizations are an effective tool for the nursing profession to influence healthcare policy, protect and educate nurses, and provide the highest quality care possible to the public that we serve. The many professional nursing organizations provide a variety of foci to match the interests of nurse members. For example, the ANA is the largest of all professional nursing organizations, with a membership of approximately 150,000. The ANA's focus is primarily to nursing as a profession across the board (ANA, 2007). In contrast, there are many specialty nursing organizations that support the interests of nurses who practice in specific clinical environments. Examples of specialty organizations include the Oncology Nursing Society (ONS), the Emergency Nurses Association (ENA), and the Academy of Medical-Surgical Nurses (AMSN). There are also professional nursing organizations that are focused on specific roles of nurses. Examples of these include the American College of Nurse Midwives (ACNM), the American Association of Colleges of Nursing (AACN), the National Association of Clinical Nurse Specialists (NACNS), and the American Organization of Nurse Executives (AONE).

The Mission and Impact of Professional Organizations

Professional nursing organizations provide the opportunity for nursing as a profession to impact nursing practice, health policy, and healthcare standards. There are multiple facets to these membership organizations that contribute to changes in the profession and in healthcare policy. Individual membership in nursing associations also helps each nurse to be better informed about their specific practice area and the profession of nursing. Participation in these same organizations also facilitates leadership development, collaboration, and networking opportunities for each member that potentially can result in career advancement (Box 5-1).

To fulfill their mission, nursing organizations further the development of nursing standards of practice, expand the body of knowledge through research and evidence-based practice, and promote nurses' general welfare in the workplace. Nursing organizations also provide **continuing nursing education**, the continued development of nursing as a profession, and legislative and political advocacy for nurses and those we serve. To match the purpose and objectives of each organization with the expectations of the individual nurse member, the organization's mission statement must be examined. The next section will discuss mission statements.

> **KEY TERM**
>
> **Continuing nursing education:** Ongoing education that nurses take part in after they've achieved basic preparation and licensure.

Mission Statements

Each professional organization has a mission statement, which clearly indicates the organization's primary purpose(s) and drives the development of several priority objectives for that specific organization. For example, the American Association of Critical-Care Nurses (AACN) has as part of its mission statement, ". . . provides and inspires leadership to establish work and care environments that are respectful, healing and humane" (AACN, n.d.). It follows that one of AACN's priority issues is healthy work environments. The National

---

BOX 5-1   FOCUS OF PROFESSIONAL NURSING ORGANIZATIONS

- Nursing as a profession
- Specialization to a clinical population
- Role function within nursing
- Collective bargaining
- Political advocacy and lobbying
- Healthcare policy

Student Nurses' Association (NSNA) has as its mission, "To mentor students preparing for initial licensure as registered nurses, and to convey the standards, ethics, and skills that students will need as responsible and accountable leaders and members of the profession" (NSNA, n.d.). This statement makes it clear what the objectives of the organization are so that members can have an expectation that they will gain information to help them take the first steps toward professional practice and leadership.

When deciding which professional organization(s) to join, each nurse must determine whether his or her objectives for professional membership match those of the organization (Box 5-2). Organizational memberships are an added professional expense and it is important that each nurse maximizes the opportunities presented by that organization. If there is not similarity in objectives, the member can be disappointed. It is important to have conversations with other nurses in the specialty to determine which professional organizations they belong to and for what reasons. Most of the professional nursing organization websites have abundant information about not only the mission of the organization, but also strategic direction, recent activities, and member benefits. This information is very useful in finding the best match to support the nurse's own career objectives.

Local, National, and International Impact

Professional nursing organizations have national headquarter offices in various parts of the country. Most of the organizations' main activities are implemented from these national offices. Many of the professional nursing organizations also have local affiliates or chapters. For example, the Association of Women's Health, Obstetric and Neonatal Nurses (AWHONN) has 52 sections. The ANA has 54 constituent member associations. Some of the professional nursing organizations have international chapters. Sigma Theta Tau is an example of a professional nursing organization with an international presence in 90 countries with a total of 431 chapters worldwide. The vision of Sigma Theta Tau is to "create a global community of nurses who lead in using knowledge, scholarship, service and learning to improve the health of the world's people" (Sigma

---

BOX 5-2   DECISIONS FOR JOINING PROFESSIONAL ORGANIZATIONS

Each nurse when deciding which professional organization(s) to join must determine if his/her objectives for professional membership are congruent with those of the organization.

Theta Tau, n.d.b.). True to the vision, the organization is actively engaged in several global initiatives and has international members on its editorial advisory boards.

Varied Professional Organizations: Clinical, Political, and Regulatory Focus

Nursing as a profession provides many career options. In the United States, there are more than 200 specialties within nursing. Career options are also widely diversified not only by these many specialty opportunities, but also by role functions. For example, there are nurse researchers, nurse faculty, nursing care providers, clinical nurse specialists, nurse informaticists, and administrators, to name just a few. Overlaid on each nurse's role function is usually at least one, or perhaps a few, clinical foci. Nurses may choose to be geriatric nurse practitioners, pediatric researchers, or providers of nursing care in labor and delivery. There are professional nursing organizations to support unique role functions, such as the National Association of Clinical Nurse Specialists (NACNS), the National Nursing Staff Development Organization (NNSDO), and the American Association of Nurse Attorneys (AANA). There are also several nursing research societies—the Southern Nursing Research Society, (SNRS), Midwest Nursing Research Society (MNRS), Western Nursing Research Society (WNRS), and Eastern Nursing Research Society (ENRS)—whose purpose is to promote nursing research. There are also nursing organizations that support both a clinical focus and a role, including the National Association of Pediatric Nurse Practitioners (NAPNAP) and the American Pediatric Surgical Nurses Association (APSNA). Many nursing organizations are structured around a specific specialty area and build within their mission political, advocacy, regulatory, and professional purposes. The Association of Women's Health, Obstetric and Neonatal Nurses (AWHONN), for example, provides numerous forms of educational resources and standards of care to support the clinical practice of these specialty nurses. This organization also advocates for women and infants in many different venues including testifying in national and state legislative forums. AWHONN also has competency measurements for the specialty (e.g., fetal monitoring and perinatal medication administration) that support regulatory needs.

Clinical

Part of the mission of a **nursing specialty organization** is to enhance the health of patients in their care. Connection to a specialty organization ensures up-to-date clinical practice information for the specific population of patients that the nurse cares for, helping him or her to optimize the quality of care delivered. To fulfill this purpose, the nursing organizations may create a wide variety of practice and educational resources. These resources can take many forms including standards of practice, evidence-based practice guidelines, research projects, protocols, educational seminars, and practice and scholarly journals. Many of these resources have migrated to online formats and webinars in an effort to reduce cost to the members and/or their organization, and to provide easy and timely access for busy nursing professionals with difficult scheduling needs. Continuing nursing education is often included in the resources to assist members in maintaining needed contact hours for licensure and specialty credentialing (Box 5-3). A few organizations, such as the Oncology Nursing Society and the American Association for Critical Care Nurses, offer specialty credentialing.

A few nursing professional organizations are aligned with certifying organizations to affiliate as independent entities of the association. As an example, the Oncology Nursing Society (ONS) offers a member discount for **certification** with the Oncology Nursing Certification Corporation (ONS, n.d.). This both encourages oncology nurses to belong to their professional organization and provides a certification standard and measurement for the specialty of oncology nursing. The American Association of Critical-Care Nurses (AACN) has a similar offering through a credentialing arm known as the AACN Certification Corporation (AACN, 2007).

KEY TERM

Certification: A designation earned by a person to ensure that he or she is qualified to perform a task or job.

Political

Nursing as a profession has a responsibility to society, with a specific aim to improve the health of the nation. Professional nursing organizations fulfill the obligation of nursing to support improved health outcomes in national and global environments in several different ways. Many international and national organizations support work at the state level through local chapters, sections, or some form of alliance. On a broader level, an organization like the American Nurses Association will represent the views and needs of its members in various policy-making arenas. Through ANA's political and legislative program (Box 5-4), the organization has

---

BOX 5-3   TYPES OF PRACTICE AND EDUCATIONAL RESOURCES FROM PROFESSIONAL NURSING ORGANIZATIONS

- Standards of practice
- Evidence-based practice guidelines
- Research project protocols
- Seminars
- Practice and scholarly journals
- Webinars
- Continuing nursing education credits
- Specialty credentialing

taken action on such issues as adequate reimbursement for healthcare services, access to health care, and appropriate nurse staffing ratios (ANA, 2007).

In some cases, nursing organizations will also fulfill their political responsibility by advocating for nurses or for those for whom they provide care. Through its patient advocacy plan, the American College of Nurse-Midwives has been active in promoting a national dialogue on the rising rate of cesarean sections. To support the certified nurse-midwife membership, the organization has supported professional liability reform in state and federal legislation to establish damage limits and other important components of liability reform (ACNM, 2007).

Regulatory

Specialty organizations also have a responsibility to support regulatory efforts in the areas of both healthcare reform and professional practice. ACNM, as mentioned previously, has several initiatives in healthcare reform. Recently, another issue of interest has been to support changes to federal regulations within the Emergency Medical Treatment and Labor Act (EMTALA) that permit midwives to discharge women without a physician signature (ACNM, 2007).

The National Council of State Boards of Nursing (NCSBN) is an entity with significant importance in the regulatory area for nurses. NCSBN is a not-for-profit organization whose membership comprises the boards of nursing in the 50 states, the District of Columbia, and four U.S. territories—American Samoa, Guam, the Northern Mariana Islands, and the Virgin Islands. The purpose of the NCSBN is to provide an organization through which boards of nursing act and counsel together on matters of common interest and concern affecting the public health, safety, and welfare, including the development of licensing examinations in nursing (Box 5-5) (NCSBN, n.d.). NCSBN develops the NCLEX-RN and NCLEX-PN examinations

---

BOX 5-4   POLITICAL FUNCTIONS OF THE ANA

Through ANA's political and legislative program, the organization has taken action on such issues as adequate reimbursement for health care services, access to health care, and appropriate nurse staffing ratios (ANA, 2007).

BOX 5-5   REGULATORY FUNCTION OF THE NSBN

The purpose of the NCSBN is to provide an organization through which boards of nursing act and counsel together on matters of common interest and concern affecting the public health, safety, and welfare, including the development of licensing examinations in nursing (NCSBN, 2007).

and therefore has a large role in the regulation of nursing licensure in the United States. (See Chapter 4 for more information about the NCLEX-RN examination.)

Membership and Involvement

After deciding which organization may best support their career journey, nurses must fully understand what opportunities might exist within that selection. There are many directions including leadership possibilities at the local and national level, task forces and committees, liaison activity with other organizations, authorship, research, and public policy.

Membership rates in professional nursing organizations have had a varied pattern of rise and fall depending on the individual organizations, with some experiencing steady increase whereas others have membership challenges.

Membership

Nurses represent the largest number of healthcare workers in the United States; however, as mentioned earlier, only about 10 percent belong to the American Nurses Association (Deleskey, 2003). Similar percentages of nurses are often seen in specialty organizations. There is a very high rate of nonparticipation by nurses in their professional organizations.

A few studies have investigated what influences nurses to join their professional nursing organizations. These studies are frequently carried out by the organizations themselves in an attempt to identify better strategies for recruitment and design of member benefits. Deleskey (2003) surveyed perianesthesia nurses and found that the most significant factors that prompted nurses to join were self-improvement, education, new ideas, programs, professionalism, validation of ideas, improvement of the profession, personal work improvement, and maintenance of professional standards. A study of nursing home administrators compared those who belonged to a long-term care professional organization with those who did not. This large-scale study of 4,220 nursing homes linked membership with a higher quality of care in nursing homes. The research suggests that quality of care in the nursing home is improved when the administrator is assisted by a professional association as a resource (Castle & Fogel 2002).

A few studies suggest the most likely reasons why nurses do not join professional associations. Early studies by Booth (1999), Lamb-Merchanick and Block (1984), and Rapp and Collins (1999) found the primary reason was cost. Lack of information about the organization and time to be involved in member activities, and lack of employer support were also cited in the study.

Recently, the rising interest in reaching **magnet status** has increased the interest of healthcare organizations and therefore employers in supporting nurses' participation in professional associations. Magnet status is recognition for healthcare organizations provided by the American Nurses Credentialing Center based on the quality of nursing care provided and the presence of a workplace culture that encourages the enhancement of professional nursing practice. One of the 14 Forces of Magnetism that the organization must meet is professional development. Organizations must document the number of nurses who belong to professional associations, are certified in their areas of practice, and maintain a record of continuing education. The pursuit of magnet status should likely accentuate healthcare organizations' support for professional development, including joining professional organizations. Nurses are likely to find increased financial and time support within magnet organizations and magnet-pursuing organizations.

> **KEY TERM**
>
> **Magnet status:** A designation by the American Nurses Credentialing Center (ANCC) that recognizes healthcare organizations that provide nursing excellence.

Membership Opportunities

Professional organizations continue to try various recruitment and retention approaches for membership. Some have established mentoring programs. Many provide student and first-time discounts. There is a wide array of creative perks to enhance member benefit appeal, including journal publications, discounts in retail stores and websites, free practice resources, discounts to annual meetings and on all resource purchases, and online continuing nursing education contact hours. There are also new member recognitions and receptions at annual meetings. Recognizing that time is a precious commodity for all nurses, organizations are now providing webinars and annual meeting DVDs and CD-ROMs so that information can be more widely disseminated in readily accessible formats any time of day.

Professional nursing organizations are continuing to enhance member benefits, recognizing the importance of tangibles to justify the nurse's expenditure (Box 5-6). The tangible member benefits are only a portion of the value of professional association membership, however. Many of the most significant benefits of membership are the intangibles that the individual member gains from

---

BOX 5-6   MOTIVATORS TO JOIN NURSING ASSOCIATIONS

- Self-improvement
- Education
- New ideas
- Programs
- Professionalism

- Validation of ideas
- Improvement of the profession
- Personal work improvement
- Maintenance of professional standards

(Deleskey, 2003)

participating in the organization's activities and networks. The intangible benefits encompass everything from a voice in critical forums on the most important professional or healthcare issues to opportunities that provide professional development and potential career growth. Professional nursing organizations provide a rich network of contacts for practice and professional development. Members can also learn new skills by authoring resources in various formats such as online, print, or presentation. Leadership experiences are abundant in these organizations and include everything from participating as a member of a committee or task force to president of the Board of Directors (Box 5-7).

A Voice at the Table

To realize the importance of the nurse's voice at the table, imagine a representative for the insurance industry representing nursing when considering salaries for nurses. If nurses are not present, someone else would surely speak for them. The involvement of professional nursing organizations in all aspects of health care and political forums ensures that nurses will be representing the interests of nurses. By being a member of a professional organization, not only are nurses supporting the ability of professional associations to participate in these important forums, but in some cases, the nurse her- or himself has the opportunity to provide specific testimony and be the voice at the table. Nurses can be called on to provide expert information on anything related to practice and the profession. An example is testifying in the local or national legislature on universal access to care. Testimony on length of stay for cesarean section or mastectomy patients has recently been a legislative issue for nursing.

KEY TERM

Evidence-based guideline: "... [A] statement that is based on the scientific literature, explicitly documents the process used to develop the statement, and grades the strength of the evidence used in making clinical recommendations" (American Association of Chest Physicians, 2007).

Task Forces and Work Groups

Many times, professional associations need members with specific expertise to represent them not only in groups external to the organization, but also in groups or task forces within the association. These small groups of expert members may develop standards of practice for a specialty, for example. They may also create **evidence-based guidelines** or develop a position statement. Depending on the structure of governance within the organization, designated small groups may

BOX 5-7   MEMBERSHIP IN PROFESSIONAL NURSING ORGANIZATIONS

- Information about nursing practice and the profession
- Leadership development

- Collaboration and networking opportunitie
- Career and job advancement
- Continuing nursing education

be advisory panels that make recommendations for the strategic direction of the association. In any of these situations, members have the opportunity to play a key role in setting practice or direction for the organization. The members in these groups also have the advantage of networking with other experts in the field through their participation in these activities and becoming a nationally known expert in the field over time.

Leadership

Members of a professional organization have abundant leadership opportunities. Often, nursing organizations are seeking volunteer members for a myriad of positions. Organizations need volunteer members to help plan events such as annual or regional meetings. Chair positions are available for task forces and committees at both the national and local levels. Participating initially at the local level is an excellent way to become involved and to learn more about the organization. Such involvement can then naturally lead to participation at the national level. Members can progress from local or chapter leaders to eventually becoming a member of the Board of Directors. Although time consuming, leadership activities provide tremendous opportunity for recognition and also become very important for future job promotion, not only in present positions but also for future career possibilities.

Liaison Activity

Frequently, nursing organizations require someone with a specific expertise to represent their particular interest to other organizations. For example, each specialty group may send a representative to the American Association of Colleges of Nursing (AACN) to discuss implementation of the clinical nurse leader role or the Doctorate for Nursing Practice. The National Council of State Boards of Nursing (NCSBN) might request certain specialty and broad-based organizations like the ANA to participate in the dialogue about clinical nurse specialists. Liaison activity often extends beyond nursing associations to other health care–related entities. The March of Dimes, for example, may request representation from AWHONN or ACNM on issues related to prevention of preterm labor or standards of care for mothers with preterm labor. The possibilities are as diverse as the healthcare environment; leadership opportunities for members of professional nursing organizations are immense.

Authorship

Professional associations provide many resources to their members and others. The wide selection of journals is largely authored within the associations. Authors submit their manuscripts to editors for publication in the journals. Depending on the intended purpose of the journal, these manuscripts may be original research or practice related. Members are often solicited to author textbook and monograph resources as well. Educational resources created by a professional nursing organization are most often written by a membership group, and this is an opportunity for new authors to be mentored in publishing. The writing opportunities are many for members who choose to share their practice innovations and new research findings.

Summary

A large number of professional nursing associations exist that are aligned with many important purposes within the nursing profession, including clinical, political, and regulatory foci. The individual nurse should examine each organization's mission statement and determine whether it is congruent with his or her own practice values. There is a nursing organization to meet the needs of any individual nurse, and these organizations can be matched to specialty, role function, or nursing in general, as is the case with the American Nurses Association.

Professional nursing organizations provide many important functions that sustain the profession and provide professional development and opportunity. Associations provide many services including professional journals, continuing education, certification, networking, and specialty standards (DeLeskey, 2003). Organizations also provide input to active political forums and represent their members' views in various healthcare and political arenas.

Only about 10 percent of nurses belong to a professional nursing association. It is imperative that nurses participate actively in their nursing organization to ensure the best for themselves as a profession and the best health outcomes for their patients.

Key Terms

- **Certification:** A designation earned by a person to ensure that he or she is qualified to perform a task or job.
- **Continuing nursing education:** On-going education that nurses take part in after they've achieved basic preparation and licensure.
- **Evidence-based guideline:** ". . . [A] statement that is based on the scientific literature, explicitly documents the process used to develop the statement, and grades the strength of the evidence used in making clinical recommendations" (American Association of Chest Physicians, 2007).
- **Magnet status:** A designation by the American Nurses Credentialing Center (ANCC) that recognizes healthcare organizations that provide nursing excellence.
- **Membership:** The state of being a member or person in a group, in this case, a professional nursing organization.
- **Nursing specialty organization:** A professional nursing organization that has a particular clinical focus.
- **Professional nursing organization:** A collective entity of nurse members that has as its purpose enhancement of some element of patient care or the nursing profession.
- **Standards of practice:** The criteria against which professional practice is measured.

Reflective Practice Questions

1. Select an organization that you are currently involved in or interested in joining following graduation. How does the mission match your philosophy of care and professional development needs?
2. What motivates a nurse to join a professional organization? What are some of the more common barriers that lead nurses to choose not to make the investment and become a member?
3. What would be the impact to the profession of nursing if nursing associations began to disappear because of declining membership?
4. What would be the potential impact to patients if nursing associations no longer existed?
5. What are some of the intangible benefits for nurses to join professional nursing organizations?
6. What can each nurse gain by participating as an active member or a leader of a professional nursing organization?

References

American Association of Chest Physicians. (2007). *Evidence-based clinical practice guidelines*. Retrieved August 4, 2007, from http://chestnet.org/education/guidelines/current-Guidelines.php.

American Association of Critical Care Nurses. (n.d.). *Certification*. Retrieved July 29, 2007, from http://www.aacn.org.

American Association of Critical Care Nurses. (2007). *Mission*. Retrieved May 22, 2007, from http://www.aacn.org/AACN/membership.nsf.

American College of Nurse Midwives (2007). Professional Liability Update. Retrieved April 6, 2007 from http://midwife.org/professional_liability.cfm.

American Nurses Association. *About the American Nurses Association*. Retrieved May 16, 2007, from http://www.nursingworld.org/about.

Booth, D. (1999). Arkansas Louisiana Nurses Association workplace advocacy/membership survey. *Pelican News, 55,* 31–33.

Castle, N. G., & Fogel, B. S. (2002). Professional association membership by nursing facility administrators and quality of care. *Health Care Management Review, 27*(2), 7–17.

Deleskey, K. (2003). Factors affecting nurses' decisions to join and maintain membership in professional associations. *Journal of PeriAnesthesia Nursing, 18*(1), 8–17.

Lamb-Merchanick, D., & Block, D. E. (1984). Professional membership recruitment: A marketing approach. *Nursing Economics, 2,* 398–402.

National Council of State Boards of Nursing. (n.d.). *About NCSBN*. Retrieved August 2, 2007, from http://www.ncsbn.org/about.htm.

National Student Nurses Association. (n.d.). *About us*. Retrieved July 29, 2007, from http://www.nsna.org/about_us.asp.

Nursing Organizations Alliance. *Member organizations*. Retrieved May 14, 2007, from http://www.nursing-alliance.org/member.cfm.

Oncology Nursing Society. (n.d.). *ONCC*. Retrieved July 29, 2007, from http://www.ons.org/about/index.html.

Rapp, L. A., & Collins, P. A. (1999). Reasons why nurses do or do not join their professional nursing organizations. *Nursing News, 2,* 1–8.

Sigma Theta Tau. (n.d.b.). *Membership*. Retrieved May 20, 2007, from http://www.nursingsociety.org/about/overview.html.

Wakefield, M. (1999). Nursing's future in health care policy. In E. Sullivan (Ed.), *Creating nursing's future* (pp. 41–50). St. Louis, MO: Mosby.

White, M. J., & Olson, R. S. (2004). Factors affecting membership in specialty nursing organizations. *Rehabilitation Nursing, 29*(4), 131–137.

Interprofessional Issues: Collaboration and Collegiality

Pamela B. Koob

LEARNING OUTCOMES

After reading this chapter you will be able to:

- Discuss the importance of interprofessional collegiality.
- Describe ways that individuals in different health professions can work together to improve patient outcomes.
- List three specific actions that you might undertake to resolve inter-professional differences.
- Explain why interprofessional differences occur and ways that you might head them off before they occur.
- Examine the significance of collegiality and collaboration in today's healthcare environment.

Introduction

Collegiality and **collaboration** are specifically noted by the American Nurses Association (ANA) in its standards of professional performance, *Nursing: Scope and Standards of Practice*. Six standards of practice and nine standards of professional performance are listed in the document. The standards refer to the expected performance and behaviors of a professional. Collaboration includes **communication**, consultation, documentation, and appropriate

Collegiality: Sharing authority and responsibility to reach a prescribed goal or outcome. Power and responsibility are shared, and mutual respect and collaboration are desired.

Collaboration: Working jointly with other healthcare professionals in a collegial manner. A process whereby healthcare professionals work together to improve patient/client outcomes.

referrals (Box 6-1). Collegiality involves sharing knowledge and skills, giving constructive feedback, improving and enhancing practice, and contributing to and supporting learning within the work environment (Kearney-Nunnery, 2001).

Collaboration

Collaboration can be defined as working actively with other healthcare professionals in a collegial manner. Such work is intrinsic and vital to success in nursing practice today. When one works collaboratively, there is an implication that there is cooperation with other healthcare professionals and that a team effort is involved in this work. Further, working collaboratively implies an even distribution of power.

A team that works collaboratively is nonhierarchical. Power is shared and each individual's input is valued equally. In such cases, titles and roles are insignificant. Everyone's voice is important and is heard. As a nurse, you will be involved in many such team efforts. In fact, you will often be placed "in charge" of a team or be designated as the leader of a particular group. Thus, it is vital that you learn to work collaboratively and respectfully with others (Kearney-Nunnery, 2001).

In 1992, the American Nurses Association defined collaboration as follows:

Collaboration means a collegial working relationship with another health care provider in the provision of (to supply) patient care. Collaborative practice requires (may include) the discussion of patient diagnosis and cooperation in the management and delivery of care. Each collaborator is available to the other for consultation either in person or by a communication device, but need not be physically present on the premises at the time the actions are performed. The patient-designated health care provider is responsible for the overall direction and management of patient care (ANA, 1992).

Later, in 1998, the ANA released an executive summary related to collaboration as an intrinsic part of nursing.

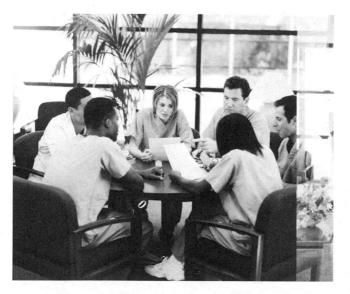

A group of doctors and nurses collaborating on a discharge plan for a client. *Source:* © Photos.com

---

BOX 6-1

In 2003, the Institute of Medicine identified essential precursors to collaboration. These were (Kearney-Nunnery, 2001):

- Individual clinical competence
- Mutual trust and respect
- Shared understanding of goals and roles
- Effective communication
- Shared decision making
- Conflict management

In the document, they wrote the following points(ANA, 1998):

- Nurses and physicians are working together and independently assessing, diagnosing, and caring for consumers preparing patient histories, conducting physical and psychosocial assessments, and reviewing and discussing their cases to determine the changing health status of each client.
- To provide effective and comprehensive care, nurses, physicians, and other health care professionals must collaborate with each other. No group can claim total authority over the other.
- The different areas of professional competence exhibited by each profession, when combined, provide a continuum of care that the consumer has come to expect.

Interprofessional Healthcare Teams

Kearney-Nunnery (2001) points out that the healthcare team is an example of ideal collaboration. Interdisciplinary teams may include nurses from different specialties, nurse practitioners, physical therapists, psychologists, social workers, and physicians. Cooperation, along with the collaboration, leads to achievement of specific goals, personal rewards for those involved, and improved outcomes for clients. In a true collaborative effort, responsibility is shared and "turfs" are not created.

Ten million people work in the healthcare industry. This is approximately 3.3 percent of the current population. The President's Advisory Commission on Consumer Protection and Quality in the Health Care Industry reported in 1998 that it was essential to harness the talents of all these individuals to achieve a unified mission. In 2003, the Institute of Medicine recommended that action be taken to support interdisciplinary collaboration and practice. Healthcare delivery systems are becoming more interdisciplinary and integrated. Thus, collaboration must be an effective means of improving client outcomes, and all healthcare workers involved in such teams must participate professionally and fully for the betterment of the client. Collegiality and collaboration between professionals is vital for effective team functioning and attainment of established goals (Kearney-Nunnery, 2001).

In today's world it is vital that interdisciplinary collaboration be a major focus of the provision of health care for the desired outcomes of client care to occur. According to Bourgeault and Mulvale (2006), there is a "renewed interest in collaborative models of health care delivered by 'interdisciplinary teams' of providers across several health care systems" (p. 481). Traditionally, there has not been extensive interdisciplinary collaboration among nurses, physicians, physical therapists, pharmacists, and other healthcare professionals (see Box 6-1). Only recently has the concept become more accepted, and progress is being made among these major disciplines.

Collaboration in Healthcare Today

There are many phenomena that promote as well as some that impede collaboration and the interdisciplinary team approach to healthcare delivery. Nurses have often been advocates for clients and sought interaction with other healthcare professionals for the betterment of the client and to achieve desired outcomes for the client. In the past, nurses may have been met with resistance from their colleagues because nurses have not always been perceived as having the power and influence to really make a difference in client-centered outcomes. However, as will be reported in this chapter, the healthcare environment has shifted to a model of collaborative practice where the nurse is a valued member and the client and his or her family are viewed as the center of the model.

The renewed move toward collaborative practice has come about as a result of physician shortage, cost containment, consumer demand, and industry and nursing goals for the best possible client health outcomes. Nurses have traditionally sought ways to provide exemplary care to their clients. Advances in technology and shifting of care to mid-level providers such as nurse practitioners,

---

BOX 6-2

Common interprofessional team members include:

- Nurses
- Physicians
- Nurse practitioners
- Dieticians
- Social workers
- Case managers
- Psychologists
- Pastoral care, ministers, rabbis, and priests

- Occupational therapists
- Physical therapists
- Dentists
- Speech and language therapists
- Researchers
- Billing and finance representatives
- Ethics committee representatives
- Infection control nurses

physician assistants, dieticians, and pastoral care counselors have also contributed to variations in today's interprofessional practice.

As healthcare models have changed and continue to change rapidly, the need for changes in our traditional roles has never been more apparent. Changes in the healthcare industry have focused on a shift from cure of illness to renewed focus on health promotion and early screening and detection. Today, the idea that care is client-centered and client-directed requires that many healthcare professionals collaborate for the betterment of the client. Thus, there have been changes in job descriptions as well as in the expectations for the registered nurse that are designed to improve client care and quality of life while controlling costs. Nurses are assuming responsibilities in mutual partnership with clients and their families and other healthcare professionals in a variety of settings.

Today, nurses work closely with interprofessional team members, and the ability to work collegially in teams is a major part of the nurse's job expectations. Nurses frequently are called upon to coordinate and integrate plans of care for clients. Nurses are required to have not only knowledge, but also excellent communication skills, good management skills, time management skills, and professional accountability. In addition, excellent clinical skills are vital. Nurses should be prepared to function as the designated leader of the team when the need arises. Collegiality and trust must be established and maintained with the team members throughout the plan of care for the client.

The use of teams to work for the betterment of clients has been shown to improve outcomes for clients. Frequently, team members have unequal power or status, but they work together in ways that a single individual is incapable of doing. Outcomes have included improved client care, decreased cost, decreased length of stay, and higher client satisfaction (Bourgeault & Mulvale, 2006). Interdisciplinary teams work together in a collaborative manner to provide optimal delivery of patient care as well as supporting cost-effective care. As noted earlier, however, some issues related to interdisciplinary care and collaboration include defining who contributes what to the plan, territoriality, and shifts that may be present related to power.

It is important to match the right person with the right task and use each individual's talents to the greatest good for the client. Staff in the team setting, such as ICU, the medical-surgical unit, or the obstetric unit, should be cultured to target the clients' needs and focus on coordinating care and enhancing collaboration. However, turf wars still may occur, and concerns about accountability, abuse of power, and other issues also can occur with the use of teams.

Shortages of Healthcare Professionals

In the United States, there are 2,900,000 registered nurses, 100,000 nurse practitioners (NPs), and 50,000 physician assistants (PAs). There is a registered nursing shortage, and this is only expected to worsen over the next 5–10 years, peaking in 2014, when most of the older baby boomers will be retired or retiring. Although the number of registered nurses appears large, not all of these nurses are working and certainly not all of these are working at the bedside. It is vital that qualified individuals are recruited and retained in nursing. Because there is a current nursing shortage, which is only expected to worsen, enrollments in nursing programs have increased and nursing programs are working diligently to increase student enrollments and graduation rates. Many programs offer special initiatives for nursing students and work very hard to make courses more accessible and student-friendly. For example, many programs have coursework online. In some instances, students live a long distance from campus and travel occasionally to a site to be "checked off" regarding certain clinical skills.

There is also a shortage of primary care providers, such as family practitioners and general practitioners. Together they comprise only 11 percent of the physician population. Thus, the provision of primary care has fallen to other physicians, such as gynecologists, pediatricians, and internists, and other providers such as nurse practitioners and PAs. Concurrent with the increased emphasis on primary care in the United States has been an increase in nurse practitioner and physician assistant programs, and the tasks involved in primary care have become the basis of their practices. With the renewal of primary care initiatives, collaboration has become the cornerstone of this field. Most regulatory boards of nursing have specific rules governing the practice of NPs, and the majority of them require collaboration (Bourgeault & Mulvale, 2006). Learning how to provide primary care and be involved in the collaboration of the provision of primary care has become another focus of nursing school curricula.

Collaborative Practice Models

Accomplishing collaboration begins with developing and organizing a collaborative team consisting of different professionals from the healthcare arena. Anyone involved with client care should be involved or represented on the team. The team requires administrative support to become successful and everyone on the team buying into the concept and process of the team. Networking, sharing, systems analysis, and the true integration of the nurses on the front line are also requirements for success (Mawdsley & Northway, 2007). When there is effective nurse–physician collaboration, nurses are better satisfied with their jobs, retention is higher, and patient outcomes improve.

As has been noted, the overall objectives of collaboration are excellent client care outcomes and satisfaction. Further, the issue of containing costs has been addressed briefly. When collaboration works for the benefit of all, cost saving should certainly be an outcome. Teams that work together collaboratively provide greater diversity and a broad range of expertise. Research has shown that such teams do save money and they also improve efficiency and prevent errors.

According to Blais, Hayes, Kozier, and Erb (2006, p. 218), the following objectives should be included in a collaborative practice model:

- Provide client-directed and client-centered care using a multidisciplinary, integrated, participative framework.
- Enhance continuity across the continuum of care, from wellness and prevention, to prehospitalization through an acute episode of illness, to transfer or discharge and recovery or rehabilitation.
- Improve client(s) and family satisfaction with care.
- Provide quality, cost-effective, research-based care that is outcome driven.
- Promote mutual respect, communication, and understanding between client(s) and members of the healthcare team.
- Create a synergy among clients and providers, in which the sum of their efforts is greater than the parts.
- Provide opportunities to address and solve system-related issues and problems.
- Develop interdependent relationships and understanding among providers and clients.

As has been stated previously, one needs to remember that collaborative practice can include any member of the healthcare team. This can certainly be the nurse and the physician, but also the social worker, case manager, physical therapist, dietitian, psychologist, nurse's aide, and others as well. Collaborative healthcare teams are capable of providing and/or ensuring the highest quality of client health care compared to what one or two healthcare professionals can do on their own.

Blais, Hayes, Kozier, and Erb (2006, p. 219) include the following in an effective collaborative model:

- Common purpose and goals
- Clinical competence of each provider
- Interpersonal competence
- Humor
- Trust
- Valuing and respecting diverse, complementary knowledge

The Nurse as a Collaborator

In the nursing profession, it is widely known that nurses have collaborated with many other healthcare professionals to provide the highest quality care to the client. Nurses have collaborated on many issues, including making changes to enhance client care, ethical issues concerning clients, financial concerns of the client, and a variety of other issues pertinent to the profession and betterment of the client. The primary goal of nurses and the nursing profession is to provide the best and highest quality care to all clients, regardless of their race, religion, ethnicity, sex or sexual orientation, or, importantly today, their ability to pay. These ethical values shape the involvement of the nurse in the collaborative practice model.

Collaboration allows and promotes autonomy, professionalism, self-confidence, and improved patient outcomes. Nurses who are functioning as team leaders have the opportunity to bring about improved patient outcomes as they share information with other healthcare professionals about clients. Professional nurses who participate in collaboration and active problem-solving can use insights obtained from other professional healthcare workers to enhance and provide excellent client care.

There are definite benefits to working collaboratively with others. Such benefits include improved client care, which is more client-focused; better-educated clients; client involvement in decision making; overall improved quality; cost savings; decreased lengths of stay; and the emergence of collegial relationships. Working together in a collaborative fashion improves the work environment as well. Typically, in work environments where there is collegiality and collaboration, there is increased job satisfaction and decreased turnover in nursing staff. Thus, there are advantages to such partnerships for the nurse, client, team members, and the involved institutions of care.

Blais, Hayes, Kozier, and Erb (2006, p. 220) have delineated some specific aspects of the nurse's role as collaborator:

- With clients:

  - Acknowledges, supports, and encourages clients' active involvement in healthcare decisions
  - Encourages a sense of clients' autonomy and an equal position with other members of the healthcare team
  - Helps clients set mutually agreed-upon goals and objectives for health care
  - Provides client consultation in a collaborative fashion

- With peers:

  - Shares personal expertise with other nurses and elicits the expertise of others to ensure quality client care

- Develops a sense of trust and mutual respect with peers that recognizes their unique contributions

- With other healthcare professionals:

  - Recognizes the contribution that each member of the interdisciplinary team can make by virtue of his or her expertise and view of the situation
  - Listens to each individual's views
  - Shares healthcare responsibilities in exploring options, setting goals, and making decisions with clients and families
  - Participates in collaborative interdisciplinary research to increase knowledge of a clinical problem or situation

- With professional nursing organizations:

  - Seeks out opportunities to collaborate with and within professional organizations
  - Serves on committees in state (or provincial), national, and international nursing organizations or specialty groups
  - Supports professional organizations in political action to create solutions for professional and healthcare concerns

- With legislators:

  - Offers expert opinions on legislative initiatives related to health care
  - Collaborates with other healthcare providers and consumers on healthcare legislation to best serve the needs of the public

Communication Skills

In order to function collaboratively, it is vital that nurses have excellent communication skills, which has been previously addressed. Further, there needs to be mutual respect and trust among those working together collaboratively. Nursing professionals need to be able to accept constructive criticism in a professional manner, as well as provide it to others in a constructive communication style.

Nurses must also be able to negotiate and make collaborative decisions. Combining the prerequisite clinical skills, knowledge, and expertise, decision making is part of the repertoire of a nursing professional. In a collaborative environment, decision making is a team effort. This requires trust, respect and consideration of others' opinions, and clinical expertise. It

> **KEY TERM**
>
> **Communication:** "All the cognitive, affective and behavioral responses that can be used to convey a message to another person" (Watson, 1979, p. 33). Communication can be verbal, such as through one's words, how these words are expressed, the tone used in expressing these words, and their pace, clarity, timing, and relevance. Communication can also be nonverbal, where words are not used, but meanings or expressions are communicated via body language, facial expressions, and the use of touch, space, and/or sound. Communication can be varied through the aspect of one's culture as well. Further, how a nurse communicates can be greatly influenced by his or her appearance.

is important to remember that the client is always the first priority. Keeping this in mind, working collaboratively with others is focused in the right direction.

Another important aspect of working collaboratively and collegially is that of conflict management. Role conflict can easily occur when working in a team. Individuals can all have different expectations and goals that may not be consistent with those of other team members. If expectations differ from one or several team members' expectations, role conflict can occur. It becomes important to keep an open mind, trust your team colleagues, explore barriers that may be present or perhaps invisible, and discuss each other's beliefs and experiences to reach compromises that enhance the quality of patient care. It may become necessary to call in a negotiator in some cases, but hopefully, this will not occur often. Nursing professionals should have the skills, education, and experience to resolve conflicts in a professional and respectful manner.

Related Nursing Theory and Research

When discussing collaboration in nursing, it is beneficial to highlight the writings of Virginia Henderson, whose theory is central to interprofessional practice. Henderson first published her *Textbook on the Principles and Practices of Nursing* (co-authored with Bertha Harmer) in 1955, followed in 1966 by *The Nature of Nursing*. Henderson also had many additional publications relevant to nursing practice. She defined the unique function of nursing in 1955 and described nursing's relationship to the client as well. Henderson's conceptualization of nursing included assisting sick or well individuals as their needs indicated. She viewed the nurse as a partner with the client and, if needed, a substitute for the client. Thus, it would seem appropriate to acknowledge her contribution to nursing's need to collaborate with other healthcare professionals. Henderson viewed the nurse as one who would seek assistance, advice, or support from whomever would be the most appropriate professional individual so as to promote and attain the most beneficial goals for the client (Blais et al., 2006). Henderson (1991) defined collaboration as "a partnership relationship between doctors, nurses, and other health care providers with patients and their families" (p. 44).

In Canada, intensive care unit (ICU) collaborative teams have been established to provide "patient advocacy at its best" (Mawdsley & Northway, 2007, p. 11). Some goals of the initial collaborative team approach included improvement of the use of red blood cell transfusions, reduction of harm due to administration of high-risk medications, prevention or early management of sepsis, reduction of cardiac arrests by using teams, and reduction of the overall incidence of central venous catheter–related infections. These goals were established at two children's hospitals to improve client outcomes through the Canadian ICU collaborative approach. Many of the goals were actually related to work that physicians initially perform, but that become the nurse's purview once the procedure is completed.

CONTEMPORARY PRACTICE HIGHLIGHT 6-1

TEAMBUILDING IN COLLABORATIVE PRACTICE

In today's healthcare environment, multiple issues are involved in interprofessional practice. Some professionals are territorial with regard to their practice and find it difficult to integrate input or suggestions from other professionals, although they realize the goal of all healthcare professionals must be improved patient outcomes. Others in the healthcare professions welcome discussion and collaboration to meet this goal. As a professional nurse, you will find that the ability to work with all types of individual practitioners will assist you in meeting your professional goals as well as provide you with the skill to deal with and address adversities and provide the best client care possible.

The children's hospitals described by Mawdsley and Northway (2007) used collaboration to accomplish their goals. These authors stressed that there are common threads to collaboration success, including nurses becoming involved in frontline change, nurses championing the changes, nurses insisting on system change for patient safety, and the support of administration.

Rieck (2007) reported on nurse–physician collaboration in a review of findings of multiple studes to examine the attitudes of nurses and physicians in the medical-surgical patient care setting. In her literature review, Rieck found that nurses in the United States, Israel, Italy, and Mexico desire nurse–physician collaboration more than do physicians. Physicians in the studies were less aware of the importance of collaboration between nurses and physicians than nurses were. However, when collaboration is in place, patient care quality is improved.

In her review, Rieck found that nurses, who were predominantly female (91 percent) with an average age of 33.5 years, agreed or strongly agreed with statements on the Jefferson scale of Attitudes toward Physician–Nurse Collaboration. Physicians, who were predominantly male (86 percent) with an average age of 34.5 years, mostly agreed with the statements about collaboration. The findings were compared between the two groups, using t-tests, and were not found to be statistically significant. Breaking the scale down to some of its important attitudes, nurses strongly agreed that interprofessional relationships should be a part of education, and physicians agreed. Another three-item scale addressed nurses' autonomy, with nurses strongly agreeing that this was important and physicians agreeing. A two-item scale addressed physician dominance. "A score of 4 indicates disagreement with the need for a collaborative relationship. A score of 6 indicates agreement and a score of 8 strong agreement with the role of collaboration. Nurses scored 5.1 and physicians scored 4.6, showing a more neutral stance toward collaboration"

(p. 121). This study reviewed by Rieck demonstrated that nurses have more positive attitudes toward collaboration, shared education, teamwork, and autonomy. Findings related to physicians were neutral for both groups.

In 2001, Hojat et al. reported on attitudes toward nurse–physician collaboration. A total of 639 nurses and physicians working in the United States and Mexico were administered an attitude scale. Results indicated that U.S. physicians and nurses had more positive attitudes toward collaboration than did their Mexican colleagues and again, as noted earlier, nurses expressed a more positive attitude toward collaborating with physicians. This study also investigated the attitudes of female physicians versus male physicians regarding collaboration, and the opinions of female physicians did not differ significantly from males. Hojat et al. recommended that medical and nursing schools should add "interprofessional education" to their curricula to promote the roles of collaborator for professionals. Such educational inclusion would lead to more positive attitudes regarding collaborative practice.

Summers, Marton, Barbaccia, and Randolph (2000) researched collaboration in a primary care setting with chronically ill seniors. The collaborative team consisted of a primary care physician (PCP), a nurse, and a social worker. Five hundred forty-three patients in 18 private offices were included in the study. Half the group received care from the team and the other half received care only from the PCP, which was the control group. The PCP group was hospitalized more frequently than those clients in the team group. Hospital readmission for the team group was less than that of those in the PCP group. Primary care physician group visits also increased in the control group and decreased in the team group. Seniors in the team group were also more active socially than those in the PCP

CONTEMPORARY PRACTICE HIGHLIGHT 6-2

ENHANCING CARE OUTCOMES THROUGH INTERPROFESSIONAL PRACTICE

You are working on an oncology unit caring for a 52-year-old woman admitted for pain management for terminal Stage IV breast cancer. She has recently left her executive position for a medical leave because she is unable to perform the responsibilities of her job. She is married and has two daughters, ages 14 and 20, who still live at home. Consider the various members of the interprofessional team that would contribute to the highest level of care for this client and her family during the hospitalization stay. Prior to discharge, what interprofessional members should be included to enhance outcomes and quality of life for this client and her family? How would you partner with the client to ensure she was the central member of the interprofessional team?

control group. Thus, this study revealed that hospital admissions, physician visits, and healthcare costs can be reduced using a collaborative approach to care.

Summary

The healthcare setting is changing daily with vast opportunities and needs for interprofessional healthcare teams. In today's healthcare environment, the population is aging and persons with chronic health conditions are increasingly common. In hospitals, nursing homes, and home health settings, the acuity level of the clients requires that nurses, physicians, social workers, dietitians, psychologists, and other healthcare professionals work together to provide the best, highest quality care. The collaborative practice model will enhance and improve client outcomes while decreasing or sustaining costs. As the government and healthcare institutions strive to reduce costs and yet improve client outcomes, nurses must function as collaborators and interprofessional healthcare team members.

The National Instititue of Health (NIH) represents all disciplines of healthcare providers collaborating to achieve improved public health of the nation. The mission of the NIH is to improve the health and quality of life of all citizens. Nursing professionals have a major role to play in reaching this goal. Today clients are more knowledgeable and they seek a more holistic form of healthcare delivery. Working with others in a collegial and collaborative fashion is vital to safe, client-driven, and cost-effective care. Nurses must be educated and prepared to be active participants on the healthcare team with the client, the client's family, and a variety of other healthcare professionals.

Key Terms

- **Collaboration:** Working jointly with other healthcare professionals in a collegial manner. A process whereby healthcare professionals work together to improve patient/client outcomes.
- **Collegiality:** Sharing authority and responsibility to reach a prescribed goal or outcome. Power and responsibility are shared and mutual respect and collaboration are desired.
- **Communication:** "All the cognitive, affective and behavioral responses that can be used to convey a message to another person" (Watson, 1979, p. 33). Communication can be verbal, such as through one's words, how these words are expressed, the tone used in expressing these words, and their pace, clarity, timing, and relevance. Communication can also be nonverbal, where words are not used, but meanings or expressions are communicated via body language, facial expressions, and the use of touch, space, and/or sound. Communication can be varied through the aspect of one's culture as well. Further, how a nurse communicates can be greatly influenced by his or her appearance.

Reflective Practice Questions

1. After reading the preceding information regarding collaboration and collegiality, how do you see your own role as a collaborator?
2. Have you been a member of a collaborative team, or an observer? What issues, if any, did you see regarding power and the sharing or lack of sharing of power? How was this or could this have been better resolved?
3. Review the collaborative model described in this chapter. Is there anything you feel does not "fit" or anything that you as a professional nurse would add?
4. Describe a situation that involved role conflict or decision making on your part. What was the most difficult aspect of your role? How did you handle the situation? What would you have done differently?

References

American Nurses Association. (1992). *House of delegates report: 1992 convention. Las Vegas, Nevada.* Kansas City, MO: Author, 104–120.

American Nurses Association. (1995). *Nursing's policy statement.* Washington, DC: Author.

American Nurses Association. (1998). Collaboration and independent practice: Ongoing issues for nursing. *Trends and Issues, 3*(5).

Blais, K. K., Hayes, J. S., Kozier, B., & Erb, G. (2006). *Professional nursing practice: Concepts and perspectives* (5th ed.). Upper Saddle River, NJ: Pearson Prentice Hall.

Bourgeault, I. L., & Mulvale, G. (2006). Collaborative health care teams in Canada and the USA: Confronting the structural embeddedness of medical dominance. *Health Sociology Review, 15*(5), 481–494.

Henderson, V. A. (1991). *The nature of nursing: Reflections after 25 years.* New York: National League for Nursing.

Hojat, M., Nasca, T., Cohen, M., Fields, S., Rattner, S., Griffiths, M., et al. (2001). Attitudes toward physician–nurse collaboration: A cross-cultural study of male and female physicians and nurses in the United States and Mexico. *Nursing Research, 50*(2), 123–128.

Kearney-Nunnery, R. (2001). *Advancing your career.* Philadelphia: F.A. Davis.

Mawdsley, C., & Northway, T. (2007). The Canadian ICU collaborative: Patient advocacy at its best. *Canadian Association of Critical Care Nurses, 18*(1), 11–13.

Rieck, S. (2007). Critique of "Nurse–physician collaboration: A comparison of the attitudes of nurses and physician in the medical-surgical patient care setting." *MedSurg Nursing, 16*(2), 119–121.

Summers, L., Marton, K., Barbaccia, J., & Randolph, J. (2000) Physician, nurse, and social work collaboration in primary care for chronically ill seniors. *Archives of Internal Medicine, 160*(12), 1825–1833.

Watson, J. (1979). *Nursing: The philosophy and science of nursing.* Boston: Little Brown.

The Global Nursing Workforce

Mary E. Riner

LEARNING OUTCOMES

After reading this chapter you will be able to:

- Identify how globalization is influencing the nursing workforce.
- Describe issues involved in the distribution of nurses globally.
- Discuss the correlation between the global burden of disease and the nursing workforce.
- Analyze factors influencing mobility of nurses across borders.
- Evaluate policy strategies for addressing the global shortage of nurses.
- Examine ways nursing education programs can internationalize curricula.

Introduction

To understand the global nursing workforce, we need to understand the broader issue of globalization. **Globalization** refers "to the interconnectedness of countries through cross-border flows of goods, services, money, people, information and ideas; the increasing openness of countries to such flows; and the development of international rules and institutions dealing with cross-border flows" (McMichael & Beagelhole, 2003, p. 8). Nurses cross

Globalization: Increased interconnections among people of different countries that facilitate the exchange of goods, services, money, people, information, and ideas across national borders.

borders for a variety of reasons including basic and advanced education, temporary travel and work, and permanent change of residence. Nurses also provide care to foreign-born persons who are now living in a new country, which requires cross-cultural, bi-national healthcare competency. Whether it is nurses or their patient populations who cross national borders, nurses, educators, and healthcare administrators need to be knowledgeable about and appreciate the increasing complexity of issues involved in nursing's contribution to promoting the health and welfare of our global population.

Millennium Development Goals: Eight goals set by the United Nations for the year 2015 for improving the health and well-being of the global population.

Global Nursing Workforce

Ensuring the availability of an appropriately prepared nursing workforce is an issue of importance within the global community, not just within the nursing profession. The scarcity of nurses, and qualified health personnel overall, has been highlighted as one of the biggest obstacles to achieving the **Millennium Development Goals** (MDGs; World Health Organization [WHO], 2004; see Box 7-1). Set for the year 2015 by the United Nations, the eight MDGs are an agreed-upon set of goals for improving the health and well-being of the global population that can be achieved if all countries work together. Four of the MDGs focus specifically on health and include eradicating extreme poverty and hunger; reducing child mortality; improving maternal health; and combating HIV/AIDS, malaria, and other diseases. Figure 7-1 shows the relationship between the density

Figure 7-1
Density of Health Workers and Probability of Survival. World Health Organization. (2006). *Source: The World Health Report 2006 – Working Together for Health.* Retrieved from http://www.who.int/whr/2006/en/ on July 31, 2007.

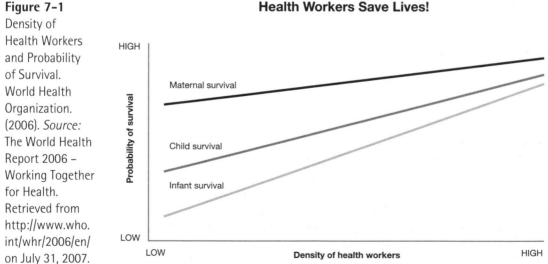

Health Workers Save Lives!

Maternal survival

Child survival

Infant survival

Probability of survival — HIGH / LOW

Density of health workers — LOW / HIGH

BOX 7-1   MILLENNIAL DEVELOPMENT GOALS WITH TARGETS

Goal 1: Eradicate extreme poverty and hunger
- Halve, between 1990 and 2015, the proportion of people whose income is less than $1 a day
- Halve, between 1990 and 2015, the proportion of people who suffer from hunger

Goal 2: Achieve universal primary education
- Ensure that, by 2015, children everywhere, boys and girls alike, will be able to complete a full course of primary schooling

Goal 3: Promote gender equality and empower women
- Eliminate gender disparity in primary and secondary education, preferably by 2005, and in all levels of education no later than 2015

Goal 4: Reduce child mortality
- Reduce by two-thirds, between 1990 and 2015, the under-5 mortality rate

Goal 5: Improve maternal health
- Reduce by three-quarters, between 1990 and 2015, the maternal mortality rate

Goal 6: Combat HIV/AIDS, malaria, and other diseases
- Have halted by 2015 and begun to reverse the spread of HIV/AIDS

Goal 7: Ensure environmental sustainability
- Integrate the principles of sustainable development into country policies and programs and reverse the loss of environmental resources
- Halve, by 2015, the proportion of people without sustainable access to safe drinking water and basic sanitation
- By 2020, achieve a significant improvement in the lives of at least 100 million slum-dwellers

Goal 8: Develop a global partnership for development
- Address the special needs of the least developed countries, landlocked countries, and small island developing states
- Deal comprehensively with developing countries' debt
- In cooperation with developing countries, develop and implement strategies for decent and productive work for youth
- In cooperation with pharmaceutical companies, provide access to affordable essential drugs in developing countries
- In cooperation with the private sector, make available the benefits of new technologies, especially information and communications

Source: United Nations. (2006). *The millennium development goals report.* Retrieved April 13, 2007, from http://unstats.un.org/unsd/mdg/Resources/Static/Products/Progress2006/MDGReport2006.pdf.

of healthcare workers and the probability of survival globally. This highlights the need for an adequate supply of well-educated healthcare workers to promote health and well-being. Four additional MDGs focus on social and physical environments associated with achieving improved health. They include achieving universal primary education, promoting gender equality and empowering women, ensuring environmental sustainability, and developing a global partnership for development (United Nations, 2006).

Global Burden of Disease

The varying levels of health among countries can be viewed in the context of understanding the global supply and distribution of healthcare workers. Figure 7-2 shows the relationship between the global burden of disease and the density of healthcare workers, according to the six country regions established by the World Health Organization (WHO). The **global burden of disease (GBD)** is a term developed by the WHO and World Bank to measure the total loss of health resulting from diseases and injuries (WHO, n.d. b). The GBD is used to understand and compare the impact of health problems among countries and regions of the world. The supply and distribution of nurses as the largest group of healthcare workers is important. Health care is labor intensive, and the availability of a sufficient well-qualified and motivated nursing workforce is a key determinant of effective health services delivery.

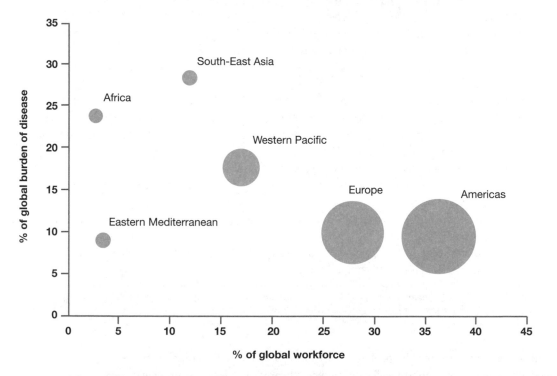

Figure 7-2 Distribution of health workers by level of health expenditure and burden of disease, by WHO region. *Source:* World Health Organization. (2006). The World Health Report 2006 – Working Together for Health. Retrieved from http://www.who.int/whr/2006/en/ on July 31, 2007.

Global Definition of Nurse and Nursing

The International Council of Nurses (ICN) estimates that there may be more than 12 million nurses worldwide (ICN, n.d.). Although the varying definitions of *nurse* in countries around the globe make it difficult to establish an accurate estimate of nurses, it is useful to identify a widely accepted definition used for regulating practice. According to the WHO, a nurse is "a person who has completed a programme of basic nursing education and is qualified and authorized in his/her country to practice nursing in all settings for the promotion of health and prevention of illness, care of the sick and rehabilitation" (WHO, n.d. a). According to the ICN:

> Nursing encompasses autonomous and collaborative care of individuals of all ages, families, groups and communities, sick or well and in all settings. Nursing includes the promotion of health, prevention of illness, and the care of ill, disabled and dying people. Advocacy, promotion of a safe environment, research, participation in shaping health policy and in patient and health systems management, and education are also key nursing roles. (ICN, n.d.)

As one example of defining nursing using a global perspective, Box 7-2 describes characteristics of nursing and midwifery developed jointly by the WHO and Sigma Theta Tau International.

BOX 7-2   GLOBAL CHARACTERISTICS OF NURSING AND MIDWIFERY GRADUATES

Programme Graduate Characteristics: In completing nursing or midwifery, graduates will be generalists who: are qualified at the Bachelor's level; are clinically competent across settings; able to provide culturally relevant care; use evidence and effective communication in practice; demonstrate leadership and critical, analytical thinking; are health advocates able to enter into effective partnerships; and demonstrate ethical practices and beliefs. These graduates have achieved an academic credential; meet eligibility for licensure examination where required; value life long learning and community service; and are expected to continually update and maintain their competence.

The success of nursing and midwifery graduates is measured through licensure exams where required, performance based assessment, delivery of safe quality care, feedback from consumers, employers and stakeholders, demonstrated ability to work collaboratively in teams and the ability to form partnerships in addressing global health needs on a local level. An additional measurement of graduate success is the individual's career progression and advancement (e.g. seeking advance degrees, publications, presentations, and funded research).

Source: World Health Organization and Sigma Theta Tau International. (2006). *Developing global standards for initial nursing and midwifery education: interim report of the proceedings.* Retrieved July 31, 2007, from http://www.nursing society.org/about/WHO_interim_report.pdf

Distribution of the Nursing Workforce

Understanding healthcare workforce distribution issues is important for ensuring effective resource development for educating nurses around the world; monitoring their distribution within countries and across country borders; and influencing policies related to the social, political, economic, and healthcare system designs that affect nursing. The shortage of nurses and other healthcare workers is being called a "human resources crisis in health" in the *High Level Forum on the Health MDGs* (High Level Forum, 2004).

The *World Health Report 2006—Working Together for Health* (2007) contains an expert assessment of the current crisis in the global health workforce and reveals an estimated shortage of almost 4.3 million doctors, midwives, nurses, and support workers worldwide (WHO, 2007). The shortage is most severe in the poorest countries, especially in sub-Saharan Africa, where health workers are most needed. Contemporary Practice Highlight 7-1 illustrates the severity of one particular healthcare

---

CONTEMPORARY PRACTICE HIGHLIGHT 7-1

Sub-Saharan Africa has 10 percent of the world's population yet is home to more than 60 percent of all people living with HIV/AIDS—an estimated 25.4 million people according to the UNAIDS program (the Joint United Nations Programme on HIV/AIDS). In light of this, nurses and midwives are increasingly being asked to provide care for persons with HIV/AIDS.

Two dilemmas exist for the nursing workforce in this area. First, occupational exposure is a significant problem, due to the high prevalence of HIV among hospitalized patients and the lack of protective equipment such as sharps containers, gloves, goggles, and impermeable gowns. This is causing nurses not only to seek employment abroad, but also to leave nursing within their own countries and work in private hospitals and clinics and in the rapidly expanding AIDS programs funded by foreign donors.

A second dilemma is that nurses and midwives are the primary healthcare providers for most of the population in sub-Saharan Africa, yet they have received little training and support to provide AIDS care and treatment. Specifically nursing faculty, nursing students, and practicing nurses are not being provided with current WHO and United Nations practice guidelines to implement evidence-based practice such as the prevention of mother to child transmission (PMTCT) guidelines. The result of the weak health systems infrastructure is that popular perceptions persist in many places that the healthcare system has little to offer persons living with HIV/AIDS.

Implications for the nursing workforce in countries with weak healthcare system infrastructures are that populations receive ineffective or no care and many nurses leave the nursing workforce for other work in-country or migrate to practice nursing in another country.

Source: Raisler, J., & Cohn, J. (2005). Mothers, midwives, and HIV/AIDS in sub-Saharan Africa. *Journal of Midwifery & Women's Health, 50*(4), 275–282.

issue, HIV/AIDS, in Africa and how it is affecting the nursing workforce. Africa has been hit the hardest by the crisis; according to the report, the continent bears 24 percent of the GBD but has only 3 percent of the healthcare workforce and 1 percent of the world's financial resources. The density of the global healthcare workforce is shown in Figure 7-3. The report identified 57 countries that cannot meet a widely accepted basic standard for healthcare coverage by physicians, nurses, and midwives—36 of these "critical countries" are in sub-Saharan Africa (see Figure 7-4).

Global Shortage of Registered Nurses

Nursing shortages are reported to be an increasing challenge in many industrialized and developing countries and have been at the forefront of international health policy debate since the late 1990s (Buchan, 2000; Chanda, 2002; Martineau, Decker, & Bundred, 2002; Organization for Economic Co-operation and Development [OECD], 2002a). Staff shortages and **geographic maldistribution** are being reported in many countries. The tendency for nurses to practice in affluent urban and suburban areas—a phenomenon known as geographic maldistribution—creates barriers to care for people living in rural and inner-city areas. These shortages

KEY TERM

Geographic maldistribution: The tendency for nurses to practice in affluent urban and suburban areas rather than in rural and inner-city areas.

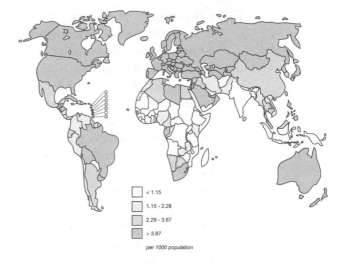

Figure 7-3 Density of healthcare workers. *Source:* World Health Organization. (2006). The World Health Report 2006 – Working Together for Health. Retrieved from http://www.who.int/whr/2006/en/ on July 31, 2007.

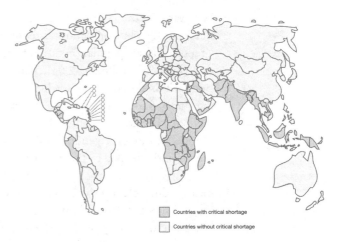

Figure 7-4 Countries with a critical shortage of health service providers (doctors, nurses, and midwives). *Source:* World Health Organization. (2006). The World Health Report 2006 – Working Together for Health. Retrieved from http://www.who.int/whr/2006/en/ on July 31, 2007.

relate to increased demand for health care, the aging of the nursing population in these countries, and difficulties experienced in some countries in recruiting home-based new entrants to nursing in the face of increased competition from other career opportunities (Buchan, 2002).

Although there is no universal definition of a nursing shortage, there is increasing evidence of nurse supply/demand imbalances in many countries. Using the country regions of the globe established by the WHO, Table 7-1 shows the ratios of physicians, nurses, and midwives per 100,000 population. Skill mix and staff mix vary among organizations, systems, and countries, and there is no single "optimal" mix of nurses and other healthcare staff to which all countries can aspire (Buchan & Calman, 2004).

Many countries are struggling to provide a minimum level of nurse staffing. The nurse:population ratio is an indication of the nurses available to care for the general population. Figure 7-5 shows the distribution by the WHO regions of the globe. Further analysis within the Pan American Health Organization region is shown in Figure 7-6. The ratio is one way of describing the accessibility and availability of nurses to provide patient care services.

The global distribution of the nursing workforce can also be viewed from the perspective of differences in nurse:population ratios according to country development and region of the globe. Figure 7-7 shows the average nurse:population ratios based on the country's development status, and Box 7-3 provides additional information related to the global distribution of the nursing workforce. For example, the United States, with a reported nurse:population ratio of 773 nurses to 100,000 population, is reporting nursing shortages. So is Uganda, with a reported nurse:population ratio of approximately 6 nurses per 100,000 population (Buchan & Calman, 2004). This variance among countries must be understood within the context of the healthcare system of each country. For example, in the United States the healthcare system operates within a market-driven environment of a developed country. This allows healthcare systems to employ a greater number of nurses. Uganda is a developing country whose healthcare system is funded and operated by the national government.

From a country-level policy perspective, a shortage is usually defined and measured in relation to that country's own historical staffing levels, resources, and estimates of demand for health services. This means the focus is on the difference between the past and present availability of nurses to fill existing positions and competitive salaries. If a country perceives there is a lack of new nurses graduating from educational programs, it may choose to increase national funding for nursing education. It is the gap between the reality of current availability of nurses and the aspiration for some higher level of provision, however defined, that is the "shortage."

TABLE 7-1 SELECTED CATEGORIES OF HEALTH WORKERS PER 100,000 POPULATION

Region	Physicians	Nurses	Midwives
Africa	17	71	20
Americas	212	414	n/a
South-East Asia	45	59	3
Europe	327	663	42
Eastern Mediterranean	96	159	n/a
Western Pacific	157	186	13

Buchan & Calman (2004). *The Global Shortage of Registered Nurses: An Overview of Issues and Action.* Retrieved from http://www.icn.ch/global/shortage.pdf on July 26, 2007.

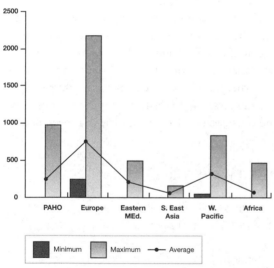

Figure 7-5 Nurse:population ratio (100,000 HAB) – min, max, and average by WHO region. *Source:* Buchan & Calman (2004). *The Global Shortage of Registered Nurses: An Overview of Issues and Action.* Retrieved from http://www.icn.ch/global/shortage.pdf on July 26, 2007.

Figure 7-6 PAHO subregions: nurse:population ratio. *Source:* Buchan & Calman (2004). *The Global Shortage of Registered Nurses: An Overview of Issues and Action.* Retrieved from http://www.icn.ch/global/shortage.pdf on July 26, 2007.

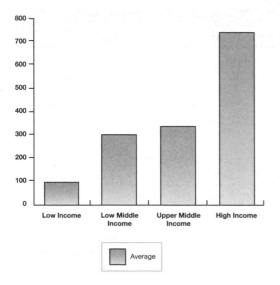

Figure 7-7 Average nurse:population ratios by World Bank development status of countries. *Source:* Buchan & Calman (2004). *The Global Shortage of Registered Nurses: An Overview of Issues and Action.* Retrieved from http://www. icn.ch/global/shortage.pdf on July 26, 2007.

Global Nursing Mobility Trends

One response to nursing shortages has been increasing international mobility and migration of nurses. In a report on nurse mobility, Buchan, Parkin, and Sochalski (2003) describe economic and working condition issues influencing migration that is increasing among professional and skilled workers (Castels, 2000; OECD, 2000). The number of people migrating has doubled from 75 million in 1965 to an estimated 150 million in 2000 (Institute of Medicine [IOM], 2000 [as cited in Buchan et al., 2003]). **International migrants** are defined as those individuals who live in countries other than their birth country for longer than a year. In parallel to the general migration, recently there has been growth in migration of skilled and qualified workers (OECD, 2000, 2002b).

Nurse migration across country borders is regulated through varying mechanisms in each country around the globe. Data available on migration indicates that some countries tend to be source countries whereas others are destination countries. Data from professional registers, employment records, and censuses of selected countries has been used to

---

BOX 7-3   GLOBAL DISTRIBUTION OF NURSING WORKFORCE

- At the country level, the reported nurse:population ratio varies in different countries from less than 10 nurses per 100,000 population to more than 1,000 nurses per 100,000, a variation of more than one hundredfold.
- The average ratio in Europe, the region with the highest ratios, is 10 times that of the lowest regions, Africa and South-East Asia.
- The average ratio in North America is 10 times that in South America.
- The average nurse:population ratio in high-income countries is almost eight times greater than in low-income countries.
- The low availability of nurses in many developing countries is exacerbated by geographical mis-distribution—there are even fewer nurses available in rural and remote areas.

Source: Buchan, J., & Calman, L. (2004). *The global shortage of registered nurses: An overview of issues and action.* Retrieved July 26, 2007, from http://www.icn.ch/global/shortage.pdf.

examine the scale of the movement of nurses. Information about migration of nurses is primarily supplied by national and state licensure or registration agencies. Although this data varies from each source country in terms of how it is collected, what is collected, and the reliability and completeness of the data, we can draw some insights into nurse migration patterns in selected countries. This is especially significant in understanding how the inflow of nurses into countries complements the existing native-educated nurse workforce. In the following sections, nurse migration information from four countries that tend to be destination countries for large numbers of nurses from many countries is presented. The four countries are Australia, Ireland, the United Kingdom, and the United States.

> **KEY TERM**
>
> **International migrants:** Individuals who reside in countries other than those of their birth for more than one year.

Australia

Australia allows nursing registration at the state level after the candidate has first been screened and approved by the Australian Nursing and Midwifery Council (ANMC, 2007). There are three entry routes for foreign-educated nurses to practice nursing in Australia: 1) permanent residence through migration; 2) long-term temporary migration, with visas granted for 1–4 years; and 3) working holiday visas for shorter time periods with a maximum period of 1 year. The main source countries for nurses applying for registration in Australia include the United Kingdom and New Zealand. Australia has established an arrangement with nine other countries that have mutually recognized qualifications and therefore "meet the requirement for registration without having to undertake a competency based assessment programme" (ANMC). In addition, nurses from New Zealand are covered by the Trans-Tasman Mutual Recognition Act of 1997, which facilitates flows between Australia and New Zealand (Nurses and Midwives Board of New South Wales, 1997).

Ireland

All nurses practicing in Ireland are registered with An Bord Altranais, the nursing and midwifery registration authority. Under arrangements established through the European Union/European Economic Area (EU/EEA), nurses from European countries are eligible to have their registration applications considered in Ireland. Although Ireland has traditionally been an exporter of nurses, it is now facing a shortage and has become an active recruiter of nurses. Registration data highlights rapid growth in inflow of nurses in recent years, with the Philippines, the United Kingdom, Australia, South Africa, and India being main sources (Buchan et al., 2003). Of the newly registered nurses in 2006, 32 percent were from Ireland, 18 percent from the EU, and 50 percent from other countries (An Bord Altranais, 2007).

United Kingdom

All nurses practicing in the United Kingdom must be registered with the Nursing and Midwifery Council (NMC), the professional regulatory authority. Applicants with general nursing qualifications from the other countries of the EU/EEA have the right to practice in the United Kingdom because of mutual recognition of qualifications across the EU. Nurses from all countries outside the EU/EEA must apply to the NMC for verification of their qualifications. There has been a strong upward trend in inflow of nurses from other countries in recent years. For the 2005–06 year initial registrants were from the following areas: 66 percent were from England, Scotland, Wales, and Northern Ireland; 6 percent were from EEA countries; and 28 percent were from countries outside the EU/EEA. The top non-EEA source countries were India, the Philippines, and Australia (NMC, n.d.).

United States

In the United States, registration and licensing of individual nurses are the responsibilities of the state-level nurse registration boards. Each board operates independently and, with more than 50 states and territories, it is very difficult to obtain a complete accounting of foreign nurses registered in the United States. There is one national data source, however: a sample survey of RNs conducted every 4 years by the U.S. Department of Health and Human Services (USDHHS). In 2004 the top three source countries where nurses received their initial nursing education were the Philippines, Canada, and the United Kingdom. One indicator of where nursing shortages likely exist in the United States is the top states employing foreign-educated nurses. The top three are California, Florida, and New York. Sectors with greater recruitment efforts can be determined by reviewing the primary places of employment for foreign-educated nurses, which are the hospital, nursing home/extended care facility, nursing education, and community/public health (USDHHS, n.d.). Table 7-2 shows the statistical data for graduates of foreign nursing schools taking the certification program exam in the United States. The number of first-time test takers between 2003 and 2006 was the lowest in 2006 and the highest in 2003.

Impact of Mobility on Source Countries

Migration from source countries can sometimes have a positive impact on the source country. Buchan, Parkin, and Sochalski (2003) identify the following three key areas of positive impact: 1) the return of migrant workers with new skills, knowledge, and experiences; 2) remittance of income earned abroad to support family members; and 3) links between migrants and their source country being established and maintained through networks. These international networks can facilitate the exchange of information and expertise among migrant workers, their international employers, and relevant organizations and professionals in the country of origin (Baptiste-Meyer, 2001, in Buchan, Parkin and Sochalski, 2003).

TABLE 7-2   UNITED STATES CERTIFICATION PROGRAM STATISTICAL DATA FROM THE COMMISSION ON GRADUATES OF FOREIGN NURSING SCHOOLS (CGFNS INTERNATIONAL)

	First Time Test Takers	Pass Rates	Repeat Test Takers	Pass Rates	Total Test Takers	Passed	
2006	12,258 (67.6%)	4,983 (72.0%)	5,870 (32.4%)	1,937 (28.0%)	18,128 (100.0%)	6,920 (100.0%)	Philippines, India, Nigeria, Taiwan, People's Republic of China, Ukraine, Iran
2005	13,959 (64.9%)	5,626 (70.5%)	7,543 (35.1%)	2,357 (29.5%)	25,637 (100.0%)	7,983 (100.0%)	Philippines, India, Nigeria, People's Republic of China, Kenya
2004	16,889 (65.9%)	7,124 (74.7%)	8,748 (34.1%)	2,413 (25.3%)	25,637 (100.0%)	9,537 (100.0%)	Philippines, India, Nigeria, People's Republic of China, Kenya
2003	14,235 (58.4%)	5,441 (60.3%)	10,142 (41.6%)	3,578 (30.7%)	24,377 (100.0%)	9,019 (100.0%)	Philippines, India, Nigeria, People's Republic of China, Kenya

Source: Commission on Graduates of Foreign Nursing Schools (CGFNS International). (n.d.). Certification Program Statistical Data. Retrieved July 24, 2007, from http://www.cgfns.org/sections/about/

For example, networks can increase the source country's capacity to address complex problems like HIV/AIDS, such as when nurses link with pharmaceutical companies willing to provide medications at reduced cost. When nurses return to their native country to practice and take up positions in administration, education, or research, the benefit received from exposure to the global community may be referred to as "brain circulation" (Kirk, 2007). However, when loss of qualified nurses becomes excessive, it can lead to a brain drain resulting in a severe reduction in the availability and quality of services. A diminished supply of workers in the source country may push wages up, putting added pressure on the country's economy (Baptiste-Meyer, 2001).

Impact of Mobility on Destination Countries

Some of the positive effects for receiving countries of an increased supply of nurses include allowing healthcare agencies to meet the demand for services, stimulating innovation capacity, and disseminating knowledge internationally (Guellec & Cervantes, 2001). An additional supply of nurses is particularly valuable in light of the aging population and nurse workforce in many industrial countries. A common misperception is that international nurses may take jobs away from the native population. However, Stalker's (2000) research indicates migrant workers tend to fill positions at the very top and the very bottom of the employment ladder.

Factors Affecting Migration of Nurses

KEY TERM

Push factors: Those factors that make it difficult to receive a basic or advanced education in nursing or to practice in the nurse's native country.

KEY TERM

Pull factors: Those factors that make migration to another country more attractive for education or practice than staying in the nurse's native country.

Push and Pull Factors

A variety of factors influence mobility trends between countries; these can be divided into push factors and pull factors. **Push factors** are those that make it difficult to receive education or practice in a native country; **pull factors** are those that make migration to another country attractive for education or practice. The main push factors stimulating workers to cross national borders include relatively low pay and poor employment conditions in source countries, with an additional pull factor of active recruitment by some industrialized countries (Buchan et al., 2003). Box 7-4 identifies push and pull factors affecting the migration of nurses.

BOX 7-4 MAIN PUSH AND PULL FACTORS IN INTERNATIONAL NURSING MOBILITY

PUSH FACTORS	PULL FACTORS
• Low pay (absolute and/or relative)	• Higher pay (and opportunities for remittances)
• Poor working conditions	• Better working conditions
• Lack of resources to work effectively	• Better resourced health systems
• Limited career opportunities	• Career opportunities
• Limited educational opportunities	• Provision of postbasic education
• Impact of HIV/AIDS	• Political stability
• Unstable/dangerous work environment	• Travel opportunities
• Economic instability	• Assist in aid work

From: Buchan, J., Parkin, T., & Sochalski, J. (2003). *International nurse mobility: Trends and policy implications.* Geneva: World Health Organization.

Economic Factors

Economic push factors associated with migration include high general unemployment rate in the country; unstable economic conditions; poor pay; overproduction of nurses for positions available; lack of competitive incentives in the public sector; work pressures such as long work hours, poor resources, and a high ratio of patients per nurse; and lack of opportunities for career development (Lorenzo, 2002 [as cited in Buchan et al., 2003]; Pan American Health Organization [PAHO], 2001; Xaba & Philips, 2001 [as cited in Buchan et al., 2003]). Pull factors include high nurse vacancy rates in many industrial countries, national wage and benefit policies and enforcement, and higher salaries.

Social Factors

Social push factors include undervaluing of nursing by family, low status of nursing in the country, a preference for urban and city life, escalating crime rates in the country, and the impact of HIV/AIDS (Lorenzo, 2002 [as cited in Buchan et al., 2003]; PAHO, 2001; Xaba & Philips, 2001 [as cited in Buchan et al., 2003]). Pull factors include increased status of nursing in industrial countries, stable social structures that provide for increased safety, and community quality of life.

Healthcare System Factors

Lorenzo (as cited in Buchan et al., 2003) believes the structure, design, and management of healthcare systems within countries influence nursing education availability, workforce supply, and the scope of practice. Financial resources devoted to the healthcare sector influence the size and capacity of the nursing workforce. Healthcare system factors, including political push factors affecting nurse migration, include nonenforcement of existing laws that control and monitor nursing supply and demand, the absence of comprehensive human resource planning in health, and inadequate networking and collaboration among institutions and agencies responsible for production and utilization of nursing human resources. Pull factors include active, targeted, international recruitment drives by destination countries because nurses are knowledge workers with a skill set in strong demand (Buchan et al., 2003).

Professional Practice Factors

Control over professional practice is a fundamental aspect of nursing. Professional push factors influencing migration include lack of emphasis on independent nursing practice, perceived weakness of nursing leadership to advocate for nurses, inability to influence policy-making bodies, inadequate networking and collaboration between nurses involved in production, inadequate utilization of nurses, failure to shift from traditional roles to innovative and entrepreneurial roles (Lorenzo, 2002 [as cited in Buchan et al., 2003]), lack of involvement in decision making, limited opportunities for professional development, lack of support for supervisors, lack of job tenure (PAHO, 2001), and few opportunities for career development (Xaba & Philips, 2001 [as cited in Buchan et al., 2003]). Pull factors include professional governance structures within regulatory and voluntary nursing organizations in industrial countries, and adoption of professional practice models that engage nurses in decision making.

Policy Interventions to Address the Nursing Workforce Distribution

Policy interventions can be used to proactively manage the supply, distribution, development, and mobility of nurses both in-country and through global migration. International recruitment of nurses is a symptom of global shortages of nurses, but the underlying problems can only be solved by local-level and country-level improvement in the status of nursing and in the planning and management of the nursing workforce.

The Human Resources for Health conceptual framework shown in Figure 7-8 was developed by the WHO to assist in managing human resources. It can be useful in visualizing the complex set of factors involved in developing policy approaches to managing the nursing workforce at any geographic level. In this framework, the healthcare system must be understood within a country's cultural, sociodemographic, economic, and geographic orientation. These broader issues can have a powerful impact on the design of a national healthcare system. Both health and nonhealth policies shape the specific structures of healthcare delivery. The healthcare system is further shaped by financial resources designated for health care, stakeholders who develop rules and regulations, and power issues within the healthcare market. The demand for labor and how the range of providers are educated and employed are aspects of

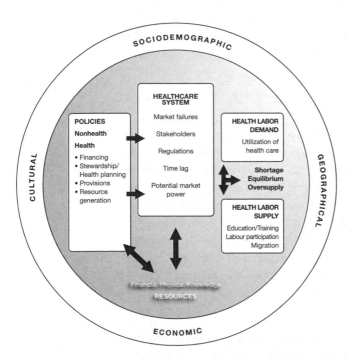

Figure 7-8 Human Resources for Health Conceptual Framework. Buchan & Calman (2004). *The Global Shortage of Registered Nurses: An Overview of Issues and Action.* Retrieved on July 26, 2007 from http://www.icn.ch/global/shortage.pdf

the labor supply. Understanding that nurse migration occurs within the features of the healthcare system and national environment can assist in appreciating the complexity of managing migration from both the source and destination country perspectives.

Workforce Planning

The WHO (2007) has created a strategy for addressing the workforce planning needs that uses a "working lifespan" approach. It did so by focusing on strategies related to the stage when people enter the workforce, the period of their lives when they are part of the workforce, and the point at which they make their exit from it. This road map of training, sustaining, and retaining the workforce offers a worker perspective as well as a systems approach to strategy (Figure 7-9). The entry period focuses on preparing the workforce through strategic investments in education and effective and ethical recruitment practices. The workforce period focuses on enhancing worker performance through better management of workers in both the public and private sectors. The final exit period addresses migration and

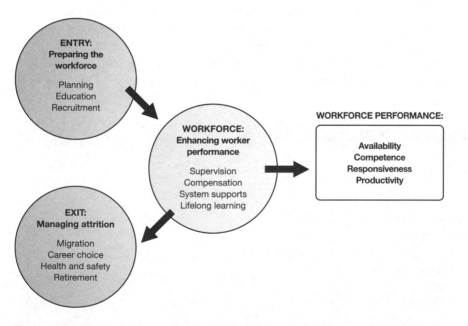

Figure 7-9 Working Lifespan Strategies for Performance Management. *Source:* World Health Organization. (2006). *The World Health Report 2006 – Working Together for Health.* Retrieved on July 31, 2007 from http://www.who.int/whr/2006/en/

attrition to reduce wasteful loss of human resources. This comprehensive model can be useful at multiple levels of technological and policy support.

Recruitment

International recruitment has increasingly become a "solution" to the nursing skill shortage in some countries. This has included large-scale active recruitment of nurses, doctors, and other professionals in addition to the natural migration flow of individuals moving across borders for a range of personal reasons (Buchan et al., 2003). Examples of recent initiatives to facilitate international recruitment of nurses include regional coordination of international recruitment for National Health Service in England, national coordination of clinical placements for overseas nurses in Ireland, provision of language skills training in Norway, and in the United States the relaxation of immigration requirements and opportunity to take the U.S. licensing examination in the nurse's home country (Buchan et al., 2003).

The ethical issues involved in recruiting nurses from developing countries are serious and of considerable concern to the nursing profession and the public. These issues include recruiting nurses needed to meet the critical healthcare needs of developing countries, recruiting nurses who were educated at the expense of the national government, and creating a national brain drain of professional workers.

Key principles on the ethical recruitment of nurses have been identified by several major nursing organizations. Two reports highlight these principles: the ICN position statement, *Ethical Nurse Recruitment* (2001), and the *Commonwealth*

BOX 7-5 ETHICAL NURSE RECRUITMENT

Key principles of the International Council of Nurses position statement:
- Transparency
- Fairness
- Mutuality of benefits for the countries involved
- Credible nursing regulation
- Effective human resources planning and development
- Access to full employment
- Good faith contracting
- Equal pay for work of equal value
- Access to grievance procedures
- Safe work environment
- Effective orientation/mentoring/supervision
- Freedom of movement

Source: International Council of Nurses. (2001). *Ethical recruitment of nurses position statement.* Geneva: Author.

Code of Practice for International Recruitment of Health Workers (Commonwealth Health Ministers, 2003). Key principles for ethical nurse recruitment included in the ICN position statement are shown in Box 7-5.

In 2005 the International Council of Nurses invited 50 global representatives to come together to discuss initiatives that could be implemented to address the world-wide shortage in the nursing workforce and the imbalances that exist in developing countries. The participants included government representatives, policy analysts, and professional nursing organization representatives, among others. Box 7-6 describes the global and individual country priorities and actions that were developed as an outcome of this meeting. Examples of identified priorities included focusing attention on ethical recruitment, infrastructure development, and human resource planning and management.

BOX 7-6   HIGH-LEVEL CONSULTATION ON THE GLOBAL NURSING WORKFORCE

Some fifty representatives of governments, employers, donors, trade unions, policy analysts, planners, researchers, and professional nursing organizations from all regions of the world met in Geneva, Switzerland, March 14–16, 2005, at the invitation of the International Council of Nurses to identify priorities and actions to deal with the critical imbalance and shortage in the nursing workforce worldwide.

Participants called on global and national partners to take immediate action along the following lines:

Action at the global level
- Increase resources to support the development of comprehensive human resource strategies.
- Explore using global health funds to strengthen human resource delivery infrastructures, including education.
- Form strategic alliances between governments, donors, agencies, educators, regulators, unions, and associations.
- Build capacity in the area of human resource planning and management.
- Build national self-sufficiency to manage domestic issues of supply and demand.
- Support an international code for ethical recruitment, effective monitoring of international flows, regulation and independent monitoring of international recruitment agencies, and respect for international labor instruments.
- Improve access to high-quality technical assistance.

Action at the country level
- Consider the range of nursing personnel required to meet national health needs.
- Embrace new models of care, with an emphasis on primary care, and new technologies.
- Address issues of skill mix and the delegation/devolution of some tasks to other workers.
- Improve workloads and working conditions.

Source: Florence Nightingale International Foundation. (n.d.). *The global nursing review initiative: Policy options and solutions.* Retrieved July 31, 2007, from http://www.fnif.org/global.htm.

Deployment and Performance

The Joint Learning Initiative, a global workforce consortium of more than 100 health leaders, believes that mobilization and strengthening of human resources for health, a neglected yet critical issue, is central to combating health crises in some of the world's poorest countries and for building sustainable health systems in all countries (Global Equity Initiative, 2004). The WHO (2007) proposes that effective strategies to boost nurses' and other healthcare workers' performance are critical for four reasons:

1. Strategies designed to increase performance will be likely to show results sooner than strategies to increase numbers.
2. The possibilities of increasing the supply of healthcare workers will always be limited.
3. A motivated and productive workforce will encourage recruitment and retention.
4. Governments have an obligation to society to ensure that limited human and financial resources are used as fairly and as efficiently as possible.

Health workforce performance is critical because it has an immediate impact on health service delivery and ultimately on population health. The WHO (2007) has identified four dimensions of workforce performance that are considered to be foundational across disciplines, countries, and systems of organizing and financing care. Table 7-3 shows the dimensions with a brief description and possible performance indicators useful in assessing progress in improving workforce productivity and quality of care of the framework. This simple yet comprehensive framework can be used to accommodate varying levels of complexity as needed within a healthcare system.

Although research about what makes nurses perform differently is progressing, globally three factors can be identified that influence their work. The WHO (2007) recognized the following three broad groups of factors that influence all workers and can be applied to nurses. First are the characteristics of the population being served. It is simpler to increase immunization coverage or adherence to treatment for tuberculosis or HIV infection where the population understands the benefits and has the motivation and resources to seek services. Second, characteristics of healthcare workers themselves are influential in performance. This includes the nurses' own sociocultural background, knowledge, experience, and motivation. Last are the characteristics of the healthcare system and the wider environment that determine the conditions under which nurses work. These include the inputs available to nurses to do their jobs; how the healthcare system is organized; how the workers are paid, supervised, and managed; and factors such as their personal safety. Multiple strategies have been identified that can be important levers in improving the performance of nurses (see Figure 7-10). These strategies are based

TABLE 7-3   DIMENSIONS OF HEALTH WORKFORCE PERFORMANCE AND PERFORMANCE INDICATORS

Dimension	Description	Possible Indicators
Availability	Availability in terms of space and time: encompasses distribution and attendance of existing workers	• Staff ratios • Absence rates • Waiting time
Competence	Encompasses the combination of technical knowledge, skills, and behaviors	• Individual: prescribing practices • Institutional: readmission rates; live births; cross-infections
Responsiveness	People are treated decently, regardless of whether or not their health improves or who they are	• Patient satisfaction; assessment of responsiveness
Productivity	Producing the maximum effective health services and health outcomes possible given the existing stock of health workers, reducing waste of staff time or skills	• Occupied beds; outpatient visits; interventions delivered per worker or facility

World Health Organization. (2007). World Health Report 2006—working together for health. Retrieved from http://www.who.int/whr/2006/en/index.html on July 31, 2007.

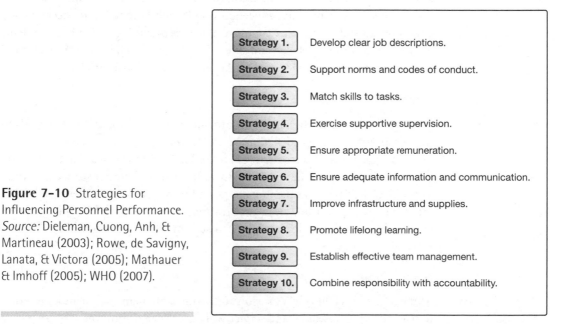

Figure 7-10 Strategies for Influencing Personnel Performance. *Source:* Dieleman, Cuong, Anh, & Martineau (2003); Rowe, de Savigny, Lanata, & Victora (2005); Mathauer & Imhoff (2005); WHO (2007).

Strategy 1.   Develop clear job descriptions.

Strategy 2.   Support norms and codes of conduct.

Strategy 3.   Match skills to tasks.

Strategy 4.   Exercise supportive supervision.

Strategy 5.   Ensure appropriate remuneration.

Strategy 6.   Ensure adequate information and communication.

Strategy 7.   Improve infrastructure and supplies.

Strategy 8.   Promote lifelong learning.

Strategy 9.   Establish effective team management.

Strategy 10.   Combine responsibility with accountability.

on experience and research on low- and middle-income countries (Dieleman, Cuong, Anh, & Martineau, 2003; Mathauer & Imhoffm, 2005; Rowe, de Savigny, Lanata, & Victora, 2005).

The WHO established the Global Health Workforce Alliance in 2007 to address healthcare worker shortages. The charge to the Alliance is to reinvigorate efforts to invest in healthcare worker education and training. The initial work includes studying the scope of financial and technical supports needed to address the substantial healthcare worker gap, the links between training institutions and universities in developed and developing nations, and the use of technology to promote distance learning, among other topics. According to the WHO, finding ways to rapidly and effectively scale up healthcare worker education demands urgent attention, innovative solutions, new funding, and political will (American Public Health Association, 2007).

Nursing Education and the Global Nursing Workforce

Educational institutions around the world have an opportunity to contribute to preparing a global nursing workforce through a variety of mechanisms. Foundational to this is valuing the preparation of nurses to work across borders both temporarily and permanently, as well as valuing the preparation of nurses knowledgeable in providing nursing care in their native country but who are now working as nurses outside their native country. Nursing educational institutions have the opportunity and responsibility in the current global context to thoughtfully integrate international dimensions in all areas of the curriculum and educational experience. This includes becoming culturally competent in receiving and educating students from other countries as well as preparing native-born students with global health knowledge and skills. The outcome will be a faculty, alumni, and organization prepared to provide health care in a global society.

Institutional Support

To ensure broad institutional support, the university mission statement needs to include an international education, research, and service statement. This serves to focus educational and research resources. The availability of a university international office to provide resources to support international students is vital. This office often serves as the initial contact for international students regarding recruitment, application, visas, registration, and housing. The office can also be instrumental in developing financial support through various internal and external mechanisms.

School Support

At the school level, having a mission and vision statement that includes international education, research, and service will emphasize commitment to preparing a global nursing workforce. Nursing schools will also find it important to have an international unit that is charged with facilitating the educational experiences of international students and visiting scholars. This unit may also serve to develop, recruit, fund, and sponsor student study abroad, service learning, and exchange programs.

Development of a globally focused faculty can be supported through travel grants, institutional partnership development, formal and informal preparation in another country's culture and healthcare system, binational or multinational research collaboratives, and appointment, promotion, and tenure systems that reward international work. An orientation for international work, on how to adapt teaching–learning strategies for international students, and on how to prepare nursing students for international experiences and supervise them in the field will assist in preparing faculty.

Internationalizing the Curriculum

Research indicates international students in general need to receive knowledge and technical skills relevant to the needs in their countries of origin (Ogilvie, Paul, & Burgess-Pinto, 2007). In addition, curriculum placed within a context of global and country trends in epidemiology, healthcare systems, and society can increase the global health knowledge of all students, both foreign-born and native-born. Exposure to and involvement in international partnerships for faculty and student research, teaching, and service can also internationalize the curriculum. Developing local partnerships with international residents and organizations locally to provide learning experiences encourages the nursing school to actively partner with the community with the intent of preparing graduates for promoting the health of a culturally diverse population.

Technology is increasingly being used for binational and multinational education offerings. Computer-mediated conferencing commonly is used to promote collaborative learning, including student learning across distance. McKenna and Samarawickrema (2003) used computer-mediated conferencing with graduate students in three countries to enhance student learning. Kahn et al. (2007) used "real-time" videoconferencing in preparing medical, dental, and nursing students from Mexico and the United States for an international collaborative service-learning experience. It was used to introduce culturally important aspects of the students' lives to each other through sharing of photos by the students.

Creating an Internationally Valuing Environment

International students are well served through a strong mentoring program. In a study of international doctoral students conducted by Ryan, Markowski, Ura, and Liu-Chiang (1998), key factors important to a successful education experience included identifying community resources to meet basic needs for adaptation to a foreign country; redesigning teaching and learning strategies for international students; preparing faculty, clinical agency staff, patients, and other students to accept and become actively involved with the international students; and developing faculty–student relationships that promote mentoring and foster professional role development. A survey of U.S. doctoral schools found the challenges to educating international students to include language, communication, financing, and support systems (Carty, O'Grady, Wichaikhum, & Bull, 2002). Academic issues that need to be addressed for international students include language abilities, writing skills and referencing, different cognitive and learning styles, and academic performance and success (Ogilvie et al., 2007).

Increasing opportunities for faculty and students to engage in international experiences within the nursing curriculum increases their preparation as global citizens. Infusing the educational environment with experiences of global significance in the local community, bringing visiting scholars to class, and developing enrichment opportunities like lunchtime talks, cultural hours, and showing videotapes depicting international cultures are all ways to internationalize the curriculum.

International Nursing Organizations

International nursing education is of importance to multiple stakeholders around the globe. Weblinks to organizations related to global nursing workforce can be found in Box 7-7. In an effort to address common educational preparation issues, facilitate the supply of nurses and nurse educators, and influence important policy issues, international nursing organizations have established organizations or task forces. The WHO has collaborating centers around the globe whose purpose is to provide equitable access to an adequately educated, skilled, and supported nursing and midwifery workforce to meet health needs. Box 7-8 provides a brief overview of the mission and mandate of these collaborating centers.

The Global Alliance on Nursing Education and Scholarship (GANES) was established in 2005 to improve patient care through nursing education and ensure a robust global supply of highly educated nurses. GANES is committed to enhancing the educational preparation of registered nurses, expanding opportunities for nursing education, and addressing student enrollment concerns, including the growing shortage of nurse faculty. GANES members include the American Association of Colleges of Nursing (AACN), the Canadian Association of Schools of Nursing (CASN), the Council of Deans and Heads of United Kingdom University Faculties and Health Professions (CoD), and the Council of Deans of Nursing and Midwifery (Australia and New Zealand) (CDNM).

BOX 7-7   GLOBAL NURSING WORKFORCE WEBLINKS

Global Alliance on Nursing Education and Scholarship (GANES):
   http://www.aacn.nche.edu/Education/GANES.htm

National League of Nursing:
   http://www.nln.org/getinvolved/AdvisoryCouncils_TaskGroups/global.htm

Commonwealth Health Ministers. (2003). Commonwealth Code of Practice for International Recruitment of Health Workers:
   http://www.thecommonwealth.org/shared_asp_files/uploadedfiles/{7BDD970B-53AE-441D-81DB-1B64C37E992A}_CommonwealthCodeofPractice.pdf

The Global Nursing Review Initiative: Policy Options and Solutions of the Global Nursing Workforce Project:
   http://www.icn.ch/global/

Florence Nightingale International Foundation:
   http://www.fnif.org

International Council of Nursing:
   http://www.icn.ch/abouticn.htm

Burdett Trust for Nursing:
   http://www.burdettnursingtrust.org.uk

International Centre on Nursing Migration:
   http://www.intlnursemigration.org

Organisation for Economic Co-operation and Development:
   http://www.oecd.org/document/54/0,2340,en_2649_37407_1935094_1_1_1_37407,00.html

Global Health Trust:
   http://www.globalhealthtrust.org/Publication.htm

World Bank:
   http://www.worldbank.org

World Health Organization, Health Services Provision:
   http://www.who.int/en/

Nursing and Midwifery, World Health Organization:
   http://www.who.int/hrh/nursing_midwifery/en/

BOX 7-8 WHO COLLABORATING CENTERS IN NURSING AND MIDWIVERY

MISSION

To provide equitable access to an adequately educated, skilled, and supported nursing and midwifery workforce to meet health needs.

MANDATE

Nursing and midwifery are recognized by the Member States as an important component of health development that requires strengthening in order to contribute effectively to improving population health outcomes. Supported by several World Health Assembly resolutions—WHA42.27, WHA45.5, WHA47.9, WHA48.8, and, most recently, WHA54.12 on strengthening of nursing and midwifery services—WHO is responding to country efforts in a variety of ways, including:

- providing policy and technical advice;
- facilitating capacity-building and collaborative partnerships;
- supporting the enhancement of evidence generation for decision-making.

The aim of any healthcare system is effective delivery of health services. Nurses and midwives globally form the largest category of health workers and provide up to 80% of direct patient care. In many developing countries, they are front-line health workers who play a central role in health services delivery. An efficient nursing and midwifery workforce is therefore a priority for any health program.

Source: WHO Web site.

In 2004 the National League of Nursing (NLN) and the National League for Nursing Accrediting Commission (NLNAC) established the Joint NLN/NLNAC Task Force on Creating a Global Nursing Education Community. The purpose of this task force is to address issues related to the development and advancement of global nursing education and faculty. NLN hosts a facilitated electronic discussion with nurse educators in and outside the United States about significant issues in nursing education.

The Honor Society of Nursing, Sigma Theta Tau International (STTI) has as its mission the goal of enhancing global health. Membership in STTI is invitational and is based upon academic and leadership achievements. In its continuing mission to improve nursing care worldwide through scholarship and practice, STTI establishes alliances with international healthcare organizations, supports global nursing initiatives, collaborates with nurses worldwide, and connects with members on an international level.

The International Council of Nurses is a federation of national nurses associations (NNAs) representing nurses in more than 128 countries. Founded in 1899, ICN is the world's first and widest-reaching international organization for healthcare professionals. Operated by nurses for nurses, ICN works to ensure quality nursing care for all, sound health policies globally, the advancement of nursing knowledge, and the presence worldwide of a respected nursing profession and a competent and satisfied nursing workforce. The goals of the ICN are "to bring nursing together worldwide, to advance nurses and nursing worldwide, and to influence health policy" (ICN, n.d.).

Summary

The global nursing workforce is well positioned to make a significant contribution to the health and well-being of the global population. The MDGs focus on problems that are amenable to nursing intervention. In order to achieve the full potential of their contributions to global population health, the nursing workforce must be effectively managed at the country, state, and local levels. The factors pushing nurses to leave nursing practice within their home countries must be improved through more effective workforce planning and development, education of an appropriately prepared workforce, deployment of existing nursing and other healthcare workers, and effective retention practices. Although nurses leave their native countries for a wide variety of reasons, employers seeking to recruit nurses internationally must be held accountable for ethical recruitment practices so that both source and destination countries are able to benefit.

Nursing education programs are preparing both foreign-born and native-born students to function in a global health environment. Skillful mentoring of international students is critical to a successful education experience. In addition, internationalizing the curriculum at home allows native-born students to knowledgably care for culturally diverse populations both locally and globally.

Key Terms

- **Geographic maldistribution:** The tendency for nurses to practice in affluent urban and suburban areas rather than in rural and inner-city areas.
- **Global burden of disease:** A term developed by the World Health Organization and World Bank to measure the total loss of health resulting from diseases and injuries.
- **Globalization:** Increased interconnections among people of different countries that facilitate the exchange of goods, services, money, people, information, and ideas across national borders.
- **International migrants:** Individuals who reside in countries other than those of their birth for more than one year.
- **Millennium Development Goals:** Eight goals set by the United Nations for the year 2015 for improving the health and well-being of the global population.
- **Pull factors:** Those factors that make migration to another country more attractive for education or practice than staying in the nurse's native country.
- **Push factors:** Those factors that make it difficult to receive a basic or advanced education in nursing or to practice in the nurse's native country.

Reflective Practice Questions

1. Should nurses from countries with an existing shortage of nurses be discouraged from migrating to practice nursing in another country?
2. How well have your educational experiences prepared you to practice nursing in a global society? What actions can you undertake to further increase your knowledge of global nursing workforce issues?
3. How do you envision the Millennial Development Goals established by the United Nations (2006) impacting your nursing practice?

References

American Public Health Association. (2007). *WHO establishes global task force to address health worker shortage.* Washington, DC: The Nation's Health.

An Bord Altranais. (2007). *Registration statistics.* Retrieved July 23, 2007, from http://www.nursingboard.ie/en/statistics_article.aspx?article=d863df67-a4af-4b34-a211-b00a38cb95ab#EACAAA

Australian Nursing Council. (2007). *Information for registered nurses regarding visas and immigration to Australia.* Retrieved July 23, 2007, from http://www.australianaustralia.com/page/Nurses_ANC/257

Baptiste-Meyer, J. (2001, July–August). The brain drain: New aspects of the south/north exodus. *The Courier ACP-EU.*

Buchan, J. (2000). Planning for change: Developing a policy framework for nursing labour markets. *International Nursing Review, 47*(4), 199–206.

Buchan, J. (2002). Global nursing shortages. *British Medical Journal, 324,* 751–752.

Buchan J., & Calman, L. (2004). *The global shortage of registered nurses: An overview of issues and action.* Geneva: International Council of Nurses.

Buchan, J., Parkin, T., & Sochalski, J. (2003). *International nurse mobility: Trends and policy implications.* Geneva: World Health Organization.

Carty, R., O'Grady, E. T., Wichaikhum, O., & Bull, J. (2002). Opportunities in preparing global leaders in nursing. *Journal of Professional Nursing, 19*(2), 70–77.

Castels, M. (2000). International migration at the beginning of the twenty-first century: Global trends and issues. *International Migration, 165,* 269–283.

Chanda, R. (2002). Trade in health services. *Bulletin of the World Health Organization, 80,* 158–163.

Commission on Graduates of Foreign Nursing Schools (CGFNS International). (n.d.). *Certification program statistical data.* Retrieved July 24, 2007, from http://www.cgfns.org/sections/about/

Commonwealth Health Ministers. (2003). *Commonwealth code of practice for the international recruitment of health workers.* Retrieved July 24, 2007, from http://www.thecommonwealth.org/shared_asp_files/uploadedfiles/{7BDD970B-53AE-441D-81DB-1B64C37E992A}_CommonwealthCodeofPractice.pdf

Dieleman, M., Cuong, P. V., Anh, L. V., & Martineau, T. (2003). Identifying factors for job motivation of rural health workers in North Viet Nam. *Human Resources for Health, 1,* 10.

Florence Nightingale International Foundation. (n.d.). *The global nursing review initiative: Policy options and solutions.* Retrieved July 31, 2007, from http://www.fnif.org/global.htm

Global Equity Initiative. (2004). Human resources for health: Overcoming the crisis. *Lancet, 364,* 1984–1990.

Guellec, D., & Cervantes, M. (2002). International mobility of highly skilled workers: From statistical analysis to policy formation. In OECD Proceedings (Ed.), *International mobility of the highly skilled* (pp. 71–99). Paris: Organization for Economic Co-operation and Development.

High Level Forum, World Health Organization. (2004). *High level forum on the health MDGs. Summary of discussions and agreed action plan.* Geneva: World Health Organization.

International Council of Nurses. (n.d.). About ICN. Retrieved May 28, 2008, from http://www.icn.ch/abouticn.htm

International Council of Nurses. (n.d.). *ICN definition of nursing.* Retrieved April 6, 2007, from http://www.icn.ch/definition.htm

International Council of Nurses. (2001). *Ethical recruitment of nurses position statement.* Geneva: Author.

International Council of Nurses. (2006). *The global nursing shortage: Priority areas for intervention.* Geneva: Author.

Kahn, H., Stelzner, S. M., Riner, M. E., Soto-Rojas, A. E., Henkle, J., Veras-Godoy, H. A., et al. (in press). Use of online technologies in an international, multidisciplinary, service-learning experience. *Service-eLearning: Educating for citizenship in a technology-rich world.* Jossey-Bass.

Kirk, H. (2007). Towards a global nursing workforce: The "brain circulation." *Nursing Management, 13*(10), 26–30.

Martineau, T., Decker D., & Bundred, P. (2002). *Briefing note on international migration of health professionals: Leveling the playing field for developing country health systems.* Liverpool, England: Liverpool School of Tropical Medicine.

Mathauer, I., & Imhoff, I. (2006). Health worker motivation in Africa: The role of non-financial incentives and human resource management tools. *Human Resources for Health, 4*, 24.

McKenna, L. G., & Samarawickrema, G. (2003). Crossing cultural boundaries: Flexible approaches and nurse education: A case study. *Computers, Informatics, Nursing, 21*(5), 259–264.

McMichael, T., & Beaglehole, R. (2003). The global context for public health. In R. Beaglehole (Ed.), *Global public health: A new era.* Oxford, England: Oxford University Press.

Nurses and Midwives Board of New South Wales. (1997). *Trans Tasman mutual recognition act 1997.* Retrieved July 31, 2007, from http://www.nmb.nsw.gov.au/Mutual-Recognition/default.aspx

Nursing and Midwifery Council. (n.d.). *Statistical analysis of the register 1 April 2005 to 31 March 2006.* Retrieved July 24, 2007, from http://www.nmc-uk.org/aFrameDisplay.aspx?DocumentID=2593

Ogilvie, L. D., Paul, P., & Burgess-Pinto, E. (2007). International dimensions of higher education in nursing in Canada: Tapping the wisdom of the 20th century while embracing possibilities for the 21st century. *International Journal of Nursing Education Scholarship, 4*(7), 1.

Organization for Economic Co-operation and Development. (2000). *Trends in international migration.* Paris: Author.

Organization for Economic Co-operation and Development. (2002a). *International migration of physician and nurses: Causes, consequences and health policy implications.* Paris: Author.

Organization for Economic Co-operation and Development. (2002b). *International mobility of the highly skilled.* Paris: Author.

Pan American Health Organization. (2001). *Report on technical meeting on managed migration of skilled nursing personnel.* Bridgetown, Barbados: Pan American Health Organization Caribbean Office.

Raisler, J., & Cohn, J. (2005). Mothers, midwives, and HIV/AIDS in sub-Saharan Africa. *Journal of Midwifery & Women's Health, 50*(4), 275–282.

Rowe, A. K., de Savigny, D., Lanata, C. F., & Victora, C. G. (2005). How can we achieve and maintain high-quality performance of health workers in low-resource settings? *Lancet, 366*, 1026–1035.

Ryan, D., Markowski, K., Ura, D., & Liu-Chiang, C. (1998). International nursing education: Challenges and strategies for success. *Journal of Professional Nursing, 14*(2), 69–77.

Stalker, P. (2000). *Workers without frontiers: The impact of globalization on international migration.* Boulder, CO: Lynne Rienner.

United Nations. (2006). *The millennium development goals report.* Retrieved April 13, 2007, from http://unstats.un.org/unsd/mdg/Resources/Static/Products/Progress2006/MDGReport2006.pdf

U.S. Department of Health and Human Services. (n.d.). *The registered nurse population: Findings from the 2004 National Sample Survey of Registered Nurses.* Retrieved July 23, 2007, from http://bhpr.hrsa.gov/healthworkforce/rnsurvey04/tables.htm

World Health Organization. (n.d. a). *European observatory on health systems and policies.* Retrieved April 6, 2007, from http://www.euro.who.int/observatory/Glossary/TopPage?phrase=N

World Health Organization. (n.d. b). *Global burden of disease.* Retrieved July 8, 2008, from http://www.who.int/trade/glossary/story036/en/

World Health Organization. (2004). *A guide to rapid assessment of human resources for health.* Retrieved July 31, 2007, from http://www.who.int/hrh/tools/en/Rapid_Assessment_guide.pdf

World Health Organization. (2007). *World health report 2006—Working together for health.* Retrieved July 8, 2008, from http://www.who.int/whr/2006/overview/en/index.html

World Health Organization & Sigma Theta Tau International. (2006). *Developing global standards for initial nursing and midwifery education: Interim report of the proceedings.* Retrieved July 31, 2007, from http://www.nursingsociety.org/about/WHO_interim_report.pdf

The Culture of Safety

Patricia Ebright

LEARNING OUTCOMES

After reading this chapter you will be able to:

- Describe the historical evolution of the current focus and approach toward patient safety in health care.
- Describe components of a framework for understanding work in complex environments.
- Explain the relationship among human factors, work complexity, and the evolution of adverse events in health care.
- Identify critical components of an effective culture of safety and the challenges in moving toward an improved culture of safety in health care.
- Apply research findings on nursing work complexity to designing safer practice environments.
- Describe the new accountabilities in the approach to patient safety for healthcare leaders, educators, and practitioners.

History of the Patient Safety Movement

The nursing profession has a rich history of developing standards, education, and approaches to nursing care that reflect an emphasis on

patient safety and quality. Therefore, it cannot be said that before the release of the Institute of Medicine report (IOM, 2000) on **medical error** and patient safety, nurses were not aware of incidents where patients may have been injured or killed by **mistakes** in the application or omission of medical interventions. Starting in the early 1980s, however, a series of events leading up to the IOM report drew attention to the injury and deaths resulting from medical error. Beginning with the establishment of the Anesthesia Patient Safety Foundation in 1984 for improvement of perioperative patient safety (Silker, 2006), several activities preceded the current focus and extraordinary shift in approach to patient safety in health care. These activities included reports of findings from physician studies on the large numbers of preventable disabling injuries and deaths identified from medical records in the 1990s (e.g., Leape, 1994); regulatory and legislative activities led by The Joint Commission (TJC, 2001) requiring hospital compliance with monitoring, investigation, and reporting of errors; and the creation of national organizations focused on patient safety (e.g., the National Patient Safety Foundation in 1998 and the National Quality Forum in 1999).

It was the magnitude of the problem of medical errors that was not appreciated by most healthcare providers until the IOM report was released in 2000. According to this report, tens of thousands of Americans die each year from errors in medical care and hundreds of thousands are injured, or almost injured, during their care. The IOM report served as a wake-up call that more needed to be done to prevent harm to patients and to improve quality of care. Some leaders in the healthcare industry realized that traditional approaches to safety and quality would no longer be sufficient to respond to the improvements necessary based on the outcomes reported in the IOM report. For example, in *Crossing the Quality Chasm: A New Health System for the 21st Century* (IOM, 2001), the authors called for fundamental change in the healthcare system focused on six goals for improvement. These six goals can be found in Box 8-1.

Influenced and led by recommendations from subsequent IOM committee reports that were focused specifically on safety (IOM, 2004, 2006), healthcare leaders searched for solutions from industries other than health care. This search resulted in the adoption of strategies used by other industries such as the airline, aerospace, and nuclear industries to prevent high-stakes failures and reduce the harm resulting from error. Learning from expert resources outside health care, a major change in thinking occurred as to why healthcare errors happen, the role of the individual in error generation, and the roles that healthcare providers and leaders play in increasing and sustaining patient safety.

BOX 8-1   IOM GOALS FOR HEALTH CARE

Health care should be:
- *Safe:* Patients should not be harmed by care that is intended to help them.
- *Effective:* Care should be based on scientific knowledge and offered to all who could benefit, and not to those not likely to benefit.
- *Patient-centered:* Care should be respectful of and responsive to individual patient preferences, needs, and values.
- *Timely:* Waits, and sometimes harmful delays in care, should be reduced for both those who receive care and those who give care.
- *Efficient:* Care should be given without wasting equipment, supplies, ideas, and energy.
- *Equitable:* Care should not vary in quality because of personal characteristics such as gender, ethnicity, geographic location, and socioeconomic status.

Source: Institute of Medicine. (2006). *Crossing the quality chasm: A new health system for the 21st century.* Washington, DC: National Academies Press.

Healthcare leaders learned that to make sustainable improvements in patient safety, their focus had to switch from individual healthcare providers and workers to the **complex systems** in which they work, and to the complexity as well as limitations within the individuals themselves. The new focus for understanding error turned from the traditional approach to patient safety that demanded perfect individual performance in imperfect situations, to understanding the imperfect situations in which imperfect performers work. This shift in focus from the individual to the multiple complex systems and processes throughout an organization has been a formidable challenge that healthcare leaders, including nurses, have been addressing since 2000.

Although numerous regulatory and legislative efforts have been established to move the healthcare industry forward with respect to safety and quality, changing an industry **safety culture** from one that has been characterized as a "blame" culture to a "non-blame" culture has been much more difficult than originally anticipated. How we respond to errors and to those involved, what we expect from those involved, what we do to learn from errors, and even how we plan and design to prevent or limit future errors reflects the degree to which we have shifted our emphasis from individuals to systems for making

KEY TERM

Complex systems: Systems in which work includes both cognitive and physical demands and is characterized by dynamism, large numbers of parts and connectedness between parts, high uncertainty, and risk (Woods, 1988).

KEY TERM

Safety culture: Shared values and beliefs in an organization that interact with the organizational structures and systems and produce behavioral norms surrounding work (Reason, 1997).

KEY TERM

Reporting system: A safety information system that collects, analyzes, and disseminates information about near misses, adverse events, and safety systems (Reason, 1997).

improvements in safety. Healthcare organizations vary widely in their growth toward the recommendations set forth by the IOM reports. Recent legislative and regulatory efforts have begun to move the safety and quality work forward.

Regulatory and Legislative Focus on Patient Safety

Legislative action and changes in the focus of accrediting bodies since 2000 reflect the important impact of the IOM reports. In response to the IOM reports, at least 22 states initiated medical error **reporting systems** in an effort to improve patient safety by 2005. And in July 2005, Congress overwhelmingly voted to pass the Patient Safety and Quality Improvement Act. This legislation was designed to encourage states to participate in a national medical error database, and protects the confidentiality of individuals who report errors and the organizations involved in the errors. Starting with Minnesota in 2003 (Minnesota Department of Health, 2007), individual states have continued to enact legislation to require healthcare organizational reporting of serious errors and public disclosure. Contemporary Practice Highlight 8-1 identifies other organizations and agencies that have initiated changes in criteria, standards, and funding priorities in response to the increased emphasis on improving patient safety.

The remainder of this chapter will describe the new approach to patient safety that health care is taking to make improvements based on learning from other industries, and the implications this new approach has for nursing practice. The cultural changes needed to move these new approaches forward are an important

---

CONTEMPORARY PRACTICE HIGHLIGHT 8-1

FOCUSING ON PATIENT SAFETY

The criteria for The Joint Commission now include annual updated lists of Patient Safety Goals (TJC, 2007) that healthcare organizations must achieve to receive a successful accreditation review. The Institute for Healthcare Improvement (IHI) has sponsored multiple clinically focused improvement initiatives to jumpstart realization of patient outcomes through specific quality and safety guidelines that have resulted in thousands of lives saved. The National Patient Safety Foundation (NPSF) and the Agency for Healthcare Research and Quality (AHRQ) fund research on patient safety and potential interventions for reaching patient safety outcomes. The following organizations also have responded to the 2000 IOM report with some type of call for new efforts to improve patient safety: Department of Health and Human Services (DHHS), Centers for Disease Control and Prevention (CDC), Center for Medicare and Medicaid Services (CMS), Leapfrog Group, and Healthgrades.

focus of the ongoing efforts because patient safety depends on changes in practice and accountabilities at all levels of healthcare organizations, including regulatory, legislative, and consumer groups.

The New Look of Patient Safety

Human factors science is focused on human performance, the interaction of humans in different situations, and its application to errors in healthcare environments and with technology. Healthcare and human factors researchers have developed an approach to patient safety based on work by Reason (1990), called New Look, to explain how things go wrong in healthcare situations (Cook, Woods, & Miller, 1998). One major hypothesis of New Look is that events are not the result of a single failure of an unreliable component (such as an individual), but rather the result of multiple failures in the intended defenses of a system. Proponents of **New Look** argue that progress toward improving patient safety can occur only when five principles that underlie productive work toward improving safety are appreciated by the providers in a healthcare system (see Box 8-2).

> **KEY TERM**
>
> **Human factors:** Sets of human-specific physical, mental, and behavioral properties, as well as the science of how people interact with tasks, machines (or computers), and the environment with the consideration that humans have properties that demonstrate limitations and capabilities. (Wikipedia, n.d.)

> **KEY TERM**
>
> **New Look:** An approach to patient safety based on understanding and adaptation of the evolution of failure, as described by James Reason (Cook, Woods, & Miller, 1998).

BOX 8-2   NEW LOOK PRINCIPLES FOR IMPROVING PATIENT SAFETY

1. Safety is made and broken in systems, not by individuals. Adverse events result from the way work is designed and the interaction of components of the system.
2. Progress on safety begins with understanding technical work. Our current understanding of real work is naïve and incomplete, leading to the development of performance rules that are impossible to apply in a complex, heterogeneous, and rapidly changing world. Progress in safety depends on understanding how technical and organizational factors play out in real work.
3. Productive discussions of safety avoid confounding failure with error. Failure results from a breakdown in systems, whereas error is usually assigned to humans and relates to a social process for attributing cause.
4. Safety is dynamic and not static; it is constantly renegotiated. Complex, ever-changing systems require that people change and adapt constantly. However, adaptation is often based on inadequate information and only partly successful. Understanding this dynamic is the foundation for understanding safety. Increasing complexity makes safety harder to achieve.
5. Trade-offs are at the core of safety. Complex work environments will always be characterized by uncertainty, discontinuities, and missing information. Understanding how people cope with these challenges will increase understanding of safety.

Source: Woods, D., & Cook, R. I. (1998). *Characteristics of patient safety: Five principles that underlie productive work.* Chicago: CtL.

Using Reason's Swiss Cheese Model to Explain Failure

According to the New Look, and as shown in Figure 8-1, **layers of defense** exist at all levels of an organization and provide boundaries around which decisions are developed and implemented. Typical healthcare organizational defenses include, but are not limited to, policies and procedures, standard care guidelines, chain of command processes for communication and decisions, budget and resource allocations, report and hand-off mechanisms, competency standards, and technology. **Latent conditions**, or **gaps**, are discontinuities in the layers

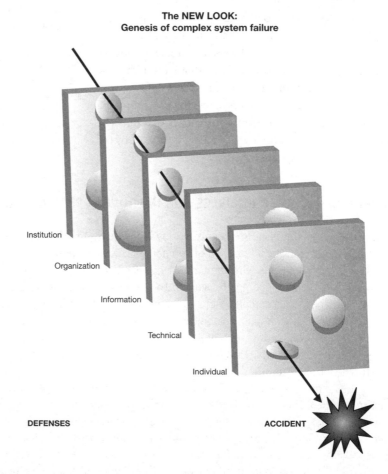

The NEW LOOK:
Genesis of complex system failure

Institution

Organization

Information

Technical

Individual

DEFENSES

ACCIDENT

Figure 8-1 Genesis of Complex System Failure. *Source:* © Reprinted with permission from Cook, R. (1997). The New Look: Genesis of complex system failure. Modified from Reason, 1991.

of defenses in the work environment. For example, a gap exists when a specific patient situation does not exactly fit a policy and procedure for medication administration (an institutional boundary related to rules), and following the policy or procedure would not be in the best interest of the patient. Another example of an existing gap is the lack of available personnel on a busy unit for one specific shift (an institutional boundary related to budget) that does not provide enough staff with the necessary competencies and experience required to provide care for the unit's acuity level and number of patients.

Neither of these situations represents an overt failure in itself, but each constitutes a type of gap or latent condition that threatens the continuity of care and, when combined with other gaps, may lead to a **near miss** (any process variation that did not affect the outcome but for which a recurrence carries a significant chance of a serious adverse outcome) or **adverse event** (untoward incidents, therapeutic misadventures, iatrogenic injuries, or other adverse occurrences directly associated with care or services provided within the jurisdiction of a medical center, outpatient clinic, or other facility; TJC, 2001). Adverse events may result from acts of commission or omission (e.g., administration of the wrong medication, failure to make a timely diagnosis or institute the appropriate therapeutic intervention, adverse reactions or negative outcomes of treatment, etc.). Some examples of more common adverse events include patient falls, medication errors, procedural errors/complications, completed suicides, parasuicidal behaviors (attempts/gestures/threats), and missing patient events.

Active failures are errors and violations due to acts performed by workers (e.g., nurses) closest to the sharp end of the system (e.g., patient care) that impact system safety most directly (Reason, 1997). What we have learned over the past 20 years in safety is that most active failures are consequences of latent conditions and not principle causes of accidents (Reason). For example, using a situation discussed above, inadequate staffing (system gap or latent condition) for a specific shift may result in a nurse who is responding to time pressures to by-pass checking all patient identifiers (active failure) before administering the wrong medication. The latent condition of inadequate staffing was a significant contributor to the error.

KEY TERM

Latent conditions: Error-producing factors like poor design, gaps in supervision, undetected system failures, lack of training, and the like arising from the decision-making levels (blunt end) of organizations that combine with active failures to result in adverse events (Reason, 1997).

KEY TERM

Gaps: Another term for latent conditions or error-producing factors (Cook, Woods, & Miller, 1998).

KEY TERM

Near-miss event: Any process variation that did not affect the outcome in a given event, but for which a recurrence carries a significant chance of a serious adverse outcome (TJC, 2001).

KEY TERM

Adverse events: Untoward incidents, therapeutic misadventures, iatrogenic injuries, or other adverse occurrences directly associated with care or services provided within the jurisdiction of a medical center, outpatient clinic, or other facility (The Joint Commission [TJC], 2001).

KEY TERM

Active failures: Errors and violations caused by acts performed by workers (e.g., nurses) closest to the sharp end of the system (e.g., patient care) that impact system safety most directly (Reason, 1997).

Trade-offs: Decision resolutions that involve conflicting choices between highly unlikely but highly undesirable events and highly likely but less catastrophic ones (Cook & Woods, 1994).

Sometimes system gaps (or latent conditions) have been around for a very long time and go unrecognized by the organization. They have become part of the "routine" work. As a result, implementation of new processes may unintentionally disrupt the effectiveness of existing bridges, as well as create new gaps in the system. For example, introduction of time-consuming processes surrounding one new technology that requires increased nurse monitoring and treatment of the patient, as well as maintenance of the technology, may cause disruptions in other aspects of patient care that lead to decision **trade-offs** (decision resolutions that involve conflicting choices between highly unlikely but highly undesirable events and highly likely but less catastrophic ones). Trade-offs are made by nurses and other healthcare providers "between interacting or conflicting goals, between values or costs placed on different possible outcomes or courses of action, and between the risks of different errors" (Cook & Woods, 1994, p. 279) and more serious adverse patient outcomes. Again, using the situation discussed above, the nurse who administered the wrong medication to a patient was dealing with time pressures that required decisions about multiple and competing work requirements. She trusted that the medication was the correct drug, dosage, route, time, and for that patient and didn't follow all checks because she had retrieved it from that patient's medication supply. She was then able to more rapidly respond to another nurse's request for help in another room. She "traded off" doing a complete check to be responsive to the need of another colleague and patient. Nurses and other direct care practitioners in current healthcare environments demonstrate resilience every day by anticipating and recognizing, and then coping with or bridging, multiple gaps. Examples are nurses who increase their "checking" of the care provided by the technician with whom they have not previously worked rather than rely on reported information, or nurses who develop their own sophisticated system of readily available handwritten notes to track medication and treatments every shift. Bridging gaps is not exclusive to nurses. Other examples of bridging gaps include physicians who always look for the "reliable, competent" nurse with whom they have worked before to discuss patient status rather than risk receiving unreliable information from nurses they do not know.

Leape and Berwick (2005) explained that health care lags behind other industries in safety because of its reliance on individual performance as the key to improvement. Other industries have reduced errors by understanding that people do make mistakes in changing environments and that the way to be safer is to design systems so that it is difficult to make a mistake and easy to recover from mistakes that do occur. And in fact, the New Look approach champions the individual as the resilient factor and solution for reaching safety in complex systems and as an essential participant in efforts that have the potential for making progress in patient safety.

Complexity of Work at Point of Care Delivery (the Sharp End)

KEY TERM

Sharp end: Frontline personnel at the operations point of the organization; for example, at the point of patient care in a healthcare organization (Reason, 1997).

A major barrier to making progress in safety and quality is the failure to appreciate the complexity of work (Woods, 1988). Researchers argue that understanding how people anticipate, detect, and bridge gaps in real work contexts is necessary for making improvements in patient safety (Cook, Render, & Woods, 2000). Healthcare workers actually create safety daily in the presence of multiple latent conditions or gaps and are the resilient factor for preventing accidents in complex systems.

As Figure 8-2 illustrates, nurses and other healthcare workers at the point of care delivery (the **sharp end** and lower point of the triangle in Figure 8-2) are involved in constantly evolving situations. Supported, and constrained, by

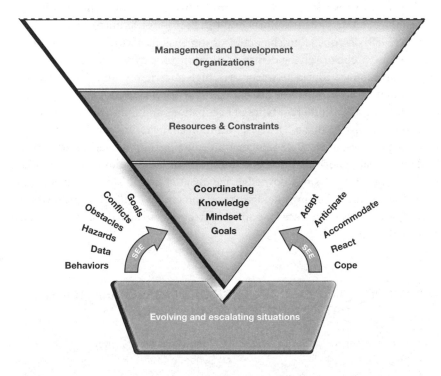

Figure 8-2 Work at the Sharp End Model. *Source:* © Reprinted with permission from Woods D. D., Johannesen L. J., Cook R. I., Sarter N. B. *Behind Human Error: Cognitive Systems, Computers, and Hindsight.* Dayton, Ohio: Human Systems Ergonomic Information and Analysis Center, WPAFB; 1994.

KEY TERM

Blunt end: Levels of strategic and other top-level decision-making persons or groups in an organization that impact the work at the point of care delivery (the sharp end) (Reason, 1997).

organizational resources and layers of defense from above (the **blunt end**), healthcare workers continuously manage workloads using their knowledge, immediate perceptions, and own goals to handle situations in the presence of multiple goal conflicts, obstacles, hazards, ambiguous and inadequate or missing data, and behaviors (the system complexities on the left side of the model) surrounding care situations. For example, unpredictability, missing knowledge, clumsy technology, and constant change are a few of the multiple features of the current healthcare environment that confront healthcare practitioners. To prevent things from going wrong, practitioners act by anticipating, reacting, accommodating, adapting, and coping (the worker resiliency on the right side of the model) to bridge gaps constantly while compromising among multiple competing goals to make trade-off decisions in the midst of a changing environment.

The cognitive work required in complex work environments can be very demanding, and despite best efforts result in decisions leading to adverse events. Woods (1988) described four characteristic dimensions of complex environments that increase problem-solving demands and difficulty: dynamism, large numbers of parts and connectedness between parts, high uncertainty, and risk. In research on complexity of work and decision making, Klein (1998) identified common characteristics across different types of occupations and industries that influence decision making (see Box 8-3). These common characteristics include time pressures, high stakes, inadequate information (missing, ambiguous, or erroneous), ill-defined goals, poorly defined procedures, dynamic conditions, people working in teams, and stress. Using knowledge, paying attention to shifts in current situational states, and balancing interacting and sometimes conflicting goals, workers in complex worlds make decisions and act, creating and actually increasing safety most of the time.

BOX 8-3   COMPLEX WORK ENVIRONMENTS: CHARACTERISTICS THAT INFLUENCE DECISION MAKING

- Time pressures
- High stakes
- Inadequate information
- Ill-defined goals

- Poorly defined procedures
- Dynamic conditions
- Teamwork
- Stress

Source: Klein, G. (1998) *Sources of power: How people make decisions.* Cambridge: MIT.

Human Limitations and Complexity

Human factors explain why we cannot expect perfect performance in complex work environments. An important aspect in developing an understanding about getting the best performance within the complexity described earlier is an explicit acceptance of the simple fact that humans are limited in the amount of information and complexity of tasks they are able to manage effectively and safely. Human beings are not perfect. Researchers report that during situations with multiple tasks, human limitations result from a variety of factors that affect "cognitive function in dynamic evolving situations, especially those involving the management of workload in time and the control of attention" (Cook & Woods, 1994, p. 270). Humans demonstrate limitations related to memory capacity, attention span, distractions, biases, physical capability, and performance in the presence of fatigue, negative emotions, and/or illness.

Cook and Woods (1994) identified two major human performance problems related to changes in attentional dynamics during certain situations—loss of situation awareness and fixation. **Loss of situation awareness** refers to failure to maintain accurate tracking of the multiple and changing interactions between parts of processes or systems. Maintaining situation awareness in complex situations would represent the ability to scrutinize and refine expectations based on new information and/or contextual aspects of a situation, or to demonstrate what Langer and Piper (1987) defined as **mindfulness**. **Fixation** refers to failure to revise the assessment of a situation as new information becomes available. Avoiding fixation in complex situations is desirable. If individuals avoid fixation, they are demonstrating **sensemaking**, or the ability to reconstruct and interpret incoming information anew in ambiguous, complex, and evolving situations (Klein, Moon, & Hoffman, 2006). Nurses and other healthcare providers are constantly taking in new information in clinical care settings that require that they demonstrate sensemaking to accurately interpret the meaning of the information and the impact it will have on decisions they need to make about patient care.

Fallibility is part of the human condition. Reason (1990) described three basic error types that are uniquely human and complicate human performance given the best of situations.

Slips and lapses (execution errors) are defined as "errors which result from some failure in the execution and/or

> **KEY TERM**
>
> **Loss of situation awareness:** Failure to maintain accurate tracking of the multiple and changing interactions between parts of processes or systems (Cook & Woods, 1994).

> **KEY TERM**
>
> **Mindfulness:** The ability to scrutinize and refine expectations based on new information and/or contextual aspects of a situation (Langer, 1989).

> **KEY TERM**
>
> **Fixation:** Failure to revise the assessment of a situation as new information becomes available (Cook & Woods, 1994).

> **KEY TERM**
>
> **Sensemaking:** The ability to reconstruct and interpret incoming information anew in ambiguous, complex, and evolving situations (Klein, Moon, & Hoffman, 2006).

> **KEY TERM**
>
> **Slips and lapses:** Execution failures or "errors which result from some failure in the execution and/or storage of an action sequence, regardless of whether or not the plan which guided them was adequate to achieve its objective" (Reason, 1990, p. 9).

storage of an action sequence, regardless of whether or not the plan which guided them was adequate to achieve its objective" (p. 9). A simple example might be when you inadvertently place an ointment instead of toothpaste on your toothbrush, having grabbed the wrong tube. These are reflex skills that go awry due to unconscious error. Any break in a routine or distraction can precipitate a slip. Reason states that the differences between slips and lapses are that slips are usually observable events whereas lapses may only involve memory and be evident only to the person experiencing the lapses. Both slips and lapses generally occur during the performance of a routine skill or behavior.

Mistakes (planning failures) occur when there are "deficiencies or failures in the judgmental and/or inferential processes involved in the selection of an object or in the specification of the means to achieve it" (Reason, 1990, p. 9). Mistakes occur in situations related to a new or unfamiliar situation or a lack of understanding of the problem due to limited availability of information. Mistakes generally occur after identification of a problem situation.

In addition to these specific human factors, other contributors that may affect human performance are the following: environmental factors including heat, cold, noise, visual stimuli, motion, distractions, and lighting; physiologic factors including fatigue, sleep loss, alcohol, drugs, and illness; and psychological factors including competing activities and emotional states such as boredom, fear, anxiety, frustration, and anger. Given the characteristics of complex work environments within health care and the variety of factors represented by the sharp end/blunt end model, it is reasonable to expect that human limitations would further complicate a healthcare practitioner's ability to maintain mindfulness and demonstrate continuous sensemaking in every situation. For example, nurses and other healthcare practitioners who are distracted frequently during work may not be able to maintain an accurate, complete, and updated picture of the current work environment and patient situations. Healthcare environments have been referred to as "environments prone to distraction." It is the failure to appreciate the contribution of complexity in our healthcare environments and human limitations of practitioners that remains one of the largest barriers in efforts to improve patient safety.

Hindsight Bias and Blame

Before the IOM released its report in 2000, traditional healthcare review of adverse events or accidents usually started at the point of the accident and included only investigation of the person(s) and details surrounding the immediate outcome. Monitoring focused on the actions and expertise of the persons involved in the outcome and on the effects and errors that followed. In the past, remedial action was directed most often toward the staff person involved in the adverse event. Although the approach to adverse event investigation has moved to a broader search for possible latent conditions or gaps, what continue to be underappreciated in many investigative reviews are the multiple environmental latent conditions, or gaps, that enabled the immediate situation characteristics to arise. This is due in part to the hindsight bias that characterizes all reviews of accidents.

> **KEY TERM**
>
> **Hindsight bias:** The natural tendency for humans looking back from an accident to consistently overstate what could have been anticipated in foresight and to see only a simplified path of decision making related to the specific accident (Fischoff, 1975).

Hindsight bias is the natural tendency for humans looking back from an accident to consistently overstate what could have been anticipated in foresight and to see only a simplified path of decision making related to the specific accident (Fischoff, 1975). What is lost in hindsight are all of the complex human and environmental factors and unavoidable trade-offs that contributed to the experience of the person involved in the actual situation. As a result of using hindsight bias, people close to adverse events are often counseled, inflexible policies and procedures remain or are rewritten to increase enforcement, and realistic alternative plans for dealing with the effect of the complexity in future situations may not even be considered.

Failure to recognize the paralyzing impact of hindsight bias in the aftermath of an accident may be one of the largest barriers to making system improvements that could prevent future accidents. Lost as a result of hindsight bias is important learning not only about system gaps that could be redesigned and eliminated from the organization, but also about potential system supports that might be appropriate to implement given normal human limitations that contributed to the event, as well as direction for increasing individual resiliency for responding to future similar complex situations.

Patient Safety Culture

Clear awareness of the effect of hindsight bias on learning and purposeful efforts toward avoiding the tendency to simplify explanations after near-miss and adverse events are core organizational behaviors that represent a patient safety culture for improving and providing safe patient care. These and additional characteristics of effective patient safety cultures that are essential for learning from near-miss and adverse events are listed in Box 8-4.

One of the most difficult aspects of health care's shift to the new approach to patient safety has been consistent application of the nonpunitive method to accident investigation. The traditional focus on the individual as the object of blame at the point of the adverse event has been a formidable target for change. Contributors to this difficulty are our human tendency for hindsight bias, as well as the catastrophic human suffering that may occur as a result of some medical adverse events. Dr. Richard Cook, an anesthesiologist and leader in patient safety

---

BOX 8-4 CHARACTERISTICS OF EFFECTIVE PATIENT SAFETY CULTURES

- Acknowledgement of human limitations
- Awareness of the effect of hindsight bias on learning
- Avoidance of the tendency to simplify explanations of near-miss and adverse events
- Commitment on the part of management to non-punitive, problem-solving approaches to accident investigation, and modeling these approaches
- Facilitation of open communication and involvement of front-line workers for learning and problem-solving
- Design of formal systems of follow-up, communication, and training after new learning, and before intended changes are developed and implemented

Sources: Cooper, M. D. (2000). Towards a model of safety culture. *Safety Science, 36,* 111–136; Zohar, D. (1980). Safety climate in industrial organizations. Theoretical and applied implications. *Journal of Applied Psychology,* 65(1), 96–102.

---

research, explains this blame response as a social phenomenon that "feels good," separates us from the event, and enables us to move past it quickly, thinking we have figured out what caused the event (personal communication, 2004). Unfortunately, this reaction diverts us from the very thing that will help to prevent future events—learning about what enabled it to occur in the first place, and what could be done to prevent the possibility of later occurrences.

In acknowledging human limitations we have had to change our expectations about healthcare worker accountabilities related to patient safety. Whereas we used to expect that individual nurses and other healthcare providers would perform perfectly in all situations, we now know that the complexity of healthcare work prevents what we might define as perfect performance in all situations. New areas of accountabilities for patient safety that must be accepted by healthcare providers, including nurses, include speaking up about barriers to safe care practices, sharing stories about details of what happened surrounding a near-miss or adverse event, demonstrating non-blame and supportive behaviors with co-workers after an event, and participating in problem-solving to improve systems to prevent future events. Cook argues that unless there was intent by the individual worker to cause harm, there is no place for blame in event investigation. Even an adverse event involving an inexperienced worker or a poorly performing worker is most often the result of system inadequacies that allowed the worker to be present in the situation in the first place. Managing poor performance is critical to patient safety, but should be managed proactively and separately from investigations of near-miss and adverse events.

As a result of the discomfort that healthcare managers and leaders feel with non-blame and non-punitive language, alternative approaches have arisen to guide them through decision making regarding follow-up actions after near-miss and adverse events. One such approach is the Just Culture Algorithm (Marx & Griffith, 2007). Further information and discussion related to the Just Culture Algorithm can be found at http://www.justculture.org. The authors support human fallibility as a reason for medical adverse events, but also lead users through decision making regarding the distinctions among systems failure, reckless conduct, and at-risk behavior. Marx and Griffith suggest that the Just Culture Algorithm, if used properly, offers a consistent organizational process and approach for application of a non-punitive response to adverse events.

Research on Nursing Work Complexity

To understand human performance in complex systems that results in failure or adverse events in healthcare situations, researchers must focus on studying the function of the system in which healthcare providers are embedded, including complexities and hazards at the sharp end, how providers cope with system gaps, and how system gaps are created or avoided through operational changes (Cook & Woods, 1994; Cook et al., 2000; Woods, 1988). This section presents research on nursing work and descriptions of factors characteristic of nursing work environments, factors that influence registered nurse (RN) decision making, and RN strategies for managing workflow in providing patient care.

A comprehensive search of the literature in 2000 revealed no research focused on the complexity of the healthcare system and its relationship to nurses' work in actual work situations. Using frameworks developed by human performance researchers, nurse researchers have subsequently conducted studies to describe registered nurse work (e.g., Ebright, Patterson, Chalko, & Render, 2003; Ebright, Urden, Patterson, & Chalko, 2004; Potter et al., 2005).

Guided by the sharp end/blunt end framework, Ebright, Patterson, Chalko, and Render (2003) conducted a study of RNs working on acute care units in one large urban healthcare facility. The purpose of the study was to identify contributors to work complexity, strategies used to manage complexity for desired outcomes, and factors affecting cognitive work leading to clinical and workload management decisions. Data were collected through direct observations of individual RNs working on nine different units, followed by individual interviews using **cognitive task analysis** techniques. Analyses of the data resulted in descriptive data that included numbers of interruptions, sources of interruptions, travel patterns, types of clinical care provided, and the types of knowledge, cues, and other factors that influenced specific decision making during the situations observed. Recording all activities of an individual nurse in sequence, thereby avoiding limitation of the data by using preselected categories, provided rich representations of the

KEY TERM

Cognitive task analysis: A technique for interview data collection and analysis to describe the cognitive work and influencing factors surrounding situations that led to and resulted in decisions.

KEY TERM

Stacking: The cognitive process of maintaining a work-to-be-done activities list, and the organizing and reprioritizing of activities as situations in care or workflow evolve (Ebright, Patterson, Chalko, & Render, 2003).

actual complex flow of RN work. Figure 8-3 represents the sharp end of the sharp end/blunt end framework with consistently recurring patterns of work complexities, work strategies, and influencers of decision making identified across nine different RNs and units studied.

Contributors to work complexity patterns included missing equipment, interruptions, waiting for access to needed systems and resources, lack of time to complete interventions that were judged necessary to reach desired outcomes, and inconsistencies in how information was communicated or could be relied on for access if needed. RN work strategy patterns included anticipating or forward thinking, proactively monitoring patient status to detect early warning signals, strategic delegation and hand-off decisions to maintain flow of workload, individually constructed workflow sheets to track care and document (memory aid), and a cognitive strategy for moving on to other activities to prevent down time when not able to complete something due to waiting for processes or inability to access resources (**stacking**).

Coordinating Knowledge, Mindset, and Goals

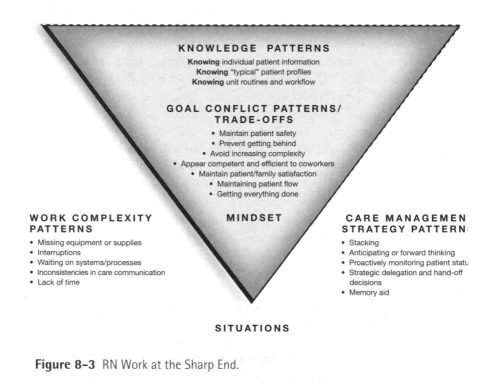

KNOWLEDGE PATTERNS
Knowing individual patient information
Knowing "typical" patient profiles
Knowing unit routines and workflow

GOAL CONFLICT PATTERNS/ TRADE-OFFS
• Maintain patient safety
• Prevent getting behind
• Avoid increasing complexity
• Appear competent and efficient to coworkers
• Maintain patient/family satisfaction
• Maintaining patient flow
• Getting everything done

WORK COMPLEXITY PATTERNS
• Missing equipment or supplies
• Interruptions
• Waiting on systems/processes
• Inconsistencies in care communication
• Lack of time

MINDSET

CARE MANAGEMEN STRATEGY PATTERN
• Stacking
• Anticipating or forward thinking
• Proactively monitoring patient statu
• Strategic delegation and hand-off decisions
• Memory aid

SITUATIONS

Figure 8-3 RN Work at the Sharp End.

Potter et al. (2005) described the cognitive work of seven RNs on an acute care unit from direct observation and interview. The researchers found the average number of stacked activities across RN lists of activities to be completed over one shift to be 11, with the maximum number of activities for an RN at any one time to be 16. Ebright and colleagues have modified their original definition of stacking to include the cognitive work of stacking that includes the organizing and reprioritizing of activities as situations in care or workflow evolve. This definition is similar to the cognitive work in sensemaking of immediate and changing situations.

Ebright, Patterson, Chalko, and Render (2003) found several factors that influenced RN decision making during patient care, as represented in Figure 8-3. Two major categories of factors were knowledge considered in the decision making and goal conflicts that arose in the midst of providing care. Three patterns of knowledge were identified: knowledge about individual patients, typical patient disease profiles, and unit workflow routines. The patterns of goal conflict or the simultaneous and sometimes competing goals trying to be reached, but difficult to reach, in a timely or as expected manner were the following: maintaining patient safety, preventing getting behind, avoiding increasing complexity, appearing competent and efficient to patients/families and co-workers, and maintaining patient/family satisfaction. Having to choose work on one goal at the expense of another is when nurses make trade-offs, as discussed earlier.

Figure 8-4 represents one individual RN's work over a period of 7 hours. The data were collected by directly observing the nurse and recording all activities in sequence, including interrupting and medication administration during that time period. The unpredictability and obvious lack of linearity in being able to complete even one medication administration task without interruption is apparent. The important contribution of this representation is that it demonstrates to those who are not nurses or no longer work at the sharp end that it is in the midst of this complex environment that nurses strive to maintain mindfulness and continuous sensemaking as they do their best to provide safe care.

Using cognitive task analysis techniques to collect detailed stories from nurses with less than one year of experience about actual near-miss and/or adverse events resulted in similar data regarding the factors contributing to RN work complexity and the multiple influencers of decision making (Ebright, Urden, et al., 2004). In addition, common characteristics surrounding the events were identified across RN participants and situations. For example, in all cases the RNs were anticipating, getting ready for, or performing some procedure or activity for the very first time since starting work on the unit. Distraction, anxiety, or both seemed to be a factor contributing to the near-miss or adverse event, even if the event was not related to the "first time" performance. In all cases, the RNs described being time constrained and feeling pressured to complete, or get ready for, some activity. In a majority of the cases, some type of hand-off of patient information

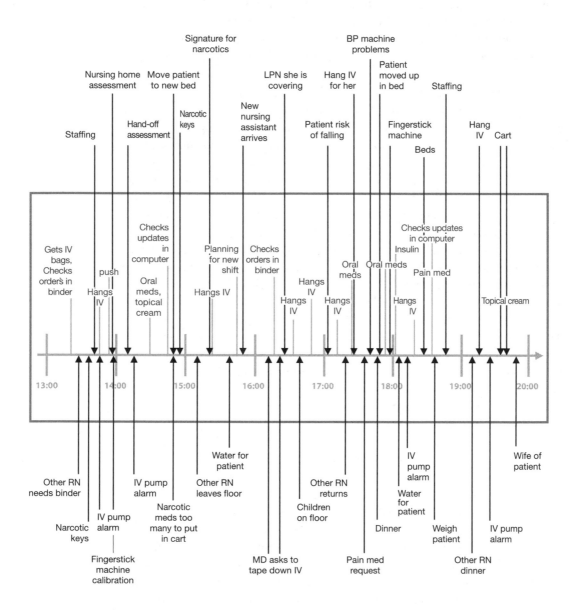

Figure 8–4 RN Work Complexity. *Source:* © Reprinted with permission from Patterson, E. (2003). Nursing work complexity.

was judged incomplete or not as helpful as it could have been. And the social pressure to perform well, whether self-imposed or originating from other RNs, was a factor influencing decision making in the majority of cases.

The researchers concluded that increasing knowledge about the complexities of actual work situations involving newer RNs and what puts them at risk for error is essential. Clinical unit strategies for managing RN anxiety generated from social pressure to perform well and/or from anticipation of performance of new activities would be a place to start for supporting new nurses.

Implications of the New Look Approach to Patient Safety

Healthcare Organizations

Given the new learning about complexity and human factors, and the futility of patient safety improvement efforts that focus on only individuals without consideration of the complex systems in which they work, most healthcare organizations are involved in major efforts to change. Making decisions that result in safe care in all situations requires practitioners who are supported by systems that account for human limitations and operations decision makers who understand work at the sharp end and how changes will impact that work. Improvement in patient safety will occur only through an effective culture of safety that is characterized by encouragement of open and honest communication about failures and learning from the reporting and investigations that follow. Creating and maintaining these characteristics is difficult given our traditional approaches to failure. Box 8-5 identifies some

---

BOX 8-5   HEALTHCARE ORGANIZATIONAL EFFORTS TO CREATE SAFER CARE ENVIRONMENTS

- Identify and reduce system gaps that contribute to complexity.
- Redesign physical structures, technology, and process and procedural designs to streamline real work at the point of care and account for human limitations.
- Increase access to real-time information to support decision making through better use of informatics technology.
- Develop non-punitive error reporting structures to encourage practitioners to speak up about near-miss and adverse events.
- Develop formal disclosure processes and patient/family supports for informing about adverse event occurrences.
- Develop formal processes for support of practitioners involved in adverse events.
- Implement leadership activities to increase leaders' understanding of work and their visibility to sharp end workers to build trust in openness and learning.
- Educate employees throughout the organization about human factors and system failure.

of the current activities and efforts by healthcare organizations to move toward safer environments.

The accountability in practice for RNs is no longer to perform perfectly in imperfect situations. We have learned that perfection is not possible in most situations. However, given our new approach, the new accountabilities for RNs are to identify barriers to providing safe patient care, speak up about near misses and adverse events, participate in problem-solving for system changes or gap elimination, and keep up-to-date on required educational offerings about changes, new processes, procedures, and technologies. For managers and administrators, the new accountabilities are to facilitate an environment where open and honest communication is encouraged, rewarded, and utilized in improving systems of care, and to involve sharp end workers in designing and implementing change. Despite these necessary steps, overcoming the tendency to blame and engage in hindsight bias, along with the legal and economic challenges inherent in publicly reporting adverse events, will continue to be formidable obstacles as health care moves forward in efforts to improve safety.

Nursing Education

Nursing education programs have begun to redesign curricula based on the learning about complex systems, advances in technology, and the changing role of the nurse in health care. Essential knowledge for RNs to perform successfully in healthcare settings is that which prepares them as knowledge workers, system thinkers, and complex system managers. The knowledge that enables RN performance in each of these roles is necessary for a most critical aspect of RN functioning based on research that describes stacking in their work.

Stacking, or the decision making that results in RNs organizing and prioritizing activities (the decisions about what to do and when to do it), depends on nurses' ability to access relevant information, maintain situation awareness or mindfulness in the midst of unpredictability, and manage with accurate sense-making as situations change. Although the healthcare organizations in which students or RNs work have some responsibility for designing supports into processes and systems, the constantly changing patient status and human behaviors of practitioners and patients/families will always demand the nurse have the knowledge and skills for managing and adapting to this complexity for safe patient outcomes. Box 8-6 contains proposed content and teaching/learning strategies considered to be important for incorporation into nursing education curricula to facilitate student acquisition of the requisite knowledge and skills for managing complexity in the healthcare environment. Contemporary Practice Highlight 8-2 provides information about Quality and Safety Education for Nurses (QSEN), an initiative dedicated to increasing the nursing profession's commitment to patient safety and quality.

BOX 8-6   PROPOSED NURSING CURRICULUM: COMPLEX SYSTEM CONTENT AND TEACHING/LEARNING STRATEGIES

- Complex system theory content
- Creative teaching/learning strategies for understanding complex system characteristics
- Simulations representing multiple contextual demands and challenges
- Stacking and stacking management principles and content to guide decisions and strategies about workflow
- Clinical debriefings that incorporate workload management strategies as well as individual patient case studies
- Conversations about and modeling of a culture of open and honest communication about:
  - System complexity contributions to near misses and errors in student/faculty clinical experiences
  - Realistic expectations of novice abilities in managing complex healthcare environments
  - Student/novice accountability for seeking assistance in new and/or uncomfortable experiences

---

CONTEMPORARY PRACTICE HIGHLIGHT 8-2

QUALITY AND SAFETY EDUCATION FOR NURSES (QSEN)

Quality and Safety Education for Nurses (QSEN) is an initiative funded by the Robert Wood Johnson Foundation with the goal of fostering commitment to the IOM-recommended quality and safety competencies within the nursing profession. One of the QSEN's priority actions has been to define and disseminate quality and safety competencies for nursing. These competencies and further information about QSEN's goals and activities can be found at http://www.qsen.org.

In addition to curricular implications resulting from learning about patient safety, there are new accountabilities for nursing faculty who teach and work with students in healthcare organizations. These include speaking up about system complexity in clinical settings to the appropriate person in charge of operations, role modeling for students appropriate communication strategies leading to system improvements, and role modeling non-blame language and the search for learning following near-miss and adverse events.

Summary

Several key events in the healthcare industry including legislative and regulatory factors have led to the current focus on patient safety in health care. One overall framework called New Look, adapted from the work of James Reason, provides a context for understanding the evolution of failure in health care despite our best intentions and focus on quality and safety. The sharp end/blunt end model explains work in complex systems, the contribution of complex environmental and human limitations on cognitive work, and the resulting decision making at the point of patient care.

Developing an effective patient safety culture has become the goal of healthcare institutions across the United States. And yet a huge challenge to these efforts is the traditional healthcare approach to medical error that includes the hindsight bias reaction of simplifying situations surrounding an adverse event. Recent research findings on the complexity of nursing work describe contributors to the complex work of nursing, strategies that nurses use to deal with the complexity, and the factors that influence decision making at the point of care. As a result of the new approach to patient safety, organizations, nursing educators, and nurses all have new accountabilities for making improvements in patient safety.

Key Terms

- **Active failures:** Errors and violations caused by acts performed by workers (e.g., nurses) closest to the sharp end of the system (e.g., patient care) that impact system safety most directly (Reason, 1997).
- **Adverse events:** Untoward incidents, therapeutic misadventures, iatrogenic injuries, or other adverse occurrences directly associated with care or services provided within the jurisdiction of a medical center, outpatient clinic, or other facility (The Joint Commission [TJC], 2001).

  Blunt end: Levels of strategic and other top-level decision-making persons or groups in an organization that impact the work at the point of care delivery (the sharp end) (Reason, 1997).

  Cognitive task analysis: A technique for interview data collection and analysis to describe the cognitive work and influencing factors surrounding situations that led to and resulted in decisions.
- **Complex systems:** Systems in which work includes both cognitive and physical demands and is characterized by dynamism, large numbers of parts and connectedness between parts, high uncertainty, and risk (Woods, 1988).
- **Fixation:** Failure to revise the assessment of a situation as new information becomes available (Cook & Woods, 1994).
- **Gaps:** Another term for latent conditions or error-producing factors (Cook, Woods, & Miller, 1998).
- **Hindsight bias:** The natural tendency for humans looking back from an accident to consistently overstate what could have been anticipated in foresight and to see only a simplified path of decision making related to the specific accident (Fischoff, 1975).

  Human factors: Sets of human-specific physical, mental, and behavioral properties, as well as the science of how people interact with tasks, machines (or computers), and the environment with the consideration that humans have properties that demonstrate limitations and capabilities (Wikipedia, n.d.).

  Latent conditions: Error-producing factors like poor design, gaps in supervision, undetected system failures, lack of training, and the like arising from the decision-making levels (blunt end) of organizations that combine with active failures to result in adverse events (Reason, 1997).
- **Layers of defense:** Organizational safeguards in place to prevent anticipated injury, damage, or failure (Reason, 1990).
- **Loss of situation awareness:** Failure to maintain accurate tracking of the multiple and changing interactions between parts of processes or systems (Cook & Woods, 1994).
- **Medical error:** Failure of a planned action to be completed as intended, or the use of a wrong plan to achieve an aim (Institute of Medicine [IOM], 2000).

- **Mindfulness:** The ability to scrutinize and refine expectations based on new information and/or contextual aspects of a situation (Langer, 1989).
- **Mistakes:** Planning failures—"deficiencies or failures in the judgmental and/ or inferential processes involved in the selection of an object or in the specification of the means to achieve it" (Reason, 1990, p. 9).
- **Near-miss event:** Any process variation that did not affect the outcome in a given event, but for which a recurrence carries a significant chance of a serious adverse outcome (TJC, 2001).
- **New Look:** An approach to patient safety based on understanding and adaptation of the evolution of failure, as described by James Reason (Cook, Woods, & Miller, 1998).
- **Patient safety:** Freedom from accidental injury (IOM, 2000).
- **Reporting system:** A safety information system that collects, analyzes, and disseminates information about near misses, adverse events, and safety systems (Reason, 1997).
- **Safety culture:** Shared values and beliefs in an organization that interact with the organizational structures and systems and produce behavioral norms surrounding work (Reason, 1997).
- **Sensemaking:** The ability to reconstruct and interpret incoming information anew in ambiguous, complex, and evolving situations (Klein, Moon, & Hoffman, 2006).
- **Sharp end:** Frontline personnel at the operations point of the organization; for example, at the point of patient care in a healthcare organization (Reason, 1997).
- **Slips and lapses:** Execution failures or "errors which result from some failure in the execution and/or storage of an action sequence, regardless of whether or not the plan which guided them was adequate to achieve its objective" (Reason, 1990, p. 9).
- **Stacking:** The cognitive process of maintaining a work-to-be-done activities list, and the organizing and reprioritizing of activities as situations in care or workflow evolve (Ebright, Patterson, Chalko, & Render, 2003).
- **Trade-offs:** Decision resolutions that involve conflicting choices between highly unlikely but highly undesirable events and highly likely but less catastrophic ones (Cook & Woods, 1994).

Reflective Practice Questions

1. What factors were found to contribute to nursing work complexity in recent research on nursing work? What factors in your work environment contribute to work complexity?
2. Think of an adverse event involving a nurse or nurses in your workplace.

You may or may not have been involved in the event. Were your RN colleagues' verbal and/or non-verbal reactions to the event reflective of an effective safety culture as described in this chapter?

3. In the adverse event you recalled in question 2, what human factors contributed to the adverse event?

4. In the recalled event from question 2, what work process or system design change might decrease the risk of the adverse event happening again?

5. Describe what you personally are accountable for in relation to improvement after awareness of an adverse event. What could you have, or did you, contribute to learning from the event described in question 2?

References

Cook, R. I., Render, M., & Woods, D. D. (2000). Gaps in the continuity of care and progress on patient safety. *British Medical Journal, 320*, 791–794.

Cook, R. I., & Woods, D. D. (1994). Operating at the sharp end: The complexity of human error. In M. E. Bogner (Ed.), *Human error in medicine* (pp. 255–310). Hillsdale, NJ: Lawrence Erlbaum.

Cook, R. I., Woods, D. D., & Miller, C. A. (1998). *Tale of two stories: Contrasting views of patient safety*. Chicago: National Patient Safety Foundation.

Cooper, M. D. (2000). Towards a model of safety culture. *Safety Science, 36*, 111–136.

Ebright, R., Patterson, E., Chalko, B., & Render, M. (2003). Understanding the complexity of registered nurse work in acute care settings. *Journal of Nursing Administration, 33*(12), 630–638.

Ebright, R., Urden, L., Patterson, E., & Chalko, B. (2004). Themes surrounding novice nurse near-miss and adverse event situations. *Journal of Nursing Administration, 34*(11), 531–538.

Fischoff, B. (1975). Hindsight does not equal foresight: The effect of outcome knowledge on judgment under uncertainty. *Journal of Experimental Psychology: Human Perception and Performance, 1*, 288–299.

Institute of Medicine. (2000). *To err is human: Building a safer health system*. L. T. Kohn, J. M. Corrigan, & M. S. Donaldson (Eds.). Washington, DC: National Academies Press.

Institute of Medicine. (2004). *Keeping patients safe: Transforming the work environment of nurses*. Washington, DC: National Academies Press.

Institute of Medicine, Committee on Identifying and Preventing Medication Errors. (2006). *Preventing medication errors: Quality chasm series*. Washington, DC: National Academies Press.

Institute of Medicine, Committee on Quality of Healthcare in America. (2001). *Crossing the quality chasm: A new health system for the 21st century*. Washington, DC: National Academies Press.

The Joint Commission. (2001). Definitions. *Joint Commission Perspectives on Patient Safety, 1*(6). Retrieved August 19, 2007, from http://www.jcrinc.com/827/

The Joint Commission. (2007). *2008 patient safety goals*. Retrieved August 19, 2007, from http://www.jointcommission.org/PatientSafety/NationalPatientSafetyGoals/

Klein, G. (1998). *Sources of power: How people make decisions*. Cambridge, MA: MIT.

Klein, G., Moon, B., & Hoffman, R. F. (2006). Making sense of sensemaking I: Alternative perspectives. *IEEE Intelligent Systems, 21*(4), 70–73.

Langer, E. J., (1989). *Mindfulness.* Reading, MA: Addison-Wesley.

Langer, E. J., & Piper A. (1987). The prevention of mindlessness. *Journal of Personality and Social Psychology, 53,* 280–287.

Leape, L. (1994). Error in medicine. *Journal of the American Medical Association, 272,* 1851–1857.

Leape, L. L., & Berwick, D. M. (2005). Five years after to err is human: What have we learned? *Journal of the American Medical Association, 293,* 2384–2390.

Marx, D., & Griffith, S. (2007). *The just culture algorithm.* Retrieved July 25, 2007, from http://www.justculture.org/algorithm.aspx

Minnesota Department of Health. (2007). *Background on Minnesota's adverse health events reporting law.* Retrieved July 25, 2007, from http://www.health.state.mn.us/patient-safety/ae/background.html

Potter, P., Wolf, L., Boxerman, S., Grayson, D., Sledge, J., Dungan, C., et al. (2005). Understanding the cognitive work of nursing in the acute care environment. *Journal of Nursing Administration, 35*(7/8), 327–335.

Reason, J. (1990). *Human error.* Cambridge, MA: Cambridge University Press.

Reason, J. (1997). *Managing the risks of organizational accidents.* Burlington, VT: Ashgate.

Silker, E. (2006). *APSF history overview.* Retrieved August 19, 2007, from http://apsf.org/about/brief_history.mspx

Wikipedia. (n.d.). *Human factors.* Retrieved July 25, 2007, from http://en.wikipedia.org/wiki/Human_factors

Woods, D. (1988). Coping with complexity: The psychology of human behavior in complex systems. In L. P. Goodstein, H. B. Andersen, & S. E. Olsen (Eds.), *Tasks, errors and mental models* (pp. 128-148). New York: Taylor & Francis.

Woods, D. D., & Cook, R. I. (1998). *Characteristics of patient safety: Five principles that underlie productive work.* Chicago: CtL.

Woods, D. D., Johannesen, L. J., Cook, R. I., & Sarter, N. B. (1994) *Behind human error: Cognitive systems, computers, and hindsight.* Wright-Patterson AFB, OH: Crew Systems Ergonomic Information and Analysis Center (CSERIAC).

Zohar, D. (1980). Safety climate in industrial organizations. Theoretical and applied implications. *Journal of Applied Psychology, 65*(1), 96–102.

Performance Outcomes in Healthcare

Beverly S. Farmer

LEARNING OUTCOMES

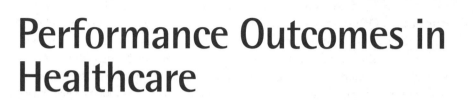

After reading this chapter you will be able to:

- Define performance outcomes and what effect they have on nursing practice and health care.
- Define quality in health care.
- Discuss historical factors that have led to the emphasis on quality outcomes measures in health care.
- Explain the effects of regulatory and accreditation agencies in improving performance outcomes of health care.
- Define core performance measures.
- Describe nursing performance indicators and discuss how they are "nursing sensitive."
- List different agencies that have developed nursing performance outcomes and what measurement tools are used to determine these outcomes.
- Analyze how pay-for-performance may affect the quality of health care.

Introduction

Public interest in and demand for performance outcomes have proliferated in the last decade. This chapter will explain what performance indicators are and how each regulatory organization uses these indicators as predictors of health-care quality. Quality outcomes and measures are complex. Agencies, both federally mandated and privately run, measure healthcare quality. This chapter will examine specific measurements for each of these agencies. There is not one consistent measurement tool or organization that has all the answers. The history of why performance measures are considered such an important part of healthcare measurement is explored as well as how other industry standards have helped define healthcare quality. Healthcare indicators and nursing-specific indictors will be presented to analyze the correlation of quality care measures with improved quality outcomes.

Performance Outcomes

In the landmark report published in 1999, *To Err Is Human: Building a Safer Health System,*" the Institute of Medicine reported that 44,000–98,000 Americans die each year as a result of medical errors. This makes medical errors the eighth leading cause of death in the United States. As consumers and the public become more aware of these statistics, the increased demand for improvement has become critical to the healthcare industry. Consumers no longer tolerate complacency in healthcare improvements. **Performance outcomes** are the measure of a quality organization. Performance outcomes can measure an organization's performance or measure client care outcomes, depending on the measurement tool. Within healthcare organizations, performance outcomes that are nurse sensitive have become an important determinant in the quality of the organization.

Standards and outcomes can be developed and made available in a variety of ways. Standards can be developed and used by public regulatory processes or through private voluntary processes. These standards may determine licensure, such as with the Center for Medicare and Medicaid Services (CMS), or accreditations through The Joint Commission. Standards measure consistency and uniformity and they also set expectations. The process of developing standards can set the expectations for the organizations and health professionals that are affected by the standards. The publication and dissemination of the standards help healthcare consumers to set expectations as well. Expectations for performance play an important role in establishing norms and facilitating improvements in outcomes. Examples of healthcare outcomes are shown in Table 9-1.

Health care is changing infinitely faster than it ever has before. One of the reasons that these changes are occurring is the continually expanding proliferation of

TABLE 9-1 EXAMPLES OF HEALTHCARE OUTCOMES QUALITY MEASURES

Measure	Example
Mortality	Infant death rate
Physiologic measures	Blood pressure
Clinical events	Stroke
Symptoms	Difficulty breathing
Functional measures	Walking a designated distance

information. Information that in the past was either not measured or not made public has become easily accessible to the general public. Information is easily accessible for patients to pick a surgeon and look at the statistics of how many surgeries he or she may have performed, what percentage of patients developed postoperative infections, or how many patients had other complications. The public can use the Internet or printed material to find and compare hospitals within a given area to determine which has the best outcomes for a given diagnosis or which quality awards have been given to a particular hospital. Although this information is available to the public, there is a wide variance in the accuracy of this information. Consumers must learn how to navigate the information to make informed decisions.

Defining Quality

The public does not routinely choose a restaurant because it just satisfies the customer. Many people look for a restaurant that has a competitive advantage such as great service, better prices, delicious food, or better than expected ambiance. The same strategies can be used for people to choose a healthcare provider or hospital. Some use the argument that third-party payers have more choice than an individual, but it does not take long for a physician or healthcare organization with poor performance outcomes to become highlighted and not be chosen by the third-party payer. It is easy for a person to use the Internet to find information about a physician or hospital. This is a much newer concept to the business of health care than to other businesses, which have been compared publicly for many years. New tools and resources for assessing and improving healthcare quality are available, and others continue to be rapidly developing (Sidebar 9-1).

SIDEBAR 9-1

The quality of health care is determined by how well a doctor, hospital, health plan, or other provider of health care keeps its members healthy or treats them when they are sick. High quality health care means doing the right thing at the right time, in the right way, for the right person, and getting the best possible results.

Consumers want quality. A frequently used definition of quality is "meeting or exceeding the customers' expectations." For some people quality health care means seeing their doctor or nurse practitioner right away, being treated courteously by the staff, and having the provider spend time with them (Sidebar 9-2). Although these things are important, clinical performance measures should be the most important outcome measure when determining whether a healthcare professional or organization is a quality provider of health care.

Measuring quality through performance outcomes is one way to determine quality in health care. There are many agencies, organizations, and individuals that measure healthcare quality; there is no one way to determine the quality of healthcare. Becoming aware of how data is collected, analyzed, and reported is a key aspect of using quality measures to make informed decisions.

The Institute of Medicine (IOM) defines quality as the degree to which health services for individuals and populations increase the likelihood of desired health outcomes and are consistent with current professional knowledge. Good quality means providing clients with appropriate services in a technically competent manner, with good communication, shared decision making, and cultural sensitivity.

In today's healthcare environment, the meticulous collection and meaningful portrayal of relevant quality data and information are equally vital to healthcare organizations, practitioners, purchasers, and the public. It is through the use of reliable performance data that healthcare organizations and individual practitioners are able to determine priority areas for quality improvement, and purchasers and consumers can make informed decisions about accessing and purchasing healthcare services. Yet, as inextricably linked as the use of performance data is to quality improvement and informed decision making, there is decidedly little cohesion among the myriad performance measurement efforts underway today, and there is most notably no national strategy to coordinate and systematize the collection, aggregation, and dissemination of performance measurement data to interested stakeholders (Sidebar 9-3). Indeed, there has been little public policy discussion of—or even a recognized need for—such a national strategy (Joint Commission). The following section explains the historical evolution of quality measures in health care. Understanding the history and where we have been should assist the healthcare industry to formulate a more consistent national strategy for performance data in the future.

The History of Quality Measures in Health Care

Quality is not a new concept. From early civilization it has been important to the survival of humans. Plato has even been credited with inventing the term *quality*. The modern quality movement began in the United States during the late 1920s with the work of Walter Shewhart. Shewhart provided great insight into the collection, analysis, and presentation of data in the quality discipline. He developed control charts that provide a statistical basis for separating variation. In the 1950s Japan emerged as an economic power in response to the emphasis on quality in the writings of W. Edwards Deming, Joseph Juran, and Armand Feigenbaum. Deming advocated improving the system rather than criticizing workers when things went wrong as well as focusing on the processes that needed to be improved. He is also credited with creating the Deming Cycle (Plan-Do-Study-Act). Joseph Juran was instrumental in introducing the quality trilogy of quality planning, quality control, and quality improvement. Juran's focus was on improving the current system. Feigenbaum is credited with the concept of Total Quality Management (TQM).

In the early 1980s the United States recognized and put into practice the works of Deming, Juran, and Feigenbaum. The concepts of these early scholars were embraced by the manufacturing industry, but the healthcare industry did not initially visualize the impact that could be made on health care. During the 1990s, healthcare organizations finally began applying these authors' principles.

Another innovation in quality was Six Sigma, a set of practices perfected by Bill Smith at Motorola in 1986. Six Sigma manages process variations that cause defects and systematically works toward managing variations to eliminate the defects. Bill Smith did not invent Six Sigma; rather he applied methodologies that have been available since the 1920s developed by pioneers like Shewhart, Deming, Juran, Isikawa, and many others. The tools used in Six Sigma programs are actually a subset of the quality disciplines that have used quality control, TQM, and Zero Defects. Many prominent healthcare organizations have adopted the Six Sigma tools as their approach for quality improvement and innovation.

Many other individuals have contributed to the knowledge of quality management. Although each has provided distinct knowledge to the study of quality, there is a consistent link throughout their contributions and ideas.

> **KEY TERM**
>
> **Quality management:** A method for ensuring that all the activities necessary to design, develop, and implement a product or service are effective and efficient with respect to the system and its performance.

Regulatory and Accrediting Agencies

There are many regulatory and accrediting bodies that are driving the use of performance outcomes within health care. These bodies share many similarities in the defining of performance outcomes, but the methods of measurement or the process for collecting information may be different. By understanding the purposes and the focus of these organizations, it is much easier to interpret the information and use it appropriately. The following sections highlight the focuses of the primary regulatory and accrediting agencies.

Center for Medicare and Medicaid Services (CMS)

The **Center for Medicare and Medicaid Services (CMS)** is a U.S. federal agency that administers Medicare, Medicaid, and the State Children's Health Insurance Program. It provides information for health professionals, regional governments, and consumers in regard to how an organization meets the standards set by the CMS. The CMS has a set of rules and regulations that contains the minimum health and safety requirements that hospitals must meet to participate in the Medicare and Medicaid programs. These rules are known as the Conditions of Participation, and every healthcare organization must meet these guidelines in order to be reimbursed for care provided to Medicare clients.

The CMS gives deemed status to some accrediting agencies, which certifies that the accreditation meets the standards set forth by the CMS. In order for a healthcare organization to participate in and receive payment from the Medicare or Medicaid programs, it must meet the eligibility requirements for program participation, including a certification of compliance with the Conditions of Participation, or standards, set forth in federal regulations. This certification is based on a survey conducted by a state agency on behalf of CMS. However, if a national accrediting organization has and enforces standards that meet or exceed the federal Conditions of Participation, CMS may grant the accrediting organization "deeming" authority and deem each accredited healthcare organization as meeting Medicare and Medicaid certification requirements. The accredited healthcare organization would then have deemed status and would not be subject to Medicare's survey and certification process.

CMS is working in conjunction with the Hospital Quality Alliance (HQA), a public-private collaboration on hospital performance measurement and reporting. This collaboration includes the American Hospital Association, the Federation of American Hospitals, and the Association of American Medical Colleges. It is supported by the Agency for Healthcare Research Quality (AHRQ), CMS, and other organizations such as the National Quality Forum, The Joint Commission, the American Medical Association, the Consumer-Purchaser Disclosure Project, the AFL-CIO, AARP, and the U.S. Chamber of Commerce. Through this initiative, a robust, prioritized, and standardized set of hospital quality measures has been refined for use in voluntary public reporting. As the first step, Hospital Compare, a new website/webtool, was developed to publicly report valid, credible, and user-friendly information

about the quality of care delivered in the nation's hospitals (www.cms.hhs.gov/
hospitalqualityinits/25_hospitalcompare.asp).

State Departments of Health

State departments of health regulate healthcare organizations in each state.
Each state's department has the responsibility of overseeing all healthcare organizations to ensure they provide safe care and follow the conditions of participation as outlined by the CMS. States also license healthcare workers including
physicians, nurses, and pharmacists. Many state health departments collect and
provide performance information about specific healthcare providers or organizations. This information is then made available to the public. Table 9-2 contains an example of one Indiana hospital's number of discharges, length of stay,
and cost, from the website of the Indiana State Department of Health.

TABLE 9-2	DESCRIPTIONS AND SELECTED DATA ON FREQUENT ALL PATIENT REFINED DIAGNOSIS RELATED GROUP (APR-DRGS)			
APR-DRG	Description	Number of Discharges	Average Length of Stay (Days)	Average Total Charges ($)
678	Neonate, bwt >2499g, born here, normal nb & nb w other probs	70,203	1.69	$925
372	Vaginal delivery	58,139	1.64	$2,986
430	Psychoses	23,171	13.01	$8,567
89	Simple pneumonia & pleurisy	22,387	5.13	$6,586
127	Heart failure & shock	21,656	5.43	$7,243
370	Cesarean section	16,582	3.16	$5,892
358	Uterine & adnexa proc for Ca in situ & non-malignancy	15,470	2.71	$6,914
88	Chronic obstructive pulmonary disease	14,841	5.31	$6,708
96	Bronchitis & asthma	14,652	3.12	$3,889
296	Nutritional & misc metabolic disorders	13,314	4.24	$4,854

Source: Indiana State Department of Health.

Joint Commission: The Joint Commission is the nation's predominant standards-setting and accrediting body in health care. The Joint Commission's comprehensive accreditation process evaluates an organization's compliance with quality and safety standards and other accreditation requirements.

The Joint Commission

The Joint Commission, an independent, not-for-profit organization, evaluates and accredits nearly 15,000 healthcare organizations and programs in the United States. Its standards focus not simply on an organization's ability to provide safe, high-quality care, but on its actual performance as well. Standards set forth performance expectations for activities that affect the safety and quality of patient care. If an organization does the right things and does them well, there is a strong likelihood that its clients will experience good outcomes. The Joint Commission develops its standards in consultation with healthcare experts, providers, measurement experts, purchasers, and consumers. The results of the survey for accreditation may be accessed on The Joint Commission Web site. Figure 9-1 shows an example of the information that is available at http://www.jointcommission.org/.

For clinicians and clients, outcomes research provides evidence about benefits, risks, and results of treatments so they can make more informed decisions. For example, one group of researchers studied the outcomes of clients with pneumonia, a common cause of hospitalization in elderly people. They developed a way for clinicians to determine which patients with pneumonia can be treated safely at home, an option that not only reduces Medicare costs but also is preferred by many clients and their families. In areas such as cancer, where outright cure is often not the only goal, outcomes research has provided information to help patients make choices that will improve their quality of life.

Outcomes researchers can identify potentially effective strategies they can implement to improve the quality and value of care. AHRQ-sponsored outcomes studies, for example, have shown that even when treatments are known to be effective, many people who could benefit from them are not getting them. Beta-blocker medication, given after myocardial infarction, can reduce mortality; blood-thinning medication can prevent strokes; and thrombolytic ("clot-buster") therapy given immediately after a heart attack can reduce the damage from the attack. Yet in each case, many eligible clients are not getting these treatments (Sidebar 9-4). By identifying and addressing the barriers to better care—for example, through development of a tool to help providers know which clients with suspected myocardial infarction will benefit from thrombolytic treatment—AHRQ researchers have helped translate these findings into practical strategies to improve care at the bedside (http://www.ahrq.gov/clinic/outfact.htm).

SIDEBAR 9-4

Many eligible clients are still not receiving the treatment that has been demonstrated in AHRQ studies to be the most effective.

Accreditation Decision: Accredited		Decision Effective Date: August xx, 2005	
This organization is in full compliance with all applicable standards Special Quality Awards: 2004 Hospital Quality Alliance Participant			
National Patient Safety Goals and National Quality Improvement Goals		**Compared to other Joint Commission Accredited Organizations**	
		Nationwide	**Statewide**
Home Care	2005 National Patient Safety Goals *(see details)*	⊘	N/A
Hospital	2005 National Patient Safety Goals *(see details)*	⊘	N/A
	National Quality Improvement Goals		
Reporting Period: **Jan 2006 - Dec 2006**	Heart Attack Care † *(see details)*	⊖	⊖
	Heart Failure Care † *(see details)*	⊕	⊕
	Pneumonia Care *(see details)*	⊕	⊘
Medicare/Medicaid Certification-Based Long Term Care	2005 National Patient Safety Goals *(see details)*	⊘	N/A
Pathology and Clinical Laboratory	2007 National Patient Safety Goals *(see details)*	⊘	N/A

Figure 9–1 Sample Joint Commission Accreditation Status.

CONTEMPORARY PRACTICE HIGHLIGHT 9-1

AGENCY FOR HEALTHCARE RESEARCH AND QUALITY (AHRQ)

Not only are regulatory and accrediting bodies involved in patient safety and quality, but many government and private sector organizations also have a clear interest in the performance outcomes of healthcare organizations. One such organization is the **Agency for Healthcare Research and Quality (AHRQ)**. The goal of AHRQ is to improve the health and health care of all Americans by supporting and conducting research that provides evidence-based information on healthcare outcomes, quality, cost, use, and access to care. In addition, the AHRQ works with a wide variety of partners to ensure that the results of research are brought to the point of care, and available for use by federal, state, and local policy makers.

Historically, clinicians have relied primarily on traditional biomedical measures, such as the results of laboratory tests, to determine whether a health intervention is necessary and whether it is successful. Researchers have discovered, however, that when they use only these measures, they miss many of the outcomes that matter most to patients. Hence, outcomes research also measures how clients function, their experiences with care, and quality of life.

The Institute for Healthcare Improvement (IHI)

The **Institute for Healthcare Improvement (IHI)** is a not-for-profit organization leading the improvement of health care throughout the world. IHI was founded in 1991 and is based in Cambridge, Massachusetts. IHI's work is funded primarily through their own fee-based program offerings and services, and also through the generous contributions of a distinguished group of foundations, companies, and individuals (www.ihi.org/IHI/About).

The Institute for Healthcare Improvement's (IHI) 5 Million Lives Campaign targets a reduction of five million instances of harm from December 2006 through December 2008. The campaign continues the six interventions of the 100,000 Lives Campaign and adds six more. The campaign's aim is to support the reduction of medical harm, so defined: "Unintended physical injury resulting from or contributed to by medical care (including the absence of indicated medical treatment), that requires additional monitoring, treatment, or hospitalization, or that results in death." The goal of a reduction of five million incidents of harm in two years is based on an estimate that 40 to 50 incidents occur per 100 admissions, for a total of 15 million incidents of medical harm each year in the United States (http://www.ncbi.nlm.nih.gov/pubmed/17724944). Table 9-3 shows the initiatives of this campaign.

The Leapfrog Group was formed in 1998. A group of large employers came together to discuss how they could work together to use the way they purchased health care to have an influence on its quality and affordability. They recognized that there were problems in the healthcare marketplace. Employers were spending billions of dollars on health care for their employees with no way of assessing its quality or comparing healthcare providers. The founders realized that they could take "leaps" forward with their employees, retirees, and families by rewarding hospitals that implement significant improvements in quality and safety. Funding to set up Leapfrog came from the Business Roundtable (BRT) and The Leapfrog Group was officially launched in November 2000. Leapfrog is supported by the BRT, The Robert Wood Johnson Foundation, Leapfrog members, and others (Sidebar 9-5).

Healthcare providers are faced with an increasingly challenging regulatory environment. They need to demonstrate their quality of care to JCAHO and CMS, as well as to a range

TABLE 9-3   INSTITUTE FOR HEALTHCARE IMPROVEMENT CAMPAIGN INITIATIVES

1. **Deploy Rapid Response Teams** … at the first sign of patient decline
2. **Deliver Reliable, Evidence-Based Care for Acute Myocardial Infarction** … to prevent deaths from heart attack
3. **Prevent Adverse Drug Events (ADEs)** … by implementing medication reconciliation
4. **Prevent Central Line Infections** … by implementing a series of interdependent, scientifically grounded steps
5. **Prevent Surgical Site Infections** … by reliably delivering the correct perioperative antibiotics at the proper time
6. **Prevent Ventilator-Associated Pneumonia** … by implementing a series of interdependent, scientifically grounded steps
7. **Prevent Harm from High-Alert Medications** … starting with a focus on anticoagulants, sedatives, narcotics, and insulin
8. **Reduce Surgical Complications** … by reliably implementing all of the changes in care recommended by SCIP, the Surgical Care Improvement Project
9. **Prevent Pressure Ulcers** … by reliably using science-based guidelines for their prevention
10. **Reduce Methicillin-Resistant Staphylococcus aureus (MRSA) infection** … by reliably implementing scientifically proven infection control practices
11. **Deliver Reliable, Evidence-Based Care for Congestive Heart Failure** … to avoid readmissions
12. **Get Boards on Board** … by defining and spreading the best-known leveraged processes for hospital Boards of Directors, so that they can become far more effective in accelerating organizational progress toward safe care

Source: Institute for Healthcare.

of pay-for-performance and quality-improvement initiatives such as the Leapfrog Hospital Rewards Program and the American Heart Association's Get with the Guidelines program.

The **Hospital Quality Initiative (HQI)**, like other CMS quality initiatives, consists of many facets. Its goals are to improve the care provided by the nation's hospitals and to provide quality information to consumers and others. CMS has several efforts in progress to provide hospital quality information to consumers and others and improve the care provided by the nation's hospitals. These activities build upon previous CMS and Quality Improvement Organizations (QIO) efforts on behalf of Medicare beneficiaries and other adults to promote the best medical practices associated with certain clinical conditions. One way that these outcomes are reported is through the Core Measures. These measures represent wide agreement from

KEY TERM

Core measures: Used to measure the quality of care provided by a hospital and its providers for clients with a specific diagnosis such as heart failure, pneumonia, or acute myocardial infarction. These measures are determined by the Center for Medicare and Medicaid Services (CMS), The Joint Commission, and the American Hospital Association.

CMS, the hospital industry, and public sector stakeholders such as the Joint Commission on Accreditation of Healthcare Organizations (JCAHO), the National Quality Forum (NQF), and the Agency for Healthcare Research and Quality (AHRQ). The hospital quality measures currently listed on Hospital Compare have gone through years of extensive testing for validity and reliability by CMS and the QIOs, the Joint Commission, the HQA, and researchers. The hospital quality measures are also endorsed by the National Quality Forum, a national standards-setting entity.

Core Measures

Institute of Medicine (IOM). In 2001, the Institute of Medicine released "Crossing the Quality Chasm: A New Health System for the 21st Century." This landmark report put the spotlight on the issue of poor healthcare quality. The report called for changes to our healthcare system and for collaboration between government and the medical community. Thus in 2003 Congress enacted the Medicare Modernization Act and in 2005 the Deficit Reduction Act, both containing provisions that call upon hospitals to report clinical care data measuring performance. In 2003 hospitals began publishing their performance data on 21 clinical quality measures of care provided to patients admitted for myocardial infarction, heart failure, pneumonia, and surgical care infection prevention. Each hospital submits the data to CMS to receive a score for each of these measures, which represents the percent of cases in which the hospital provided the recommended care. CMS then publishes hospitals' performance data. This allows the public to observe how a hospital is performing relative to other hospitals on each of the 21 measures. This data is published quarterly. An example of Core Performance Measures is in Table 9-4.

All of the Hospital Core Quality Measures used by The Joint Commission and CMS are endorsed by the National Quality Forum (Sidebar 9-6). These measures are also utilized for the "Hospital Quality Alliance: Improving Care through Information" initiative, a voluntary public reporting initiative led by the American Hospital Association, the Federation of American Hospitals, and the Association of American Medical Colleges. This initiative is supported by The Joint Commission, CMS, NQF, Agency for Healthcare Research and Quality, American Federation of Labor and Congress of Industrial Organizations, and AARP (formerly American Association of Retired Persons).

KEY TERM

Institute of Medicine (IOM): Provides a vital service by working outside the framework of government to ensure scientifically informed analysis and guidance. The IOM's mission is to serve as an adviser to the nation to improve health. The IOM provides unbiased, evidence-based, and authoritative information and advice concerning health and science policy to policy makers, professionals, and leaders in every sector of society, and to the public at large.

SIDEBAR 9-6

Currently, Hospital Core Quality Measure sets are for acute myocardial infarction (AMI), heart failure (HF), pneumonia (PN), and Surgical Care Improvement Project (the surgical infection prevention measures were transitioned into SCIP). In addition, The Joint Commission has core measure sets for pregnancy and related conditions (PR) and children's asthma care (CAC).

TABLE 9-4   CORE PERFORMANCE MEASURES

Performance measure	2002	2003	2004	2005	2002–2005 improvement (percentage points)
Heart attack care composite	86.9%	89.8%	91.5%	90.0%	3.1%
Providing smoking cessation advice	66.6%	76.2%	84.2%	92.1%	25.5%
Prescribing ACE inhibitor/ARB at discharge	75.8%	78.5%	79.9%	83.6%	7.8%
Prescribing a beta blocker at discharge	87.3%	90.3%	92.5%	94.8%	7.5%
Prescribing a beta blocker at arrival	85.0%	88.2%	90.0%	92.2%	7.2%
Prescribing aspirin at discharge	92.0%	93.7%	94.5%	95.6%	3.6%
Providing aspirin at arrival	93.0%	94.3%	94.7%	95.4%	2.4%
* Providing thrombolytic therapy within 30 minutes of arrival	N/A	N/A	N/A	38.6%	N/A
* Providing PCI balloon therapy within 120 minutes of arrival	N/A	N/A	N/A	68.3%	N/A
*** Inpatient Mortality see below					
Heart failure care composite	59.7%	66.3%	71.2%	76.0%	16.3%
Providing smoking cessation advice	42.2%	56.8%	69.7%	83.8%	41.6%
Providing discharge instructions	30.9%	42.4%	49.6%	59.2%	28.3%
Providing left ventricular function assessment	81.5%	84.5%	87.5%	90.8%	9.3%
Prescribing ACE inhibitor/ARB at discharge	74.2%	75.8%	76.3%	83.0%	8.8%
Pneumonia care composite	72.3%	76.1%	79.9%	81.0%	8.7%

(continues)

TABLE 9–4 CORE PERFORMANCE MEASURES *(continued)*

Performance measure	2002	2003	2004	2005	2002–2005 improvement (percentage points)
** Inpatient Mortality see below					
Providing smoking cessation advice	37.2%	50.2%	65.5%	80.0%	42.8%
Providing pneumococcal screening & vaccination	30.2%	37.6%	48.8%	62.8%	32.6%
Measuring oxygen in the bloodstream	95.0%	97.2%	98.6%	99.3%	4.3%
Taking a blood test before giving antibiotics	82.0%	82.3%	82.2%	83.1%	1.1%
* Providing antibiotics within four hours of arrival	N/A	N/A	N/A	74.5%	N/A
* Providing antibiotics to intensive care unit patients within 24 hours of arrival	N/A	N/A	N/A	50.1%	N/A
* Providing antibiotics to non-intensive care unit patients within 24 hours of arrival	N/A	N/A	N/A	83.9%	N/A

Currently, Hospital Core Quality Measure sets are for acute myocardial infarction (AMI), heart failure (HF), pneumonia (PN), and Surgical Care Improvement Project (the surgical infection prevention measures were transitioned into SCIP). In addition, The Joint Commission has core measure sets for pregnancy and related conditions (PR) and children's asthma care (CAC).

CMS, along with its sister agency, AHRQ, is in the final stages of developing a standardized survey of patient perspectives of their hospital care, known as Hospital CAHPS (HCAHPS). Information from this survey will be publicly reported on Hospital Compare in the future. Public reporting of standardized measures on patients' perspectives of the quality of hospital care will encourage consumers and their providers to discuss their care and to make more informed decisions on how to get the best hospital care, as well as increase the public accountability of hospitals.

Nursing Performance Indicators

Nurses, as the principal caregivers in any healthcare system, directly and profoundly affect the lives of clients and are critical to the quality of care they receive. Today's nurses practice in an environment that challenges the core of their contribution to quality. Client acuity and shorter lengths of stay, the nursing shortage, changing technology, and expansion of public and community health services must be addressed in the context of quality care. Higher client expectations have produced a greater demand for quality, and mounting financial pressures require nursing to examine the balance of quality and cost.

Nursing care is critical to the quality of client care and the success of any healthcare delivery system. Given the importance of nursing care, the absence of standardized nursing care performance measures is a major void in healthcare quality assurance and work system performance. The need for such measures is intensified by the national nursing shortage. Furthermore, as new ways to deliver client-centered care are developed, standardized ways to measure the performance of care delivered by healthcare teams will be essential to evaluating the effectiveness of these new practices. The following section describes specific initiatives to measure nursing performance.

National Database for Nursing Quality Indicators (NDNQI)

In 1994, the American Nurses Association (ANA) launched the Safety & Quality Initiative to explore and identify the empirical linkages between nursing care and patient outcomes (Sidebar 9-8). The Nursing Care Report Card for Acute Care

SIDEBAR 9-7

Nurses directly and profoundly affect the lives of clients and are critical to the quality of care they receive.

KEY TERM

National Database of Nursing Quality Indicators (NDNQI): The American Nurses Association (ANA) established the National Database of Nursing Quality Indicators (NDNQI) in 1998. It is maintained by the Kansas University Medical Center School of Nursing. Participating hospitals use the database to collect and report unit-specific data. Members receive relevant national comparative data and annual trended comparisons. Nursing-sensitive indicators reflect the structure, process, and outcomes of nursing care.

TABLE 9-5   NURSING-SENSITIVE INDICATORS FROM NDNQI

- Patient Falls
- Patient Falls with Injury
  - Injury Level
- Pressure Ulcer Rate
- Hospital-acquired Pressure Ulcer Rate
- RN Satisfaction
- Nursing Hours per Patient Day
  - RN Hours per Patient Day
  - LPN Hours per Patient Day
  - Unlicensed Assistive Personnel Hours per Hours per Patient Day
- Staff Mix
  - RN
  - LPNs
  - UAP
  - Percent Agency Staff
- RN Education/Certification
- Pediatric Pain Assessment, Intervention Reassessment (AIR) Cycle
- Pediatric Peripheral Intravenous Infiltration
- Psychiatric Physical/Sexual Assault
- Patient Population—Adult or Pediatric
- Hospital Category (teaching, non-teaching, etc)
- Type of Unit
- Number of Staffed Beds Designated by the Hospital

New Indicators Undergoing Development
- Restraints
- Practice Environment
- Nursing Turnover
- Nursing Musculoskeletal Injuries

(ANA, 1995) proposed 21 measures of hospital performance with an established or theoretical link to the availability and quality of nursing services in acute care settings.

Nursing-sensitive indicators (Table 9-5) reflect the structure, process, and outcomes of nursing care. The structure of nursing care is indicated by the supply of nursing staff, the skill level of the nursing staff, and the education/certification of nursing staff. Process indicators measure aspects of nursing care such as assessment, intervention, and RN job satisfaction.

Client outcomes that are determined to be nursing sensitive are those that improve if there is a greater quantity or quality of nursing care (e.g., pressure ulcers, falls, and intravenous infiltrations).

Some client outcomes are more highly related to other aspects of institutional care, such as medical decisions and institutional policies (e.g., frequency of primary C-sections, cardiac failure), and are not considered "nursing-sensitive."

The National Quality Forum (NQF) is a not-for-profit membership organization created to develop and implement a national strategy for healthcare quality measurement and reporting. A shared sense of urgency about the impact of healthcare quality on patient outcomes, workforce productivity, and healthcare costs prompted leaders in the public and private sectors to create the NQF as a mechanism to bring about national change. NQF is leading an effort to understand more fully the extent to which nurses contribute to improved patient safety and healthcare outcomes and promote nursing care quality.

Nursing is the largest healthcare profession in the United States. Nursing constitutes the largest operational expense in any healthcare system.

TABLE 9-6   NQF 15 NATIONAL VOLUNTARY CONSENSUS STANDARDS FOR NURSING-SENSITIVE CARE

Category	Measure
Patient-Centered Outcome Measures	1. Death among surgical inpatients with treatable serious complications (failure to rescue) 2. Pressure ulcer prevalence 3. Fall prevalence 4. Falls with injury 5. Restraint prevalence (vest and limb only) 6. Urinary catheter-associated urinary tract infections for intensive care unit patients 7. Central line catheter-associated bloodstream infection rate for ICU and high-risk nursery (HRN) 8. Ventilator-associated pneumonia for ICU and HRN
Nursing-Centered Intervention Measures	9. Smoking cessation counseling for acute myocardial infarction 10. Smoking cessation counseling for heart failure 11. Smoking cessation counseling for pneumonia
System-Centered Measures	12. Skill mix 13. Nursing care hours per patient day 14. Practice environment scale-nursing work index 15. Voluntary turnover

Nursing is the largest healthcare profession in the United States, with nurses serving as the principal caregivers in hospitals and other institutional care settings. Nursing time constitutes the single largest operational expense in any healthcare delivery system (Sidebar 9-9). However, considering nursing as an organized service and nurses as individual caregivers are critical to optimal healthcare system performance, little attention has been directed toward developing nursing care performance measures. The National Quality Forum (NQF) has endorsed 15 nurse-sensitive measures through its formal Consensus Development Process. This is the first-ever set of national standardized performance measures to assess the extent to which nurses in acute care hospitals contribute to client safety, healthcare quality, and a professional work environment. These consensus standards can be used by consumers to assess the quality of nursing care in hospitals, and they can be used by providers to identify opportunities for improvement of critical outcomes and processes of care. Furthermore, these standards can be used by purchasers to create incentives and reward hospitals for better performance.

SIDEBAR 9-9

Nursing is the largest healthcare profession in the United States. Nursing constitutes the largest operational expense in any healthcare system.

KEY TERM

Magnet status: The Magnet Recognition Program, established by the American Nurses Credentialing Center in 1993, recognizes healthcare organizations that demonstrate excellence in nursing practice and adherence to national standards for the organization and delivery of nursing services.

SIDEBAR 9-10

There are 14 forces of magnetism that must be achieved by an organization prior to becoming designated a magnet hospital.

KEY TERM

Pay-for-performance: An emerging movement in healthcare insurance. Providers under this arrangement are rewarded for meeting pre-established targets for delivery of healthcare services.

TABLE 9-7   FORCES OF MAGNETISM AS DESIGNATED BY AMERICAN NURSES

- Quality of nursing leadership
- Organizational structure
- Management style
- Personnel policies and programs
- Professional models of care
- Quality of care
- Quality improvement
- Consultation and resources

American Nursing Credentialing Center (ANCC) Magnet Recognition Program. Another measure of nursing performance is **Magnet status**. The Magnet designation is awarded by the American Nursing Credentialing Center Magnet Recognition Program to a healthcare organization that has demonstrated an environment of excellence for nursing practice and client care (Sidebar 9-10). Research shows that Magnet hospitals have better client outcomes and a higher level of client and nurse satisfaction compared to non-Magnet hospitals. To achieve this status of excellence, a team of professionals with experience in quality indicators, nursing administration, and nursing care evaluates a hospital's nursing services, clinical outcomes, and client care delivery systems. The forces of magnetism are listed in Table 9-7.

There are 14 forces of magnetism that must be achieved by an organization prior to becoming designated a magnet hospital. Magnet recognition involves the entire hospital but the focus is based on nursing care and nursing satisfaction. As healthcare costs continue to rise the government is looking at ways to reward those individuals and organizations that are consistent in having positive performance outcomes. Pay-for-performance strategies for achieving system-wide improvements in healthcare quality and patient safety are being introduced into the healthcare arena as a strategy to reward good performance outcomes. It promotes structured incentives for practitioners and providers to achieve benchmarks of performance. The hope is that by offering positive rewards—both for reaching thresholds of performance and for making continuous strides in improving the quality of health care—high-quality health care will be delivered on a consistent basis. This approach acknowledges the reality that financial rewards are among the most powerful tools for bringing about behavior change.

However, pay-for-performance programs are operating in a complex reimbursement environment that often creates barriers to reaching the goal of consistent, high-quality care for all patients. For example, payment systems frequently do not recognize the nuances of care delivery, nor do they always pay fairly for important aspects of care, such as activities that support patient education, continuity of care, or integration of services. Many new programs that are seeking to harness payment policy to drive quality and safety goals are either already operative or in development. However, alignment of payment policies to support the provision of safe, high-quality care is a complex undertaking. Such policies and programs must be credible, minimize unintended negative consequences, and most importantly, be transparent and attentive to ethical considerations. It is important to recognize as well that non-financial incentives can also drive positive behavior changes.

Pay-for-performance programs are largely untested. It is important that these programs be well-designed, make every effort to encompass all affected stakeholders for whom the incentives must be aligned, and be designed and implemented in a manner that maintains and continually promotes trust among all of the participating parties. Just as important, the broad-scale implementation and success of these programs must coincide with the timely creation and deployment of an electronic health infrastructure that facilitates the collection, transmittal, and analyses of the performance data that will drive these programs. The design of these programs and ongoing efforts to evaluate their effectiveness should eventually provide the bases for understanding how best to use financial and other incentives to leverage continuous improvement in the safety and quality of health care.

Pay-for-performance programs are largely untested. Further research needs to be conducted to evaluate the effectiveness of the programs (Sidebar 9-11).

Alignment of payment program incentives to support the provision of safe, high-quality care is a complex undertaking, for it must simultaneously achieve fair reimbursement for necessary services, promote desired behavior change, and avoid unintended consequences. In the end, new payment policies and programs must work to the advantage of the client and support the provision of client-centered care.

> **SIDEBAR 9–11**
>
> Pay-for-performance programs are largely untested. Further research needs to be conducted to evaluate the effectiveness of the programs.

Summary

Nursing must become more transparent in the performance outcomes that are specific to nursing care and translated at the bedside to improved outcomes. Measurement of outcomes is profoundly impacting healthcare delivery and reimbursement. The measurement of performance outcomes of nursing care through organizations such as NQF and Magnet demonstrate quality is based on what the client's outcomes show as a direct result of care. Government, both state and federal, are using the data from organizations to compare and choose which individual practitioners and organizations are providing quality.

As performance outcomes become more refined and there is more consensus in the methodology of the data collection, even more emphasis will be placed on these outcomes. Choice of healthcare providers will be based on the clinical performance outcomes. In the past there has been a strong emphasis on financial outcomes and while these outcomes continue to be a driving force in healthcare, more emphasis will be placed on safety and the clinical outcomes of clients. It is important to note that the financial and clinical outcomes are not mutually exclusive. More and more organizations are realizing better financial outcomes as the performance outcomes improve in patient care.

Key Terms

- **Agency for Healthcare Research and Quality (AHRQ):** The health services research arm of the U.S. Department of Health and Human Services (DHHS), complementing the biomedical research mission of its sister agency, the National Institutes of Health. AHRQ is a home to research centers that specialize in major areas of healthcare research such as quality improvement and patient safety, outcomes and effectiveness of care, clinical practice and technology assessment, and healthcare organization and delivery systems.
- **Center for Medicare and Medicaid Services (CMS):** A U.S. federal agency that administers Medicare, Medicaid, and the State Children's Health Insurance Program. It provides information for healthcare professionals, regional governments, and consumers in regard to how an organization meets the standards set by the CMS.
- **Core measures:** Used to measure the quality of care provided by a hospital and its providers for clients with a specific diagnosis such as heart failure, pneumonia, or acute myocardial infarction. These measures are determined by the Center for Medicare and Medicaid Services (CMS), The Joint Commission, and the American Hospital Association.
- **Institute of Healthcare Improvement (IHI):** A not-for-profit organization seeking to improve health care around the world. IHI's work is funded primarily through fee-based program offerings and services, and also through the support of a group of foundations, companies, and individuals. The IHI conducts the 5 Million Lives Campaign.
- **Institute of Medicine (IOM):** Provides a vital service by working outside the framework of government to ensure scientifically informed analysis and guidance. The IOM's mission is to serve as an adviser to the nation to improve health. The IOM provides unbiased, evidence-based, and authoritative information and advice concerning health and science policy to policy makers, professionals, and leaders in every sector of society, and to the public at large.
- **Joint Commission:** The Joint Commission is the nation's predominant standards-setting and accrediting body in health care. The Joint Commission's comprehensive accreditation process evaluates an organization's compliance with quality and safety standards and other accreditation requirements.
- **Leapfrog Group:** A voluntary program aimed at mobilizing employer purchasing power to alert the U.S. health industry on "leaps" in healthcare safety, quality, and customer value so they will be recognized and rewarded. Among other initiatives, Leapfrog works with its employer members to encourage transparency and easy access to healthcare information as well as providing rewards for hospitals that have a proven record of high-quality care.
- **Magnet status:** The Magnet Recognition Program, established by the American Nurses Credentialing Center in 1993, recognizes healthcare organizations

that demonstrate excellence in nursing practice and adherence to national standards for the organization and delivery of nursing services.

- **National Database of Nursing Quality Indicators (NDNQI):** The American Nurses Association (ANA) established the National Database of Nursing Quality Indicators (NDNQI) in 1998. It is maintained by the Kansas University Medical Center School of Nursing. Participating hospitals use the database to collect and report unit-specific data. Members receive relevant national comparative data and annual trended comparisons. Nursing-sensitive indicators reflect the structure, process, and outcomes of nursing care.
- **Pay-for-performance:** An emerging movement in healthcare insurance. Providers under this arrangement are rewarded for meeting pre-established targets for delivery of healthcare services.
- **Performance outcomes:** A predetermined set of goals that are met consistently when the same standards of care are given.
- **Quality management:** A method for ensuring that all the activities necessary to design, develop, and implement a product or service are effective and efficient with respect to the system and its performance.

Reflective Practice Questions

1. Recollect a client you have cared for who experienced a myocardial infarction. How did the Core Quality Measures translate at the bedside for nursing care and overall healthcare toward better outcomes for this client?
2. Compare and contrast the different agencies that are driving the use of performance outcomes in healthcare.
3. How does having magnet status at a hospital affect client performance outcomes? How does magnet status impact the autonomy and satisfaction of nurses?
4. Do you agree or disagree with the concept of *pay-for-performance*? Give rationale to support your stand.

References

Agency for Healthcare Research and Quality. (2004). Guide to Health Care Quality. Retrieved August 3, 2007, from http://www.ahrq.gov

Agency for Healthcare Research and Quality. n.d. The Outcome of Outcomes Research at AHCPR: Final Report. Retrieved August 15, 2007, from http://www.ahrq.gov/clinic/outcosum.htm

ANCC. (2006). Magnet Hospitals. Retrieved August 28, 2007, from http://www.nursingworld.org/ancc/magnet

Barry, R., Murcko, A., & Brubaker, C., (2002). *The Six Sigma book for healthcare: Improving outcomes by reducing errors.* Chicago, IL: Health Administration Press.

Collins, James C. (2001). *Good to great: Why some companies make the leap...and others don't.* New York: Harper Collins.

Indiana State Department of Health

Institute of Healthcare Improvement. (2006). 5 Million Lives Campaign. Retrieved September 19, 2008, from http://www.ihi.org/IHI/Programs/Campaign

Institute of Medicine. (2001). *Crossing the quality chasm: A new health system for the 21st century.* Washington, DC: National Academy Press Publisher.

Institute of Medicine. (1999). *To err is human: Building a safer health system.* Washington, DC: National Academy Press Publisher.

National Quality Forum. (2007). Nursing care quality at NQF. Retrieved August 5, 2007, from http://www.qualityforum.org/nursing

National Quality Forum. (2007). Nursing performance measurement and reporting: A status report. Retrieved August 5, 2007, from http://www.qualityforum.org

National Quality Forum. (2007). Tracking NQF-endorsed consensus standards for nursing-sensitive care. Retrieved August 3, 2007, from http://www.qualityforum.org/nursing

O'Leary, D. Improving America's hospitals: A report on quality and safety. (2005). Retrieved August 5, 2007, from http://www.jointcommissionreport.org

Sower, V. Quality management text manuscript. (2006). Retrieved July 30, 2007, from http://www.shsu.edu/_mgt_ves/mgt481/Chapter1.pdf

Sower, V., Duffy, J., et al. (2001). The dimensions of service quality for hospitals: Development and use of the KQCAH scale. *Health Care Management Review*, 26, 47–59.

chapter 10

Healthcare Delivery

Patricia Gail Colo Braun and Beverly A. Mendes

LEARNING OUTCOMES

After reading this chapter you will be able to:

- List different types of healthcare delivery systems.
- Discuss a variety of reimbursement plans in healthcare delivery.
- Define family and discuss how family and societal changes impact healthcare delivery.
- Identify key challenges facing healthcare providers in the delivery of care today.
- Enhance awareness of the cultural, ethnic, and financial needs of individuals seeking health care.
- Compare and contrast common inpatient and outpatient settings for care delivery.
- Analyze current viewpoints and formulate your own on the issues that impact healthcare delivery today as well as in the future.

Introduction

In today's world of changing healthcare delivery systems, managed care, and capitation, the nursing profession has been called to transform the delivery of the client's care to coordinate with the specific care delivery system. The nursing profession needs to be acquainted with the concepts of insurance programs, managed care, and the needs of uninsured clients to make decisions about how to reduce costs, deliver quality care, and ensure client satisfaction (Ellis & Hartley, 2004). The outcomes of managed care and the rising number of Americans who are uninsured or underinsured have influenced the profession of nursing to respond to healthcare reform measures. Critical thinking and care decisions in partnership with clients and their families are vital to address health outcomes within complicated and expensive delivery system models.

Nursing has evolved from a profession focused on treating illness to one that underscores disease prevention, holistic care, and health promotion through client empowerment. As a discipline, nursing is embedded in the art and science of caring for individuals to regain, maintain, or improve their health, to prevent illness, and to sustain comfort, respect, and dignity. The healthcare system is also a business-oriented enterprise, however, and the practice of nursing is embedded within this context. Therefore, the primary purpose of this chapter is to describe the U.S. healthcare delivery system in terms of reimbursement plans; issues of access, quality, and cost; and common settings for inpatient and outpatient care.

Healthcare Delivery

A **healthcare delivery system** is a mechanism for providing services that meet the health needs of individuals. Healthcare institutions must manage their operating costs and be fiscally responsible in all decisions regarding revenue and expenditures. Nurses and other care providers are continually seeking cost-effective strategies to deliver quality services to clients. In turn, consumers are demanding improved accessibility to quality health services that are affordable.

Over the last several years the healthcare system in the United States has changed the ways in which reimbursement for delivery of services occurs. In the past, healthcare costs were reimbursed to providers as fee-for-service through the client's Medicare or Medicaid coverage, indemnity insurance plan, or self-payment options as arranged by the client and provider. Traditional fee-for-service health care has gradually become less prevalent as cost-saving healthcare options such as **managed care** have become the norm. Managed care health insurance has become the most frequent type of health insurance coverage in the United States. With healthcare costs constantly

KEY TERM

Healthcare delivery system: A mechanism for providing services that meet the health needs of individuals.

KEY TERM

Managed care: Administrative control over primary healthcare services for a defined client population.

SIDEBAR 10-1 INCENTIVES TO PROVIDE CARE AT A LOWER COST

Healthcare providers are faced with an increasingly challenging regulatory environment. Alternative delivery systems have been established over the last decade. These have grown because of an incentive to provide care at a lower cost. Examples of cost-saving measures include increased outpatient surgeries, decreased length of hospital stays, and enhanced home healthcare services. A major restructuring of hospital workforces and cost-cutting systems have been implemented in response to decreased reimbursement rates.

on the rise, managed care health insurance has offered a more affordable option to traditional fee-for-service plans (DeNavas-Walt, 2006).

Healthcare Financing

It is generally concluded that health care in the United States is too expensive. Indeed, healthcare costs have been slowly increasing over the last 25 years (Holahan & Ghosh, 2005). Many factors contribute to the increase in healthcare costs. Hospital spending is one of the major contributing factors, partially due to higher prices being paid for hospital services and a frequent rise in hospital wage rates. Hospital organizations have gained a significant amount of negotiating leverage over health plans and have used this leverage to demand rate increases. These situations have resulted in third-party payers as well as consumers taking political action and demanding quality health care balanced with a reduction of healthcare costs.

Since the early 1980s the basic approach for reimbursing hospitals, physicians, and long-term care providers of services has been restructured. This trend has resulted in government, public sectors, and private insurance payers creating varied reimbursement plans to healthcare providers and institutions for their healthcare delivery. A complex blend of private and public mechanisms has arisen to affect how Americans pay for health care. Health insurance covers a wide array of healthcare financing methods including the social insurance of Medicaid, the self-insurance plans of employers, and the managed care programs of health maintenance organizations (HMOs) and preferred provider organizations (PPOs).

Medicare and private health insurance play a vital role in influencing the direction and structure of our nation's healthcare system. After Medicare, private health insurance has been the most prevalent source of financing for the U.S. healthcare system. Health insurance is a mechanism created to help protect against risk and against potential substantial financial loss from a catastrophic illness. A person protected by insurance against a specific risk is called the insured.

Insured clients pay for a portion of their health care themselves. Persons not covered by either private or government-supported health financing programs are called uninsured.

Private Health Insurance

Private health insurance may be acquired by an individual or a group. Group insurance measures the risk for the insured group, resulting in lower premiums for each member. Indemnity commercial health insurance reimburses healthcare providers through a fee for each health service provided to the insured person. The traditional method for reimbursement was retrospective; the amount of insurance paid was based on the service received. This type of insurance also provided catastrophic coverage, thus paying for major medical events like an automobile accident or major surgery.

Managed Care Organizations

Currently healthcare coverage is more likely to be administered by a managed care organization. Managed care is a system that controls the utilization and cost of services by limiting unnecessary treatment (Shi & Singh, 2003). Healthcare delivery under a managed care organization is designed to affect the operation and structure of the healthcare system and thus affect the use of services by the consumer. Managed care attempts to control costs by controlling access to unnecessary care.

The primary care physician or primary nurse practitioner is the gatekeeper in the managed care system. This provider has the coordinating role for the client's healthcare needs by being responsible for all primary care for the client and determining when referral to specialists is necessary. The goal of this gatekeeper concept is to reduce the client's use of resources and self-initiated use of specialty services and to ensure overall coordination without duplication of care.

Health Maintenance Organizations

A health maintenance organization (HMO) is a prepaid health plan that delivers comprehensive health care to members through designated providers, has a fixed monthly payment for healthcare services, and requires members to be in a plan for a specified period of time, usually one year. HMOs are a type of group healthcare practice that provides basic and supplemental health maintenance and treatment services to voluntary enrollees who prepay a fixed periodic fee that is set without

---

KEY TERM

Managed care organization (MCO): Receives a predetermined capitated payment for each client enrolled in the program.

SIDEBAR 10-2

The term *managed care* describes administrative control over primary healthcare services for a defined client population. The managed care organization (MCO) or healthcare system receives a predetermined capitated payment for each client enrolled in the program. The MCO accepts the financial risk for the provision of client care. The client is required to use only primary care physicians, and referrals to specialists must be approved by the organization.

regard to the amount or kind of services received. All health care is obtained from hospitals, physicians, and other providers participating in the HMO.

A preferred provider organization (PPO) may be organized by a group of physicians and nurse practitioners, an outside entrepreneur and insurance company, or a company with a self-insurance plan. The PPO is the insurance industry's response to the growth of HMOs. Contractual arrangements are made by PPOs with providers for the delivery of healthcare services on a discounted fee schedule (Shi & Singh, 1998).

Government Insurance Plans

Public financing of healthcare services accounts for roughly 46 percent of the total expenditures of health care in the United States. Medicare and Medicaid are well-established programs. Similar to Social Security, **Medicare** is a healthcare entitlement program for persons over the age of 65 years and for some chronically ill persons. Individuals have contributed toward Medicare via taxes. People are entitled to the benefits regardless of their income and assets. **Medicaid** is a "welfare" program in which the amount of benefits depends on a person's income and assets. Medicare and Medicaid purchase government-funded services from the private sector (Shi & Singh, 1998).

> **KEY TERM**
>
> **Medicaid:** A grant program or government insurance plan providing partial healthcare services for indigent people.

> **KEY TERM**
>
> **Medicare:** Similar to Social Security, Medicare is an entitlement program. Individuals have contributed toward Medicare via taxes. People over the age of 65 years and some chronically ill persons are entitled to the health benefits regardless of their income and assets.

Medicare was enacted in 1965 as Title XVIII of the Social Security Act. Healthcare services are provided for those disabled persons who are eligible for Medicare Part A, which pays for hospitalization and some skilled care posthospitalization. Medicare Part B coverage has a monthly premium for people desiring supplemental insurance. Medicare recipients can also participate in a managed care organization.

Medicaid is a grant program providing partial healthcare services for indigent people. The federal government provides matching funds to the states on the basis of the per-capita income in each state. By law, the federal matching dollars cannot be less than 50 percent or more than 83 percent of the total state Medicaid program costs.

A prospective payment system (PPS) is a payment system in which the amount paid for a specific service is predetermined. This system was implemented for short stay inpatient hospitalizations (Medicare Part A) in the mid-1980s under the Social Security Act of 1983. The predetermined reimbursement amount is set according to the diagnosis-related groups (DRGs), a system of classification or grouping of clients according to medical diagnosis. Payment is based on diagnosis and date of discharge rather than length of stay per diem. It also is based on a range set for "bundled services" (Kovner & Jonas, 2002).

Another form of payment is a capitation system. In this system, payment for healthcare services is based on an arrangement between the purchaser of care and the provider; the provider receives a flat fee to provide a defined level for care. The provider therefore theoretically has an investment in keeping the enrollee healthy.

Economic and Quality Concerns

Changing economic conditions contribute to the rise in economic healthcare costs. Softer labor markets, increasing unemployment rates, and lower profit margins drive employers to control the company's increased insurance premium expenses through insurance buy-down programs that reduce employee benefits and increase employee costs. "The large benefits buy-down in 2002 was driven by low cost sharing changes as a result of a large increase in network Preferred Provider Organization (PPO) deductibles and increases in drug co-payment amounts" (Strunk, Ginsburg, & Gabel, 2002, p. 307).

Recent healthcare cost data provides evidence that managed care's ability to constrict payment rates for the use of

SIDEBAR 10-3

To become leaders in health care, nurses must understand the healthcare system and the issues that impact how care is provided and reimbursed. Under managed care contracts, pressure exists on hospitals and physicians to use resources more efficiently and decrease hospital admissions for clients. In a managed care system, what role should nurses have in decisions on care delivery for clients and their families?

CONTEMPORARY PRACTICE HIGHLIGHT 10-1

HEALTH PROMOTION AND ILLNESS PREVENTION

Health promotion attempts to modify a client's knowledge, attitudes, and skills to adopt behaviors leading to a healthier lifestyle, thus achieving a higher level of wellness on any point on a continuum from health to illness. Illness prevention involves the use of immunizations and medications that prevent disease or detect disease in its earliest, most treatable stages. Diagnosis and treatment of illness will continue to be a major element of the healthcare system. Nurses, as health promoters and educators, play a vital role in health promotion. Clients and their families can be empowered with knowledge that may have a lifelong impact.

- What is the importance of health promotion to you as a nurse?
- Is health promotion only for those people who have insurance?
- How do politics, culture, and various reimbursement plans shape the outlook of health promotion for clients and healthcare providers?

hospital services has decreased. According to the most recent trends in private health care, costs are back to where they were before managed care began to dominate the health insurance landscape (Strunk et al., 2002).

Issues Affecting Healthcare Delivery: Changes in Society and Families

Healthcare delivery and access to healthcare providers are challenged by the evolving changes in the health-promotion model, demographics of society, and family structure. The major purposes of health care are to promote wellness and prevent illness and disability. *Disease prevention* activities are focused on the individual, the family, and/or the community. Services are aimed at caring for an individual after a disease or disability has developed. *Health promotion* is centered on prevention, advocating self-care; the interactive nature of family, culture, and community; continuity; and collaboration of care. Traditionally the U.S. healthcare system concentrated on disease prevention rather than health promotion; however, within the past decade it has engaged in more health-promoting behaviors.

Changes in the composition of a population are important for the planning of healthcare services. The age of the population, the contribution of family support systems, and health problems of specific groups affect the need for specific services. The aging population in the United States has created a demand for services for older adults. The U.S. Bureau of the Census predicted that in the year 2010 approximately 40 million Americans will be age 65 years or older. People 85 years or older are the fastest growing group of the U.S. population.

Families are a group of individuals that interact together, share common beliefs and values, care and relate to each other, and share strengths and weaknesses. Families are connected by their relationship with each other, and they may change structurally over time. Families function to meet goals. These goals are achieved over time and are influenced by trends in families or evolving health needs as the family grows and changes. Although the traditional family as we know it (mother at home, father, children) is still intact, single-parent families, divorced parents with both parents working, live-in partners, and homosexual partners that may have children challenge traditional healthcare delivery and call for more unique and creative ways to deliver and access care. In 1980, 77 percent of children in a home were living with both parents. In 2003, only 68 percent of children

KEY TERM

Family: A group of individuals that interact together, share common beliefs and values, and care and relate to each other. Families are connected by their relationship with each other and they may change structurally over time.

in the United States living at home were living with both parents (America's Children, 2007). Thus, healthcare delivery has changed to take into account the changing structure of family and society. Home visits, evening/weekend appointments/clinics, and email communication are examples of how changes in family structure are influencing healthcare delivery and access for today's families.

Healthcare access and delivery also have changed because urban living has become more common as U.S. cities have expanded. Family support systems have declined as the United States has evolved from a rural economy with large families to a nation of city residents with small families often a long distance from their family of origin. (See Chapter 18 for more on urban healthcare issues.)

The issues related to our changing society and family structure are different today as compared to even the last decade. A family seeking prenatal care for an adolescent or a family 40 years or over experiencing their first pregnancy has very unique needs. Families who have a child with a chronic condition or illness face day-to-day challenges that often require a wide variety of specialization from healthcare providers. Coordination of care for a child with a chronic condition can be complex. As the child grows and develops, it is important for the nurse to enlarge the circle of providers to include school and other community-based agencies. The delivery system for the child and family can include a wide variety of agencies and locations such as neighborhood centers or parishes. (See "Parish Nursing" later in this chapter.)

Vulnerable Populations

The United States can be described as a country of diversity that includes different vulnerable populations including ethnic minority groups, the poor, those with a variety of religious beliefs, and immigrants. These groups diversify further by gender, race, and social class. A wide range of disparities in education and income levels associated with vulnerable populations affect access to health care and opportunities for health-promotion activities (see Chapter 13). The changing ethnic composition of the United States is creating a demand for a healthcare system that is more responsive to minorities and the needs of the vulnerable. Hispanics, Muslims, and Asians are among the minority ethnic and religious groups whose presence is noticeably increasing in the United States. There is a growing demand for healthcare providers who speak languages other than English and understand the health needs of a multiethnic society.

In the 21st century, ethnic minorities are estimated to make up 28.2 percent of the U.S. population and are expected to climb to 37 percent by the year 2025 (U.S. Census Bureau, 1999). The economic, social, and political issues that result from these growing populations will impact these groups' access to health care and services that are affordable. Healthcare personnel, especially in nursing, also need to become more diversified to meet the health needs of the growing body of people with diverse ethnic backgrounds requiring care.

Vulnerable populations include the uninsured, the working poor who do not receive adequate health benefits, and the underinsured. These groups receive less than adequate health care, often receiving too little too late. Limited access to preventive care often results in crisis visits to emergency rooms and urgent care centers. The underserved often receive little primary prevention or continuity of care for chronic conditions (see Chapter 13). The underserved also often receive their health care from the public sector and through local, state, and federal funding. This places a great strain on healthcare services in communities, adding to the burden of disease costs (Institute of Medicine, 2003). Over one-third of the U.S. public is uninsured or underinsured. The U.S. government and the voting public are examining various universal healthcare programs. It is possible that forthcoming legislation would enact a national health insurance plan in the future.

> **SIDEBAR 10-5**
>
> Vulnerable populations include the uninsured, the poor, the working poor who do not receive adequate health benefits, and the underinsured. Economic, social, and political issues of vulnerable populations need to be addressed in the healthcare system and delivery models.
>
> Vulnerable populations often receive little preventative care, resulting in them seeking care in a health crisis.

> **SIDEBAR 10-6**
>
> Nursing needs to promote diversity within the profession.

The inequitable distribution of wealth is a contributing factor to the uneven distribution of health care. Many Americans living in poverty are the victims of social and environmental harms such as drug addiction, acquired immunodeficiency syndrome (AIDS), crime, and chronic illness. Their children also suffer from addiction and low birth weight with consequential mental and physical problems. The need for health services for vulnerable populations is strongly tied to the poor economic conditions of the communities in which they reside.

Crossing the Quality Chasm

Major changes in the structure of the U.S. healthcare system, including the increasing influence of market forces, changes in payment and delivery systems, and welfare reform, have significant implications for healthcare delivery. Federal, state, and local public health agencies must strengthen their efforts to address access to quality services. Globally, health care is threatened by a convergence of powerful trends: increasing demand, rising costs, uneven quality, and misaligned incentives. If ignored, these trends will overwhelm healthcare systems, creating massive financial burdens as well as health problems for current and future generations.

Crossing the Quality Chasm, a New Health System for the 21st Century was developed by the Committee of Quality of Health Care in America, Institute of Medicine (IOM, 2001) to create strategies for fostering greater accountability for quality of care. The report identified important areas of research that should be pursued to facilitate improvements in quality. The major focus is centered upon the personal healthcare delivery system, specifically, the provision of preventive, acute, chronic, and end-of-life health care for individuals.

Presently, patient safety has emerged as the most urgent issue. In its report, *To Err Is Human: Building a Safer Health System*, the Institute of Medicine (1994) discovered that tens of thousands of Americans die each year due to errors in health care, and hundreds of thousands suffer or barely escape from nonfatal injuries that a truly high-quality care system would largely prevent. The IOM Committee of Quality of Health Care in America's narrative on safety tells a disturbing story about the quality of U.S. health care—multiple widespread shortcomings combined with the lack of quality resources. The patient safety report was a cry for action to make care safer and to improve the U.S. healthcare delivery system as a whole, in all its quality dimensions.

CONTEMPORARY PRACTICE HIGHLIGHT 10-2

CANADA'S IMPACT ON HEALTH PROMOTION

The term *health promotion* was coined in a 1974 report by Canadian Health Minister Marc Lalonde (MacDonald, 1992). This classic report ignited the concept of healthcare promotion, policy development, and new strategies for health professionals to practice. Health promotion initiatives grew worldwide when the World Health Organization began a campaign for global public health. Canada has worldwide recognition for health promotion and has presented its theoretical frameworks to other countries.

Comparatively, the United States was not a leader in the initial health promotion movement. The United States created *Healthy People 2000*, followed by *Healthy People 2010*, to provide a type of national framework for the health of all Americans (U.S. Department of Health and Human Services [USDHHS], 2000; U.S. Public Health Service, 1990). The latest document, *Healthy People 2010* (http://www.health.gov/healthypeople/), is intended to improve the health of all people in the United States in the first decade of the 21st century. Individual health and community health are linked, creating a healthy community and improving the overall health status of the nation. The two main goals are to increase quality and years of healthy life and to eliminate health disparities. The 2010 edition includes 28 focus areas with 467 objectives. The document is separated into four major areas: 1) promoting healthy behaviors, 2) promoting healthy and safe communities, 3) improving systems for personal and public health, and 4) preventing and reducing diseases and disorders.

- Compare and contrast the Canadian National Health System with the insurance and managed care industry in the United States. Analyze the advantages and disadvantages of both.

Healthcare Delivery Settings

The healthcare system is designed to provide comprehensive health services for the individual, family, and community. The following sections will discuss common delivery settings: hospitals, rural hospitals, psychiatric facilities, extended care facilities, rehabilitation, hospice, home care, parish nursing, and adult day care centers.

Hospitals

Hospitals are institutions for the medical and nursing care of ill and injured persons requiring complex services with a high risk of complications. Hospital services are appropriate when intensive monitoring is necessary for the detection or prevention of complication from an injury or illness. Hospitals offer an array of inpatient and outpatient services for acute and subacute conditions. Services include emergency, rehabilitative, and skilled nursing care. Some hospitals serve multiple purposes in a community.

General hospitals offer a wide range of medical, surgical, obstetrical, pediatric, and emergency services. A community hospital serves a specific location in an area of a city or a suburban or rural community. Rural hospitals are often limited in the scope of their services compared to urban hospitals. Poor economic conditions, isolated rural areas, weather conditions, limited availability of transportation, and long distances affect rural residents' access to health care. Rural hospitals have difficulty recruiting healthcare providers such as pediatricians, obstetricians, internists, and nurses.

Large urban hospitals provide a full complement of services including state-of-the-art technological care by specialists. Tertiary hospitals are large medical centers that provide highly sophisticated care and maintain extensive research and teaching programs. Tertiary care centers attract consumers of care from larger geographical areas.

Hospitals are classified as either public or private. Public hospitals are owned by agencies of the federal, state, or local government. Federal hospitals are maintained for special groups of federal beneficiaries such as military and government personnel, veterans, and Native Americans. State governments limit themselves to operating hospitals intended to safeguard public health by treating mental illness and contagious disease. Private hospitals are owned and operated by corporations or charitable organizations. As health care grew to be one of the largest industries in the United States, multi-hospital chains developed in response. The change in reimbursement methods and the need to constrain costs while still providing a variety of healthcare services forced cost

SIDEBAR 10-8

Nurses must recognize the importance of a competitive environment. Consumers of health care are more informed than ever before and have high expectations for services.

constraints that allowed large corporations to be at a market advantage over smaller single-hospital systems.

Rural Primary Care Hospitals

Many rural hospitals in the United States have been forced to close due to economic failure and a shortage of primary care providers and nurses. Major changes in the healthcare delivery system and the impact of local economies and occupational foundations have altered distribution, recruitment, and retention factors in nursing. Healthcare reform has prompted innovative approaches for major tertiary centers to establish affiliations or mergers with rural hospitals. Nurse practitioners are serving a valuable need in rural communities, where they use medical protocols or work under collaborative agreements with staff physicians. Rural hospitals in remote areas provide life-sustaining treatment for inpatient care, and acutely ill or injured clients prior to being transferred to an acute care or tertiary center.

Psychiatric Care Facilities

Clients with mental health and behavioral problems such as depression, anxiety, violent behavior, and eating disorders often require special counseling and treatment in psychiatric facilities. Hospitalization involves a short length of stay for treatment with the intent to transfer to outpatient treatment centers. Clients are referred for community follow-up at clinics or with counselors at discharge.

The number of public and private psychiatric facilities and the number of beds devoted to inpatient psychiatric facilities have decreased over the past two decades. New treatment methods, consumer protection laws, and issues of cost are responsible for the change from inpatient care to community care. The result of the shift to community care and the client's right to refuse treatment has contributed to an increased number of homeless people who have difficulty managing their mental illness and adhering to their medication regimens.

Extended Care Facilities

Extended care facilities provide nursing, custodial, and intermediate medical care for clients recovering from an acute or chronic illness or disability. Hospitals are focused on early discharge practices, so elderly patients as well as younger clients are often admitted to extended care facilities. Often younger clients have sustained a trauma due to an accident and require rehabilitative or supportive care prior to discharge home. Intermediate care facilities, also known as skilled nursing facilities (SNFs), are part of the system of care. They provide skilled care by a licensed nursing staff. Clients often require wound care, long-term ventilator management, intravenous fluids, and physical rehabilitation.

More than half of the financial support for 24-hour patient coverage in extended care originates from public funds such as Medicaid and Medicare. Medicare covers 100 days of SNF treatment, with the dollar amount covered decreasing after the first 20 days. According to Lueckenotte (2000), the client's diagnosis should be appropriate for the therapy received.

Additional care options for seniors include assisted-living facilities, residential care, and retirement centers. Assisted-living arrangements offer services associated with a resident's activities of daily living. Residential care services offer assistance with meals and medicine. Retirement centers foster self-care so residents can maintain their own lifestyle while having some services available for those who require them.

Long-term care is closely regulated through licensure and certification requirements. For clients who are unable to care for themselves and have no expectation of improvement, the only source of public funding for long-term care is Medicaid.

SIDEBAR 10-10

Clients with a chronic illness and disabilities have long-term care needs across their life span. Continuing care is offered in nursing homes, nursing centers, group homes, retirement communities, adult day care, and senior centers.

Rehabilitation

Rehabilitation goals are centered on restoration of function, maintenance of the remaining levels of physical and mental function, and prevention of further deterioration. Rehabilitation activities are beneficial for a wide range of health problems—such as stroke, joint replacement, burns, and spinal cord injury—that occur in persons with an acute or chronic illness or for a time-limited basis. Rehabilitation services also are utilized by clients with past illnesses or injuries that have left them with residual physical or mental impairments that affect their ability to function normally. People are living longer with chronic illness and often need rehabilitation services.

Palliative Care

Supportive care consists of nursing, medical, psychological, and social services aimed at helping the client manage chronic illness, disability, or terminal illness when rehabilitation or restoration is not a realistic goal. This care is offered in a hospital, nursing home, hospice, or client home setting to meet the physical, emotional, spiritual, and cultural needs of the client and the family. Major efforts are concentrated on helping the client to achieve or maintain the highest level of functioning, permitting the greatest degree of independence and participation in the community.

SIDEBAR 10-11

Specialized rehabilitation services, such as cardiovascular and pulmonary programs, have emerged to assist clients and families in adjusting to new challenges. Lifestyle modification focuses on helping the client to live at the highest level of function and quality of life. Nurses and other members of the healthcare team often visit clients in their homes to help the client gain the maximum level of independence.

SIDEBAR 10-12

Family dynamics, cultural practices, and spiritual values are essential assessments when forming care partnerships with the client and family in their home.

SIDEBAR 10-13

Home care reimbursement is covered by government insurance plans such as Medicare and Medicaid, by self-payment, and by private insurance.

Hospice

Hospice incorporates special services that address the unique needs of dying people and their families. Medical, spiritual, legal, financial, and family support services are provided. Hospice is a system of family-centered care that embraces the client together with the family as the unit of care. Hospice often allows clients to remain at home with comfort and dignity. Care may vary from specialized care in the home to care in a nursing home, hospital, freestanding hospice, or home health agency. Many hospice programs also offer respite care provided in the agency to promote family and caregiver relief, which is vital to preserve the health of the primary caregivers and family.

Home Healthcare Services

Home healthcare services are provided to individuals and families in their home to promote, maintain, or restore health, or to maximize their level of independence while minimizing the effects of disability and illness (Stanhope, 2000). Home care provides an array of allied professional and paraprofessional services and assistive equipment to clients and families in their homes for health maintenance, education, illness prevention, diagnosis and treatment, palliation, and rehabilitation. Nursing care is the major service offered by Medicare home care. Home services also include physical, occupational, speech, and respiratory therapy. Home care agencies also provide skilled nursing care such as wound care and ostomy management.

Parish Nursing

Parish nursing began almost 30 years ago. It was originated by a Lutheran pastor, Dr. Granger Westberg, in 1985. Parish nursing has expanded from the original six nurses working with Dr. Westberg to more than 3,000 nurses in a parish setting today (Dochterman McCloskey & Bulechek, 2004). Parish nurses are found throughout the United States and represent most religious denominations. They provide a holistic focus to the ongoing care of children and families while respecting spiritual and religious needs.

The role of the parish nurse is very independent and innovative. Community based, the parish nurse focuses on members of his or her church community. The parish nurse promotes health and healthy lifestyles for the members of the church community in which they serve. Depending on the size of the parish or church community, the parish nurse may serve one church or several churches in his or her community. A key element is that the parish nurse is in the immediate environment to maintain a caring relationship with children, the elderly, and other family members.

The health ministry and practices of a nurse assuming the parish nurse role are governed by *Scope and Standards of Parish Nursing Practice*. These standards were established in 1998 by the American Nurses Association (ANA) and the Health Ministry Association and provide a description and standardization of common practices and characteristics of a parish nurse. They also help to establish practice guidelines for nurses in a faith ministry. This guide also outlines the scope of parish nursing and direction for documentation using systems such as the North American Nursing Diagnosis Association (NANDA) and Nursing Outcome Classification (NOC) system.

Parish nursing is growing in local communities, states, and nationally as well as internationally. Parish nurses, also called faith, congregational, or church nurses, are making significant contributions to families in congregations throughout the world. The parish nurse provides continuity of care at the community grass-roots level to improve holistic health outcomes.

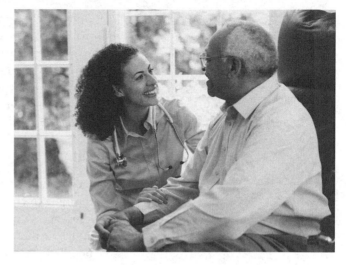

A nurse and patient talk during a home visit. *Source:* © Corbis Collection/Alamy Images

KEY TERM

Parish nurses: Promote holistic health and healthy lifestyles for the church community members they serve.

SIDEBAR 10-14

Parish nurses are innovative and independent in their community roles, providing care to parish members and their families.

Adult Day Care Centers

Adult day care centers are part of a system that may be associated with a hospital, nursing facility, or independent center. A range of health and social services are provided to specific client populations who live alone or with family in the community. They allow family members who are care providers to continue their lifestyles and employment and still provide home care for their relatives. Older adults receive physical rehabilitation, daily counseling, or supervision. Clients with chemical dependency requiring rehabilitation often attend day centers. Healthcare costs are reduced because the client receives care and services during the day while still living at home.

Respite care is a service that provides temporary relief to informal caregivers such as family members who care for children, psychiatric clients, or frail older adults. Home respite care provides temporary homemaker or home health services. Adult day care is a type of respite care. The caregiver is able to leave the home for errands or well-needed social time while a responsible person stays in the home to care for the loved one.

Summary

Changes and trends in the care of individuals and families will continue to challenge healthcare systems. Nurses need to address access, quality, safety, and the cost of health care within the business context of the delivery systems. Vulnerable populations, the uninsured, and the underinsured will continue to impact delivery systems. Scarcity and lack of resources and poor access to the healthcare delivery system are challenges that must continue to be addressed. A wide variety of innovative healthcare roles and delivery systems will continue to evolve to provide quality care in a wide variety of diversified environments. The nursing profession needs to be informed of the concepts of insurance programs, managed care, reimbursement plans, and government programs. Nurses need to clarify their own viewpoints on health issues and be involved in future policies and legislation regarding the healthcare delivery system.

Key Terms

- **Family:** A group of individuals that interact together, share common beliefs and values, and care and relate to each other. Families are connected by their relationship with each other and they may change structurally over time.
- **Healthcare delivery system:** A mechanism for providing services that meet the health needs of individuals.
- **Home health services:** An array of allied professional and paraprofessional services and assistive equipment provided to clients and families in their homes.
- **Hospice:** Incorporates special services that address the unique needs of dying people and their families. Medical, spiritual, legal, financial, and family support services are provided.
- **Managed care:** Administrative control over primary healthcare services for a defined client population.
- **Managed care organization (MCO):** Receives a predetermined capitated payment for each client enrolled in the program.
- **Medicaid:** A grant program or government insurance plan providing partial healthcare services for indigent people.
- **Medicare:** Similar to Social Security, Medicare is an entitlement program. Individuals have contributed toward Medicare via taxes. People over the age of 65 years and some chronically ill persons are entitled to the health benefits regardless of their income and assets.
- **Parish nurses:** Promote holistic health and healthy lifestyles for the church community members they serve.
- **Respite care:** A service that provides temporary relief to informal caregivers such as family members who care for children, psychiatric clients, or frail older adults.

Reflective Practice Questions

1. Is access to affordable healthcare delivery more effective with the managed care model? How have the various delivery systems impacted the quality and cost of health care?
2. Reflect on the multiple influences responsible for changes in healthcare delivery. Analyze the advantages and disadvantages of private insurance, Medicaid, Medicare, private self-payment systems, and universal or national health systems.
3. Do you believe health care is a privilege or a right? Should all people have access to the same healthcare services regardless of ability to pay or citizenship status?
4. What changes do you see in your community that are redefining the family as a structure in society? Identify access and care issues for families in your community.

5. What efforts can be made to deliver quality health care to those who cannot afford it? Is the answer a national or universal healthcare program?

6. What are some variables in delivering quality health care to a diversified population in your community? How would you encourage the community members to become involved in the community health services?

7. What are some of the challenges that individuals from diverse cultures and ethnic backgrounds face when entering the nursing profession?

8. Is it good to have competition in the healthcare environment? Does this limit services to those most in need?

9. Does a competitive healthcare environment promote quality of care?

10. How can family dynamics be assessed so that a healthcare provider can assist and support families in making critical decisions in health care?

11. How is home care delivery influenced by the client's type of insurance?

12. How does the term *parish nurse* reflect the role of this type of healthcare provider?

References

America's Children, *Key national indicators of well-being.* 2007. Retrieved July 26, 2008 from http://childstats.gov/americaschildren/highlights.asp

American Nurses Association. (1998). *Scope and standards of parish nursing practice.* Washington, DC: Author.

Committee on Quality of Health Care in America & Institute of Medicine (2001). *Crossing the quality chasm: A new health system for the 21st century.* Washington, DC: National Academy Press.

DeNavas-Walt, C. (2006). *Income, poverty, and health insurance coverage in the United States: 2005.* U.S. Census Bureau, Current Population Reports, P60-231. Washington, DC: U.S. Government Printing Office.

Dochterman McCloskey, J. C., & Bulechek, G. M. (Eds.). (2004). *Nursing intervention classification (NIC)* (4th ed.). St. Louis, MO: Mosby.

Ellis, J. R., & Hartley, C. L. (2004). *Nursing in today's world: Trends, issues and management.* Philadelphia: Lippincott Williams & Wilkens.

Hoffman, E. B. (2006, November). Retrieved October 17, 2007, from http://22/smshhs.gov/Medicare

Holahan & Ghosh, 2005

Institute of Medicine. (1994). *Defining primary care: An interim report.* Washington, DC: National Academy Press.

Institute of Medicine. (2000). *To err is human: Building a safer health system.* Washington, DC: National Academy Press.

Kovner, A. R., & Jonas, S. (2002). *Health care delivery in the United States.* New York: Springer.

Lueckenotte, A. (2000). *Gerontologic nursing* (2nd ed.). St. Louis, MO: Mosby.

MacDonald, G. (1992). Health promotion: Discipline or disciples? In *Health promotion: disciplines and diversity* (pp.). New York: Routledge.

Singh, D. A., & Shi , L. (2003). Delivering Health Care in America. Sudbury, MA: Jones and Bartlett Publishers.

Stanhope, M. (2000). Community health nursing in home health and hospice care. In M. Stanhope (Ed.), *Community health nursing: Process and practice for promoting health* (5th ed.). St. Louis, MO: Mosby.

Strunk, B. C., Ginsburg, P. B., & Gabel, J. R. (2002, August). *Tracking health care costs: Growth accelerates again in 2001.* Retrieved July 14, 2008, from http://content.health affairs.org/cgi/content/abstract/hlthaff.w2.299v1

U.S. Census Bureau, 1999. *Statistical abstract of the United States.* Retrieved July 25, 2008 from http://www.census.gov/prod/2001pubs/statab/sec01.pdf

U.S. Department of Health and Human Services. (2002). *Healthy people 2010.* Washington, DC: Government Printing Office.

U.S. Public Health Service. (1990). *Healthy people 2000. National health promotion and disease prevention objectives.* Washington, DC: Government Printing Office.

chapter

11

Evidence–Based Nursing Practice

Mary Reid Nichols and Nena R. Harris

LEARNING OUTCOMES

After reading this chapter you will be able to:

- Describe and differentiate between evidence-based practice (EBP) and evidence-based nursing (EBN).
- Describe the principles of evidence to guide clinical practice.
- Synthesize the components of EBP.
- Analyze and provide examples of the different types of evidence that currently guide practice.
- Discuss the process of EBP.
- Describe the levels of evidence and critically appraise research findings.
- Understand the Stetler Model of Research Utilization.
- Use specific clinical examples to apply research evidence.

Introduction

Evidence-based practice (EBP) is foundational for excellent clinical practice, in the development of practice guidelines, and in making decisions about diagnostic testing and changes in treatments or procedures (Klardie, Johnson, McNaughton, & Meyers, 2004). EBP begins with a clinical question (e.g., "What is the best way to reduce the severity of neonatal lung

Evidence-based practice (EBP):
The process of problem solving using the best research evidence in clinical decision making for patient care. It is a combination of a systematic search for and critical appraisal of the most relevant research available to answer a specific clinical question, with the clinician's own clinical expertise and patient values and preferences included.

Evidence-based nursing (EBN):
Clinical decision making by nurses that is a combination and integration of the best research evidence; it also includes the nurse's clinical expertise and patient values and preferences about a specific type of care.

disease?") and advances to identify and evaluate the best research available to answer the question (e.g., "Prenatal steroids reduce the severity of neonatal lung disease") (Cochrane Collaboration, 2001).

Of concern is that EBP principles have been adopted by only about 15 percent of clinicians, despite data that indicate quality healthcare outcomes can improve up to 28% improvement when EBP is used to guide practice (Duffy, 2005; Fineout-Overholt, Levin, & Melnyk, 2005). Nurses need to know what defines **evidence-based nursing (EBN)** and evidence-based practice. How does a nurse know that specific evidence will benefit patient care? To understand how EBP is an essential element of EBN and clinical practice, components and defining attributes, principles, and types of EBP will be addressed in this chapter. This chapter also will explore the background, history, applications, and process of EBP. Examples of data sources for EBP as well as a discussion about issues in contemporary practice will be included. The role of the nurse in applying research findings to practice will be examined, and implications for nursing education, research, and practice also will be addressed.

What Is Evidence-Based Health Care and Evidence-Based Practice?

Evidence-based health care, conducted with caring and with an awareness of the patient and family's preferences and values, helps nurses and other healthcare providers to make better clinical decisions that ensure optimal patient outcomes (Pravikoff, Tanner, & Pierce, 2005). *Evidence-based practice (EBP)* is a problem-solving approach to clinical care that incorporates the diligent use of current best evidence from well-designed studies and clinical expertise (Melnyk & Fineout-Overholt, 2005). EBP is based on clinical decision making that includes the patient's clinical state, the specific clinical setting, and the patient's circumstances (Haynes, Devereaux, & Guyatt, 2002). Optimal care, based on the best available evidence, results in improved patient care outcomes, which is a major goal of many professional and healthcare organizations as well as policy-making bodies and federal agencies (Fineout-Overholt, Melnyk, & Schultz, 2005). Each clinician is required to solve clinical problems, and the goal is that research evidence will be used to guide clinical practice (Banning, 2005). Evidence can be derived from published research findings or clinicians can personally conduct research. For the clinician, conducting research may involve conducting a small clinical study to develop clinical protocols or it could mean assisting with larger clinical trials that test the efficacy of a clinical protocol on a large number of patients (Mohide & Cocker, 2005). For nurses, Klardie, Johnson, McNaughton, and Meyers (2004) suggested that research evidence is the basis for implementing change in nursing practice and is based on the nursing process. Nurses can choose to participate in any or all of the steps shown in Table 11-1 to change nursing practice. DiCenso, Guyatt, and Ciliska's (2005) model in Table 11-1 illustrates the process of change in practice using research evidence.

EBP refers to clinical decisions based on the best research evidence, such as that found in **randomized controlled trials (RCTs)**, and is considered to be foundational evidence for best practice; however, EBP also includes clinical expertise and patient values (Ciliska, 2006; DiCenso et al., 2005). EBP uses a hierarchy of evidence (from 1 = highest level of evidence to 5 = lowest level of evidence) to guide decision making; this hierarchy will be discussed later in this chapter. Kirkbaum, Baumbusch, Shultz, and Anderson (2007) indicated that the newest developments in EBP updates and continuing education are based on the results of the latest RCTs where significant statistical results from research findings are the basis for practice guidelines.

EBP, supported empirically by RCTs, is best utilized to answer what specific treatment will work best for a specific condition. An example of EBP is the well-known and groundbreaking zidovudine (AZT) efficacy and safety clinical trial during which it was found that all human immunodeficiency virus (HIV)-infected pregnant women who received AZT during pregnancy did not transmit HIV to their fetus (Connor et al., 1994).

The clinical application of EBP has five benefits according to Kennedy and Carr (2006), which are listed in Table 11-2.

TABLE 11-1   STEPS TO IMPLEMENT CHANGES IN NURSING PRACTICE

- Assess the need for a change in practice.
- Ask an answerable research question.
- Synthesize best available evidence.
- Stimulate inquiry/discussion.
- Design a change in practice.
- Implement practice change.
- Evaluate practice change.

Source: DiCenso, A., Guyatt, G., & Ciliska, D. (2005). *Evidence-based nursing: A guide to clinical practice.* St. Louis, MO: Mosby.

KEY TERM

Randomized controlled trial (RCT): Experimental research that is the strongest design to support a cause and effect relationship. Subjects are randomly assigned to a treatment group or a control group.

TABLE 11-2   BENEFITS OF EVIDENCE-BASED PRACTICE

1. Foundation for practice guidelines, diagnostic testing, and changes in treatments or procedures
2. Eliminates unnecessary treatment or procedures
3. Evaluates research findings to find treatments or procedures that are effective and/or are cost-effective
4. Helps to standardize care
5. Assists with evaluating clinical outcomes

Source: Kennedy, H. P., & Carr, K. C. (2006). Using evidence to support clinical practice. In K. D. Schulling & F. E. Likis (Eds.), *Women's gynecologic heath* (pp. 41–63). Sudbury, MA: Jones and Bartlett.

TABLE 11-3 COMPONENTS OF EBP

- Research evidence, evidence-based theories, expert opinions
- Evidence obtained from patient assessment, physical exam, availability of resources
- Clinical expertise and experience
- Patient preferences and values

Source: Melnyk, B. M., & Fineout-Overholt, E. (2005). *Evidence-based practice in nursing and health care: a guide to best practice.* Philadelphia: Lippincott.

Melnyk and Fineout Overholt (2005) have also identified four essential components of EBP that are foundational to evidence-based clinical decision making (see Table 11-3).

Nurse clinicians need to understand, use, and apply the concept of EBP in order to provide excellent patient care. EBP is based on research findings to guide clinical decision making about patient care. Excellent patient care is based on research evidence and can be used to create clinical guidelines to standardize patient care (Belcher & Vonderhaar, 2005). In addition, nurses need to obtain and keep current with the most up-to-date information about new research findings and to maintain professional competence. EBP is becoming more evident in clinical practice and in clinical education (Eisenberg, 2001; Guyatt & Drummond, 2001; Sackett et al., 2000). With the increased emphasis on EBP, contemporary nursing education now focuses on an exploration of evidence from RCTs as well as from other naturalistic studies where concepts are explored in the context of clinical management of patients (Banning, 2005). Nurse clinicians at the bedside are in an excellent position to contribute to nursing knowledge and improve patient care by identifying clinical problems, collecting data for nursing research studies, and then applying research findings in the clinical care setting (Ayers & Coeling, 2005).

As a result of methodologically rigorous review of the best evidence on a specific topic, evidence-based clinical practice guidelines have been developed to guide clinical practice. This has improved quality of care, provided a more streamlined patient care process, and improved patient outcomes (Grimshaw & Russell, 1993; Grimshaw et al., 1995). Cochrane used the findings from thousands of low-birth-weight and preterm infants that resulted in infant mortality as an exemplar for EBP. Based on supporting evidence from RCTs, it was concluded by the meta-analysis that prenatal steroids reduce the severity of neonatal lung disease in high-risk women and reduce preterm infant mortality from 50 percent to 30 percent (Cochrane Collaboration, 2001).

History and Background of Evidence-Based Practice

Florence Nightingale (1957) applied evidence to practice in the 19th century. *Notes on Nursing*, originally published in 1859, was an early version of EBP. Nightingale's method was to rigorously monitor all nursing care for the effectiveness of patient outcomes. From the mid-19th century until the mid-20th century, however, clinical decisions were primarily based on expert opinion and clinical experience. In the 1960s, a British epidemiologist, Dr. Archie Cochrane, was responsible for introducing the notion of EBP, asserting that effective patient care required empirically based interventions. Beginning in 1972, Cochrane's publications were critical of the medical profession because there were few **systematic reviews** of evidence for making healthcare policy and clinical patient care decisions (Enkin, 1992). Cochrane believed that only RCTs were sufficient evidence for making medical decisions (Cochrane Collaboration, 2001). Until his death in 1988, Cochrane was a staunch advocate for EBP, and as a result had a profound influence on how modern patient care and healthcare policy decisions are made.

> **KEY TERM**
>
> **Systematic review:** Summary of evidence obtained by researchers on a specific topic or clinical problem. It uses a step-by step rigorous process to identify, synthesize, and evaluate research studies to answer a specific clinical question and to make conclusions about best evidence.

During the late 1970s, research utilization was found in much of the nursing literature. Estabrooks (1998) described research utilization as using "research findings in all aspects of one's work as a registered nurse" (p. 19). EBN is more than research utilization; it includes evidence-based nursing skills, as described by DiCenso et al. (2005) (see Table 11-4).

The Process of Evidence-Based Practice

EBP is a continuum from a clinical question (Contemporary Practice Highlight 11-1) about best practice to finding and evaluating the best research that answers the clinical question (Kennedy & Carr, 2006). Melnyk and Fineout-Overholt (2005) identified five key steps of EBP, as shown in Table 11-5.

TABLE 11-4 EVIDENCE-BASED NURSING SKILLS	TABLE 11-5 KEY STEPS OF EVIDENCE-BASED PRACTICE
1. Define the patient problem. 2. Determine the information needed by searching the literature. 3. Select the best evidence. 4. Categorize the evidence. 5. Synthesize clinical application. 6. Determine the balance between advantages and disadvantages. 7. Implement and evaluate clinical decision based on patient values.	1. Ask the "burning clinical question." 2. Collect the best and most relevant evidence. 3. Critically evaluate the evidence. 4. To make a clinical decision or change, incorporate all evidence with one's own clinical experience, patient preferences, and values. 5. Evaluate the change or clinical practice decision.
Source: DiCenso, A., Guyatt, G., & Ciliska, D. (2005). *Evidence-based nursing: A guide to clinical practice.* St. Louis, MO: Mosby.	*Source:* Melnyk, B. M., & Fineout-Overholt, E. (2005). *Evidence-based practice in nursing and health care: A guide to best practice.* Philadelphia: Lippincott.

A systematic step-by-step approach can be used to examine the "burning clinical question" mentioned in step 1. The following sections will step through an example regarding the clinical question of best practices to prevent unplanned pregnancies in adolescent women.

PICO format

P = patient population (i.e., adolescent women)

I = intervention of interest (abstinence education)

C = comparison intervention (oral contraceptives)

O = outcome (prevention of pregnancy)

Ciliska, D. (2005). Educating for evidence-based practice. *Journal of Professional Nursing, 21*(6), 345–350; Melnyk, B. M., & Fineout-Overholt, E. (2005). *Evidence-based practice in nursing and health care: A guide to best practice.* Philadelphia: Lippincott.

Step 1

The clinical question should be asked in the PICO format; PICO stands for population, intervention, comparison intervention, and outcome (Ciliska, 2005; Melnyk & Fineout-Overholt, 2005). The PICO format will answer the following questions:

1. Who are the patients, clients, or individuals of a particular age, gender, community, or group (e.g., adolescent women)?

2. What interventions have answered the specific clinical question (e.g., abstinence education)?

3. Is there a comparison with another intervention (e.g., oral contraceptives)?

4. What are the consequences of the intervention (e.g., pregnancy prevention)?

Step 2

The search for best evidence (Guyatt & Rennie, 2002) is achieved by conducting systematic reviews or meta-analyses on empirical evidence. The evidence is evaluated by the type of evidence and ranges from highest (level 1 evidence) to lowest (level 7 evidence). The seven levels of evidence known as the rating system for the hierarchy of evidence was developed by Guyatt & Rennie (2002) and Harris et al. (2002), and is shown in Table 11-6.

TABLE 11-6   RATING SYSTEM FOR HIERARCHY OF EVIDENCE

Level 1 evidence: Systematic review or meta-analysis of all RCTs, or EBP

Level 2 evidence: Obtained from at least one well-designed RCT

Level 3 evidence: Obtained from a well-designed controlled trial without randomization

Level 4 evidence: Obtained from well-designed case-control and cohort studies without randomization

Level 5 evidence: Obtained from systematic reviews of descriptive and qualitative studies

Level 6 evidence: Obtained from a single descriptive or qualitative study

Level 7 evidence: Obtained from the opinion of authorities and/or reports of expert committees

Source: Guyatt, G., & Rennie, D. (2002). *Users' guides to the medical literature.* Chicago: AMA Press; Harris, R. P., Helfand, M., Woolf, S. H., Lohr, K. N., Mulrow, C. D., Teutsch, S. M., et al. (2001). Current methods of the U.S. Preventative Services Task Force: A review of the methods. *American Journal of Preventive Services, 20*(Suppl. 3), 21–35.

CONTEMPORARY PRACTICE HIGHLIGHT 11-1

CLINICAL QUESTIONS

Melnyk and Fineout-Overholt (2005) identified the best evidence to guide clinical practice in the specialty areas of emergency and trauma care, adults and critical care, and adults in primary care. The following examples highlight contemporary practice issues and researchable clinical questions. Examine each clinical scenario listed below and create your own "burning clinical question." You can also search literature databases to obtain the most current evidence in order to guide your practice.

Emergency and Trauma Care

Issues

- *Predictors of adult patients surviving cardiopulmonary arrest*
- *Predictors of outcomes in children sustaining out-of hospital cardiopulmonary arrest*

Examples of Clinical Questions

- What are predictors of survival?
- What is the level of evidence for these predictors?
- What is the role of various interdisciplinary team members to enhance survival?
- What special skills or education are needed for the nurse to implement the evidence-based care or protocol?
- What is the role of the nurse in acting as an advocate for the family?

Issue

- *The effectiveness of psychological interventions to prevent post-traumatic stress disorder (PTSD) following traumatic events*

Examples of Clinical Questions

- What interventions have been tested to prevent PTSD?
- Would these interventions fit with the patients' values in my clinical setting?
- What is the cost to implement these interventions?
- What special skills or education are needed for the nurse to implement the evidence-based care or protocol?

Adults and Critical Care

Issues

- *Readiness for weaning from mechanical ventilation*
- *Effect of routine nursing interventions on tissue oxygenation*
- *Effectiveness of health professionals' education on smoking cessation*

Examples of Clinical Questions

- What physical assessment and laboratory parameters have been tested to assess readiness to wean the patient from mechanical ventilation?
- Would the routine nursing interventions on tissue oxygenation be the same in my clinical setting?
- What special skills or education are needed for the nurse to implement the evidence-based care or protocol to wean the patient from mechanical ventilation?
- What educational interventions have the best success for smoking cessation?
- Do the educational interventions have different effectiveness for men vs. women and for adults vs. adolescents? What is the level of evidence for each population?

Evidence-based nursing (EBN) is at the core of the knowledge base for professional nursing practice. EBN includes evidence-based practice to make clinical decisions and improve nursing practice. Evidence-based nursing (EBN) encompasses a broader approach than EBP. EBN, based on the nursing model of decision making and clinical judgment, is central to the knowledge base for nursing practice. Nursing decisions are often based on the effectiveness of nursing interventions that can sometimes, but not always, be evaluated only by RCTs (Fleming, 2007). The nursing practice model is based on empirical evidence and the evaluation of clinical practice and its effects on the patient or client. The best evidence in nursing incorporates relevant clinical research and also focuses on the safety, effectiveness, and cost-effectiveness of nursing interventions. EBN also takes into consideration available resources, accurate ways to measure nursing interventions, the strength of cause and effect relationships, and the perceived meaning of the patient's experiences (DiCenso et al., 2005).

EBN follows the principles of EBP and includes the four elements of evidence-based decision making for nursing care: best research evidence, clinical expertise, patient preferences in their specific situation, and available resources for nursing assessment and interventions (DiCenso et al., 2005). EBN additionally considers ethical and cultural aspects, psychosocial issues, and family considerations in clinical care decisions (Fleming, 2007). Fleming also noted that the goal of evidence-based health delivery of care is quality care with cost restraint.

The following example helps clarify the differences between EBP and EBN. Several RCTs may offer evidence that use of tap water for wound cleansing is as effective as using normal saline (Fernandez, Griffiths, & Ussia, 2002). EBP would take account of the evidence that the use of tap water to cleanse acute wounds reduces infection and that several randomized controlled studies concluded that there was no difference in the infection and healing rates in wounds cleansed with tap water compared with other solutions (Fernandez et al.). However, EBN will also take into consideration the impact of this intervention on each individual, the family caregivers (e.g., Is using tap water uncomfortable compared to normal saline in wound cleansing?), and economics both in the hospital and at home (e.g., Which method of wound cleansing is more cost-effective?) and evaluate the effectiveness and patient acceptance of the treatment as well as outcomes associated with quality of life (similar outcomes as far as wound healing and infection rates). In summary, EBP uses RCTs to decide the effectiveness of a treatment, whereas EBN also uses evidence to establish clinical practice guidelines that help to standardize patient care that guides clinical decision making and optimal, cost-effective patient care (Belcher & Vonderhaar, 2005).

It is important to note that in the past, clinical practice was based more on levels 6 and 7, and the goal is to now base clinical decisions on levels 1–5.

Step 3

Critical appraisal of research answers the following questions, developed by Kennedy and Carr (2006), when critically appraising or evaluating empirical evidence:

- *Results of the study:* What were the study results?
- *Validity of results:* Do the results seem valid?
- *Comparable patient group:* Do the subjects compare to the kinds of patients in my practice?

Step 4

This step, integrating the evidence, synthesizes and compares the evidence from the literature with the clinician's expertise, a clinical assessment of the patient, and available healthcare resources.

Step 5

Evaluating the effectiveness of the intervention is achieved by asking how effective the treatment or the clinical decision was with a particular patient in a particular setting.

Evidence-based nursing helps nurses to ask important clinical questions, differentiate between strong and weak research evidence, clearly understand research study results, sort out the risks and benefits of clinical management options, and apply specific evidence to individual patients to improve clinical outcomes

---

BOX 11-1   TYPES OF EVIDENCE

Step 1: The clinical question: Is the use of tap water for wound cleansing as effective as using normal saline?

Step 2: The search for best evidence: Using the Cochrane Library and EBSCO Publishing resources, there is evidence that the use of tap water and saline to cleanse acute wounds reduces infection.

Step 3: Critical appraisal of research: Several randomized controlled studies have concluded that there is no difference in the infection and healing rates in wounds cleansed with tap water compared with other solutions.

Step 4: Integrating the evidence: Consider the impact of this intervention on each individual and the family: Is using tap water comfortable and acceptable compared to normal saline in wound cleansing? Consider the economic impact both in the hospital and at home: Which method of wound cleansing is more cost-effective?

Step 5: Evaluate the effectiveness of the intervention: Similar outcomes of wound healing and infection rates occur when using either tap water or saline for wound cleansing.

TABLE 11-7 EXAMPLES OF RECENT SYSTEMATIC REVIEWS AND CORRESPONDING LEVEL OF EVIDENCE

Level	Example	Explanation
Level 1: Likely reliable evidence	• Prenatal steroids reduce the severity of neonatal lung disease but increase the rate of Cesarean delivery (reported in *Lancet*, 2006;367:1913–1919). • Diphenhydramine (Benadryl) is more effective than desloratadine (Claritin) or placebo for seasonal allergic rhinitis (reported in Annals of *Allergy Asthma Immunology*, 2006;96:606–614).	Systematic review or meta-analysis of all randomized controlled trials (RCTs), or evidence-based practice (EBP)
Level 2: Mid-level evidence	• Vitamin K appears to reduce postmenopausal fracture rates and was evaluated in a systematic review of 13 studies, one of which was a well-designed RCT (found in *Archives of Internal Medicine*, 2006;166:1256–1261).	Obtained from at least one well-designed RCT
Level 3: Lacking direct evidence	• A systematic review of 14 controlled trials that were not randomized determined that exercise improves glycemic control in Type 2 diabetes (found in *Cochrane Database System Review*, 2006[3]:CD002968).	Obtained from a well-designed controlled trial without randomization

KEY TERM

Meta-analysis: The summarization of the results of several quantitative studies critically reviewed, synthesized, and evaluated to answer a specific clinical question about the effectiveness of an intervention across multiple studies in different settings.

KEY TERM

Descriptive studies: Research conducted in order to describe characteristics of selected variables or a certain phenomenon.

KEY TERM

Qualitative study: A descriptive type of research in which variables are not quantified numerically to describe a phenomenon of interest. Data are obtained through open-ended questions or interviews.

(DiCenso et al., 2005). As stated earlier, the strongest research evidence comes from the systematic reviews and **meta-analyses** of randomized controlled trials (RCTs). When RCTs are not available, evidence from nonrandomized **descriptive** and **qualitative studies** as well as expert opinions and evidence-based theories may guide clinical decisions (Melnyk & Fineout-Overholt, 2005). Note that the authors for each research study described the level of evidence (Contemporary Practice Highlight 11-2) based on the analysis and evaluation of the studies.

Applying Research Findings to Practice

Several models can be applied to improve clinical decision making. For example, as noted by Kennedy and Carr (2006), to successfully integrate research findings into practice, it is necessary to follow the five sequential phases of the Stetler Model of Research Utilization (2001). The five phases of this model and questions to ask are as follows:

CONTEMPORARY PRACTICE HIGHLIGHT 11-2

EXAMPLES OF LEVEL 1: LIKELY RELIABLE EVIDENCE

- Anticholinergics reduce asthma-related hospital admission (found reported in *Thorax*, 2005; 60:740–746). This was based on 32 RCTs that included 3,611 patients and 10 trials that included 1,786 children and adolescents.

  The practice implications: Multiple doses of inhaled ipratropium (an anticholinergic) compared to beta2-agonists may reduce the rate of hospital admissions in adults and children with moderate to severe asthma.

- Selective serotonin reuptake inhibitors (SSRIs) have onset efficacy for depression as early as 1 to 6 weeks (reported in *Archives of General Psychiatry*, 2006; 63:1217–1223). Based on 28 RCTs with a total of 5,872 patients.

  The practice implications: There is no significant advantage of SSRIs at 1 week; however, after 2–6 weeks there was a 79 percent increased chance of remission of depression among those receiving an SSRI compared with those receiving placebo.

Based on this level of evidence, consider how you might change your practice:

- How would you implement this information in education programs for community members with asthma?
- What type of education and suicide assessment should be used for a patient with depression who has been on SSRIs for 1 week?

- *Preparation phase:* What are the purposes, priorities, and measurable outcomes related to the identified problem?
- *Validation phase:* What evidence will be selected to synthesize and critique evidence? Personally, what is the applicability to my clinical setting?
- *Comparative evaluation/decision-making phase:* What research findings will be used or selected? Where do the collected findings belong as far as the hierarchy of evidence? How will findings be applied? Does a study need to be proposed and conducted?
- *Transition application phase:* How will this information be shared? What strategies for change need to be developed?
- *Evaluation phase:* What is the feasibility on a short-term and long-term basis? What are the cost benefits? What resources are available?

Also, in addition to the levels of research evidence discussed earlier, evidence is evaluated by the quality of the study—good, fair, or poor—and the net benefit to the patient—substantial, moderate, small, or negative (Kennedy & Carr, 2006). Recommendations for application of research findings and guidelines are based on the U.S. Preventive Services Task Force's (1996) list of the strength of recommendations shown in Table 11-8.

TABLE 11-8 RECOMMENDATIONS FOR USE OF RESEARCH EVIDENCE IN CLINICAL PRACTICE

The 5 Phases of The Stetler Model of Research Utilization

1. Preparation
2. Validation
3. Comparative Evaluation/Decision-Making
4. Translation Application
5. Evaluation

Source: Harris, R. P., Helfand, M., Woolf, S. H., Lohr, K. N., Mulrow, C. D., Teutsch, S. M., et al. (2001). Current methods of the U.S. Preventative Services Task Force: A review of the methods. *American Journal of Preventive Services,* 20(Suppl. 3), 21–35.

KEY TERM

Case-control studies: Research that retrospectively compares the characteristics of one individual with certain medical conditions to another who does not have the medical condition.

Clinical Application Examples

The scientific literature for nursing as well as other health disciplines has dramatically increased the current body of knowledge. The state of the science can be examined in the literature and reviewed for the level of evidence for clinical application. The following are a few key examples in various nursing specialty fields where evidence is substantiating a change in the way nurses practice. Moore, Anderson, and Bergman (2003) found that skin-to-skin contact between mother and baby at birth reduces crying, improves mother–baby interaction, keeps baby warmer, and helps women breastfeed successfully. This may be characterized as Level 2 evidence (likely effective) and was based on the analysis of 1,925 mother–baby pairs in at least two clinical trials with more benefits demonstrated than adverse effects. This intervention would be *strongly recommended* because there is good evidence of improved health outcomes and the benefits outweigh harm.

Thompson, Rivara, and Thompson (1999) found that the use of helmets resulted in a 63–88 percent reduction in head and facial injuries in bicyclists of all ages involved in all types of crashes including those involved with motor vehicles. Although the conclusions were based on five well-conducted **case-control studies**, not randomized controlled trials, this evidence supports the consideration to *strongly recommend* (good evidence of improved health outcomes, benefits outweigh harm) the application of research findings to clinical practice through safety education on helmet use for individuals and communities.

Gillespie and colleagues (2003) assessed interventions designed to prevent the incidence of falls in elderly people (either living in the community or in institutional or hospital care). Based on 21,668 subjects, the authors concluded that interventions to prevent falls are likely to be effective and are now available; however, less is known about their effectiveness in preventing fall-related injuries in seven clinical trials. This would likely be a *recommended* intervention (fair evidence of improved health outcomes, benefits outweigh harm).

From Clinical Questions to Evidence

Barrett (2002) noted that clinical questions provide the basis for research, and research provides a way to evaluate the effectiveness and safety of clinical practice.

Research starts with a clinical question about a clinical problem from everyday clinical practice, patient care practices, interventions, and cost-effective quality care (Contemporary Practice Highlight 11-3). Additionally, social issues can influence research questions based on gender, race, poverty, and healthcare disparities. These research questions translate into research aims or purposes for a research study with two primary criteria: clinical significance and a gap in current knowledge (National Institutes of Health, 2001). Priorities for funding in nursing

---

CONTEMPORARY PRACTICE HIGHLIGHT 11-3

CLINICAL QUESTIONS IN WOMEN'S HEALTH

Sakala (2007) listed recent systematic reviews from the Cochrane Database and included the following women's health questions as examples of researchable clinical questions:

- What are the differences in ad libitum or demand/semi-demand feeding versus scheduled interval feeding for preterm infants?
- Is elective cesarean section delivery at term becoming more common and requested by women for non-medical reasons?
- What is the effectiveness of self-help and guided self-help interventions for eating disorders?
- What is the effectiveness of surgical treatment of fibroids on subsequent fertility?
- Does calcium supplementation during pregnancy prevent hypertensive disorders and related problems?
- Are mechanical devices for urinary incontinence effective in women?
- Are spinal manipulation interventions effective for primary and secondary dysmenorrhea?
- What is the effectiveness of screening for family and intimate partner violence?

Select several questions of interest to you and consider the following:

- Do you have a passion for this clinical issue that would continually motivate you to find the answer?
- How would you establish what is already known on this clinical question?
- Is this clinical question consistent with the research priorities of the National Institute of Nursing Research?
- How would you motivate other nurses and physicians to become involved on your research team on the investigation of this clinical question?
- What would it cost to investigate this clinical question?

research can be found within the National Institute of Nursing Research (NINR) pathways, and health promotion and disease prevention objectives in *Healthy People 2010* (U.S. Department of Health and Human Services, 2004).

Selected Data Sources

There are many data sources for systematic reviews of evidence. The following are some frequently used primary sources:

- *Clinical Evidence (http://www.clinicalevidence.com):* Identifies important clinical questions, and then answers them through a systematic search for randomized controlled trials, summarizing the best evidence. A key disadvantage of this site is that information is generally limited to treatment-related conditions. There is a cost for a subscription, but a free trial is available.
- *The Cochrane Collaboration (http://www.cochrane.org):* Cochrane Reviews are available by subscription to the Cochrane Library, but review abstracts are available at no charge.
- *Database of Abstracts of Reviews of Effects (DARE):* Includes recent abstract entries assessing the quality of systematic reviews. DARE abstracts are available without charge.
- *DynaMed (http://www.dynamicmedical.com):* Systematically surveys original research reports, journal review services, systematic review sources (such as Clinical Evidence and the Cochrane Library), drug information sources, and guideline collections. There is a fee, but a free trial is available.
- *Agency for Healthcare Research and Quality (AHRQ) (http://www.ahrq.gov):* Provides a public resource for clinical practice guidelines in collaboration with the American Medical Association and the American Association of Health Plans.
- *Essential Evidence Plus (http://www.essentialevidenceplus.com):* A search engine that allows you to search multiple databases, including Essential Evidence Plus (http://www.essentialevidenceplus.com/) (concise evidence-based summaries selected for clinical relevance and validity from more than 100 journals), Cochrane Database abstracts, selected guidelines, clinical decision rules, diagnostic test calculators, and the complete "Griffith's 5-Minute Clinical Consult." There is a subscription cost, but a free trial is available.
- *UpToDate (http://www.uptodate.com):* A collection of well-referenced reviews. It contains specialty-focused information and includes multiple specialties. There is a subscription cost, but a free trial is available.
- *Cumulative Index of Nursing and Allied Health Literature* (CINAHL) *(http://www.cinahl.com), Medline (http://medline.cos.com/)*, and *PsycINFO* are all extensive common search engines for nursing, medicine, and psychology literature.

- *SearchMedica Primary Care (http://www.search-medica.com):* A new generation of medical search engines. It contains an EBM and meta-analysis category for access to EBP information.
- *Association of Women's Health, Obstetric, and Neo-natal Nurses (AWHONN) (http://www.awhonn.org/awhonn):* Includes nursing clinical practice guidelines, which include topics such as breast-feeding support, neonatal skin care, and nursing management of the second stage of labor.
- *Registered Nurses Association of Ontario (RNAO) (http://www.rnao.org):* Developed a toolkit to enhance the use of clinical practice guidelines.
- *Sigma Theta Tau International (http://www.nursingsociety.org):* Its publication, *Woldviews on Evidence-Based Nursing*, provides systematic reviews to guide nursing practice in many clinical areas.
- *Academic Center for Evidence-Based Nursing (ACE) (http://www.acestar.uthscsa.edu):* At the University of Texas Health Science Center at San Antonio, it offers annual national EBP continuing education (CE) conferences for nurses and other healthcare professionals.

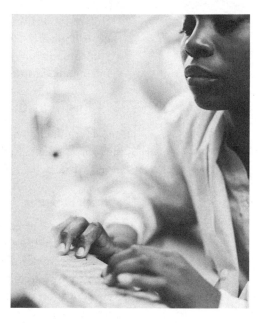

Nurse working on a computer.
Source: © Photos.com

- *Center for Research and Evidence-Based Practice (CREP) (http://www.son.rochester.edu/son/research/centers/research-evidenced-based-practice):* At the University of Rochester (New York) School of Nursing, it also offers annual national EBP CE conferences for nurses and other healthcare professionals. The annual national/international conference focuses on best evidence to guide practice in specific areas: care of high-risk children and youth, acute/critical care, care of older adults, and psychiatric/mental health care.
- *The Joanna Briggs Institute (Adelaide, Australia) (http://www.joannabriggs.edu.au)* and *the Sara Cole Hirsch Institute for Best Nursing Practice at Case Western Reserve School of Nursing (http://fpb.case.edu/HirshInstitute):* Two additional sources to find information about EBN and EBP.

Sakala (2007) also identified the peer-reviewed journal (*Implementation Science*) as a source for open online access to content relating to methods to promote the transition of research findings into practice. Also, online tutorials that teach the five steps of EBP are available at Middlesex University in London and at the University of Rochester Medical Center.

Web-based information on the formulation of searchable and answerable questions can be found from the following Web sites:

- University of Illinois College of Medicine at Peoria (http://www.uic.edu/depts/lib/lhsp/)
- Studentbmj.com (http://studentbmj.com)
- *International Medical Student's Journal.*

EBN's Implications for Education, Research, and Practice

The goal for nursing science and nursing knowledge is that EBP will become part of the professional culture of nursing through education, research, and practice (Rycroft-Malone et al., 2004).

Nursing Education

Informatics is a required skill in nursing education for professional access to well-designed research. Information literacy is an essential component of EBP because it enhances the nurse's ability to use the best available research literature to ensure optimal patient outcomes (Tanner, Pierce, & Pravikoff, 2004). Undergraduate nursing education programs will continue to implement improved course outcomes that will focus on incorporating research evidence to guide clinical practice (Ferguson & Day, 2005). Memorization of rote facts needs to be replaced with teaching the critical thinking skills required for contemporary clinical situations because evidence-based teaching prepares clinicians for EBN (Ironside & Spaziale, 2006). Students and new graduates need to have high-level thinking capabilities to ensure patient safety and high-quality patient care (Ironside, 2005).

Focusing on advanced degrees in nursing is key to preparing nurses for research and leadership in clinical practice. Nurses with advanced degrees (master of science in nursing [MSN], doctor of nursing practice [DNP], and doctor of philosophy in nursing [PhD]) will be better prepared to influence patients, other nurses, and healthcare systems. Advanced practice nurses (APNs) are also in a position to help in the design and implementation of clinical nursing research that provides the basis for the development of evidence-based clinical practice guidelines and protocols. Hopp (2005) contends that clinical nurse specialists (CNS) and other APNs can facilitate EBP as a solution to bridge the gaps among education, research, and practice. Continuing education programs for practicing clinicians also will increasingly be focused on EBP and EBN, which optimally will guide professional practice.

Nursing Research

Ayers and Coeling (2005) urged all nurses to be involved in research, either as consumers of research or as participants involved in the research process itself. Clinicians at the bedside are well-positioned to contribute to the nursing profession's body of knowledge and enhance nursing care by identifying nursing clinical problems worthy of research, being involved in data collection for nursing studies, and applying research findings to clinical care. Nurse scientists, APNs, and nurse clinicians need to work collaboratively to develop, implement, and evaluate carefully designed clinical research (Duffy, 2005). Increasing knowledge and skills associated with the EBP process provides nurse clinicians with the tools required to maintain ownership of their practices and help to transform health care (Fineout-Overholt, Melnyk, & Shultz, 2005).

Nursing Practice

Klardie and colleagues (2004) described the application of clinical practice guidelines (CPGs) as being an additional expected outcome of EBP. CPGs or **clinical care protocols** reflect the most up-to-date practice based on evidence and knowledge; the goal is to have the latest scientific knowledge available to clinicians (Weaver, Warren, & Delaney, 2005). Although there is a plethora of research demonstrating well-designed clinical intervention research, few research findings are effectively implemented in the clinical setting (Duffy, 2005).

> **KEY TERM**
>
> **Clinical care protocols:** Clinical practice guidelines (CPGs) that reflect the most up-to-date practice based on evidence for reference and knowledge with the goal of having the latest scientific knowledge available to clinicians to make decisions about care. Elements include systematic literature review, and the consensus of expert decision makers and consumers who consider the evidence and make recommendations.

Health care is said to be in crisis and in need of change (Institute of Medicine, 2005). A fundamental change in the current healthcare system is needed to close the gap between practice and patient care quality with a redesign of the healthcare system that includes policy makers, healthcare leaders, clinicians, regulators, and informed consumers (Newhouse, Dearholt, Poe, Pugh, & White, 2005). Keys are implementing EBP and strengthening clinical information systems to improve the overall quality of health care (Barnsteiner & Prevost, 2002; Klem & Weiss, 2005). Better clinical decisions and improved patient outcomes can be realized by health care that is evidence-based and provided in a caring context (Pravikoff et al., 2005). Additionally, Fineout-Overholt and colleagues (2005) stressed that the key elements of a best practice culture are EBP mentors, partnerships between academic and clinical settings, well-designed research and resources, and administrative support, all of which will foster the acceleration and adoption of EBP in education and clinical settings.

Summary

This chapter has explored evidence-based practice (EBP) and evidence-based nursing (EBN) including the background, defining attributes, components, and significance. Additionally, this chapter described methods of incorporating EBP into clinical decision making. Information was provided for a basic understanding of EBP and EBN and its application in clinical practice, how to locate and evaluate appropriate clinically relevant research literature, how to develop an understanding of resources for literature search and to evaluate research-based evidence, how to understand the levels of evidence, and how to evaluate the effects of interventions on patient outcomes.

Killeen and Barnfather (2005) posit that bachelor of science in nursing (BSN) students, agency personnel, and faculty can lead practice innovations supported by EBP. This chapter has highlighted what EBP actually means, how EBN is essential for the nursing professional, examples of evidence that guides clinical decisions, and how to integrate evidence into your clinical decision making.

As professional nurses navigate through the clinical practice arena, each clinical decision will be based not only on the best research evidence available, but also on professional experience and the client or patient values and preferences. The goal of using evidence to guide nursing practice must be based on the realization that there can be a 28 percent improvement in quality healthcare outcomes when evidence-based nursing care is utilized (Duffy, 2005; Fineout-Overholt, Melnyk, & Shultz 2005). It is essential to remember that EBN can improve patient safety, efficiency, and the effectiveness of health care.

Key Terms

- **Case-control studies:** Research that retrospectively compares the characteristics of one individual with certain medical conditions to another who does not have the medical condition.
- **Clinical care protocols:** Clinical practice guidelines (CPGs) that reflect the most up-to-date practice based on evidence for reference and knowledge with the goal of having the latest scientific knowledge available to clinicians to make decisions about care. Elements include systematic literature review, and the consensus of expert decision makers and consumers who consider the evidence and make recommendations.
- **Controlled trial:** Research in which there is a treatment group and a group that does not receive the treatment (control group) so that comparisons can be made about the effectiveness of an intervention on a specific health issue and health outcome.
- **Descriptive studies:** Research conducted in order to describe characteristics of selected variables or a certain phenomenon.
- **Evidence-based nursing (EBN):** Clinical decision making by nurses that is a combination and integration of the best research evidence; it also includes the nurse's clinical expertise and patient values and preferences about a specific type of care.
- **Evidence-based practice (EBP):** The process of problem solving using the best research evidence in clinical decision making for patient care. It is a combination of a systematic search for and critical appraisal of the most relevant research available to answer a specific clinical question, with the clinician's own clinical expertise and patient values and preferences included.
- **Meta-analysis:** The summarization of the results of several quantitative studies critically reviewed, synthesized, and evaluated to answer a specific clinical question about the effectiveness of an intervention across multiple studies in different settings.
- **Qualitative study:** A descriptive type of research in which variables are not quantified numerically to describe a phenomenon of interest. Data are obtained through open-ended questions or interviews.
- **Randomized controlled trial (RCT):** Experimental research that is the strongest design to support a cause and effect relationship. Subjects are randomly assigned to a treatment group or a control group.
- **Systematic review:** Summary of evidence obtained by researchers on a specific topic or clinical problem. It uses a step-by-step rigorous process to identify, synthesize, and evaluate research studies to answer a specific clinical question and to make conclusions about best evidence.

Reflective Practice Questions

1. Using a model such as Stetler's, how can a nurse make EBP more focused and acceptable to clinicians to successfully integrate research findings into practice?

2. How does the clinician utilize research evidence in clinical practice in specific specialty areas?

3. How does the clinician align clinical practice with research in specific clinical settings to maintain EBN strategies?

References

Agency for Healthcare Research and Quality (AHRQ). (2002). *Systems to rate the strength of scientific evidence. Fact sheet.* AHRQ Publication No. 02P0022. Rockville, MD: Author. Retrieved June 24, 2007, from http://www.ahrq.gov/clinic/epcix.htm

Ayers, D. M., & Coeling, H. (2005). Incorporating research into associate degree nursing curricula. *Journal of Nursing Education, 44*(11), 515–518.

Banning, M. (2005). Conceptions of evidence, evidence-based medicine, evidence-based practice and their use in nursing: Independent nurse prescribers' views. *Journal of Clinical Nursing, 14*(4), 411–417.

Barnsteiner, J., & Prevost, S. (2002). How to implement research-based practice: Some tried and true pointers. *Reflections on Nursing Leadership, 28*(2), 18–21.

Barrett, E. A. (2002). What is nursing science? *Nursing Science Quarterly, 15*(1), 51–60.

Belcher, J. V., & Vonderhaar, K. J. (2005). Web-delivered research-based nursing staff education for seeking magnet status. *Journal of Nursing Administration, 35*(9), 382–386.

Brucker, M. C. (2005). Providing evidence-based care: You can understand research and use it in practice! *AWHONN Lifelines, 9*(1), 46–55.

Ciliska, D. (2005). Educating for evidence-based practice. *Journal of Professional Nursing, 21*(6), 345–350.

Ciliska, D. (2006). Evidence-based nursing: How far have we come? What's next? *Evidence-Based Nursing, 9*(2), 38–40.

Cochrane, A. L. (1972). *Effectiveness and efficiency: Random reflections on health services.* London: Nuffield Provincial Hospitals Trust.

Cochrane Collaboration. (2001). *Informational leaflets.* Retrieved June 25, 2007, from http://www.cochrane.org/cochrane/cc-broch.htm#cc

Connor, E. M., Sperling R. S., Gelber R., Kiselev, P., Scott, G., O'Sullivan, M. J., et al. (1994). Reduction of maternal–infant transmission of human immunodeficiency virus type 1 with zidovudine treatment. *New England Journal of Medicine, 331*, 1173–1180.

DiCenso, A., Guyatt, G., & Ciliska, D. (2005). *Evidence-based nursing: A guide to clinical practice.* St. Louis, MO: Mosby.

Duffy, M. E. (2005). Translation research: Its relationship to evidence-based practice. *Clinical Nurse Specialist, 19*(2), 60–62.

Estabrooks, C. A. (1998). Will evidence-based nursing practice make practice perfect? *Canadian Journal of Nursing Research, 30*, 15–36.

Eisenberg, J. M. (2001). *Evidence-based medicine: Expert voices.* Washington, DC: Agency for Healthcare Research and Quality.

Enkin, M. (1992). Current overviews of research evidence from controlled trials in midwifery obstetrics. *Journal of Obstetricians and Gynecologists of Canada, 9*, 23–33.

Ervin, C. E. (2002). Evidence-based nursing practice: Are we there yet? *Journal of the New York State Nurses Association, 33*(2), 11–16.

Fawcett, J., Watson, J., Neuman, B., Hinton, P., & Fitzpatrick, J. (2001). On nursing theories and evidence. *Journal of Nursing Scholarship, 33,* 115–119.

Ferguson, L., & Day, R. A. (2005). Evidence-based nursing education: Myth or reality? *Journal of Nursing Education, 44*(3), 107–115.

Fernandez, R., Griffiths, R., & Ussia, C. (2002). Water for wound cleansing. *Cochrane Database of Systematic Reviews, 4.* Art No. CD003861. Retrieved May 25, 2008, from http://www.cochrane.org/reviews/en/ab003861.html

Fineout-Overholt, E., Levin, R., & Melnyk, B. M. (2005). Strategies for advancing evidence-based practice in clinical settings. *Journal of the New York State Nurses Association, 35,* 28–33.

Fineout-Overholt, E., Melnyk, B. M., & Shultz, A. (2005). Transforming health care from inside out: Advancing evidence-based practice in the 21st century. *Journal of Professional Nursing, 21*(6), 335–344.

Fleming, K. (2007). The knowledge base for evidence-based nursing: A role for mixed methods research? *Advances in Nursing Science, 30*(1), 41–51.

Gillespie, L. D., Gillespie, W. J., Robertson, M. C., Lamb, S. E., Cummings, R. G., & Rowe, B. H. (2003). Interventions for preventing falls in elderly people. *Cochrane Database of Systematic Reviews, 4.* Art No. CD000340. Retrieved May 26, 2008, from http://www.cochrane.org/reviews/en/ab000340.html

Graham, J. D., Harrison, M. B., Brouwers, M., Davies, B. L., & Dunn, S. (2002). Facilitating the use of evidence in practice: Evaluating and adapting clinical practice guidelines for local use by health care organizations. *Journal of Obstetric, Gynecologic, and Neonatal Nursing, 31,* 599–611.

Grimshaw, J. M., Freemantle, N., Wallace, S., Russell, I., Hurwitz, B., Watt, I., et al. (1995). Developing and implementing clinical practice guidelines. *Quality Health Care, 4*(1), 55–64.

Grimshaw, J. M., & Russell, I. (1993). Effect of clinical guidelines on medical practice: A systematic review of rigorous evaluations. *Lancet, 342*(8883), 1317–1322.

Guyatt, G., & Rennie, D. (2002). *Users' guides to the medical literature.* Chicago: AMA Press.

Guyatt, G. H., & Drummond, R. (Eds.). (2001). *Users guide to the medical literature: A manual for evidence-based practice.* Chicago: American Medical Association.

Harris, R. P., Helfand, M., Woolf, S. H., Lohr, K. N., Mulrow, C. D., Teutsch, S. M., et al. (2001). Current methods of the U.S. Preventative Services Task Force: A review of the methods. *American Journal of Preventive Services, 20*(Suppl. 3), 21–35.

Haynes, R. B., Devereaux, P. J., & Guyatt, G. H. (2002). Clinical expertise in the era of evidence-based medicine and patient choice. *ACP Journal Club, 136,* A11–A14.

Hopp, L. (2005). Minding the gap: Evidence-based practice brings the academy to clinical practice. *Clinical Nurse Specialist, 19*(4), 190–192.

Institute of Medicine. (2001). *Closing the quality chasm: A new health system for the 21st century.* Washington, DC: National Academy Press.

Institute of Medicine, 2005

Ironside, P. M. (2005). Teaching thinking and reaching the limits of memorization: Enacting new pedagogies. *Journal of Nursing Education, 44*(10), 441–449.

Ironside, P. M., & Spaziale, H. S. (2006). Using evidence in education and practice: More findings from the national survey on excellence in nursing. *Nursing Education Perspectives, 27*(4), 219–221.

Kennedy, H. P., & Carr, K. C. (2006). Using evidence to support clinical practice. In K. D. Schulling & F. E. Likis (Eds.), *Women's gynecologic heath* (pp. 41–63). Sudbury, MA: Jones and Bartlett.

Kessenich, C. R., Guyatt, G. H., & DiCenso, A. (1997). Teaching nursing students evidence-based nursing. *Nurse Educator, 22*(6), 25–29.

Killeen, M., & Barnfather, J. (2005). A successful teaching strategy for applying evidence-based practice. *Nurse Educator, 30*(3), 127–132.

Kirkbaum, S. R., Baumbusch, J. L., Schultz, A. S. H., & Anderson, J. M. (2007). Knowledge development and evidence-based practice: Insights and opportunities from a postcolonial feminist perspective for transformative nursing practice. *Advances in Nursing Science, 30*(1), 26–40.

Klardie, K. A., Johnson, J., McNaughton, M. A., & Meyers, W. (2004). Integrating the principles of evidence-based practice into clinical practice. *Journal of the American Academy of Nurse Practitioners, 16*(3), 98–105.

Klem, M., & Weiss, P. M. (2005). Evidence-based resources and the role of librarians in developing evidence-based practice curricula. *Journal of Professional Nursing, 21*(6), 380–387.

Melnyk, B. M., & Fineout-Overholt, E. (2005). *Evidence-based practice in nursing and health care: A guide to best practice.* Philadelphia: Lippincott.

Mohide, E. A., & Cocker, E. (2005). Toward clinical scholarship: Promoting evidence-based practice in the clinical setting. *Journal of Professional Nursing, 21,* 372–379.

Moore, E. R., Anderson, G. C., & Bergman, N. (2003). Early skin-to-skin contact for mothers and their healthy newborns. *Cochrane Database of Systematic Reviews, 2.* Art No. CD003519. Retrieved May 26, 2008, from http://www.cochrane.org/reviews/en/ab003519.html

National Institutes of Health. (2001). *Qualitative methods in health research.* NIH Publication No. 02-5046. Bethesda, MD: Office of Behavioral and Social Sciences Research, NIH.

Newhouse, R., Dearholt, S., Poe, S., Pugh, L. C., & White, K. M. (2005). Evidence-based practice: A practical approach to implementation. *Journal of Nursing Administration, 35*(1), 35–40.

Nightingale, F. (1957). *Notes on nursing: What it is and what it is not.* Philadelphia: Lippincott. (Originally published 1859.)

Pravikoff, D. S., Tanner, A. B., & Pierce, S. T. (2005). Readiness of U.S. nurses for evidence-based practice. *American Journal of Nursing, 105*(9), 40–51.

Sackett, D. L., Strauss, S. E., Richardson, W. S., Rosenberg, W., & Hayes, R. B. (2000). *Evidence-based medicine: How to practice and teach EBM.* New York: Churchill Livingstone.

Sakala, C. (2007). Current resources for evidence-based practice. *Journal of Midwifery and Women's Health, 52,* 77–81.

Stetler, C. B. (2001). Adapting the Stetler Model of Research Utilization to facilitate evidence-based nursing. *Nursing Outlook, 49,* 272–279.

Tanner, A., Pierce, S., & Pravikoff, D. (2004). Readiness for evidence-based practice: Information literacy needs of the nurses in the United States. *Medinfo, 11*(Pt 2), 936–940.

Thompson, D. C., Rivara, F. P., & Thompson, R. (1999). Helmets for preventing head and facial injuries in bicyclists. *Cochrane Database of Systematic Reviews, 4.* Art No. CD01855. Retrieved October 10, 2007, from http://www.cochrane.org/reviews/en/ab001855.html

U.S. Department of Health and Human Services. (2004). *About healthy people.* Retrieved June 26, 2007, from Healthy People 2010 Web site: http://www.healthypeople.gov/About/

U.S. Preventive Services Task Force. (1996). *Guide to clinical preventive services* (2nd ed.). Baltimore: Williams & Wilkins.

Weaver, C. A., Warren, J. J., & Delaney, C. (2005). Bedside, classroom, and bench: Collaborative strategies to generate evidence-based knowledge. *International Journal of Medical Informatics, 74*(11), 989–999.

chapter 12

Emergency Planning and Response

Kristi L. Lewis

LEARNING OUTCOMES

After reading this chapter you will be able to:

- Identify the specific Category A agents that may be used in a bio-terrorism event.
- Recognize the types of chemical agents that may be used in a chemical attack.
- Discuss the types of events that require emergency planning and response activities.
- Increase awareness of the role of the nurse in emergency planning and response activities.
- List three types of natural disasters that require emergency planning and response activities.
- Discuss health education practices that increase preparedness for a family to survive emergencies.

Introduction

Since the beginning of the 21st century, the world has experienced many events that have caused public health professionals to engage in **emergency planning and response (EP&R)** activities. The events of

Emergency planning and response (EP&R): Activities that are conducted before, during, and after an event that may involve extensive destruction.

September 11, 2001, the emergence of new infectious diseases such as severe acute respiratory syndrome (SARS) in 2003, the Indian Ocean tsunami in 2004, and Hurricane Katrina in 2005 brought attention to the need for better planning to prevent such events and control the aftermath. Today, concerns about the spread of an influenza strain that could kill millions and the possibility of yet another terrorist attack still remain. Although events that have resulted in high morbidity and mortality are not new, it is important to note that not until after the events of September 11th did the medical community realize that they were not prepared for terrorist attacks (Rhyne, 2005). Hurricane Katrina also highlighted the need for extensive planning and preparation for natural disasters.

EP&R can best be defined as activities that are conducted before, during, and after an event that may involve extensive destruction. EP&R activities are needed at the local, state, and federal levels. One of the main target audiences for conducting EP&R activities is healthcare professionals. Training and education are necessary to prepare the current and future workforce for developing, disseminating, and evaluating such activities. Universities and colleges are now offering courses in emergency planning and response. Many are offering certificate, undergraduate, and graduate-level degree programs to help expand the knowledge base. In response to the events of September 11th, the Association of American Medical Colleges (AAMC) made recommendations that U.S. medical schools should educate students on emergency planning and response activities as part of their school curriculum to ensure that events would be well coordinated (Parrish et al., 2005).

Although public health nurses have long been active in EP&R activities, from the planning and execution phases to the follow-up postdisaster, nurses in hospitals, acute care clinics, and mental facilities are taking on a significantly enhanced role. EP&R activities at all levels should involve more than the public health workforce, and are not just the role of public health professionals. Healthcare providers are seeing their role change to include participation in activities related to emergency planning and response. Nurses at all levels of training play a significant part in EP&R activities, and their role is rapidly being redefined.

SIDEBAR 12-1

EP&R is a growing field that requires collaboration from many disciplines including public health, medicine, public administration, social work, psychology, public planning, and nursing.

The purpose of this chapter is to provide an overview of the specific topic areas within the EP&R field. This chapter will focus on emergency planning and response as it relates to healthcare professionals; it is divided into topic areas based on events such as 1) bioterrorism events, 2) chemical emergencies, 3) radiation, 4) natural disasters, and 5) outbreaks. Mass causalities, the psychological impact, and the role of the nurse in planning and assisting with such emergencies also will be discussed.

Biological and Chemical Agent Overview

Biological and chemical events can be both intentional and unintentional. Intentional events are usually identified as terrorist attacks and can be domestic or international. The purpose of an intentional release of a biological or chemical agent is to cause harm to the general public and disruption to daily life activities that could harm the overall economy. Unintentional events are accidents that can result in the release of a biological or chemical agent.

Biological agents have been a component of terrorist attacks since the beginning of recorded history. One example of this was seen during the 14th century when Tartars catapulted plague-contaminated cadavers into a nearby city on the Black Sea. While the attack was successful, it also caused a continuation of the Black Death in Europe (Phillips, 2005). Terrorist attacks are usually either overt or covert events. During an **overt event**, those involved know about the attack as soon as it occurs, with little if any lag time. An example of an overt attack would be a chemical attack where as soon as the chemical agent is released the population exposed is aware and may start exhibiting signs and symptoms. During a **covert event**, the individuals involved are not aware for a period of time that an attack has occurred. Most biological agents used in bioterrorism events are used in covert events because signs and symptoms of exposure to a biological agent may not occur for hours or even days based on the incubation period of the agent.

One concern about biological events is that during the incubation period, an individual can be asymptomatic and yet still communicable. This could lead to secondary spread if the mode of transmission of the biological agent is person-to-person such as smallpox (Centers for Disease Control and Prevention [CDC], 2000).

The Centers for Disease Control and Prevention (CDC) has five focus areas for dealing with a biological or chemical event. The five focus areas identified by CDC are:

- Preparedness and prevention
- Detection and surveillance
- Diagnosis and agent identification
- Response
- Communication

Healthcare providers may be called upon to assist in one or more of these five areas. The role of the nurse will be discussed in more detail for each of the five EP&R topic areas of the chapter.

KEY TERM

Overt event: An attack that those involved know about as soon as it occurs, with little if any lag time.

KEY TERM

Covert event: An attack that the individuals involved are not aware of for a period of time.

SIDEBAR 12-2

Incubation period is defined as the time that lapses between when the host receives the agent and when the host presents with symptoms.

Bioterrorism Events

A biological agent is a living organism and can involve bacteria, viruses, or parasites.

There are three distinct classes of biological agents, labeled Categories A, B, and C. They vary based on the ease of mass production and the health effects if released into a population.

Category A is characterized by agents that are easy to produce and disseminate and may have a direct mode of transmission (i.e., person-to-person). Category A agents of concern include variola major (smallpox), *Bacillus anthracis* (anthrax), *Yersinia pestis* (plague), *Clostridium botulinum* toxin (botulism), *Francisella tularensis* (tularemia), filoviruses including Ebola hemorrhagic fever and Marburg hemorrhagic fever, and arena viruses that include Lassa (Lassa fever) and Junin (Argentine hemorrhagic fever) (CDC, 2000). (See Table 12-1.)

An example of a Category A **bioterrorism** event occurred less than a month after the events of September 11th when a man was admitted to a local hospital in South Florida with fever and altered mental status. The 63-year-old male was given antibiotic therapy, but died 3 days later. An autopsy later revealed inhalation anthrax (CDC, 2001a; Zinkovich, Malvey, Hamby, & Fottler, 2005). During a 2-month period, 22 cases of anthrax were identified. Five of the 22 identified cases resulted in death (CDC, 2001b). Evaluating previous bioterrorism events such as this example can assist those who must develop and implement appropriate response plans in the future. In particular, it is important to understand how the events were initially detected and the process involved in reporting them (Ashford et al., 2003). Clues to a possible biological or chemical terrorist attack include the presence of an unusual disease case such as anthrax, an unusual increase in a disease, or an unusual pattern of death.

The U.S. Army Medical Research Institute of Infectious Diseases (USAMRIID) has evaluated numerous biological agents to predict whether they could be used in a bioterrorist attack. According to experts, although there is a strategic national stockpile that includes medical supplies that should arrive within 12 hours of a disaster, localities should be prepared to use their own resources for the initial 24 hours. This means that hospitals and clinics need to purchase supplies and have them available in the event of a disaster (Martin, 2006). An all-hazards disaster plan should be in place and annual drills or tabletop exercises should be conducted to assess the feasibility of the plan.

Category B agents are relatively easy to produce and disseminate; however, not as easy as those in Category A. Although Category B agents can cause illness and death, they are far less deadly than the agents in Category A. The majority of Category B agents are transmitted indirectly. This means they are not transmitted person-to-person (direct transmission), but rather require a vector or

TABLE 12-1   BIOLOGICAL CATEGORIES, AGENTS, AND DISEASES

Category	Agents	Diseases
A	Anthrax	*Bacillus anthracis*
	Botulism	*Clostridium botulinum toxin*
	Plague	*Yersinia pestis*
	Smallpox	variola major
	Tularemia	*Francisella tularensis*
	Viral hemmorrhagic fevers	filoviruses and arenaviruses
B	Brucellosis	*Brucella* species
	Epsilon toxin	*Clostridium perfringens*
	Food safety threats	*Salmonella, Escherichia, Shigella*
	Glanders	*Burkholderia mallei*
	Melioidosis	*Burkholderia pseudomallei*
	Psittacosis	*Chlamydia psittaci*
	Q fever	*Coxiella burnetii*
	Ricin toxin	from castor beans
	Staphylococcal	enterotoxin B
	Typhus fever	*Rickettsia prowazekii*
	Viral encephalitis	alphaviruses
	Water safety threats	*Vibrio cholerae*
C	Emerging infectious diseases	Nipah virus, hantavirus

Note. From the Centers for Disease Control, Emergency Preparedness & Response website. (2007). Available at http://www.bt.cdc.gov/agent/agentlist-category.asp.

vehicle. A vector is a living organism that transmits an agent to a host, such as a human. For example, the flea is a vector for typhus fever and the tick is the vector for Rocky Mountain spotted fever. A vehicle is a nonliving object that may be contaminated with an agent and can then transmit it to a host via ingestion. For example, when contaminated with a strain of salmonella, egg salad can cause salmonellosis in a host (i.e., a human).

Category C agents are composed of newly emerging infectious agents that have the potential to be mass produced and disseminated to a large population of individuals within a geographical region. These cause diseases that have not been seen in humans or that occur in a new geographical location. With their ease in production and mass dissemination comes the risk for high levels of morbidity and mortality.

For the purposes of this chapter, the focus will be on Category A agents because they pose the greatest threat to public health.

Smallpox

Smallpox is a disease caused by the variola virus that has two distinct forms—variola minor and variola major. Variola minor is less severe than variola major, with a lower fatality rate. Variola major is the most common and severe form of variola, and can be easily spread from person to person. Nearly 30 percent of cases infected with variola major lead to death. Symptoms of smallpox include a rash with raised bumps and high fever.

Although the World Health Organization declared that smallpox was eradicated in 1977 after the last known case was identified in Somalia, it may still be a plausible threat due to its high death rate and person-to-person transmission. After the events of September 11th, smallpox vaccination was reinitiated among healthcare providers and first responders. After several months, the risk seemed to outweigh the possible benefits and vaccination was once again put on hold (CDC, 2007c). Because smallpox is spread from person to person, the main role of public health professionals and healthcare providers will be to contain the outbreak as much as possible through the early identification and isolation of cases and the quarantine of individuals who may have been contaminated but are not showing signs and symptoms of disease.

Anthrax

Anthrax, a bacterial disease caused by *Bacillus anthracis*, comes in three forms: cutaneous, inhalation, and gastrointestinal. Although all three forms of anthrax can be treated with antibiotics, the gastrointestinal and inhalation forms can cause severe illness and death. Cutaneous anthrax begins with a painless skin lesion that may progress to a black eschar. Those with cutaneous anthrax may experience symptoms such as a fever and malaise. Death from cutaneous anthrax is rare if treated with an antibiotic, but as many as 20 percent of those who are not treated may die. Inhalational anthrax, however, has a higher fatality rate even with prompt initiation of antibiotics. In the bioterrorism-related anthrax cases that occurred in 2001, 45 percent of those diagnosed with inhalation anthrax died. Individuals with inhalation anthrax present with viral-like respiratory illness, and it should be included in the differential diagnosis of those presenting with unexplained upper respiratory illness and symptoms such as fever and muscle aches. Gastrointestinal anthrax may occur after consuming raw or undercooked meat that has been contaminated with anthrax. Symptoms include severe abdominal pain, fever, nausea, anorexia, and bloody diarrhea. The death rate due to gastrointestinal anthrax is reported to be around 25 to 60 percent (CDC, 2001a).

Although anthrax is not spread person-to-person, it can be spread through handling animal products that have been infected with the bacteria or from eating undercooked meat that has been infected. Treatment recommendations for adults with anthrax should include antibiotic therapy with ciprofloxacin 500 mg po BID or doxycycline 100 mg po BID (CDC, 2001b).

Botulism

Botulism is a paralyzing disease of the muscles caused by toxin released from the bacterium *Clostridium botulinum*. On average, 110 cases are reported annually within the United States. Botulism cannot be spread person-to-person, but untreated it has a high fatality rate.

Twenty-five percent of all botulism cases are foodborne and are due to the improper preparation and storage of foods. Individuals with foodborne botulism usually present with symptoms that include drooping eyelids, difficulty in swallowing, dry mouth, abdominal pain, nausea, vomiting, and diarrhea. In September 2006, four individuals reported to area hospitals in Georgia and Florida with symptoms that included cranial nerve palsies and flaccid paralysis that resulted in respiratory failure requiring mechanical ventilation. After extensive testing, foodborne botulism was identified in the serum of all four patients. Further investigation identified the consumption of commercial carrot juice as the cause of the botulism poisoning (CDC, 2006a).

The mode of transmission of infant botulism is unclear; however, preliminary studies have identified corn syrup and honey as possible sources. Experts agree that further studies need to be conducted to evaluate risk factors including environmental exposures. Symptoms of infant botulism include poor eating with difficulty sucking, crying, neck weakness that may cause the head to flop, constipation, and respiratory distress.

Wound botulism encompasses 30 to 40 percent of all botulism cases. The primary risk factor is illicit intravenous drug use, where the transmission occurs through needle puncture sites. Individuals with wound botulism may present with neurological symptoms similar to foodborne illness, but without the gastrointestinal symptoms (CDC, 2006b, 2006c). Botulism differs from many of the other

SIDEBAR 12-5

Botulism comes in three forms: foodborne botulism, infant botulism, and wound botulism.

SIDEBAR 12-6

Infant botulism is the most common form of botulism, comprising nearly 70 percent of all botulism cases.

bioterrorism agents because the bacteria form a toxin. This toxin causes respiratory paralysis and therefore is a concern because most persons will require mechanical ventilation. Many community-level hospitals have only a few ventilators and therefore would not be able to treat a large number of clients with botulism.

Plague

Plague, caused by the bacterium *Yersinia pestis*, has three forms: pneumonic, bubonic, and septicemic. The pneumonic plague form infects the lungs and can be spread person-to-person via respiratory droplets. Symptoms of pneumonic plague mimic respiratory influenza and include fever, headache, shortness of breathe, chest pain, and cough. Bubonic plague, the most common form of plague, is transmitted by fleas and cannot be spread person-to-person. Clients with bubonic plague will present with symptoms that include enlarged and tender lymph nodes, fever, headache, and overall bodily weakness. Septicemic plague cannot be spread person-to-person and occurs when the *Yersinia pestis* bacteria multiply in the person's blood throughout the body. This bacteremia can be a secondary effect from either pneumonic or bubonic plague or it can occur alone. Symptoms include fever, chills, and shock. Rapid treatment with an antibiotic must occur within 24 to 48 hours to reduce the risk of death.

Tularemia

The incidence of tularemia in the United States is low, with approximately 100–200 cases reported annually. Tularemia is caused by the bacteria *Francisella tularensis* and occurs naturally within the United States. It is often referred to as "rabbit fever" because it can be found in mammals such as rabbits (Farlow et al., 2005). Tularemia is highly infectious and can be manufactured and disseminated as an airborne weapon. Although tularemia can be manufactured as a biological weapon, it cannot be transmitted via person-to-person contact. It can be spread through the bite of a tick that carries the agent, handling of infected animal carcasses, consumption of contaminated food, or inhalation of aerosolized particles. Signs and symptoms of tularemia include fever, chills, headaches, diarrhea, muscle and joint pain, cough, and weakness (CDC, 2003b, 2003c). Treatment for tularemia includes antimicrobial therapy, with streptomycin being the drug of choice. Other suitable drugs include gentamicin, tetracycline, and chloramphenicol (Dennis et al., 2001).

The Role of the Nurse in Bioterrorism Events

It is important for nurses to make keen observations and use deductive reasoning in evaluating clients who may have been exposed to a biological agent. In a study conducted by the Department of Health and Human Services, 75 percent of family practice physicians surveyed stated that they did not feel they were prepared to diagnose a bioterrorism-related illness in a patient (Neff, 2002). Nurses should be on alert for individuals who present with unusual symptoms that lack a clear diagnosis.

During an outbreak, nurses need to evaluate and triage clients based on symptoms and severity. In large outbreaks, clients must be triaged based on the severity of symptoms. In many cases, the nurse may be the first professional to come in contact with an exposed client. Early identification and treatment could reduce the overall morbidity and mortality that results from the attack. In addition to assessment and triage, nurses may be asked to report findings to local authorities including the public health department and provide follow-up on potential cases or contacts of confirmed cases. Samples for laboratory testing may also need to be collected and submitted with rigorous follow-up of the results with the public health department.

> **SIDEBAR 12-8**
>
> When a biological exposure is suspected, the nurse must conduct an immediate assessment and interview of clients and their family members that includes health history questions on environmental and occupational exposures.

Nurses play an important role in planning and preparing for bioterrorism events. In many health departments, hospitals, and healthcare centers, nurses are serving as leaders in developing multilevel and multidisciplinary plans for a bioterrorism event. In this leadership role, nurses are writing protocols, coordinating personnel, and providing training opportunities for staff. Many nurses also are engaging in drills to assess preparedness and resource needs during such events.

Chemical Emergencies

Chemical agents can be either manmade or derived from natural sources such as vegetation. At this point in time, **chemical emergencies** seem inevitable regardless of the intent. Through a surveillance system at the Agency for Toxic Substances and Disease Registry (ATSDR), during a 51-month period approximately 36,784 events were reported that involved the release of hazardous substances. Approximately 107 of these events involved improper disposal of hazardous waste, which resulted in 101 injuries. Most injuries were respiratory-related and many required medical care at a local hospital (CDC, 2005a).

> **KEY TERM**
>
> **Chemical emergency:** The release of some hazardous chemical agent either unintentionally, such as through an accidental industrial release, or intentionally, as in a terrorist attack.

Chemical emergencies, like biological emergencies, can be either intentional or unintentional, both with potentially disastrous outcomes. An example of an unintentional chemical emergency occurred in 2005, when two freight trains collided in Graniteville, South Carolina. The collision caused the release of nearly 11,500 gallons of chlorine gas, which resulted in 9 casualties and 529 persons with injuries needing immediate medical care. The incident prompted public health officials to study the effects of chlorine gas related to health outcomes (CDC, 2005d).

An example of an intentional chemical emergency involved the contamination of ground hamburger. In January 2003, 1,700 pounds of ground beef were recalled after 36 individuals complained of becoming ill or having family members who became ill after ingesting the product. Laboratory analysis revealed that nearly 100 people were ill after consuming ground beef. The tests verified that the beef had been contaminated with nicotine. Based on an extensive investigation it was discovered that the contamination did not occur in the processing plant, but at a single grocery store. Upon further study, investigators found that the poisoning was caused by one individual who had contaminated nearly 200 pounds of ground beef with an insecticide containing nicotine as the main ingredient (CDC, 2003d). Whether intentional or unintentional, chemical emergencies are plausible and can lead to extensive public health consequences.

Chemical agents that could be used in a terrorist attack or could be released accidentally and lead to serious public health outcomes are categorized by either the type of chemical or by the effects the chemical has on the human body. The 13 categories are the following (see Table 12-2):

- Biotoxins
- Blister agents/vesicants
- Blood agents
- Caustics (acids)
- Choking/lung/pulmonary agents
- Incapacitating agents
- Long-lasting anticoagulants
- Metals
- Nerve agents
- Organic solvents
- Riot control agents/tear gas
- Toxic alcohols
- Vomiting agents

The Role of the Nurse in Chemical Events

The role of the nurse in chemical events mirrors his or her role in bioterrorism events. Nurses play a significant role in the early identification of a chemical agent and the assessment, triage, and treatment of affected individuals.

TABLE 12-2 HAZARDOUS CHEMICALS: CATEGORY, TYPES, AND EFFECTS

Category	Types	Effects on Body
Biotoxins	Abrin Brevetoxin Colchincine Digitalis Nicotine Ricin Strychnine Tetrodotoxin Trichothecene	
Blister Agents	Distilled mustard (HD)	Severely blister the eyes, respiratory tract, and skin on contact

Vesicants	Mustard gas (H) (sulfur mustard)
	   Mustard/lewisite (HL)
	   Mustard/T
	   Nitrogen mustard (HN-1, HN-2, HN-3)
	   Sesqui mustard
	   Sulfur mustard (H) (mustard gas)
	Lewisites/chloroarsine agents
	   Lewisite (L, L-1, L-2, L-3)
	   Mustard/lewisite (HL)
	   Phosgene oxime (CX)	

Blood Agents	Arsine (SA) Carbon monoxide Cyanide chloride (CK) Hydrogen cyanide (AC) Potassium cyanide (KCN) Sodium cyanide (NaCN) Sodium monofluoroacetate	
Caustics (Acids)	Hydrofluoric acid (hydrogen fluoride)	Burn or corrode skin, eyes, and mucus membranes on contact
Choking/Lung	Ammonia	Cause severe irritation or swelling of the respiratory tract

(continues)

TABLE 12-2   HAZARDOUS CHEMICALS: CATEGORY, TYPES, AND EFFECTS *(continued)*

Category	Types	Effects on Body
Pulmonary Agents	Bromine (CA) Chlorine (CL) Hydrogen chloride Methyl bromide Methyl isocyanate Osmium tetroxide Phosgene Diphosgene (DP) Phosgene (CG) Phosphine Phosphorus, elemental, white, or yellow Sulfuryl fluoride	
Incapacitating	BZ	Alter state of consciousness (possibly cause unconsciousness)
Agents	Fentanyls Other opioids	
Long-Acting	Super warfarin	Prevent blood from clotting properly
Metals	Arsenic Barium Mercury Thallium	
Nerve Agents	Sarin (GB) Soman (GD) Tabun (GA) VX	Damage the nervous system
Organic Solvents	Benzene	Destroy tissue by dissolving essential bodily fats and oils
Riot Control	Bromobenzylcyanide (CA)	Irritate mucus membranes
Agents/Tear Gas	Chloroacetophenone (CN) Chlorobenzylidenemalononitrile (CS) Chloropicrin (PS) Dibenzoxazepine (CR)	
Toxic Alcohols	Ethylene glycol	Damage internal organs and the nervous system
Vomiting Agents	Adamsite	Cause nausea and vomiting

Source: Centers for Disease Control and Prevention.

Radiation

Radiation, a ubiquitous form of energy, can come from either man-made sources such as medical devices or natural sources such as the sun. The release of radioactive material can result in radioactive contamination and radiation exposure. Radioactive contamination is defined as radioactive particles that are on or in an object or a living organism such as humans. For example, radioactive material can be on clothing, objects, and the skin. Internal contamination can occur when the individual inhales or ingests radioactive material. Radioactive exposure, in contrast, is defined as the penetration of the body by radioactive material given off in the form of particles or waves. For example, an individual who has had an X-ray for medical diagnostic purposes has been exposed to radiation and therefore has had radioactive waves or particles penetrate their body (CDC, 2005e). In many cases, small amounts of radiation have little if any adverse health effect.

Adverse health effects have been documented, however, from exposure to large doses of radiation for a short period of time or from prolonged exposure to low doses (CDC, 2005a). Table 12-3 illustrates the leading radioactive isotopes that can be found in radiation events. Radiation events can include accidents or intentional release due to a terrorist attack. Although rare, in the past 50 years there have been approximately 10 different events where radiation was released that resulted in the contamination of either small groups with high exposure levels or low exposure among a large population of people.

Approximately 237 employees and rescue workers suffered effects related to the accidental release of radiation in April 1986 from a nuclear reactor located in Chernobyl, Ukraine (formerly the Soviet Union). Thirty workers died due to conditions related to radiation exposure and nearly 15,000 people living within the community suffered health conditions. Over the years since this event, an increase in thyroid cancer; neurological damage; respiratory, gastrointestinal, and hemopoietic diseases; and conditions related to the exposure have been documented in individuals exposed to the radiation (Agency for Toxic Substances and Disease Registry [ATSDR], 1999).

Radiation exposure can also be intentional. In fall 2006, United Kingdom officials began an investigation related to the death of Alexander Litvinenko, a former Russian spy contaminated with polonium-210 (Po-210). Traces of radioactive material were also found at a London sushi bar where Litvinenko was presumably poisoned.

With the concern of an intentional radiation event comes the worldwide concern over dirty bombs. A dirty bomb is composed of a mixture of explosives and radioactive material that can be released when the bomb explodes. Dirty bombs are often mistaken for atomic bombs such as those used in the attacks on Hiroshima and Nagasaki in World War II. Atomic bombs are much more powerful

KEY TERM

Radiation: A ubiquitous form of energy that can come from either man-made sources such as medical devices or natural sources such as the sun.

TABLE 12-3   RADIOACTIVE ISOTOPES

Isotope	Source	Effect on Body
Americium-241	Plutonium	Can cause certain cancers; if ingested, can stay in the body
Cesium-137	Nuclear fission	Can cause burns, acute radiation sickness, possibly death; exposes tissues to gamma radiation and beta particles
Cobalt-60	Linear acceleration	Skin burns, acute radiation sickness, possibly death, can cause cancer because of exposure to gamma radiation
Iodine-131	Nuclear fission	Burns to the eyes and skin; internal exposure can affect the thyroid gland possibly leading to thyroid cancer
Iridium-192	Nonradioactive iridium in nuclear reactors	Increased risk for cancer because of gamma exposure; burns, acute radiation sickness, possibly death
Plutonium-240	Uranium in nuclear reactors	Emits alpha particles; therefore, if inhaled can cause lung damage, disease, and cancer
Polonium-210	Naturally occurring at low levels	Destroys genetic materials in cells; irradiation of internal organs which can lead to death
Strontium-90	Nuclear fission	Readily incorporates into bones and teeth where it can cause cancers of the bone or bone marrow
Uranium-235	Rock, soil, and water	Skin will block alpha particles, but if ingested, can cause bone, liver, or lung cancer and kidney damage

and cause the release of large amounts of radioactive material that can spread for miles. The detonation of a dirty bomb would not cause extensive or widespread release of radioactive material. Injuries related to the explosion from a dirty bomb are the primary concern.

One effect of radiation exposure is acute radiation syndrome (ARS), also known as radiation toxicity or radiation sickness (CDC, 2005a). ARS is a characteristic result of radiation exposure where the dose is high and exposure is of short duration to the entire body. ARS has extensive physiological effects on the human body and can affect the central nervous system, cardiovascular system, and gastrointestinal system and destroy bone marrow.

ARS is identified by four clinical stages: 1) prodromal, 2) latent, 3) manifest illness, and 4) recovery or death. The prodromal stage involves symptoms such as nausea, vomiting, anorexia, and diarrhea. Those exposed can also experience confusion and loss of consciousness. The symptoms can occur within a few minutes of exposure or can occur days after the event and go on for hours, days, or weeks depending on the dosage. In the latent phase, exposed individuals may look healthy; however, destruction of bone marrow is common. In the manifest illness stage, symptoms include anorexia, fever, and malaise. In this stage, death due to infection and possible hemorrhage is likely, depending on the amount radiation exposure. In the final stage, individuals exposed to low doses of radiation for a short period of time usually recover. Death is common, however, for those who were exposed to higher levels of radiation or to low levels for an extended period of time (CDC, 2005a).

ARS is alarming, but cutaneous radiation injury (CRI) also can result after exposure to radiation. With CRI, the degree of skin damage is related to the amount and depth of radiation exposure. Symptoms of CRI can include itching, tingling, and edema. If the hair follicles are damaged, hair loss also can result. Individuals with CRI need to be monitored for infection and provided with effective pain management (CDC, 2005e).

Although the health effects of radiation exposure to adults can result in ARS and CRI, exposure to low doses of radiation in-utero has been shown to have little if any health effects on the fetus. For example, although physicians are cautious, radiation exposure to the mother from diagnostic medical procedures has been shown to have little if any negative health effects both short and long term to the fetus. However, the risk of miscarriage, severe mental retardation, and malformation can be high for those exposed to high levels of radiation (CDC, 2005a).

The Role of the Nurse in Radiation Events

The role of nurses and other healthcare providers during a radiological event is multifaceted. Although transfer of radioactive material from a contaminated client is rare, healthcare providers should evaluate any possible self-contamination prior to treating the client. After the possibility of self-contamination has been eliminated, the nurse should remove the client's clothing by cutting and rolling the clothing away from the face. Once the clothes have been removed they should be placed in a double bag, and closed and labeled as hazardous material. The next step is for the nurse to cleanse possible contaminated body areas with saline water. If facial contamination has occurred, eyes, nose, and mouth need to be flushed. Wounds may need to be covered with a waterproof dressing. Clients who are able to stand may be able to be decontaminated in a showering facility

---

SIDEBAR 12–10

Health effects of radiation exposure vary depending on the dose and the length of exposure. Health effects can vary from mild to severe and can take days, months, or years to develop. Some studies, for example, have shown that radiation may increase the risk for cancer later in life (CDC, 2005a).

(CDC, 2005e). In some situations, nurses will need to triage clients to prioritize those who need immediate treatment. Nurses should obtain a health history so that the client can be given appropriate treatment.

During most radiological events that require medical attention, the role of the nurse may involve supportive care, surveillance, treatment of secondary infections, pain management, and follow-up for mental health support. Immediately after the event, the nurse should secure the airway and closely monitor the respiratory and circulatory status, blood pressure, blood gases, and other physiological markers. Clients need to be followed or closely monitored after the initial evaluation. Nurses need to provide client education on the treatment being provided or on mechanisms to prevent secondary effects such as an infection.

Natural Disasters

After the attacks of September 11th, more emphasis has been placed on events that could be biological, chemical, or radiological, whether through accidental or intentional means. Natural disasters, however, have always occurred, causing extensive destruction and mass casualties. Natural disasters and severe weather can occur in any place with little, if any, warning.

Severe weather can include extreme heat during the summer months and extreme cold during the winter months, which may lead to ice and snowstorms. Both natural disasters and severe weather result in secondary conditions or effects that can cause or pose a health threat. Examples of a secondary effect would include a power outage from a storm or mold from a flood.

Earthquakes are an example of a natural disaster that can result in extensive destruction and mass casualties. Many feel that earthquakes are rare and that only certain geographical locations in the United States (like California) are prone to having an earthquake. Scientists, however, believe that there will be a major earthquake in the New Madrid seismic zone of the central United States (which includes Arkansas, Missouri, Tennessee, and Kentucky) sometime prior to 2035 (CDC, 2003a).

Tornadoes are another type of natural disaster that has led to the need for emergency planning and response. In March 1994 several severe thunderstorms and tornadoes occurred in several counties in the northeastern part of Alabama. Although warnings were issued, the tornado hit land only 5 minutes after being identified by the National Weather Service. The disaster resulted in over 400 individuals with injuries and 47 deaths (CDC, 1994). Each year within the United States there are approximately 1,000 injuries and an average of 51 deaths due to tornadoes (CDC, 1997). When a severe thunderstorm occurs the conditions may be favorable for a tornado (CDC, 2003a).

Tornadoes can arise quickly with little warning and within minutes can cause severe destruction and even loss of life. Although injuries can occur during the actual event, most occur in the days and weeks after the tornado. Such injuries are related to postevent cleanup activities including stepping on nails, broken glass, and other debris (CDC, 2005b).

Although tornadoes can occur with little warning, hurricanes often can be detected early, allowing for some preparation. However, even with advanced computer technology, hurricanes can change direction or gain strength quickly. Hurricanes are a type of tropical cyclone that can lead to miles of mass destruction and high levels of morbidity and mortality (Federal Emergency Management Agency [FEMA], n.d.). Annual morbidity and mortality rates due to hurricanes are hard to calculate because activity is very cyclical. During 2005, hurricane activity peaked and became the most active on record with a total of 27 storms. Hurricanes are ranked by categories ranging from one to five, with one being the lowest and usually resulting in the least severe aftermath. The categories are determined by the strength of sustained winds, amount of damage, and storm surge height. Categories three, four, and five are considered major hurricanes and require both extensive planning and response.

Severe weather is another example of natural events that can lead to adverse circumstances requiring emergency planning and coordinated response activities. Examples of severe weather can include extreme heat, extreme cold, and excessive precipitation including ice, snow, and rain. Weather that causes extremes can cause damage to property and lead to adverse health events such as severe morbidity and mortality. Extreme heat is defined by the CDC as having "temperatures that are 10 degrees or above the average high temperature for the region and last for several weeks" (CDC, 2006d).

Hyperthermia is the inability of the human body to compensate when temperatures are elevated above 98.6°F. Although heat-related illness and deaths are preventable, 8,015 individuals died in the United States from extreme heat between 1979 and 2003. This accounts for more deaths than from hurricanes, lightning, tornadoes, floods, and earthquakes combined (CDC, 2006d). Heat-related illness occurs when the body is not able to compensate and properly cool itself through sweating. In many cases sweating alone will not compensate for the overheating. When humidity is high, it may be difficult for the sweat to evaporate rapidly, thereby preventing the body from releasing heat fast enough to maintain bodily function. When body temperatures rise quickly and the body cannot compensate physiologically to cool or lower body temperatures, the human brain can be severely damaged. This can lead to a heat stroke.

SIDEBAR 12-13

According to the CDC, warning signs of a heat stroke include 1) extremely high body temperature (above 103°F); 2) red, hot, and dry skin; 3) rapid, strong pulse; 4) throbbing headache; 5) dizziness; 6) nausea; 7) confusion; and 8) unconsciousness.

Milder effects of extreme heat include heat exhaustion, heat cramps, and heat rash. Heat exhaustion is due to exposure over several days to high temperatures and the lack of proper replacement of fluids. Signs of heat exhaustion include heavy sweating, paleness, muscle cramps, tiredness, weakness, dizziness, headache, nausea or vomiting, and fainting. Heat exhaustion can lead to a heat stroke if not treated. Individuals who engage in physical activities that result in excessive sweating can develop heat cramps, a sign of heat exhaustion. Heat cramps are caused by the body's depletion of salt and moisture from dehydration. Painful cramps can result from the lack of salt and moisture primarily in the muscles (Table 12-4).

Those at risk for adverse health effects due to extreme heat include the elderly, young children, individuals with mental illness, and those with chronic illnesses. Other factors that make an individual at risk for illness or death related to extreme heat include individuals with obesity, fever, dehydration, heart disease, or who are taking prescription drugs or using alcohol (CDC, 2006d).

Although extreme heat can cause severe illness and death, extreme cold also can result in negative outcomes. Winter storms can lead to extreme cold, which can lead to adverse health conditions and even death. Health effects caused by extreme cold from winter weather may include hypothermia, household fires due to the misuse of alternate heating sources and candles, asphyxiation due to

TABLE 12-4   SYMPTOMS ASSOCIATED WITH HYPERTHERMIA AND HYPOTHERMIA

SEVERE HEAT		SEVERE COLD
Heat Exhaustion	Heat Stroke	Hypothermia
Heavy sweating	Temperature above 103 Fahrenheit	Slow pulse
Paleness	Red, hot, and dry skin	Shivering
Muscle cramps	Rapid strong pulse	Loss of color
Fatigue	Confusion	Confusion
Fainting	Unconsciousness	Memory loss
Dizziness	Dizziness	Numbness
Headache	Throbbing headache	Drowsiness
Nausea/Vomiting	Nausea/ Vomiting	Slow breathing

carbon monoxide poisoning, and motor vehicle accidents due to poor and hazardous road conditions (CDC, 2007b). One example of a health effect due to extreme cold is hypothermia, caused when the body is exposed to cold temperatures and cannot replace heat at a rate fast enough to compensate for the heat lost. Individuals exposed to extreme cold can become mentally confused, causing the individual to be unable to think clearly. Individuals in this state may not be able to find their way to a safe and warm location or be able to provide some way to warm the body either through adding clothes or starting a fire.

Health effects due to exposure to the extreme cold include hypothermia and frostbite. According to the CDC, hypothermia is defined by the core body temperature and can be classified as mild, moderate, or severe (CDC, 2007b). Signs of hypothermia include shivering, confusion, memory loss, and drowsiness (see Table 12-4). Individuals with a temperature below 95°F need immediate medical attention. Another health condition caused by extreme cold is frostbite, which is characterized by the loss of feeling and color in various areas of the body. Certain areas of the body including the nose, ears, cheeks, chin, fingers, and toes are more prone to frostbite because blood circulation is limited and the areas are likely to be exposed to the elements.

Secondary Effects of Natural Disasters and Severe Weather

After natural disasters or severe weather, power lines and gas lines can be damaged. This can result in fires or electrocution. The lack of electrical power can also lead to the use of alternative heating sources that, if not used properly, can lead to carbon monoxide poisoning. Sources of carbon monoxide (CO) include small gasoline engines, stoves, generators, and gas ranges. CO also can be produced by charcoal-burning devices such as gas grills. Signs of CO poisoning include dizziness, headache, nausea, vomiting, and confusion. CO is colorless and odorless. It can cause loss of consciousness and result in death.

Food-borne illnesses are also likely after a natural disaster when power outages are common and food may be spoiled due to a lack of refrigeration. Nurses may be asked to provide information to the public on food safety following a natural disaster. Water contamination can also occur after such events. When water contamination occurs local health officials may issue a "boil water" advisory and ask the community to boil water for 5 minutes or longer prior to consumption to reduce the risk of gastrointestinal infections. For those with a private or community well, disinfection may be required to kill any potential pathogens. Wells may be evaluated for contaminants such as fecal bacteria by local environmental health officials.

Role of the Nurse in Natural Disasters

Nurses play a significant role before, during, and after a natural disaster. Local health organizations such as health departments, hospitals, and clinics have prepared disaster plans for events such as hurricanes, tornadoes, and extreme temperatures. Nurses play an integral part in the planning process. Many nurses are developing contingency plans for clinical services in the event of a natural disaster so that client care can still be delivered to those in critical need. Others are working to ensure that resources such as supplies and personnel are available during a disaster and they can be obtained with ease and little forewarning. Prior to a natural disaster, nurses may assist or lead in developing, updating, testing, and disseminating emergency plans. Coordination of supplies and resources including personnel may fall under the role of the nurse and require extensive foresight.

During a natural disaster, nurses may need to assist with shelters that are established for those who do not have adequate housing. In shelters, nurses provide care and support during a dramatic and emotional period of uncertainty. Nurses also may be asked to assist in rescue, especially of those who may have injuries requiring immediate medical attention. The role of the nurse during such events may also include serving as a healthcare representative for community members and their families related to the event and their health.

According to the CDC, a home emergency kit should be developed that includes a flashlight with extra batteries; a battery-operated portable radio; bottled water; canned and packaged food; a manual can opener; and a first-aid kit with bandages, antibiotic ointment, and prescription medication. Personal items should also be included such as toiletries and over-the-counter medications.

Outbreaks

Outbreaks are defined as the occurrence of more cases of a particular disease than expected within a geographical location (Oleckno, 2002). The public has become more aware of outbreak events and expects follow-up through disease investigation and identification. In the spring of 2006, the Illinois Department of Public Health noticed an increase in *Acanthamoeba* keratitis (AK), an infection of the eye. After further investigation, the CDC confirmed an increase in AK cases among soft contact lens wearers who were using a specific brand of multipurpose cleaning solution. Approximately 138 cases of AK were identified (CDC, 2007a). Another national outbreak involved contaminated Peter Pan and Great Value peanut butter. By the end of the investigation, nearly 425 cases of *Salmonella* Tennessee had been identified. Investigations on how the peanut butter became contaminated are still being conducted.

In many localities, epidemiologists employed at local or state health departments will conduct outbreak investigations to identify the cause of the outbreak. Although outbreaks are common, there is always a need to conduct an investigation. Primarily, outbreak investigations are conducted to identify the etiology

or cause of the outbreak. Other reasons for conducting outbreak investigations include gaining knowledge about a specific disease or disease-causing agent (pathogen), providing
information to the general public, and evaluating intervention or prevention activities. By gaining knowledge on pathogens or diseases caused by pathogens, future outbreaks can
be avoided and current outbreaks may be better controlled to
prevent further transmission. In conducting outbreak investigations, interventions and prevention activities can be evaluated, such as hospital
protocols to prevent the spread of hospital-acquired infections. Investigations
have also provided information to the public to reduce anxiety and to increase
adherence with certain behaviors such as obtaining influenza shots or practicing
proper hand hygiene. Conducting outbreak investigations have also proven to be
beneficial to policy makers in the development of laws such as the requirement to
vaccinate all children prior to entering school.

> **SIDEBAR 12-15**
>
> Epidemiologists are public health
> scientists who work as disease
> detectives in conducting inves-
> tigations and studies to find the
> etiology or cause of an outbreak.

During outbreaks, nurses and other healthcare providers should provide information to the general public by communicating with the media. By alerting the
media about an outbreak, other cases or individuals at risk for being a possible
case can be identified and provided assistance. Working with the media can also
be beneficial in reducing anxiety among the general public.

Summary

Biological, chemical, and radiological events have occurred throughout history
and still pose a serious threat today. Natural disasters such as hurricanes, tornadoes, and severe weather have resulted in the need for better emergency planning
and preparation. The overall goal of EP&R is to provide an infrastructure so that
local, state, and federal agencies can provide assistance before, during, and after an
emergency to improve health and safety outcomes. EP&R activities are aligned to
protect the public's health through a reduction in morbidity and mass casualty.

The role of the nurse during emergency-related events is multifaceted. Nurses
may be required to triage patients based on symptoms, provide first-aid assistance, administer medications, and provide needed psychological assistance.

Although epidemiologists are employed to conduct outbreak investigations,
nurses play a significant role, and in many local health departments are labeled
"nurse epidemiologists." In addition to outbreak investigations, nurses are
needed to follow up on isolated cases of a particular communicable disease such
as hepatitis or HIV, as required by the state. Nurses assist with obtaining laboratory specimens for investigative interpretation of results. Another important task
for nurses is surveillance. Local, state, and federal health agencies conduct regular
surveillance on a number of reportable or notifiable diseases. Nurses may also be
in charge of tracking diseases within a specific area or community and reporting

those numbers to the state health department, which in turns reports regularly to the CDC.

In conclusion, nurses play a key role in emergency planning and response for a wide range of events including biological, chemical, and radiological emergencies as well as natural disasters and outbreaks. Emergency planning and response activities are conducted before, during, and after an event that may involve extensive destruction. Nurses must collaborate with other public healthcare professionals at the local, state, and federal levels to protect the safety and health of the nation and decrease morbidity and mortality during emergencies.

Key Terms

- **Bioterrorism:** The use of a biological agent to intentionally produce disease in a susceptible population.
- **Chemical emergency:** The release of some hazardous chemical agent either unintentionally, such as through an accidental industrial release, or intentionally, as in a terrorist attack.
- **Covert event:** An attack that the individuals involved are not aware of for a period of time.
- **Emergency planning and response (EP&R):** Activities that are conducted before, during, and after an event that may involve extensive destruction.
- **Overt event:** An attack that those involved know about as soon as it occurs, with little if any lag time.
- **Radiation:** A ubiquitous form of energy that can come from either man-made sources such as medical devices or natural sources such as the sun.

Reflective Practice Questions

1. Name three specific natural disasters that may cause the need for emergency planning and response activities.
2. Identify three Category A agents that may be used in a bioterrorism event.
3. What is the disaster plan at the agency where you practice? Would the personnel and supply resources sustain the community for the initial 24 hours of a disaster? How are nurses mobilized in the disaster plan? What changes would you suggest in the disaster plan?
4. Describe the role of the nurse in bioterrorism events. What training opportunities do you have in your community to prepare you for this role?
5. You are working with families with infants and young children in hurricane-prone Florida on a public health education project. You need to create a meal plan with suggested emergency food sources that would sustain the family for five days without electricity. What meals would you plan and what dry foods should the family have stored for emergencies?
6. How would you develop and prepare emergency planning and response activities for tornadoes in a trailer park for low-income families? How would you include the families in the emergency planning?
7. List some secondary events that may be involved with natural disasters.
8. What type of events might require nurses as well as other healthcare providers to engage in emergency planning and response activities?

References

Agency for Toxic Substances and Disease Registry (ATSDR). (1999). *Toxicological profile for ionizing radiation*. Atlanta, GA: U.S. Department of Health and Human Services, Public Health Service.

Ashford, D. A., Kaiser, R. M., Bales, M. E., Shutt, K., Patrawalla, A., McShan, A., et al. (2003). Planning against biological terrorism: Lessons from outbreak investigations. *Emerging Infectious Diseases, 9*(5), 515–519.

Centers for Disease Control and Prevention. (1994). Tornado disaster—Alabama, March 27, 1994. *Morbidity and Mortality Weekly Report, 43*(19), 356–359.

Centers for Disease Control and Prevention. (1997). Tornado-associated fatalities—Arkansas, 1997. *Morbidity and Mortality Weekly Report, 46*(19), 412–416.

Centers for Disease Control and Prevention. (2000). Biological and chemical terrorism: Strategic plan for preparedness and response. Recommendations of the CDC Strategic Planning Workgroup. *Morbidity and Mortality Weekly Report, 49*(RR-4), 1–13.

Centers for Disease Control and Prevention. (2001a). Update: Investigation of anthrax associated with intentional exposure and interim public health guidelines, October 2001. *Morbidity and Mortality Weekly Report, 50*(41), 889–893.

Centers for Disease Control and Prevention. (2001b). Update: Investigation of bioterrorism-related anthrax and interim guidelines for exposure management and antimicrobial therapy. *Morbidity and Mortality Weekly Report, 50*(42), 909–919.

Centers for Disease Control and Prevention. (2003a). *Being prepared for an earthquake.* Retrieved June 14, 2007, from http://www.bt.cdc.gov/disasters/earthquakes/prepared.asp

Centers for Disease Control and Prevention. (2003b). *Frequently asked questions (FAQ) about tularemia.* Retrieved July 23, 2007, from http://www.bt.cdc.gov/agent/tularemia/pdf/tularemiafaq.pdf

Centers for Disease Control and Prevention. (2003c). *Key facts about tularemia.* Retrieved July 23, 2007, from http://www.bt.cdc.gov/agent/tularemia/pdf/tularemiafacts.pdf

Centers for Disease Control and Prevention. (2003d). Nicotine poisoning after ingestion of contaminated ground beef—Michigan, 2003. *Morbidity and Mortality Weekly Report, 52*(18), 413–416.

Centers for Disease Control and Prevention. (2004a). *Facts about pneumonic plague.* Retrieved July 23, 2007, from http://www.bt.cdc.gov/agent/plague/factsheet.asp

Centers for Disease Control and Prevention. (2005a). *Acute radiation syndrome.* Retrieved July 6, 2007, from http://www.bt.cdc.gov/radiation/pdf/ars.pdf

Centers for Disease Control and Prevention. (2005b). *After a tornado.* Retrieved June 23, 2007, from http://www.bt.cdc.gov/disasters/tornadoes/after.asp

Centers for Disease Control and Prevention. (2005c). *Chemical emergencies overview.* Retrieved July 2, 2007, from http://www.bt.cdc.gov/chemical/pdf/chemical-emergencies-overview.pdf

Centers for Disease Control and Prevention. (2005d). Public health consequences from hazardous substances acutely released during rail transit—South Carolina, 2005; selected states, 1999–2004. *Morbidity and Mortality Weekly Report, 54*(3), 64–67.

Centers for Disease Control and Prevention. (2005e). *Radiation emergencies.* Retrieved July 6, 2007, from http://www.bt.cdc.gov/radiation/

Centers for Disease Control and Prevention. (2006a). Botulism associated with commercial carrot juice—Georgia and Florida, September 2006. *Morbidity and Mortality Weekly Report, 55*(40), 1098–1099.

Centers for Disease Control and Prevention. (2006b). *Botulism: Clinical description.* Retrieved July 17, 2007, from http://www.bt.cdc.gov/agent/Botulism/clinicians/clindesc.asp

Centers for Disease Control and Prevention. (2006c). *Botulism: Epidemiological overview for clinicians.* Retrieved July 17, 2007, from http://www.bt.cdc.gov/agent/Botulism/clinicians/epidemiology.asp

Centers for Disease Control and Prevention. (2006d). *Frequently asked questions about extreme heat*. Retrieved June 14, 2007, from http://emergency.cdc.gov/disasters/extremeheat/faq.asp

Centers for Disease Control and Prevention (2007a). Acanthamoeba keratitis multiple states, 2005-2007. *Morbidity and Mortality Weekly Report, 56*(21), 532–534.

Centers for Disease Control and Prevention. (2007b). Hypothermia-related mortality—Montana, 1999–2004. *Morbidity and Mortality Weekly Report, 56*(15), 367–368.

Centers for Disease Control and Prevention. (2007c). *Smallpox disease overview.* Retrieved July 17, 2007, from http://www.bt.cdc.gov/agent/smallpox/overview/disease-facts.asp

Dennis, D. T., Inglesby, T. V., Henderson, D. A., Bartlett, J. G., Ascher, M. S., Eitzen, E., et al. (2001). Tularemia as a biological weapon: Medical and public health management. *Journal of the American Medical Association, 285*(21), 2763–2773.

Farlow, J., Wagner, D. M., Dukerich, M., Stanley, M., Chu, M., Kubota, K., et al. (2005). *Francisella tularensis* in the United States. *Emerging Infectious Diseases, 11*(12), 1835–1841.

Federal Emergency Management Agency. (n.d.). *Learn about hurricanes*. Retrieved July 23, 2007, from http://www.fema.gov/hazard/hurricane/hu_about.shtm

Los Angeles County, Department of Health Services, Public Health Nursing. (2003). *Public health nursing practice model.* Retrieved July 8, 2008, from http://lapublichealth.org.

Martin, P. (2006). Establishing and sustaining healthcare operations in a contingency: A logistical perspective. *Journal of Healthcare Management, 51*(6), 407–414.

Neff, M. (2002). Survey results demonstrate need for response training to bioterrorism. *American Family Physician, 66*(77), 1140.

Oleckno, W. (2002). *Essential epidemiology: Principles and applications.* Prospect Heights, IL: Waveland Press Inc.

Parrish, A. R., Oliver, S., Jenkins, D., Ruscio, B., Green, J. B., & Colenda, C. (2005). A short medical school course on responding to bioterrorism and other disasters. *Academic Medicine, 80*(9), 820–823.

Phillips, M. B. *Bioterrorism: A brief history. Northeast Florida Medicine.* 32–35.

Rhyne, C. D. (2005). Wake-up call. *Topics in Emergency Medicine, 27*(3), 180–182.

Zinkovich, L., Malvey, D., Hamby, E., & Fottler, M. (2005). Bioterror events: Preemptive strategies for healthcare executives. *Hospital Topics: Research and Perspectives on Healthcare, 83*(3), 9–15.

Addressing Primary Prevention and Education in Vulnerable Populations

Diane Baer Wilson and Lisa S. Anderson

LEARNING OUTCOMES

After reading this chapter you will be able to:

- Define the term *vulnerable populations*.
- Identify what constitutes a health disparity.
- Discuss at least three factors that contribute to health disparities.
- Understand what health behaviors are classified as primary prevention.
- Discuss how diet, exercise, and tobacco use contribute to increased risk of developing major chronic diseases in the United States.
- Give examples showing how health behaviors are distributed in vulnerable populations.
- Identify three key approaches for educating and motivating clients to improve their health behaviors.
- Discuss challenges for improving health behaviors in vulnerable populations.

Chronic disease: A long-lasting disease that typically remains with a patient from onset to end of life and requires management of symptoms. Examples are cancer, cardiovascular disease, diabetes, and cerebrovascular disease. According to the U.S. Centers for Disease Control and Prevention, chronic disease is responsible for 7 out of 10 deaths in the United States.

Vulnerable populations: Groups that are likely to have compromised access to health care and, therefore, are more likely to have poorer health outcomes, including higher mortality rates, compared to less vulnerable groups.

Primary prevention: Actions taken to modify health behaviors such as diet, sedentary behavior, or smoking towards preventing or managing a chronic condition such as heart disease or cancer. An example is reducing one's intake of dietary fat to help lower cholesterol levels and prevent one from exceeding recommended cholesterol guidelines.

Introduction

Three **chronic diseases** account for the majority of deaths in the United States each year. Some 59 percent of Americans die annually from either heart disease, stroke, or cancer (Mokdad, Marks, Stroup, & Gerberding, 2004). However, in learning more about the populations represented in these statistics, one might be surprised at some of the trends. What research shows is that poor, underserved, and minority populations have higher death rates across all of these diseases. Further, these individuals are also less likely to have health insurance and thus, they find it more difficult to even access health care compared with more affluent groups. This chapter will identify **vulnerable populations** and provide a discussion on why they are at greater risk for poor health outcomes compared to other populations. In addition, this chapter explores the role of **primary prevention** in chronic disease risk reduction. Primary prevention refers to modifying health behaviors such as diet, sedentary behavior, or smoking towards reducing one's risk of developing chronic diseases such as heart disease, stroke, cancer and diabetes. The third part of this chapter details the role of nurses in helping individuals in vulnerable populations become educated and motivated to practice preventive behaviors in order to lower their risk of developing chronic diseases.

Defining Vulnerable Population

Socioeconomic status and poverty rates have more to do with differences in health status and mortality rates than any specific race or culture. People who live in poverty tend to be less educated, be hungry, live in substandard conditions, have less access to health care, and be more likely to practice unhealthy behaviors (Freeman, 2004). Over time, data have demonstrated that socioeconomic status is a strong and persistent predictor of health status. A landmark study, published in 1967, examined this issue in the United States and Europe, tracing back to the 17th century, and reported better health and lower mortality rates were consistently associated with higher income and higher levels of education (Antonovsky, 1967). If one looks at any of several measures, the results are consistent. For example, life expectancy in 1990 was 45.5 years in Angola, which is a very poor country, but it was 66 years in Ecuador and over 75 years in the United States, a highly developed country (United Nations Development Program, 1993).

According to the U.S. Census Bureau, some 35 million Americans (12 percent) met the criteria for being classified as "poor" and 15 percent of all Americans had no health insurance when the census was taken in 2002. More African Americans (24 percent) and Hispanics (22 percent) live below the poverty line than do Caucasians (8 percent). Likewise more African Americans (20 percent) and Hispanics (32 percent) are without medical insurance compared with Caucasians (11 percent). Research shows that individuals residing in lower-income locations have a higher death rate among both males and females (Ward et al., 2007).

People with Disabilities

Vulnerable populations may include people in additional groups such as individuals with a **disability**. Although many people with disabilities are fully functional, maintain employment, and have a high quality of life, some disabilities can make it more difficult to find employment. In addition, some disabilities may place individuals at greater risk for developing

> **KEY TERM**
>
> **Disabilities:** Physical or mental impairments that substantially limit a person from completing activities of daily living.

comorbidities. For example, an individual with diabetes who does not control his or her blood sugar levels is at greater risk for developing infection, having poor circulation, and developing heart disease. Thus, this serves as another example of a potentially vulnerable population.

Elderly and Young Children

Age is also a factor that can be associated with poor health outcomes. Both socioeconomic factors and physiological issues contribute to these groups being more at risk for poor health than individuals in other age groups. Elderly people are often on a fixed income and may not have health insurance to supplement governmental health plans; thus they may not be able to afford medical procedures and care that are not covered by Medicare. Children are particularly at risk if they either are uninsured or have inadequate coverage for medical care, because this often means they have inadequate access to medical care. Uninsured children are 70 percent more likely than insured children to require medical treatment for chronic conditions such as asthma (Crenshaw, 2007).

Physiological differences also contribute to vulnerabilities. Older people, particularly those with less body mass, and very young children do not tolerate extreme heat or cold. For example, they are the groups targeted in extreme heat warnings in the summer because they are more prone to dehydration and heat stroke. Overall, however, individuals in these age categories tend to have a weaker immune response and they are often prioritized for public health initiatives such as flu vaccine distribution, usually given in winter months.

The Interplay of Economic, Social, and Cultural Issues on Health Status

How being poor actually impacts health turns out to be a complex issue. Over the last decade, thinking has shifted from a primary focus on poverty as the prime factor related to health status to a broader focus. In reality, there is no one reason that explains why those who live in poverty are more likely to be ill and are more likely to die prematurely. However, experts have identified that the combination of social, economic, and cultural factors may result in vulnerable populations having a disproportionate burden from chronic diseases such as cancer and stroke, compared with more affluent groups (Freeman, 2004). The mechanisms by which economic, social, and cultural issues are operational and impact on health are not widely known, identifying important areas of research for social scientists, public health epidemiologists, and healthcare providers such as nurses, physicians, psychologists, and allied health professionals. The schema shown in Figure 13-1 clearly depicts the synergy among factors that, combined, increases the likelihood of experiencing poor health, poor quality of life, and compromised access to health care, often leading to health disparities.

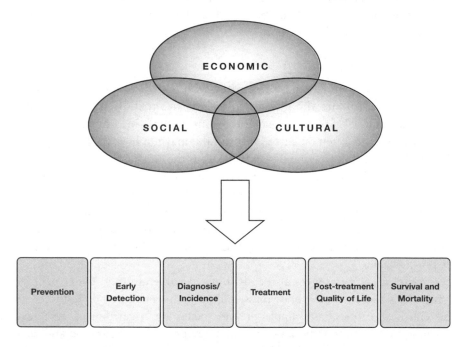

Figure 13–1 Factors that influence health disparities. *Source:* From *CA Cancer* 2004;54:78–93. Reprinted with permission from Lippincott, Williams, & Wilkins.

CONTEMPORARY PRACTICE HIGHLIGHT 13-1

HEALTH DISPARITIES ACROSS THE CANCER CONTINUUM OF CARE

The model shown in Figure 13-1 depicts the multifactorial aspects that contribute to social and health disparities. Freeman presents the inter-relatedness of economic, social, and cultural influences that together place individuals at greater risk for having a disproportionate burden of poor health care across the continuum of cancer care and suboptimal health outcomes. This model is particularly relevant for healthcare practitioners in that it emphasizes the synergy created by the intersection of multiple factors. Disparities in disease outcomes may begin with differences in each of the areas of care; thus, people in vulnerable populations may need more client education and access to healthcare practitioners, beginning with prevention (Freeman, 2004).

Health Disparities

Once evidence was found that overall mortality rates varied by education and socioeconomic status, more study was given to examining chronic disease rates in order to determine whether they also reflected differences by population groups. The term **health disparities** is used to describe groups that have a disproportionate amount of disease compared to the proportion of representation in the population. When we look at the major chronic diseases we see, for example, that African American men have higher mortality rates for prostate cancer than Caucasian men; likewise, African American women are 13 percent more likely to die from breast cancer than Caucasian women (American Cancer Society [ACS], 2007). Figure 13-2 shows cancer death rates per 100,000 for males and females across five race/ethnic groups (ACS, 2006). Similarly, African Americans have the highest occurrence of hypertension and are the racial group most likely to develop high blood pressure at a young age (CDC, 2007a). The greatest disparity occurs in those ages 40–59. Among African Americans in this age group, half have hypertension, compared to 30 percent of whites (Jones-Burton & Saunders, 2005). With a higher burden of hypertension, it is not surprising that African Americans also have a higher burden of cardiovascular disease (CVD) and stroke. Data from 2004 show that African Americans have a higher prevalence of both CVD and stroke compared to whites and Mexican Americans (Rosamond, et al., 2007). Table 13-1 shows the prevalence of stroke and CVD for three different ethnic groups.

Other racial and ethnic groups suffer disproportionately from chronic diseases such as diabetes. According to the U.S. Centers for Disease Control and Prevention (CDC), American Indians and Alaska Natives are 2.6 times more likely than

> **KEY TERM**
>
> **Health disparities:** Differences in the incidence, prevalence, mortality, and burden of disease and other adverse health conditions that exist among specific population groups.

whites to have type 2 diabetes, while Native Hawaiians are 2.5 times more likely to be diagnosed with type 2 diabetes than whites who reside in that state. African Americans and Mexican Americans have twice the risk for a type 2 diabetes diagnosis than whites (CDC, 2007b).

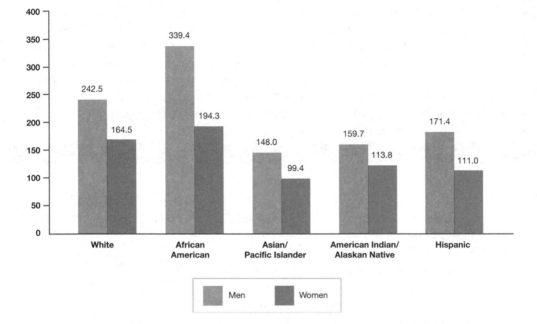

Figure 13-2 Cancer mortality per 100,000 by gender and ethnicity. *Source:* ACS Facts and Figures, 2006.

TABLE 13-1   PREVALENCE OF CARDIOVASCULAR DISEASE AND STROKE BY ETHNIC GROUP, 2005

	Prevalence (%)					
	Whites		African Americans		Mexican Americans	
Disease	Male	Female	Male	Female	Male	Female
Cardiovascular disease	37.2	35.0	44.6	49.0	31.6	34.4
Cerebrovascular disease (stroke)	2.4	2.7	4.1	4.1	3.1	1.9

Source: Rosamond, et al., 2007.

Summary of Vulnerable Populations

Overall, there is evidence that a combination of several factors including poverty, culture, and social issues contribute to individuals being at risk for poor health outcomes including developing chronic disease and lower life expectancy. This section discussed minorities, the disabled, and the very young and the elderly as examples of groups that can be considered vulnerable for inadequate medical care and thus, poorer health outcomes.

Individual Health Behaviors: Primary Prevention

Over the last decade, researchers have provided evidence linking health behaviors such as how we eat (diet), how active we are, and whether we smoke or drink to the risk of developing some of the most prevalent chronic diseases in the United States. In fact, the top three chronic diseases in the United States, heart disease, stroke, and cancer, are all fueled by **obesity** and by being physically inactive. In other words, if people would reduce their food intake and exercise in order to reach a body mass index (BMI) of 18–25 kg/m², many heart attacks, strokes, and cancer diagnoses would likely be averted. Experts estimate that 30,000 cases of cancer could be prevented through diet modifications alone (ACS, 2006). In this section of the chapter we will discuss the top preventable causes of death in the United States and how they are distributed in vulnerable populations. Preventable causes of death have also been quantified to show how much they contribute to the top diseases that account for the most deaths in the United States (Figure 13-3).

> **KEY TERM**
>
> **Obesity:** Having an excess of body fat. Obesity is clinically determined by body mass index (BMI), which is calculated by dividing a person's weight in kilograms by height in meters squared (kg/m²). A person with a BMI of 30.0 or more is defined as obese.

Obesity

Being **overweight** or obese is one of our most pressing public health issues today, and the rates of obesity are increasing. The majority of Americans are overweight; more than 65 percent of the population has a BMI greater than 25 kg/m² (Hedley et al., 2004). In 2003, U.S. Surgeon General Richard Carmona, MD, MPH, said "As we look to the future and where childhood obesity will be in 20 years, it is every bit as threatening to us as is the threat of terrorism. Obesity is the threat from within" (Ornish, 2007). Dr. Carmona was responding to the fact that an obesity epidemic has been proclaimed in the United States, based on the huge increases in the prevalence of overweight and obesity. Rates of overweight and obesity are increasing among both adults and children. In 1999–2000, 14 percent of children and teens were overweight compared to 17 percent in 2003–2004. Among adult males, 27.5 percent were obese in 1999–2000 compared to 32.2 percent of adult males in 2003–2004 (Ogden, 2006).

> **KEY TERM**
>
> **Overweight:** Having an excess of body weight that includes fat, muscle, bone, and water. Overweight is clinically determined by BMI, which is calculated by dividing a person's weight in kilometers by height in meters squared (kg/m²). A person with a BMI ranging between 25.0 and 29.9 is defined as overweight.

Causes of Obesity

Many factors contribute to becoming overweight, but they all come down to consuming more calories than are burned each day. Eating too much and being less

---

CONTEMPORARY PRACTICE HIGHLIGHT 13-2

QUANTIFYING THE CONTRIBUTION OF UNHEALTHY LIFESTYLE BEHAVIORS IN CAUSES OF DEATH IN AMERICANS

Figure 13-3 quantifies and ranks the unhealthy behaviors that significantly contribute to causes of death in the United States and how their rankings have changed since 1990. It shows that tobacco use, diet (overweight), and lack of physical exercise are the top three health habits that contribute to heart attacks, stroke, cancer, diabetes, and other physical conditions. Health behaviors are the only known non-pharmaceutical modifiable factors for reducing risk of chronic disease. Thus, there is greater focus on these issues by the healthcare industry, food manufacturers and marketers, businesses, and organizations at all levels of our society to support individuals in "practicing prevention" through smoking cessation, healthier diets, and more physical activity.

Source: Mokdad, A. H., Marks, J. S., Stroup, J. L., & Gerberding, J. L. (2000). Actual causes of death in the United States, 2000. *Journal of the American Medical Association, 291,* 1238–1245.

Actual Causes of Death in the United States in 1990 and 2000

Actual Cause	No. (%) in 1990*	No. (%) in 2000
Tobacco	400,000 (19)	435,000 (18.1)
Poor diet and physical inactivity	300,000 (14)	400,000 (16.6)
Alcohol consumption	100,000 (5)	85,000 (3.5)
Microbial agents	90,000 (4)	75,000 (3.1)
Toxic agents	60,000 (3)	55,000 (2.3)
Motor vehicle	25,000 (1)	43,000 (1.8)
Firearms	35,000 (2)	29,000 (1.2)
Sexual behavior	30,000 (1)	20,000 (0.8)
Illicit drug use	20,000 (<1)	17,000 (0.7)
Total	**1,060,000** (50)	**1,159,000** (48.2)

* Data are from McGinnis and Foege. The percentages are for all deaths.

Figure 13-3 Actual Causes of Death in the US. *Source:* From *Journal of the American Medical Association* 2004; 291: 1238–1245. American Medical Association. All Rights Reserved.

physically active are hallmarks of wealthy nations, where food is affordable, heavily marketed, and readily available. In addition, as wealth increases in a society, mundane physical tasks are becoming more automated and require less physical labor; with the prospect of robotics in the future, these patterns will only increase.

Food Consumption Patterns

Changing patterns in society and the marketplace have contributed to people consuming more calories. Americans are eating outside of the home more than ever before. Data indicate that approximately 50 percent of all food purchased is consumed outside the home (Tillotson, 2004). Fewer people cook at home,

SIDEBAR 13-1 THE OBESITY EPIDEMIC

Overweight and obesity have significantly increased among both adults and youth in the United States, and the rates continue to increase. Note the change in female Mexican Americans and African Americans shown in Figure 13-4. Overweight is a risk factor for diabetes, heart disease, stroke, and many types of cancer including breast cancer. Increases in youth overweight/obesity rates are particularly of concern because there was a parallel increase in Type 2 diabetes among youth during this time period. These increases prompted the U.S. government to identify an obesity epidemic to raise the public's awareness of the health consequences and suggest solutions across multiple domains such as business, health care, marketing, schools, churches, and individuals' health behavior choices (Flegal, 2002).

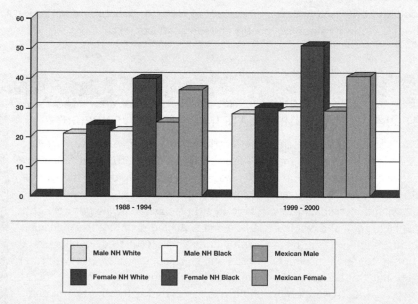

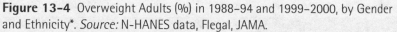

Figure 13-4 Overweight Adults (%) in 1988–94 and 1999–2000, by Gender and Ethnicity*. *Source:* N-HANES data, Flegal, JAMA.

where it is easier to have control over portion sizes and the ingredients used in cooking. Eating out often translates into eating larger portions and consuming higher levels of fat and sugar. Fast food is not only convenient, it is relatively inexpensive, making it easy for working families to go to the drive-through to pick up fast food on the ride home from work. Recently, more healthy choices have begun appearing on menus in restaurants, including fast food chains. In 2005, the McDonald's food chain stopped its "super size" designation out of pressure from individuals and health organizations concerned about obesity in children (Young & Nestle, 2007).

Food Insecurity

Some research evidence shows that individuals who regularly do not have adequate supplies of food or go hungry for periods of time may be more likely to overconsume food later in their adult years (Townsend, Peerson, Love, Achterberg, & Murphy, 2001). This is common in areas where there has been poverty or insecure economic resources. A newer term for this is *food insecurity*. In a study conducted by Wilson et al. (2004) that examined mother–daughter differences in food and dietary practices, African American women were more likely to identify "not having enough food" as a main feature in their homes growing up in rural areas, compared with Caucasian women. In addition, the younger African American women mentioned that their mothers were concerned when they lost weight, rather than perceiving a moderate weight loss as having positive health benefits. Food insecurity is now an important area of research so that more can be learned about how this may impact appetite and food patterns.

CONTEMPORARY PRACTICE HIGHLIGHT 13-3

EARLY FOOD INSECURITY: DOES IT TRANSLATE INTO ADULT OVERWEIGHT?

In searching for ways to better understand how individuals start to practice habits that may support overweight and obesity, the term *food insecurity* has been introduced. The term refers to having underlying anxiety about not having enough food and whether this issue might motivate individuals to eat more. This condition is common in underdeveloped countries and can be related to growing up in poverty; thus it can occur in any location. A qualitative study of two generations of African American women (Wilson et al., 2004) reported that food scarcity was not uncommon in their families of origin, and women relayed vivid memories of basically sitting down to meals with very little to eat and watching their mothers manage it with dignity. In a recent study conducted by Olson and colleagues over 3 years with rural women ($n = 30$), growing up in a poor household was associated with obesity and emotional eating in adulthood (Olson et al., 2007).

Food Advertising

The marketing of food is a huge part of the food industry. Food advertising is so sophisticated that it targets specific gender, age, and ethnic groups. Companies put a big focus on conducting market research so they specifically learn what appeals to various groups. Cereal manufacturers are a good example. They are very successful at marketing cereal products to kids through Saturday morning cartoons on television, so much so that these practices have come under scrutiny by federal regulators. In addition to federal regulation, private groups have acted. In 2007, the Kellogg's company announced it would phase out ads targeting children under 12 as well as stop using well-known children's characters or toys to promote products that did not meet certain nutritional guidelines (Martin, 2007). The guidelines were based on the calorie, sugar, fat, and sodium content of primarily breakfast foods. Kellogg's made its decision because of the threat of a lawsuit by two advocacy groups and some private citizens who wanted to eliminate the promotion of less healthy foods to young children (Center for Science in the Public Interest, 2007).

Cola beverage companies represent another market segment that competes so heavily that they are said to have "advertising wars." They are known for state-of-the-art ad campaigns that appeal to nearly all ages but target teens and young adults. A few companies do use health to target certain groups, such as the lean microwave dinners that appeal to women who are health and fitness conscious.

Beverage Consumption

There have been huge shifts in the U.S. consumption patterns of beverages over the last decade. Whereas milk used to be the top consumed beverage among youth in the United States, milk consumption has steadily decreased over the last decade and soft drinks and bottled water have significantly increased (Tillotson, 2004). Milk products are the highest food sources of calcium and vitamin D, essential nutrients for healthy bones and teeth. Experts are concerned about bone health in young U.S. females as they mature, given their low intake of milk and the increase in osteoporosis among older adults (Harel, Riggs, Vaz, White, & Menzies, 1998). In earlier times, carbonated sodas were an occasional treat; however, carbonated beverages now are very popular and are also very inexpensive. Restaurants often provide drink refills at no charge, which add additional calories. In addition, standard serving sizes for beverages have increased substantially. In the 1960s, a small soft drink at a restaurant was generally 8 ounces and around 80 calories. Now the standard is 12 or 16 ounces. Some convenience stores offer 24- or 36-ounce cups; a soft drink in the latter container size has 310 calories. Soft drink consumption has particularly increased among teens and youth, groups that are already suffering from overweight and obesity (Striegel-Moore et al., 2006). In a 24-hour period, beverage intake can significantly contribute to higher caloric intake and more body fat.

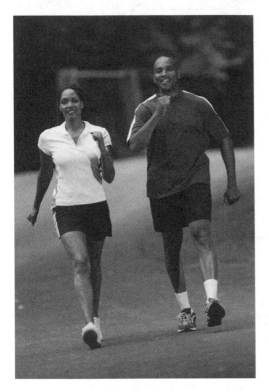

A young couple walking on a path for exercise.
Source: © Comstock Images/Alamy Images

Soft drink vending machines have become a controversial topic recently, especially those in schools, because they offer "empty calorie" beverages—beverages that contain about 1.5 ounces of sugar and no actual nutrients. Experts observe that having machines in schools sends mixed messages to students learning about health and nutrition in class during a time when obesity is at epic proportions. From 1985 to 1997, milk purchasing decreased almost 30 percent among U.S. school districts while purchases of soft drinks increased by over 1,000 percent (Nestle, 2002).

Patterns of Physical Activity

Being physically active burns more calories than sedentary behavior, and thus, is essential for weight control and obesity prevention. Physical activity as part of daily living has been reduced significantly in U.S. life in schools, places of work, and communities. Many families provide an automobile for each child of driving age. In younger children, safety may be an issue so that walking to school occurs less often as well. Use of the television and computers has been shown to take up many hours for kids and teens. However, studies show that the number of hours of television watched per day is directly correlated with overweight and obesity (Hager, 2006). Policy changes in local school districts have resulted in less physical education for students in public schools; many states have used time formally designated for physical activity for adding more courses. Data show that overall, less than 50 percent of Americans participate in moderate exercise, defined as brisk walking or bicycling at least 20 minutes three or more times per week; only 25 percent exercise at vigorous levels (American Cancer Society, 2006).

Obesity Consequences: Chronic Disease

There are many consequences of being overweight, including both psychological and physiological issues. Low self-esteem, depression, and being vulnerable to bullying are especially common in overweight children (Eissenberg, Neumark-Sztainer, & Story, 2006). Among adults, studies show that obese individuals may be discriminated against in the workplace; obese people are actually less likely to be employed than those with lower BMIs (Tunceli, Li, & Williams, 2006). Beyond these reasons, obesity is associated with early mortality and shorter life expectancy because being overweight is linked to developing chronic diseases that are the top causes of death in the United States. Although overweight has long been tied to increased risk of developing cardiovascular disease, stroke, and diabetes, more recently published data have linked obesity to cancer risk and significantly increased mortality rates. A comprehensive study (Calle, Rodriguez, Walker-Thurmond, & Thun, 2003) showed that having a higher BMI was significantly associated with higher death rates in 11 types of cancer in men and 12 types in women, including breast cancer. Obesity may account for some of the disparities that exist in overall chronic disease incidence and mortality rates.

Addressing Obesity: Solutions

Losing weight can seem like such a simple thing, particularly if you are not overweight. Even healthcare providers can be judgmental in working with overweight clients (Befort et al., 2006). However, food patterns are deeply rooted behaviors that are complex and are often steeped in family culture, religion, food preferences, and food availability as well as socioeconomic status. Thus, it is important to understand what individuals are dealing with in addressing how a client might begin to change their eating habits and level of physical activity. The last part of this chapter deals specifically with strategies that nurses and other healthcare professionals can use to teach clients how to start making changes in health behaviors when they are ready to do so.

Smoking

Although smoking rates among adults have declined over the last two decades, some 25 percent of U.S. adults still smoke today in spite of more and more legislation and policies being approved that ban smoking in restaurants, government agencies, and business offices. As early as 1930, physicians began to notice that most clients with lung cancer were smokers. It wasn't until the 1950s that definitive evidence from work by Dr. Ernst Wynder and others established that smoking was related to significant health risks including increased risk of developing lung cancer (Wynder, 1954). Today, we know that beyond lung cancer, smoking is also associated with increased risk of heart disease and stroke, as well as emphysema and chronic obstructive pulmonary disease and oral cancers. Some 400,000 premature deaths each year are related to smoking, making it the top preventable cause of death in the United States (Mokdad et al., 2004). Reducing smoking rates in the United States is a key **Healthy People 2010** objective for primary prevention of chronic diseases in the U.S. population. Table 13-2 shows the distribution of smoking behavior across adult gender and race/ethnic groups (ACS, 2007).

In the 1990s the government brought a lawsuit against the tobacco industry. The U.S. Tobacco Settlement was reached,

> **KEY TERM**
>
> **Healthy People 2010:** A statement of national health objectives designed to identify the most significant preventable threats to health and to establish national goals to reduce these threats in the next decade. Goals are set to help public health professionals, healthcare providers, and others work toward improving the health of citizens. Healthy People 2010 can be accessed at http://www.healthypeople.gov.

TABLE 13-2 PERCENTAGE OF U.S. ADULT CURRENT SMOKERS BY RACE/ETHNICITY AND GENDER

Race/Ethnicity	Males	Females
White (non-Hispanic)	25.7	23.0
African American	25.5	20.4
Hispanic/Latino	23.2	12.8
American Indian/Alaskan Native	27.4	38.6
Asian American	19.8	7.9

Source: American Cancer Society. (2007). *Cancer facts and figures 2007.* Atlanta: Author.

whereby cigarette manufacturers were shown to be dishonest in advertising as well as in targeting children. States received funding from the settlement to 1) help farmers transition from growing tobacco to growing other crops, and 2) support youth smoking prevention programs. Youth smoking continues to be common in high school students and, to some degree, among middle school students. This trend is of concern for a number of reasons; first and foremost, today's youth constitutes the next generation of smokers—most adult smokers began smoking in their youth. Years of smoking can contribute to greater difficulty in quitting in adult years. Second, research by Wilson et al. (2005) demonstrated that youth who smoke are significantly more likely to have a lower intake of milk and vegetables as well as exercise less frequently than non-smokers. These patterns were more likely in girls than boys and were evident even starting in middle school. Combining smoking with poor food intake may place youth at even higher risk of developing chronic diseases as they mature, given lower intake of protective nutrients that may offset damage from tobacco use (Wilson et al.).

It is important to assess smoking in clients when they are seen by healthcare providers for either an illness visit or a physical exam. Smoking is a very difficult habit to change and it can be easy for healthcare providers to decide that it is just too hard to address. However, it has been shown that having a healthcare provider ask patients about their smoking status and remind them of how damaging the habit is may prompt a certain percentage of clients to quit smoking, indicating that healthcare providers carry a lot of credibility when they articulate health promotion messages to clients (Whitlock, Orleans, & Pender, 2002). New models of delivering prevention messages are being tested for healthcare providers to ask about smoking and then refer clients to a "quit line" offered by some state health departments and organizations such as the American Cancer Society.

In youth, smoking can be even harder to treat because youth are often hiding their habit. Evidence shows that few traditional school-based youth smoking prevention/cessation programs have been successful (Skara & Sussman, 2003), and some experts are calling for a new paradigm for addressing youth smoking. New data have been helpful, however, in identifying predictors of youth smoking. These include peers and family members who smoke, living in a single parent family, and having a poor relationship with parents. Being close to one's parents helps to reduce the risk of youth smoking, but if the parents smoke, the protective effect is moderated (Wilson, Heckman, McClish, Obando, & Dahman, 2007).

Teaching Clients About Improving Health Behaviors

The Institute of Medicine recommended in 2000 that "a better balance is needed between the clinical approach to disease, presently the dominant public health model for most risk factors, and research and intervention efforts that address generic social and behavioral determinants of disease, injury, and disability" (Smedley & Syme, 2000, pp. 7–8). As already noted, health behavioral change is one of the most challenging issues that nurses and other healthcare professionals face. Behavior, such as lifestyle habits that include smoking, diet, and exercise, is learned over time, and, unlike an acute condition such as an infection, cannot be changed just by taking prescription medicines. Medical knowledge has led to many advances that enable us to make organ transplants, insert heart pacemakers, and map the human genome. Yet it has been recognized that medical advances that have successfully treated acute disease are not well-suited for chronic disease, which is a long-term condition that requires self-management of certain health behaviors (Bandura, 2004). The complexity of health behavior has made it difficult to understand people's motivations and encourage change that will benefit those with chronic disease. For example, why is it that some people continue to smoke after a heart attack? What makes it so difficult for many people to stick to a weight-loss diet or maintain a regular exercise program?

This third section of this chapter presents health behavior change theories and tools for assessing and addressing unhealthy behaviors in clients and in various clinical and community settings.

Major Theories of Health Behavior

There are a number of universally accepted explanations for what drives human behavior, many of which are specific to health-related behaviors. These are useful in understanding why people choose to change or continue certain habits and how best to motivate them to make healthy lifestyle changes. These explanations are known as models or theories. Although there are many, some of the most commonly used health behavior theories are 1) Social Cognitive Theory, 2) the Health Belief Model, and 3) the Transtheoretical Model.

Social Cognitive Theory

Social Cognitive Theory (SCT), developed by Alfred Bandura and first published in the 1970s, departed from the prevailing thought that environment was the main influence on behavior (Bandura, 1977, 1986). SCT instead is based on the idea that people's cognitive processes also influence their environment and that *reciprocal determinism*, or the constant interaction that occurs among people, their environment, and their behavior, is central to understanding behavior. The ideas of self-efficacy, the belief in one's ability to change a behavior successfully, along with self-control, the ability to maintain a change in behavior, are central to SCT. Thus, a client who firmly believes they can reduce fat intake in their diet is more likely to succeed in meeting this goal than one who has low confidence in his or her ability to adhere to new dietary guidelines.

Health Belief Model (HBM)

The Health Belief Model is one of the oldest models of health behavior and has been widely used to explain the adoption of several different health behaviors (Becker, 1974; Rosenstock, 1966). Based on the impact of personal beliefs on actions related to health, the HBM contains four main components: perceived susceptibility, perceived severity, perceived threat, and perceived benefits of action weighed against perceived barriers to action. According to the HBM (see Figure 13-5), clients will not consider a health-related behavioral change without first perceiving 1) that they are susceptible to a disease, 2) that the disease would have severe effects on them personally, and 3) that based on the perceived susceptibility and perceived severity, the disease is believed to be a threat. Perceiving a threat creates motivation to make changes to avoid that threat; however, final action is influenced by 4) perceived benefits of the action weighed against 5) perceived barriers to successfully taking that action.

For example, a fair-skinned woman who believes she is more susceptible to skin cancer and that the disease would affect her severely perceives sun exposure to be a threat. Her final decision to take preventive action would be based on whether she felt she could overcome the barriers to taking action (e.g., the inconvenience of wearing a hat in the sun and applying sunscreen) to realize the benefits (reduced risk of sunburn and skin cancer, and diminished effects of sun-related aging).

Transtheoretical Model

The Transtheoretical Model, or Stages of Change Theory (Prochaska & DiClemente, 1982), is an important tool for nurses and other healthcare professionals. This model is used to assess the client's readiness to change and is based on the premise that individuals are not all ready to accept immediate changes in their eating habits, food choices, and exercise routines. Instead, change occurs in stages (see Table 13-3).

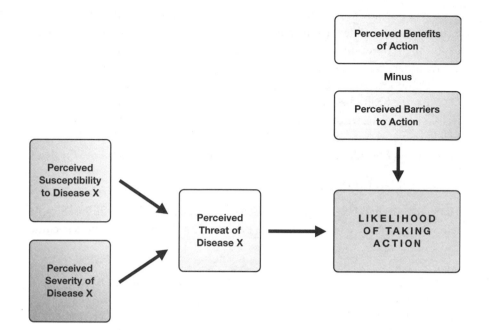

Figure 13–5 Health Belief Model. *Source:* From Kaplan, Sallis, & Patterson, *Health and Human Behavior.* Courtesy of James F. Sallis, PhD.

TABLE 13-3   STAGES OF CHANGE IN THE TRANSTHEORETICAL MODEL

Stage	Definition
Precontemplation	Individual has no intention to take action within the next 6 months.
Contemplation	Individual intends to take action within the next 6 months.
Preparation	Individual intends to take action within the next 30 days and has taken some behavioral steps in this direction.
Action	Individual has changed overt behavior for less than 6 months.
Maintenance	Individual has changed overt behavior for more than 6 months.

Source: Prochaska, J. O., Redding, C. A., & Evers, K. E. (2002). The transtheoretical model and stages of change. In K. Glanz, B. K. Rimer, & F. M. Lewis (Eds.), *Health behavior and health education: Theory, research, and practice* (3rd ed., pp. 99–120). San Francisco: Jossey-Bass.

It is important to note that some stages may last for months or years. For example, it is possible for someone to be in the precontemplation stage for years or in the preparation stage for several months. In addition, the stages do not always progress in clear succession; at any stage after precontemplation, a client may relapse and have to begin the process again.

The three health behavior theories just described represent some of the most well-known in the field, but many more exist and refinements and new developments arise as researchers continue their work. Sidebar 13-2 provides information on a few other health behavior models, including some that are newer to the field.

Client Behavioral Change

Understanding and changing health behaviors are two different things. Simply telling clients about a need to change a behavior is unlikely to succeed in eliciting

---

SIDEBAR 13-2 SPOTLIGHT ON OTHER HEALTH BEHAVIOR MODELS

Precaution Adoption Process Model (PAPM): Also based on stages of change, this model describes the stages people go through as they learn about a preventive behavior or activity (such as taking calcium to prevent osteoporosis), from lack of awareness through awareness and decision making to taking action (Weinstein & Sandman, 2002).

Human Strengths Approach: A holistic approach to health promotion based on Leddy's Theory of Healthiness, the Human Strengths Approach focuses on the role of client strengths in maintaining health and emphasizes the importance of the nurse and client as partners, with the nurse acting as a "client resource" rather than an expert who tells the client what to do (Leddy, 2006).

Revised Health Promotion Model (RHPM): This model explains the factors that influence health-promoting behaviors. Pender (1996) based this model on two other theories, Social Cognitive Theory, described in this chapter, and Expectancy-Value Theory, which is based on the concept that human behavior is rational and economical, and that people will not put time and effort into working toward goals unless they value those goals and believe them to be achievable. Pender's original Health Promotion Model (HPM) was proposed as a way to integrate nursing and behavioral science viewpoints into the factors that affect health behaviors (Pender, 1996). It differed from other models in that it did not incorporate perceived fear or threat as motivating factors and thus was deemed applicable to health behaviors for which threat is not judged to be a major motivator. The RHPM, a refinement of the original HPM, is based on three major factors that influence health-promoting behaviors: 1) individual characteristics and experiences, such as prior related behavior and personal factors; 2) behavior-specific cognitions and affect (such as interpersonal influences from family, peers, situations, or perceived barriers and perceived self-efficacy); and 3) behavioral outcome (e.g., committing to a plan of action that results in behavioral change). Health-promoting behavior is the desired outcome (Pender; Wu & Pender, 2005).

behavior change. It is necessary to educate clients to provide them with the tools they need to make change. Although it is helpful to provide clients with a tailored education program that involves more than one member of the healthcare team (e.g., nurses, physicians, dietitians, psychologists), even brief interventions by primary care practitioners have been effective for risky behaviors such as smoking (Whitlock et al., 2002). Research shows that education may also confer to clients a greater sense of control over an illness and may help to diminish feelings of helplessness, inadequacy, and insecurity (Glajchen, 1996; Whitlock et al.).

Skilled nurse educators create an environment that encourages learning with trust, respect, and acceptance. Effective education actively involves clients by helping them understand their readiness to change, establish their own goals, and evaluate their progress in terms of these goals. Nurse educators also help clients understand the factors that help to motivate them and provide support to encourage and sustain behavioral change (Redman, 2001).

Although a variety of educational approaches exist, one model that has been described by a nurse and that parallels the practice of nursing is described in Figure 13-6.

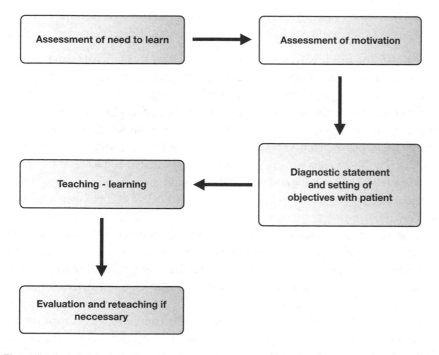

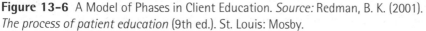

Figure 13-6 A Model of Phases in Client Education. *Source:* Redman, B. K. (2001). *The process of patient education* (9th ed.). St. Louis: Mosby.

Regardless of the model chosen, basic common steps are crucial when working with a client to encourage behavioral change. These include assessment, development, and implementation of the client-tailored program for change, and evaluation, reassessment, and revision as needed.

Assessing a Client

To provide clients with the skills and information they need to take steps toward making a change, nurses must first assess a client's knowledge, ability, motivation, confidence, and resources for making such a change. It is helpful in this process to assess a client's current stage of change along with level of motivation to make changes. Attempting a client education program without understanding client motivation can lead to failure, because unmotivated clients are much less likely to comply with the instructions nurses provide. On the other hand, highly motivated clients who are ready to take action will likely need less advice and assistance in the process. Examples of questions that can be used to assess motivation are:

- Have you ever thought about making changes in your [insert behavior; e.g., exercise habits]?
- What would you like to change about your [insert behavior] now?
- What concerns do you have about changing your [insert behavior] now?

Assessment also involves understanding the client's knowledge and level of comprehension of the diagnosis and disease, treatment, and behaviors that the client can adopt to improve his or her health. Through this assessment, the nurse can measure the scope of a client's knowledge, identifying how to tailor educational efforts to the client's needs. Given the wide access to knowledge through the Internet, many clients today may be more familiar with their condition than were clients 10–20 years ago and may require less intensive education. Other clients will have little or no knowledge of their condition and will need more information. The varying range of client knowledge makes this a crucial area to include in assessment.

Assessment also should include factors that may influence the client's ability to succeed in implementing change beyond health status and motivation. It is important for healthcare professionals to realize that a person's behaviors are influenced by the interaction of physical environment and interpersonal and intrapersonal factors (Whitlock et al., 2002). These factors are especially important when working with vulnerable populations. Therefore, assessment should address issues such as client literacy level, socioeconomic status, and physical and psychological stressors in home and work environments that may have a negative effect on client ability to change. Consideration of these factors can lead to tailored plans that will be the most helpful to the client. For example, a client with low literacy levels may require simple instruction or the inclusion of a fully literate family member or close friend to help with the **health behavior change**; or a client who lives alone or is unlikely to be supported by family members may benefit from referral to a group education setting to provide social support. A client who works long hours on the job and relies frequently on restaurant food for meals may need guidance on healthy food choices.

KEY TERM

Health behavior change: A persistent and lasting change in a person's actions. Overweight/obesity, lack of physical activity, and dietary habits are the top three preventive behaviors that health educators seek to change.

Creating and Implementing the Plan

Nurses should work together with their clients to develop and implement the behavioral change plan. A client-driven educational approach helps to create an environment that allows clients to express their feelings, questions, and concerns, facilitating the formulation of mutual goals with the nurse. Research has shown that health outcomes are often more favorable when clients believe they are informed and involved in treatment decisions and the clinician approaches the educational efforts as a partner rather than an authoritative guide (Tattersall, Butow, & Clayton, 2002; Whitlock et al., 2002). Nurse educators should aim to provide information, correct misconceptions, address feelings about the recommended change, provide support, and motivate the client to foster change. Nurses should validate the client's feelings about recommended changes by using language such as, "I know it's hard to . . .", "It must be difficult to . . .", or "I'd like to help you with . . .". In developing and discussing the plan, nurses should also show optimism about the chances for success to motivate the client ("I really think you'll be able to . . ." or "You seem confident in taking the necessary steps to achieve your goal of . . ."). The plan should also include follow-up appointments to discuss how things are going. Follow-up appointments show clients that their behavioral change is important, that the nurse educator wants to spend time helping them monitor their progress, and that any obstacles encountered will be tackled together with the nurse educator (Redman, 2001).

Goal-setting is a critical part of client-centered education. Goals are most effectively created by clients with the assistance of a healthcare professional, after examining areas needing change. Clients should focus on only a few goals at one time and they may be more or less challenging depending on the client's confidence to achieve them. Goals should be clearly defined and include specific time frames. Clients may need "cues" from the nurse or healthcare professional to identify potential challenges and barriers that could threaten their ability to achieve their goals. The nurse educator can use feedback, reflection, summary, and problem-solving skills to encourage clients to consider ways to cope with anticipated difficulties. This process will help clients be more prepared and self-assured. Clients who have confidence to handle different situations and obstacles are more likely to achieve their goals.

Evaluating, Reassessing, and Revising

Maintaining any behavior change is often difficult. Follow-up enables the nurse educator to evaluate and monitor progress, determining if the plan is appropriate. Useful questions include, "What part of the plan was most helpful?" and "What part of the plan did not work?" Such inquiries can help the nurse educator and client improve the plan, refining future goals.

Throughout the entire process, the nurse can use open-ended assessment questions that enable him or her to tailor the helping relationship to the needs of the client. Reflective statements such as, "Tell me more about . . .", "I hear you saying . . .", and summary statements are helpful to clarify and summarize what the client shares.

The Educational Environment

Nurses see clients in hospitals, offices, community clinics, other outpatient settings, and home settings. Client education can be provided one-on-one, or nurse educators may become involved in classroom settings through such venues as a hospital's community education program. The nurse educator should be aware of the unique characteristics of each setting and how the environment can enhance educational efforts. In addition, it is important for the nurse educator to communicate with other members of the healthcare team who are working with the client (e.g., dietitians, health educators, physicians) to ensure a coordinated approach toward behavioral change.

Hospital Setting

The clinical setting can offer key opportunities to initiate or reinforce a client's educational plan, given the opportunities for follow-up visits with the client. Nurses can begin counseling during hospitalization, with follow-up visits scheduled to continue through the course of outpatient treatment or therapy. Recent studies show that many clients view diet and exercise education postsurgery as an opportune time to start practicing better habits—a "teachable moment" (Rock & Demar-Wahnefried, 2002). Analysis from 143 postsurgical breast cancer clients indicated a preference for education shortly after breast surgery (Monnin, 1998). Thus, inpatient education can be an excellent beginning to the counseling process. However, time pressures in the current healthcare model may challenge doing thorough inpatient health education.

Outpatient Setting: Individual

Changing trends in the healthcare system, leading to decreased admissions and shortened length of stay in hospitals, have propelled outpatient counseling to the forefront. Because of these trends, hospitalized clients usually are those with exacerbations of their condition or severe illnesses. Therefore, during rehospitalization or an acute episode of illness, clients may not be receptive to learning. In addition, most clients require more education and follow-up than can be provided in the inpatient setting or during discharge planning sessions. Reduced time for adequate counseling and some clients' lack of readiness to learn immediately following diagnosis support the concept that client education may best be achieved outside the hospital setting (see Sidebar 13-3). This trend also underscores the need to provide printed information (e.g., brochures) for clients, and additional Web resources if clients have access to and familiarity with using the Internet.

Outpatient Setting: Group

Group education settings can be an effective place to provide client education. Nurse educators may become involved in leading group education sessions as part of their hospital's community education program, or they may recommend clients to programs to supplement their education. Education in a group setting can provide clients with social support through opportunities to share with others who are trying to change health behaviors. Learning from the experiences of others, hearing how others have overcome obstacles, and providing insight from their own experiences can provide clients with the motivation and reinforcement needed to help them follow through on their plans (Whitlock et al., 2002), in accordance with the basics of Social Cognitive Theory (Bandura, 2004). Being with others facing similar situations can remove feelings of isolation, helping clients feel that they are not alone in their struggle to change health behaviors (Pender, 1996).

A group education program should never be a substitute for a tailored, one-on-one approach through which nurses provide clients with personal support, motivation, reassessment of goals, and evaluation on progress. However, appropriate group education programs can complement individual efforts by the nurse. In referring clients to group education programs, nurses should be familiar with the program content, know its reliability and efficacy, and assess the program

---

SIDEBAR 13-3 FOCUS ON INPATIENT VS. OUTPATIENT NUTRITIONAL COUNSELING

Schiller and colleagues (1998) assessed clients' perceived benefits of nutrition counseling and examined whether counseling outcomes differed for inpatients versus outpatients, using a telephone interview 2–8 weeks after counseling.

Four hundred adult clients at two academic health centers participated in the study. Of these participants, 274 clients (69 percent) received inpatient counseling and 126 (31 percent) received outpatient counseling services. Counseling addressed individuals' diagnosis and type of diet instruction.

Telephone interviews indicated that, after speaking with a dietitian, 60 percent of all subjects were able to fully describe their prescribed diet, 57 percent of all subjects felt better emotionally, 37 percent felt better physically, and 64 percent felt in control of their condition after counseling. Outpatients and newly instructed clients demonstrated a better understanding of their diet modifications compared to inpatients ($p < 0.01$), and those previously instructed ($p < 0.05$).

logistics, such as location and time offered, with the client. It is important to follow up with the client on successive visits to determine whether the client participated or felt that barriers prevented participation.

Areas to Consider in Client Education

Multiple variables contribute to a client's ability to learn, including a client's physical condition and comfort level, length of time since and adjustment to the diagnosis, financial resources, educational level, cultural context, support system, and language barriers. The Joint Commission has specific standards for client education, including assessing client "learning needs, cultural and religious beliefs, emotional barriers, desire and motivation to learn, physical or cognitive limitations, and barriers to communication" and providing education that is appropriate to patient needs (Bass, 2005, p. 17). Clients differ in their educational backgrounds, intellectual abilities, and attitudes towards accepting responsibility for healthy behaviors (Polinsky, 1994). Some general assessment of these issues is important for optimal client education.

To be effective in educating clients, nurses and other healthcare professionals must demonstrate greater cultural competence (see chapter 14). Although defined in many ways and encompassed in several terms, cultural competence basically

---

SIDEBAR 13-4 FOCUS ON CULTURAL COMPETENCY

Many terms are used to define and refer to cultural competency. These can include cultural sensitivity, multicultural, culturally based, or ethnic identity (Resnicow, Braithwaite, Dilorio, & Glanz, 2002). The U.S. Office of Minority Health defines cultural and linguistic competency as "a set of congruent behaviors, attitudes, and policies that come together in a system, agency, or among professionals that enables work in cross-cultural situations" (Office of Minority Health, 2007b). Cultural competency is important because of the influence of culture and language on:

- Health, healing, and belief systems
- How both clients and providers perceive illness, disease, and their causes
- The behavior of clients and their attitudes toward healthcare providers
- How a provider delivers services, based on her or his own cultural background

The National Standards on Culturally and Linguistically Appropriate Services (CLAS) have been developed primarily for healthcare organizations, but individual providers are encouraged to follow the CLAS standards. The 14 standards are based on several themes that include Culturally Competent Care Standards, Language Access Services, and Organizational Supports for Cultural Competence. The standards include guidelines such as healthcare organizations providing a diverse staff representative of the demographic characteristics of their service areas, providing language assistance services to non-English-proficient clients at all times in a timely manner, and ensuring the competence of language assistance, relying on trained interpreters, if possible and agreed to by the client (Office of Minority Health, 2007a). More information on cultural competency is available by going to http://www.omhrc.gov and clicking on the "Cultural Competency" tab.

means the ability to understand and effectively relate to people from diverse groups—in terms of gender, race, age, religious background, culture, language, educational level, and socioeconomic status (Nunez & Robertson, 2005). A culturally sensitive, individualized behavior change plan can impact a client's long-term physical status, function, and quality of life. Therefore, nurses must work with other members of the healthcare team, such as dietitians, physical therapists, or speech therapists, to better tailor client health assessment and implement the most effective education plan during the initial diagnosis, the treatment phase, or long-term follow-up period (American Dietetic Association [ADA], 2003). Given the diversity of client populations, tailoring may also require allowing for client-specific cultural norms and/or providing interpreters and non-English educational materials for non-English-speaking clients. Nurses and other healthcare professionals today are often more successful in communicating with clients if they communicate clearly and also reflect empathy, self-awareness, honesty, gender sensitivity, cultural awareness, and knowledge (see Sidebar 13-5). Following are some issues that nurse educators must consider when working with an increasingly diverse client population.

Gender and Culture

Gender and culture are two additional factors that may impact on perceptions, attitudes, and the process of learning. For example, an educator may not detect the depth of depression a man with prostate cancer is experiencing. Traditional gender stereotypes may discourage some men from showing emotion or weakness. In addition, an educator may not be familiar with cultural norms that influence dietary habits among people of certain cultures. However, a sensitive

---

SIDEBAR 13-5 SPOTLIGHT ON CLIENT COMMUNICATION

Effective communication is critical to convey messages and interpret feedback. Nurses and healthcare professionals must be able to validate and empathize with both verbal and nonverbal messages. The following is some basic advice for communicating effectively with a client:

- Be warm, empathetic, and non-judgmental.
- Remember that each client is a unique individual and there is no "one size fits all" approach.
- Respect the client.
- Be sure to emphasize your confidence in the client's ability to change, to help increase the client's feel of self-efficacy.
- Make the client aware that there is more than one way to approach and maintain successful behavior change.
- Acknowledge any previous successes the client has to increase confidence and self-efficacy.

Source: Whitlock, E. P., Orleans, C. T., Pender, N., & Allan, J. (2002). Evaluating primary care behavioral counseling interventions: An evidence-based approach. *American Journal of Preventive Medicine, 22*(4), 267–284.

educator can recognize, understand, and feel comfortable with such differences and realize when, for example, it may be appropriate to include on the healthcare team a person who can offer informed insight of the client's cultural background and the impact that this background may have on the client's cooperation with the efforts of the healthcare team.

Language and Literacy

Spoken language and literacy level are critical for client understanding of prescribed health regimens and efforts to change health behaviors. Clients who are non-native speakers of English may require translators or benefit from the presence of a family member who is fluent in English. Otherwise, serious misunderstandings may occur that can impact patient care and lead to negative clinical outcomes. For instance, a prescription to take a medication "once a day" could be misinterpreted by a native speaker of Spanish with limited capability in English, because in Spanish, "once" is the number 11. A case study reporting on language barriers tells of a non-English-speaking family whose 13-year-old daughter, the only member who could speak English, was stricken with severe abdominal pain and too ill to communicate. Hospital staff told her parents, without using an interpreter, to bring the girl back immediately if her condition deteriorated, but that if there was no change, to bring her back in 3 days. The parents understood only that the girl should be brought back in 3 days and so did not react immediately when her symptoms worsened. By the time the girl was brought to the emergency department, her appendix had ruptured and she died shortly thereafter (Smith, Bussey-Jones, Horowitz, Whitehurst-Cook, & Chen, 2005).

Literacy, both general and health-specific, also is a critical factor in client education. Fully or partially illiterate clients may have difficulty understanding oral instructions or printed materials and are unlikely to be able to access resources available on the Internet. Such clients may indicate that they understand instructions even when they do not, simply to avoid looking foolish or uneducated (Bass, 2005). These clients require special approaches and may benefit from the help of a literate family member or friend. In addition, general health literacy is important to the success of client education efforts. According to the Institute of Medicine, nearly half of all adults in the United States have difficulty understanding and using health information, and those clients who are less proficient have a higher rate of hospitalization and use of emergency services (Nielsen-Bohlman, Panzer, & Kindig, 2004). Furthermore, a survey of adult literacy including health literacy found that adults age 65 or older had lower average health literacy scores than adults under age 65 (Kutner, Greenberg, Jin, & Paulsen, 2006). (See Sidebar 13-6.)

Thus, the nurse educator must be aware of a client's general literacy level and familiarity with health information before embarking on a plan for health behavior change or providing printed materials as a client resource.

SIDEBAR 13-6 FOCUS ON HEALTH LITERACY

According to a 2003 assessment of adult literacy by the National Center for Educational Statistics, most adults 16 or older in the United States (53 percent) have intermediate health literacy, which indicates reading skill that will enable them to comprehend moderately challenging literacy activities (Kutner et al., 2006). Only 12 percent were proficient, which is the highest level of literacy. Twenty-two percent had basic health literacy, and 14 percent had below basic literacy. Definitions from the survey were as follows:

- *Proficient:* Has skills needed to perform more complex and challenging literacy activities
- *Intermediate:* Has skills needed to perform moderately challenging literacy activities
- *Basic:* Has skills needed to perform simple and everyday literacy activities
- *Below Basic:* Has not more than the most simple and concrete literacy skills

Figures 13-7 and 13-8 show the distribution of health literacy levels by age and by race/ethnicity. The oldest adults had the lowest literacy levels. Hispanics had the greatest proportion with Below Basic, followed by American Indian/Alaska Natives and African Americans. Whites, those of multiracial origin, and Asian/Pacific Islanders had the highest proportion of Intermediate proficiency or higher.

For more information, visit http://nces.ed.gov/pubsearch/ and search for the document by title.

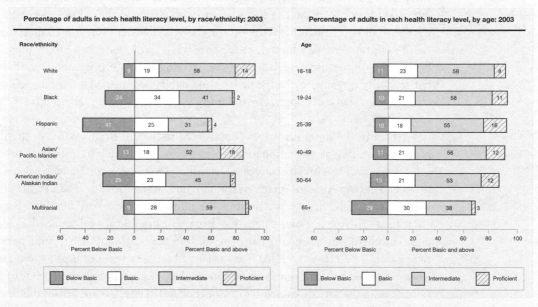

Figure 13-7 Percentage of adults in each health literacy level, by race/ethnicity: 2003.

Figure 13-8 Percentage of adults in each health literacy level, by age: 2003.

NOTE: Detail may not sum to totals because of rounding. Adults are defined as people 16 years of age and older living in households or prisons. Adults who could not be interviewed because of language spoken or cognitive or mental disabilities (3 percent in 2003) are excluded from this figure. All adults of Hispanic origin are classified as Hispanic, regardless of race. The Asian/Pacific Islander category includes Native Hawaiians. Black includes African American, and Hispanic includes Latino.

Source: Kutner, M., Greenberg, E., Jin, Y., & Paulsen, C. (2006). *The Health Literacy of America's Adults: Results from the 2003 National Assessment of Adult Literacy* (NCES 2006-483). Washington, DC: U.S. Department of Education, National Center for Education Statistics.

Personal Resources

Many healthcare providers fail to recognize the importance of understanding the whole client in achieving successful health outcomes. This is particularly true when working with certain vulnerable populations. A client facing a large number of personal stressors in his or her life that stem from living in poverty may not have the personal resources to take on the additional challenges that a health behavior change requires. In addition, if a client's physical or social home environment is inadequate in some way, it could interfere with efforts to initiate and maintain change. For example, an obese client living in a subsidized housing community who does not feel safe spending time outside is unlikely to follow advice to undertake a personal walking program. Similarly, a client advised to make dietary changes but who lacks adequate transportation to a grocery store or does not live in an area where stores offer a variety of healthy foods lacks a basic resource for initiating dietary change. Finally, the social home environment is an important factor to consider when working with clients to make health behavior change. Will family members support the changes the client is trying to make? A client's efforts to make a lifestyle change are often facilitated when family members join in on the effort, such as a spouse agreeing to try quitting smoking or an entire family agreeing to change their eating habits or undertake a regular exercise program. Lack of support from family members can deter client efforts to enact change.

Critical to personal resources is a client's socioeconomic status. A client lacking economic or educational experience may be unlikely to initiate change or even to comply with an established health regimen. An example is a case history of an elderly African American woman, non-adherent with medications for hypertension. This client saw a second-year internal medicine resident for a persistent sore throat, but had a negative throat culture and no evidence of allergies. The client was not taking her hypertension medication. Further inquiry by the resident's preceptor revealed that the client had been without heat for several weeks and used her gas oven as a heat source, sleeping in front of it to keep warm (and causing the sore throat from dry air exposure). The client explained that she did not take her hypertension medications because of the experience of a friend who had run out of hypertension medication for a few days, had a rapid rise in blood pressure leading to a stroke, and was told that not taking the pills caused the stroke. The client was therefore afraid to take her medication because she feared she would not remember to take it regularly and would also suffer a stroke. As a result of this inquiry, the physicians suggested that the client use a weekly patch for her medication, contacted a social worker to resolve the client's need for heat, and told her in the meantime to put a pan of water in the oven to provide humidity in the air. These steps resolved the sore throat and reduced the client's blood pressure (Smith et al., 2005).

Summary

This chapter provided an overview of the potential healthcare challenges for individuals from populations that may be at greater risk for developing chronic diseases and the consequences commonly seen in individuals with these diseases. In addition, it gave an overview of health behavior theories and described the main health behaviors that contribute to the top causes of death in the United States today. Finally, the chapter explained how to translate behavioral change education and motivation strategies for working with individuals and groups to enhance their abilities to practice health-promoting behavior for chronic disease risk reduction.

Key Terms

- **Chronic disease:** A long-lasting disease that typically remains with a patient from onset to end of life and requires management of symptoms. Examples are cancer, cardiovascular disease, diabetes, and cerebrovascular disease. According to the U.S. Centers for Disease Control and Prevention, chronic disease is responsible for 7 out of 10 deaths in the United States.
- **Disabilities:** Physical or mental impairments that substantially limit a person from completing activities of daily living.
- **Health behavior change:** A persistent and lasting change in a person's actions. Overweight/obesity, lack of physical activity, and dietary habits are the top three preventive behaviors that health educators seek to change.
- **Health disparities:** Differences in the incidence, prevalence, mortality, and burden of disease and other adverse health conditions that exist among specific population groups.
- **Healthy People 2010:** A statement of national health objectives designed to identify the most significant preventable threats to health and to establish national goals to reduce these threats in the next decade. Goals are set to help public health professionals, healthcare providers, and others work toward improving the health of citizens. Healthy People 2010 can be accessed at http://www.healthypeople.gov.
- **Obesity:** Having an excess of body fat. Obesity is clinically determined by body mass index (BMI), which is calculated by dividing a person's weight in kilograms by height in meters squared (kg/m^2). A person with a BMI of 30.0 or more is defined as obese.
- **Overweight:** Having an excess of body weight that includes fat, muscle, bone, and water. Overweight is clinically determined by BMI, which is calculated by dividing a person's weight in kilometers by height in meters squared (kg/m^2). A person with a BMI ranging between 25.0 and 29.9 is defined as overweight.
- **Primary prevention:** Actions taken to modify health behaviors such as diet, sedentary behavior, or smoking towards preventing or managing a chronic condition such as heart disease or cancer. An example is reducing one's intake of dietary fat to help lower cholesterol levels and prevent one from exceeding recommended cholesterol guidelines.
- **Vulnerable populations:** Groups that are likely to have compromised access to health care and, therefore, are more likely to have poorer health outcomes, including higher mortality rates, compared to less vulnerable groups.

Reflective Practice Questions

1. Discuss the difference between the terms *health disparities* and *vulnerable populations*. What are the implications for practice when a nurse is working with individuals or groups from vulnerable populations?

2. This chapter discusses the issue that causes of health disparities are "multifactorial." Explain what is meant by the term multifactorial and how these issues impact nursing practice.

3. Identify three causes of the obesity epidemic. In providing client education, which issue would you address first in working with a male client, 42 years old, who reports that he is ready to lose weight?

4. To ground an educational session focused on helping a current smoker stop smoking, which behavior change health model would you select in planning your session? Provide a rationale for your answer.

5. Name and discuss five steps for planning and delivering successful client prevention education in a women's health clinic located in an underserved area.

References

American Cancer Society. (2004). *Cancer Facts and Figures 2004.* Atlanta: Author.

American Cancer Society. (2006). *Prevention and early detection 2006.* Atlanta: Author.

American Cancer Society. (2007). *Cancer facts and figures 2007.* Atlanta: Author.

American Dietetic Association. (2003). Position paper: Integrating medical nutrition therapy and pharmacotherapy. *Journal of the American Dietetic Association, 108,* 1368–1379.

Antonovsky, A. (1967). Social class, life expectancy and overall mortality. *Millbank Memorial Fund Quarterly, 45,* 31–73.

Bandura, A. (1977). Self-efficacy: Toward a unifying theory of behavioral change. *Psychological Review, 84,* 191–215.

Bandura, A. (1986). *Social foundations of thought and action.* Englewood Cliffs, NJ: Prentice-Hall.

Bandura, A. (2004). Health promotion by social cognitive means. *Health Education and Behavior, 31,* 143–164.

Bass, L. (2005). Health literacy: Implications for teaching the adult patient. *Journal of Infusion Nursing, 28*(1), 15–22.

Becker, M. H. (1974). The health belief model and sick role behavior. *Health Education Monographs, 2,* 409–419.

Befort, C., Greiner, K., Hall, S., Pullver, K., Nolen, L., Carboneau, A., et al. (2006). Weight-related perceptions among patients and physicians: How well do physicians judge patients' motivation to lose weight? *Journal of General Internal Medicine, 21*(10), 1086–1090.

Calle, E. E., Rodriguez, C., Walker-Thurmond, K., & Thun, M. J. (2003). Overweight, obesity, and mortality from cancer in a prospectively studied cohort of U.S. adults. *New England Journal of Medicine, 24*(17), 1625–1638.

Center for Science in the Public Interest. (2007, June 14). *Kellogg makes historic settlement agreement, adopting nutrition standards for marketing foods to children.* Press release. Retrieved July 14, 2008, from http://www.cspinet.org/new/200706141.html

Centers for Disease Control and Prevention, Office of Minority Health and Health Disparities. (2007a). *Eliminate disparities in cardiovascular disease (CVD).* Retrieved July 31, 2007, from http://www.cdc.gov/omhd/AMH/factsheets/cardio.htm

Centers for Disease Control and Prevention, Office of Minority Health and Health Disparities. (2007b). *Eliminate disparities in diabetes.* Retrieved July 31, 2007, from http://www.cdc.gov/omhd/AMH/factsheets/diabetes.htm

Crenshaw, K. (2007). The laws of health: Our uninsured population. *Esquire.* Retrieved July 30, 2007, from http:/www.aces.edu/urban/metronews/

Eissenberg, M. E., Neumark-Sztainer, D., & Story, M. (2003). Associations of weight-based teasing and emotional well-being among adolescents. *Archives of Pediatric and Adolescent Medicine, 157*(8), 733–738.

Freeman, H. (2004). Poverty, culture, and social injustice: Determinants of cancer disparities. *CA: A Cancer Journal for Clinicians, 54*(2), 72–77.

Glajchen, M. (1996). Teleconferencing as a method of educating men about managing advanced prostate cancer pain. *Journal of Psychosocial Oncology, 14,* 73–87.

Hager, R. I. (2006). Television viewing and physical activity in children. *Journal of Adolescent Health, 39*(5), 656–661.

Harel, A., Riggs, S., Vaz, R., White, L., & Menzies, G. (1998). Adolescents and calcium: What they do and do not know and how much they consume. *Journal of Adolescent Health, 3,* 225–228.

Hedley, A., Ogden, C., Johnson, C., Carroll, M., Curtin, L., & Flegal, K. (2004). *Journal of the American Medical Association, 291*(23), 2847–2850.

Jones-Burton, C. J., & Saunders, E. (2005). Cardiovascular disease and hypertension. In D. Satcher & R. J. Pamies (Eds.), *Multicultural medicine and health disparities* (pp. 167–180). New York: McGraw-Hill.

Kutner, M., Greenberg, E., Jin, Y., & Paulsen, C. (2006). *The health literacy of America's adults: Results from the 2003 National Assessment of Adult Literacy* (NCES 2006-483). Washington, DC: U.S. Department of Education, National Center for Education Statistics.

Leddy, S. K. (2006). *Health promotion: Mobilizing strengths to enhance health, wellness, and well-being.* Philadelphia: F.A. Davis.

Martin, A. (2007, June 14). Kellogg to phase out some food ads to children. *New York Times.* Retrieved February 5, 2008, from http://www.nytimes.com/2007/06/14/business/14kellogg.html

Mokdad, A. H., Marks, J. S., Stroup, J. L., & Gerberding, J. L. (2000). Actual causes of death in the United States, 2000. *Journal of the American Medical Association, 291,* 1238–1245.

Monnin, S. (1993). Nutrition counseling for breast cancer clients. *Journal of the American Dietetic Association, 93,* 72–73.

Nestle, M. (2002). *Food politics.* Berkeley: University of California Press.

Nielsen-Bohlman, L., Panzer, A. M., & Kindig, D. A. (Eds.). (2004). *Health literacy: A prescription to end confusion.* Committee on Health Literacy, Board on Neuroscience and Behavioral Health, Institute of Medicine. Washington, DC: National Academies Press.

Núñez, A., & Roberston, C. (2005). Cultural competency. In D. Satcher & R. J. Pamies (Eds.), *Multicultural medicine and health disparities* (pp. 371–388). New York: McGraw-Hill.

Office of Minority Health. (2007a). *National standards on culturally and linguistically appropriate services (CLAS).* Retrieved August 3, 2007, from http://www.omhrc.gov/templates/browse.aspx?lvl=2&lvlID=15

Office of Minority Health. (2007b). *What is cultural competency?* Retrieved August 3, 2007, from http://www.omhrc.gov/templates/browse.aspx?lvl=2&lvlID=11

Ogden, C. L., Carroll, M. D., Curtin, L. R., McDowell, M. A., Tabak, C. J., & Flegal, K. M. (2006). Prevalence of overweight and obesity in the United States, 1999–2004. *Journal of the American Medical Association, 295*(13), 1549–55.

Ornish, D. The threat from within. *Newsweek.* Retrieved January 25, 2007, from http://www.newsweek.com/id/70227

Pender, N. J. (1996). *Health promotion in nursing practice.* Stamford, CT: Appleton & Lange.

Polinsky, M. (1994). Functional status of long-term breast cancer survivors: Demonstrating chronicity. *Health and Social Work, 3,* 166–173.

Prochaska, J. O., & DiClemente, C. (1982). Transtheoretical theory: Toward a more integrative model of change. *Psychotherapy: Theory, Research, and Practice, 19*(3), 276–287.

Prochaska, J. O., Redding, C. A., & Evers, K. E. (2002). The Transtheoretical Model and stages of change. In K. Glanz, B. K. Rimer, & F. M. Lewis (Eds.), *Health behavior and health education: Theory, research, and practice* (3rd ed., pp. 99–120). San Francisco: Jossey-Bass.

Redman, B. K. (2001). *The process of patient education* (9th ed.). St. Louis: Mosby.

Resnicow, K., Braithwaite, R. L., Dilorio, C., & Glanz, K. (2002). Applying theory to culturally diverse and unique populations. In K. Glanz, B. K. Rimer, & F. M. Lewis (Eds.), *Health behavior and health education: Theory, research, and practice* (3rd ed., pp. 485–509). San Francisco: Jossey-Bass.

Rock, C., & Demark-Wahnefried, W. (2002). Nutrition and survival after the diagnosis of breast cancer: A review of the evidence. *Journal of Clinical Oncology, 20*(15), 3302–3316.

Rosamond, W., Flegal, K., Friday, G., Furie, K., Go, A., Greenlund, K., et al. (2007). Heart disease and stroke statistics—2007 update: A report from the American Heart Association statistics committee and stroke statistics subcommittee. *Circulation, 115*(5), e69–e171.

Rosenstock, I. M. (1966). Why people use health services. *Millbank Memorial Fund Quarterly, 44,* 94–127.

Schiller, M. R., Miller, M., Moore, C., Davis, E., Dunn, A., Mulligan, K., et al. (1998). Clients report positive nutrition counseling outcomes. *Journal of the American Dietetic Association, 98,* 977–982.

Skara, S., & Sussman, S. (2003). A review of 25 long-term adolescent tobacco and other drug use prevention program evaluations. *Preventive Medicine, 37*(5), 451–474.

Smedley, B., & Syme, L. S. (Eds.). (2000). *Promoting health: Intervention strategies from social and behavioral research.* Washington, DC: National Academy Press.

Smith, W. R., Bussey-Jones, J., Horowitz, C. R., Whitehurst-Cook, M., & Chen, A. H. (2005). Case studies in multicultural medicine and health disparities. In D. Satcher & R. J. Pamies (Eds.), *Multicultural medicine and health disparities* (pp. 361–368). New York: McGraw-Hill.

Striegel-Moore, R. H., Thompson, D., Affenito, S. G., Franko, D. L., Obarzanek, E., Barton, B. A., et al. (2006). Correlates of beverage intake in adolescent girls: The National Heart, Lung, and Blood Institute Growth and Health Study. *Journal of Pediatrics, 14*(2), 183–187.

Tattersall, M. H. N., Butow, P. N., & Clayton, J. M. (2002). Insights from cancer client communication research. *Hematology and Oncology Clinics of North America, 16,* 731–743.

Tillotson, J. E. (2004). America's obesity: Conflicting public policies, industrial economic development, and unintended human consequences. *Annual Review of Nutrition, 24,* 617–643.

Townsend, M., Peerson, J., Love, B., Achterberg, P., & Murphy, J. (2001). Food insecurity is positively related to obesity in women. *Journal of Nutrition, 131*(6), 1738–1745.

Tunceli, K., Li, K., & Williams, L. (2006). Long-term effects of obesity on employment and work limitations among U.S. adults, 1986 to 1999. *Obesity, 14*(9), 1637–1646.

United Nations Development Program. (1993). *Human development report 1993.* New York: Oxford Press.

Weinstein, N. D., & Sandman, P. M. (2002). The precaution adoption process model. In K. Glanz, B. K. Rimer, & F. M. Lewis (Eds.), *Health behavior and health education: Theory, research, and practice* (3rd ed., pp. 121–143). San Francisco: Jossey-Bass.

Whitlock, E. P., Orleans, C. T., Pender, N., & Allan, J. (2002). Evaluating primary care behavioral counseling interventions: An evidence-based approach. *American Journal of Preventive Medicine, 22*(4), 267–284.

Wilson, D. B., Heckman, C., McClish, D., Obando, P., & Dahman, G. (2007). Parental smoking, closeness to parents, and youth smoking. *American Journal of Health Behavior, 31*(3), 261–271.

Wilson, D. B., McClellan, M., & Musham, C. (2004). From mothers to daughters: Transgenerational food and diet and communication in an underserved group. *Journal of Cultural Diversity, 11*(1), 12–17.

Wilson, D. B., Smith, B., Speizer, I., Bean, M., Mitchell, K., Uguy, S., et al. (2005). Differences in food intake and exercise by smoking status in adolescents. *Preventive Medicine, 40*(6), 872–879.

Wu, T. Y., & Pender, N. J. (2005). A panel study of physical activity in Taiwanese youth: Testing the revised Health-Promotion Model. *Family and Community Health, 28*(2), 113–124.

Wynder, E. (1954). The place of tobacco in the etiology of lung cancer. *Connecticut Medicine, 18*(4), 321–330.

Young, L. M., & Nestle, M. (2007). Portion sizes and obesity: Responses of fast food companies. *Journal of Public Health Policy, 28*(2), 238–248.

chapter 14

Cultural Diversity and Care

Joan C. Engebretson and Judith A. Headley

LEARNING OUTCOMES

After reading this chapter you will be able to:

- Compare common value orientations associated with cultures.
- Analyze components of cultural diversity.
- Describe the components and principles of cultural competence.
- Describe the influence of technology on cultural development and communication systems.
- Discuss cultural influences on beliefs and systems related to health and illness.
- Discuss the role of culture in interactions with clients.
- Identify appropriate patterns, challenges, and needs of clients in the cultural domain.

Cultural Diversity and Practices

Culture is the combination of ideas, customs, skills, arts, and other capabilities of a people or group, although as a whole, it is more complex than any one of these elements. Culture is learned from birth through language acquisition and socialization, and is the process by which an individual adapts to the group's organized way of life. This process also provides for the transmission of culture from one generation to another. Members of the cultural group share cultural beliefs and patterns of behavior that create a group identity, which has a powerful influence on behavior, usually on a subconscious level. Culture is largely tacit, meaning it is not generally expressed or discussed at a conscious level. Most culturally derived actions are based on implicit cues rather than written or spoken sets of rules.

Although many of the underlying beliefs and value systems of a culture are stable, all cultures are inherently dynamic and changing; therefore, it is difficult to generalize from one situation or time to another. Cultural practices are continually adapting to the environment, historical context, technology, and availability of resources. As a result, the context in which people live influences, and is influenced by, cultural practice. Anthropology (the study of cultures) and nursing are both based on a holistic perspective. Culture has a significant impact on health and illness behaviors, as well as patterns of response. It directly influences health behaviors such as diet and exercise. Cultural beliefs and practices also affect the types of health problems that are attended to and the actions taken to deal with them. Activities taken to promote, maintain, or restore health are all performed in a cultural context. Therefore, an understanding of the client's perceptions and the context in which he or she lives are necessary for optimal client care.

Culture also determines much of the relationship and type of communication between a client and a healthcare provider. Given that the United States is a culturally diverse nation, nurses and other healthcare providers encounter individuals and groups whose habits of health maintenance, reactions to illness or disease, and use of healthcare services may differ from their own. An awareness of and accommodation to the cultural aspects of health and illness behaviors enable one to promote health by skillfully blending professional knowledge with knowledge of the individual's or group's beliefs. **Culturally competent health care** is the delivery of health care with skill, knowledge, and sensitivity to cultural factors. With the increase of cultural pluralism in North America, it is essential that nurses develop cultural competency to deliver care.

Cultural Competency

With increasing diversity in the population, and the recognition that health disparities exist across ethnic groups, healthcare regulatory agencies recommend that cultural competency become a goal in the provision of health care. The Office of Minority Health has developed standards and recommendations that apply to the institutional level as well as to the individual provider (Office of Minority Health, n.d.). Institutions are mandated to provide adequate translation, and individual providers are encouraged to develop more culturally appropriate care.

The National Center for Cultural Competency at Georgetown University uses a conceptual framework developed by Cross, Bazron, Dennis, and Isaacs (1989) that describes a continuum from cultural destructiveness to cultural competency. Professionals seek to counter cultural destructiveness, the lowest level of the continuum, through laws such as the Civil Rights Act of 1964 (Title VI), which mandates that healthcare providers do not discriminate according to **race**, **ethnicity**, or creed. The ethic of nonmaleficence, or "do no harm," also addresses this basic level. The second level of the continuum, cultural incapacity, refers to unintentional practices that may be harmful to patients through ignorance, insensitive attitudes, or improper allocation of resources. Cultural blindness, the third level, is exemplified by treating all patients alike without accommodating cultural differences. Providing translators, developing health education aimed at specific cultural groups, and creating programs that address diverse groups' access to care are good examples of cultural precompetence, which is level four. Cultural competence, level five, is best described as an ongoing learning process for the provider who can integrate cultural knowledge into individualized patient-centered care. This eventually leads to the highest level of the continuum, cultural proficiency. Practicing in a culturally competent manner also incorporates the three aspects of evidence-based practice: best evidence from valid and clinically relevant research, the provider's clinical expertise, and the patient's values and unique preferences (Sackett et al., 2003).

Culturally competent health care must be provided within the context of a client's cultural background, beliefs, and values related to health and illness to attain optimal client outcomes. In addition to the Transcultural Nursing Society, there is a corpus of literature in nursing to learn more about cultural competence (Campinha-Bacote, 2001; Douglas, 2002; Leininger, 2001; Purnell & Paulanka, 1998; Spector, 2000).

A plethora of sensitivity training and educational programs have been implemented and curricula have been developed in nursing and other healthcare professions. Lipson and Desantis (2007) recently reviewed a number of approaches in nursing education and concluded that there is a lack of consensus on what should be taught and how it should be integrated into the curricula. A systematic review of healthcare provider education concluded that cultural competence training shows promise for improving the knowledge, attitudes, and skills of healthcare professionals (Bernal, 1996). However, there was little evidence in patient outcomes. Another systematic review conducted on professional education in mental

KEY TERM

Race: A social classification that denotes a biologic or genetically transmitted set of distinguishable physical characteristics.

KEY TERM

Ethnicity: Designation of a population subgroup sharing a common social and cultural heritage.

health care reached similar conclusions of limited evidence on the effectiveness of cultural competence training and service delivery (Beach et al., 2005).

Most educational approaches have addressed knowledge, attitudes, and skills. Knowledge has often focused on facts and characteristics about specific cultures. This "cookbook" approach has been criticized as leading to **stereotyping**. The approach of cultural sensitivity training attempts to address attitudes. What seems to be more valuable is for providers to learn a set of skills that enable them to provide quality patient care to everyone. In a literature review of cultural competence and the clinical encounter, Betancourt concluded that healthcare providers develop the skills for a patient-centered approach that does the following: 1) assesses core cross-cultural issues, 2) explores the meaning of the illness to the patient, 3) determines the social context in which the patient lives, and 4) engages in a negotiation process with the patient (Bhui et al., 2007).

Bernal has identified five components for developing cultural sensitivity: open-mindedness, awareness of one's own cultural values, understanding of differences, knowledge, and adaptation skills, which are explained below (Betancourt, 2006).

1. Awareness and acceptance of cultural differences require an open-minded attitude about other worldviews. It is important to recognize that providing care based on one's own perspective may not be in the best interest of the client. Nurses who use a nonjudgmental approach in learning about a client's cultural belief system will not only gain a wealth of information, but also readily establish mutual trust in their nurse–client relationships.

2. An awareness of one's own biases and attitudes is a step toward overcoming them. Recognition of personal cultural attitudes requires conscious effort; most people are unaware of their cultural beliefs because their beliefs are so integrated into their perception of the world. It is important to note that value awareness does not mean that one tries to eliminate values. We all need to hold values in order to live our lives. The essential aspect is to become aware of our own values, so that we can better understand the values of another.

3. It is essential to recognize basic differences among cultures without promoting the superiority of one culture over another. Often, in an effort to connect with people of other cultures, people assume that there are few differences among cultures. Although recognizing similarities may be useful for making connections, it can obscure basic differences necessary for cultural understanding. For example, a European American cannot fully understand an African American without recognizing the legacy of slavery in the African American culture.

4. One of the best ways to learn about diverse cultures is to interact with people from those cultures. However, opportunities to become immersed

in another culture are not always available. An alternative is to expose one-self to culturally focused literature, films, and music, which can enhance cultural understanding.

5. Adaptation includes the ability to articulate an issue from another's per-spective, as well as to recognize and reduce resistance and defensiveness. The ability to admit errors is important, because resolving errors when interacting with someone from another culture allows for the exploration of cultural issues that enhance understanding and communication. It is often better to risk a confrontation than to avoid the issue, which could result in continued misperception or lost opportunity for better cultural understanding.

Although the importance of developing cultural competency is now empha-sized, there is also a developing awareness that competency is always a growth process, implying that it requires more than an accumulation of facts about dif-ferent cultures (Gregg & Saha, 2006). The clinical encounter, in which cultural competency is most demanding, requires individual or family-centered care (Dreher & MacNaughton, 2002).

Cultural Diversity and Health Disparities

Despite the fact that humans are 99.9 percent identical at the DNA level, there are differences in prevalence of illness among groups. This may be explained by genetic differences; dietary, cultural, environmental, and socioeconomic factors; or a combination thereof (Collins, 2003). Health disparities in the United States exist for multiple health outcomes. For example, African Americans have the highest overall risk of developing cancer and the greatest overall risk of dying from it (Underwood, 2000). In the United States, infant mortality is inversely related to the mother's educational level. It is also highest for infants of non-Hispanic African American mothers and is lowest for those of Chinese mothers (Centers for Disease Control and Prevention [CDC], 2002). Some common issues in health disparities that have been identified are socioeconomic status, social discrimina-tion based on gender or race and ethnicity, distribution of healthcare resources, and social policies (Macinko & Starfield, 2002). Determinants of health include social conditions, environmental hazards, lifestyle and cultural practices, access to health care, and human biology and genetics. Socioeconomic status underlies three major determinants of health: access to health care, environmental exposure to health-related agents, and health behaviors (Adler & Newman, 2002a, 2002b).

Race and Ethnicity

Ethnicity refers to values, perceptions, feelings, assumptions, and physical char-acteristics associated with ethnic group affiliation. Often, ethnicity refers to nationality—a group sharing a common social and cultural heritage. In contrast, race typically refers to a biologic, genetically transmitted set of distinguishable physical characteristics. In some literature, however, race has often been misused to describe differences in people that have no basis in biology or science. Demographic data are commonly gathered with no differentiation of ethnicity or definitions of race. Both skin color and country of origin have been used to classify race. For example, many natives of India (considered racially Caucasian) have darker skin than do many natives of Africa.

Race and culture have significant relationships to illness states because biologic differences can make certain groups of people vulnerable to specific diseases. For example, genetic predisposition for sickle cell disease affects people of African and Mediterranean descent; predisposition for Tay-Sachs disease affects Ashkenazi Jews. Also, certain diseases that may be attributable to a combination of genetic predisposition and lifestyle, including nutritional patterns, are more prevalent in some groups. One example is the disproportionately high prevalence of diabetes in Native Americans and Hispanics. Some diseases are connected to lifestyle risks, such as substance abuse and human immunodeficiency virus (HIV) infection, which are related to particular social behaviors. An emerging body of information on the differences in response to pharmaceuticals by ethnic and racial groups has led to a new field of pharmacogenomics (Burroughs, Maxey, & Levy, 2002). Cultural subgroups can be attributed to multiple factors that determine values, beliefs, and behaviors. Ethnicity is the most common cultural demarcation, but intraethnic variations may be more pronounced than interethnic variations, especially in a culturally pluralistic society. Other variables that have been proposed as influencing cultural groupings are religion, socioeconomic status, geographic region, age, common beliefs, and professional orientation, such as nursing and medicine.

Factors Related to Culture

Religion is an important factor in determining the values and beliefs of a culture. Religion, an organized system of beliefs, is differentiated from spirituality, which is born out of each individual's personal experience in finding meaning and significance in life. Religious faith and the institutions derived from that faith have a powerful influence over human behavior. All religions have experiential, ritualistic, ideological, intellectual, and consequential dimensions. Religious views have historically served as a unifying force for groups of people with a set of core values and beliefs.

Socioeconomic status refers to one's social status, occupation, education, economic status, or a combination of these. Socioeconomic explanations are often discounted when determining the relationships between ethnicity or race and health status or health. It is necessary to distinguish between cultural identification and the common experience of being poor in our society. By illustration, the experience of being poor in our society is different from that of being Hispanic, and also must be further distinguished from being both poor and Hispanic. The impact of socioeconomic status on both morbidity and mortality measures of specific groups is highly significant and is related to health disparities; lower socioeconomic status groups have higher morbidity and mortality rates for various diseases (Evans et al., 1994).

The local or regional manifestations of the larger culture bring up such distinctions as rural, urban, southern, or midwestern. For example, African Americans living in the southern region of the United States may have different beliefs and behaviors than those in the northern region, based somewhat on their heritage of slavery and exposure to the civil rights movement.

The age of the individuals within a cultural group also has a profound influence on their beliefs and behaviors. Value systems are tied to historically shared events that occur in childhood; therefore, each generation develops a unique value system. For example, there is much in the popular literature about the differences among the baby boomers (people born in the late 1940s and 1950s), generation X (those born in the 1960s and 1970s), and generation Y (people born in the late 1970s and 1980s).

Common beliefs or ideologies may unite a cultural group or subculture, as well as differentiate that group from the larger culture. These value systems may be related to religion (e.g., the Amish), lifestyle (e.g., communal groups), sexual orientation (e.g., gay and lesbian groups), or political ideologies (e.g., feminist separatist groups). Social or professional orientations also often constitute a type of cultural grouping. For example, the biomedical culture of many hospitals constitutes an unfamiliar culture for many laypeople. Healthcare professionals use unique and esoteric language, as well as rituals, roles, expectations, patterns of behavior, and symbolic communication that are often alien to the layperson.

Common Myths and Errors

Errors of stereotyping are common among those who define the world by strict categories of ethnicity or race. It is also problematic to presume that all members of another culture conform to a common pattern without regard to individual characteristics or the variety found within one cultural grouping. For example, some people assume that all African Americans eat soul food or that all Hispanics are Catholic. Failure to recognize that values from a particular cultural group can vary across time and location leads to stereotyping cultures with values that no longer guide the group's thinking or behavior. Stereotyping is less obvious in some cases, such as a nurse manager assigning all Hispanic clients to the Mexican American nurse. Such action does not take into account the differences within the Hispanic group, presumes that all Hispanics are alike, and disregards the individual.

The heterogeneity of ethnic groups is often underestimated, but as mentioned earlier, the variations within ethnic groups may be as great as or greater than those between ethnic groups. For example, the Hispanic culture includes persons of Puerto Rican, Cuban, Spanish, and South and Central American origins. These people are from many different socioeconomic backgrounds and represent the Caucasian, Mongoloid, and Negroid racial groups. Sometimes Asians from different countries and backgrounds are grouped together and treated as generic Asians, an attitude that totally ignores the historical differences among Asians. Kipnis (1998) related a clinical incident that occurred in Hawaii, in which a Korean patient with a serious medical condition refused a treatment that promised a better than 50 percent chance of recovery with minimal risks. Clinical staff were puzzled by his refusal of treatment coupled with his request for life support if he experienced cardiopulmonary arrest. On further investigation, he mentioned that all his physicians were Japanese. In the early 1900s, Japan had ruthlessly tyrannized Korea, much as the Nazis in Germany tyrannized Poland prior to and during World War II. Thus, the Korean gentleman very much wanted to live, but his cultural history caused him to refuse treatment directed by the Japanese physicians.

Ethnocentrism is the tendency, usually unconscious, for individuals to take for granted their own values as the only objective reality and to look at everyone else through the lens of their own cultural norms and customs. Ethnocentric views often result from a lack of knowledge of other cultures and the presumption that one's own behavior is not influenced by culture. Many people of the dominant culture falsely assume that they have no cultural practices and beliefs. This restrictive view of the world perceives people and cultures with different beliefs and behaviors as culturally inferior. An extreme and more conscious form of ethnocentrism is xenophobia, an inherent fear of cultural differences, which often leads people to bolster their security in their own values by demeaning the beliefs and traditions of others. This attitude often takes the form of prejudice or racism.

Cultural imposition is the perception that successful cultural adaptation involves a change to the cultural views of the dominant group, regardless of an individual's cultural heritage. This posits an inherent view that the dominant culture is superior, and its values are imposed upon others.

Often disguised as equal treatment for everyone, cultural blindness ignores cultural differences as if they did not exist. This view overlooks real diversity and the importance of other perspectives. The concept of the "melting pot" assumes that, in the process of **acculturation** and assimilation, everyone takes on significant aspects of the dominant culture such

KEY TERM

Ethnocentrism: A world view based to a great extent on the socialization of individuals within their own culture, to the extent that such individuals believe that all others see the world as they do.

KEY TERM

Acculturation: The process of the adaptation or accommodation of an individual immigrant or immigrant group to a new culture.

that the original culture is largely lost. This assimilation or melting pot view is challenged by concepts of heritage consistency, which is the degree to which one maintains practices and beliefs that reflect one's own heritage.

Development of Cultural Patterns and Behaviors

Anthropologists have studied the similarities between cultures related to the universal experience of being human. Their major focus has been on the variation of ways that humans organize and structure their social world. Some of the factors that contribute to the development of cultural patterns and behavior are geography and migration, gender-specific roles, value orientations and cultural beliefs, and technological development.

Geography and Migration

Social groups evolve through interaction with the climate, as well as in conjunction with the availability of food and resources. The persistence of dietary patterns reflects the types of food available in a particular region. For example, fish constitutes a large portion of the traditional diet of people from Norway and the Philippines, whereas dairy products and meats are dominant in the food patterns of Finland and Germany.

Social organization falls in line with these geographic patterns. For example, the social structure of a fishing village differs from that of a nomadic group that hunts for food, and from that of a settled agrarian culture. Urbanization and industrialization are also important for the way society organizes and social roles develop. Social roles become patterned and often institutionalized into hierarchical structures that reflect social, economic, and political power. These social structures and roles greatly alter people's daily lives and the economics of providing for families.

Climate, environmental conditions, and political and economic factors are very important in migration patterns. Climate change, famine, political upheaval, and overpopulation have all been responsible for migration. For example, a large wave of Irish immigrants came to the United States in the late 1840s following a potato famine that was causing starvation, disease, and death in Ireland. In the 1980s, many immigrants came to the United States to flee political unrest in El Salvador. Many Vietnamese and Southeast Asians sought political refuge and opportunities in the United States following the Vietnam War. A large number of nurses seeking professional and economic opportunities moved to the mainland United States from the Philippines in the 1980s. Even in the 1990s and the early 21st century, a large number of immigrants have steadily come to the United States seeking economic opportunities.

Cultural patterns change through the sharing of ideas, beliefs, and practices that follow trade or migration. Immigrants bring cultural patterns, values, and beliefs with them. Along with their adaptation to the new host culture, they expose the host culture to a different set of cultural beliefs and practices. Both cultures assimilate aspects of the other.

The historical context of immigration is important and varies among groups. Many African Americans arrived involuntarily and endured a lengthy history of slavery. Hispanics may be immigrants seeking economic opportunity, refugees from political upheavals, or descendants of people living in the Southwest before it became a part of the United States. The fact that many Asian immigrants find it necessary to take a job with lower status than they had in their country of origin creates cultural and economic hardships for the family. In many Hispanic families, the father immigrates alone to establish a better economic future for the family. Estranged from the family, he may be at risk for such behavioral health risks as AIDS and alcohol abuse. Health issues may also arise because of low income and low self-esteem.

Acculturation is an important process in the adaptation, assimilation, or accommodation of immigrant groups to a new culture. This is sometimes referred to as hybridization. This is because in the process of adapting to a new culture, immigrants integrate the new culture into their beliefs and lifestyle and yet retain heritage consistency, maintaining pride in and adhering to their parent culture. According to the theory of orthogonal cultural identification, this process does not take place along a single continuum, but rather has numerous dimensions that operate independently from each other (Oetting & Beauvais, 1990–91). Intergenerational gaps frequently develop because the youth in a family become more quickly acculturated to the dominant society, and they may challenge the more traditional values, beliefs, and customs of their parents. This, in turn, may threaten the integrity and lines of respect in the family and roles within the family and society, particularly the role of women. Conflicts that arise from intergenerational gaps can lead to the alienation of young people and families from both the ethnic culture and the general dominant culture.

Gender Roles

All cultures develop socially sanctioned roles for each gender. Over the past century, the social role for women in the United States has undergone many changes. The role of women has expanded from its traditional focus on childbearing and child rearing to include participation in the workplace and marketplace. The feminist movement has championed this expanded role and has heightened consciousness about opportunities consistent with the American values of individualism, equality, and political freedom. Furthermore, the feminist movement has challenged the values and structures developed by elite, masculine power, such as competition, strong focus on objectives and goals, the harnessing and control of nature, principle-based ethics, and productive activities. Feminists have promoted cultural practices and organizations that espouse more feminine values such as teamwork, focus on social process, working in harmony with nature, relationship-based ethics, and social connections. As people from other cultures move into the United States, these differing values and expanded roles for women may challenge the traditional family roles. In some cases where women's roles take a more traditional position, a woman may need to get her husband's or father's permission prior to receiving medical care for herself or her children.

Women have played significant roles in the healing arts as well. Historically and cross-culturally, women have discovered and preserved information about healing herbs and plants. In the Middle Ages, women were often persecuted for their knowledge of plants and other healing arts, which were deemed mysterious and suspicious. As medicine became more scientific and moved into a professional and scientific status, women were disengaged from the official healing roles (Achterberg, 1990). Women were associated with nature, and men with developing technology to tame and control nature. Women's roles in the healing arts reflected this dichotomy. With the establishment of medical professions, women's roles even in midwifery—a traditional role for women—were reduced, and physicians took over the practice and moved it into hospitals. Women who worked in medical professions were often in non-physician roles or positions of lower power and social status, such as nurses, social workers, and physical therapists.

Basic Value Orientations and Beliefs

All cultures hold certain value orientations that are central to their cultural patterns of behavior. These values can be both implicit and explicit. They influence an individual's perception of others, direct that individual's responses to others, and reflect his or her identity. These values are the basis for understanding oneself and one's social relationships, political and economic structures, and direct and motivated behavior. These values are generally quite stable and do not change quickly. In a classic work on cultural orientations, Kluckhohn (1976) identified three categories by which cultures address universal concerns of human nature. Relationship to other persons is expressed in individual, familial, or communal orientations (Kluckhohn, 1976).

In western culture and in particular the United States, these value orientations are reflected in a strong emphasis on individualism, mastery over nature, future-focused time orientation, and an action orientation to being. This can be seen in health care when the provider sees the individual who is the patient and often ignores the impact on the family. Our mastery over nature is illustrated in our efforts to understand and cure disease and control health issues. Future orientation is reflected in our goal orientation and an emphasis on the effect our actions may have on the future. Both healthcare providers and patients expect some type of action or treatment from the clinical encounter. This reflects the shared value of an action-oriented culture. The healthcare system both influences and is influenced by the general cultural orientations. Cultural conflicts may occur when we fail to recognize that our patients hold differing value orientations.

Worldviews and cosmologies essential to Western Judeo-Christian-Islam beliefs differ from those of other world religions. Three dominant cosmology assumptions foundational to Western Judeo-Christian-Islam beliefs are monotheism, transcendence, and dualism (Engebretson, 1996). Monotheism, the belief in one god or creator who is separate from humans, contrasts with the beliefs common in many agrarian societies, whose members believe in polytheism (i.e., multiple gods with different attributes) or pantheism (i.e., the locus of the sacred in all living things). The Western view of transcendence, or relating to God as separate from humans and knowing God through prayer, supplication, and rituals, can be contrasted with the Eastern view of immanence, or finding God by looking inward and doing other spiritual exercises to discover the sacred. Finally, Western dualism, separation of material from non-material aspects of being, is in contrast to monism, or the essential unity found in both the pantheistic and Eastern belief systems. Many "new age" perspectives are exploring these issues in the context of different cultural beliefs.

CONTEMPORARY PRACTICE HIGHLIGHT 14-1

LEININGER'S (2001) THREE MODES OF INTERVENTION

Leininger (2001) identified three modes of intervention involving clinical decision making that focus on cultural practices:

1. *Cultural preservation and maintenance* refers to professional actions that retain relevant care values to support aspects of the client's culture that positively influence his or her health care.

2. *Cultural accommodation and negotiation* refers to professional actions to bridge the gap between the client's culture and biomedicine for beneficial health outcomes, by recognizing the cultural relevance of a practice and integrating it into the treatment plan, even though the cultural practice has no scientific basis.

3. *Cultural repatterning and restructuring* refers to professional actions that assist the client in making changes in, but not discarding, practices that may be harmful to his or her well-being.

You are caring for a Japanese woman with Stage II breast cancer who was admitted for a partial mastectomy. During the admission assessment, she shares with you that she knows she has cancer because she had a termination (abortion) of a pregnancy and she did not disclose this to her spouse. She also reports she is uncertain if she will take chemotherapy as recommended. She is considering performing tai chi daily instead of taking chemotherapy. Using Leininger's three modes of interventions, how would you focus your care for this client?

Technology and Culture

In contemporary Western culture, as well as in much of the world, technology is widely expanding. The development of technology impacts values, religion, politics, and the arts and sciences. Medical technology in particular has progressed in its development of intricate instruments that allow for more complex procedures, such as computer-based imaging, microsurgery, gene mapping, targeted therapies, and pharmacogenomics. The development of these technologies poses new ethical and cultural questions related to the human and social impact this technology may have. Often the use of these technologies challenges existing cultural values. Once the technology is available for use, it often becomes the fuel for ethical debates related to such issues as allocation of resources, fetal tissue transplantation and right to life, and genetic testing and right to privacy.

Technology has also held a powerful influence on culture through its use in communication, which affects not only how information is conveyed, but also what type of knowledge is valued (Postman, 1993). Traditionally, knowledge was passed on by oral means in stories, parables, and poetry. Essential knowledge (i.e., cultural wisdom associated with oral tradition) was preserved through memory, often aided by rhythm and rhyme. Many cultures today have their roots in oral traditions.

With the advent of written communication, the world became a different culture based on the type of knowledge that was conveyed and developed. Printed materials recorded information with detail, precision, and accuracy in a way that oral speech could not. The ability to read this information also facilitated discussions and formation of complex thoughts. Thus, scientific and factual information gained value, giving rise to the development of modern scholarship.

Today's electronic culture, dependent on telephones, radio, television, and computers to communicate information, has an enormous impact on the beliefs, values, and behaviors of contemporary society. In relation to health care, patients have access to a plethora of health-related information from multiple sources. This has presented new challenges for healthcare providers to help patients interpret information and make appropriate choices.

In the late 20th and early 21st centuries, people in the developed and industrialized world have been exposed to a number of different cultures, as a result of both immigration and electronic technology. Electronic media, allowing for fast and more universal dispersal of information, has promoted intercultural communication throughout the world as never before. Such communication has led to unprecedented exposure to different cultures, with results ranging from attempts to integrate diverse ideas to overt conflict and violence. Scientific and technologic advances, as well as global, political, social, and economic

SIDEBAR 14-1

Nurses must evaluate how healthcare goals are achieved when they deliver culturally competent care. How would you evaluate culturally competent care?

changes, have challenged existing cultural systems and increased the velocity of cultural change. Some cultural critics have predicted a major cultural change in the United States. Anderson (1995) describes a shift in contemporary culture as evidenced by the emphasis on the environment, religion and spirituality, and postmodern multiculturalism.

Ethnic Groups in North America

Culturally diverse groups in the United States have grown to substantial proportions of the population. In their practice, nurses are likely to encounter representatives of different cultures. General descriptions about these various ethnic groups may provide helpful orientations to the group. It is important to remember that there is much diversity within ethnicities and that in the processes of globalization and exposure to other cultures, these cultural beliefs are dynamic. Therefore, it is extremely important to avoid stereotyping. Reading about and engaging in discussions and activities with members of these cultural groups can help to avoid stereotypical interpretations of these groups and aid in developing cultural competency.

Native Americans

The indigenous peoples of the Americas number 2.5 million and live across the United States, Alaska, and the Aleutian Islands (U.S. Census Bureau, 2000). Only 5.6 percent of Native Americans are age 65 or older, compared to 14 percent of European Americans, indicating a shorter life expectancy. They cluster in tribal groups, with the largest concentrations located in the Pacific and Western mountain regions of the United States. There is considerable variation among the tribes regarding language, beliefs, customs, health practices, and rituals. Tribes or clans constitute a social unit in which members may or may not be blood relatives, and both family and clan are powerful sources of the Native American's identity and support. Largely because of the respect for the wisdom accrued with aging, elders are typically the community leaders. Value orientations center on harmony with nature, a present-time orientation, and an integration of rituals and religion into everyday life.

Many Native Americans still adhere to folk healing practices, seeking out local healers before going to a healthcare clinic. Folk healing practices may fall into the shamanic category or often be understood in a supranormal paradigm. Common health problems include diabetes, obesity, infectious disease, alcohol abuse, and diseases associated with poverty. Years of racism, dehumanization, and oppression have left a legacy in which many Native Americans may mistrust Caucasian healthcare providers.

European Americans

The largest ethnic group in North America is made up of the European Americans. According to the Census Bureau (2000), they constitute the dominant culture and comprise approximately 75 percent of the population of the United States. The largest emigrations from various regions in Europe occurred in the late 1700s, all through the 1800s, and into the first half of the 20th century. Many immigrants to the United States carried the European ideas of the Age of Reason, dominance over nature, and the belief in progress and technologic advancement. Their quest for freedom enhanced an abiding value of individualism. They were generally action-oriented, future-directed, and focused on progress and productivity. Families are an important social unit among European Americans, but the value of individualism is pervasive. Although this group is diverse, the values are usually consistent with dominant values of the culture. Therefore, members of this group may not be as aware of the role that culture plays in their lives as the members of other cultural groups.

African Americans

The 2000 U.S. Census estimated the number of African Americans in the United States to be 35 million, or 12 percent of the population. This is anticipated to increase to 61 million by 2050. One third of this population was under the age of 18 in 2000. This group is very heterogeneous and varies in economic status, religion, education, and regional background. Many African Americans are descendants of slaves who were brought to the United States; others are recent immigrants from Africa and the Caribbean islands. Within the social structure of slavery, families were dispersed and individuals were not allowed to read. Thus, a tradition of strong matriarchal family units with a rich oral tradition developed. Social organization centers on the family, kinship bonds, and the church or mosque. Some of the health disparities among African Americans may be related to the disproportional rate of poverty. Many African Americans have absorbed much of the dominant culture, but some adhere to ancestral beliefs of illness as disharmony with nature and supranormal healing rituals or folk healing. The history of slavery and the Tuskegee atrocities have made some African Americans mistrustful of receiving professional health care or participating in clinical research studies.

Asian Americans

Constituting 4 percent of the total U.S. population, or approximately 10.5 million people in 2000, Asian Americans are expected to represent 8 percent of the population by 2050 (U.S. Census Bureau, 2000). Approximately two thirds reside in the western part of the United States. This group is composed of immigrants and refugees from the Pacific Rim countries, such as China, Japan, Korea, Thailand, Laos, Vietnam, Cambodia, and the Philippines. People from Pakistan and India are often included in this group as well. There is wide diversity in language, customs, and beliefs in this group. Traditional Asian families tend to be patriarchal, revere their elders, and value achievement and honor. Certain infectious diseases, such as tuberculosis and hepatitis, are common among Asian Americans, depending on the country from which they emigrated. Stress-related diseases and suicides are high, as many do not seek mental health care because of an associated stigma and a threat to honor. Asians' traditional health practices often are oriented around the balance paradigm in which health is equated with balance and the unimpeded flow of energy, or "chi." Traditional healing includes the use of herbal preparations, and many families practice traditional dermabrasion procedures such as coining, pinching, or rubbing.

Pacific Islanders and Native Hawaiians

The Native Hawaiian and other Pacific Islander (NHPI) population constituted 874,000 individuals, or 0.3 percent of the U.S. population in the 2000 Census. Native Hawaiians are the largest subgroup (58 percent), although the majority of this group reported one or more other races as well. Nearly three fourths of this population lives in the west, with over half living in California and Hawaii. There were several differences in the way that questions about race were asked in the 2000 Census, and this was the first census in which NHPIs were separated statistically from the Asian group. Thus, comparisons are difficult, but the number of NHPIs increased approximately 9 percent since 1990 for individuals selecting a single race category.

There is great diversity in beliefs and customs. As an aggregate group, NHPIs are socioeconomically disadvantaged and underserved in terms of access to social and health services. Pacific Islanders have high rates of health-related risk behaviors, such as smoking, heavy alcohol consumption, and high fat and caloric intake, which leads to obesity. Native Hawaiians have the second highest overall cancer incidence rate and the highest age-adjusted cancer mortality rate compared to other ethnic groups, with high rates of breast, colorectal, prostate, lung, and stomach cancers (Intercultural Cancer Council, n.d.). Native Hawaiians are 2.5 times more likely to have diabetes than white residents of Hawaii of similar age. Other common illnesses among NHPIs are asthma, hypertension, and hypercholesterolemia (Hawaii Department of Health, n.d.).

Hispanic or Latino Americans

The Hispanic population in the United States includes more than 35 million people, or 12.5 percent of the U.S. population, and is predicted to reach 24 percent by 2050 (U.S. Census Bureau, 2000). The majority of these immigrants come from Mexico, with others from Puerto Rico, Cuba, and Central and South America. This is the fastest growing group in the United States. Although the Spanish language is a common factor, there is much diversity in dialects and cultural practices. This group comprises indigenous peoples of the Americas, Spanish and other European settlers, and some African-Caribbean groups. Predominant religions are Catholicism and Pentecostalism. The family and extended family are

PERSONAL VALUE SYSTEM

You are working in a prenatal clinic and caring for a Korean 17-year-old who is 8 months pregnant. The family is very ashamed of their daughter and the teen's father is insisting that the girl give the baby up for adoption. The pregnant teen says she wants to keep the baby but she does not want to offend her father. Respond to the points below as you consider a culturally competent plan of care for this teen and her family.

1. Clarify your own values, beliefs, and ideas related to your heritage.
2. Identify barriers in your own life to acceptance of cultural diversity.
3. Explore activities that will increase your awareness and acceptance of this teen and her family.
4. What resources or referrals would be helpful for this teen and her family regarding the tension over the pregnancy and decisions regarding the infant?

important, and the family unit is traditionally patriarchal. Many believe that illness may be punishment for sins or the result of witchcraft or *brujería*, meaning the "evil eye." Traditional health beliefs regarding hot and cold remedies for various maladies reflect humeral balance beliefs. Healing also incorporates many spiritual elements, such as worship of saints and use of talismans.

Impact of Culture on Health Care

Concepts of health and healing are rooted in culture. The concept of disease generally refers to the diagnostic label or categorization of a disorder that medicine treats, whereas the concept of illness incorporates the personal, social, and cultural aspects of the experience. Cultural practices influence an individual's behavior to promote, maintain, and restore health, and how, when, and whom they seek for help or treatment. Cultural beliefs, values, and practices are also extremely important in birth and death.

Nursing Applications

Six phenomena evidenced in all cultural groups have variations that are relevant to the provision of culturally competent nursing assessment and care, and are outlined below (Giger & Davidhizar, 1999). It is useful to understand these variations in clinical practice.

Communication: There are cultural variations in the expression of feelings, use of touch, body contact, gestures, and verbal and nonverbal communication. Language shapes experiences and influences perceptions and actions. Warmth and humor are two communication factors that are interpreted differently through various cultures. For example, many Asians may not overtly express their emotions, because they may fear "losing face."

Personal space: Spatial behavior refers to the comfort level related to personal space, meaning the area that surrounds a person's body. Spatial territoriality is the need to have and to control personal space. Cultures vary in the level of proximity to others that is acceptable. For example, Western culture has three zones: the intimate zone (less than 18 in.), the personal zone (18 in. to 3 ft), and the social zone (3–6 ft). Cultural background also influences aspects of objects within space, such as orderliness, cleanliness, and structural boundaries of furniture and architecture.

Time: Cultures vary in their orientation toward time, both social time and clock time. Social time refers to patterns and orientations related to the ordering of social life, whereas clock time represents an objective, ordered approach of viewing time in a linear fashion that infers causality. Some cultures orient around cyclic approaches that attach time to natural events that repeat, such as seasons or migration patterns. For example, in mystical thought, magic or ritual may negate the temporal order of causality and reverse a bad event. All cultures contain the three orientations of future, present, and past, with one being dominant.

Social organization: Families, religious groups, kinship groups, workplace groups, and special interest groups are social organizations. Families vary in structure, dynamics, roles, and organizational patterns. Kinship structures and the relative geographic location of family members have cultural implications. Religious organizations provide not only social connections, but also a context in which to understand one's relationship to the world, the cosmos, and the meaning in life.

Environmental control: Different cultures have different perceptions of the ability of an individual to control nature, the environment, and personal relationships. The locus of control may be external (i.e., an event contingent on luck or fate), internal (i.e., an event contingent on one's own behavior or characteristic), or outside (i.e., an event in harmony with nature, as in some Asian cultures). In folk medicine, for example, events are perceived as natural and unnatural. Natural events have to do with the world as God intended and the laws of nature. Unnatural events upset the harmony of nature and are outside the world of nature.

Biologic variations: In a pluralistic culture, it is important to determine those factors that are strictly biologic (i.e., genetic) and those that are ethnic adaptations related to living in a particular environment (e.g., availability of certain types of food) or in certain social conditions (e.g., socioeconomic status, lifestyle). Biologic factors to be considered are body size and structure, including variations in teeth, facial features, and skin color; variations in metabolism and

SIDEBAR 14–2

When a client requires the services of a translator, the nurse should follow these communication strategies (Degazon, 1996):

- Orient the translator to the topics to be covered, the client's situation, and the degree of accuracy required.
- Observe the client for nonverbal communication that does not match the message intended and request clarification.
- Slow down the communication process.
- Encourage the translator to let the nurse know when something is difficult to translate so that it may be reworded.
- Limit the use of medical jargon, slang, and metaphors in order to reduce the chance for error.
- Consider the impact of differences in gender, educational level, and socioeconomic status between the client and translator. This is particularly important when topics of a sensitive or personal nature are to be discussed.

enzyme production that result in drug reactions, interactions, and sensitivities; and susceptibility to disease (e.g., hypertension, diabetes, sickle cell anemia). Nutritional issues, including food preferences, habits, and patterns, as well as deficiencies such as lactose intolerance, all have medical implications.

This information is a helpful guide to thinking about cultural variations. However, no amount of factual knowledge about cultural variation can replace careful individual assessment, because there is more intracultural variation than intercultural variation.

Summary

Members of minority or varied cultural groups may distrust and fear the Western biomedical healthcare system, of which nurses are a part. The element of trust is essential to the formation of a therapeutic nurse–client relationship, so clients need to know that nurses are receptive and nonjudgmental regarding their differences. Nurses must approach cultural competency through knowledge of self and knowledge of other cultures. To develop the ability to interact with clients appropriately, nurses should clarify their personal values, recognize the healthcare system as a culture, learn about the specific culture of each client, interact and intervene in a culturally consistent manner, and elicit feedback regularly from the client and family. Skills such as listening, explaining, acknowledging, recommending, and negotiating facilitate a nonjudgmental perspective toward the client's cultural beliefs. Nurses and clients should validate their perceptions and discuss similarities and differences in their perceptions to formulate health-related goals and interventions.

Cultural competency is a dynamic, challenging process faced by all healthcare providers, regardless of their cultural background or association. The process of sharing information in a straightforward manner demystifies other cultures and, for example, makes it possible for the nurse and client to find common ground and understand the context of differences.

The nurse and patient conjointly develop an approach to address the identified concerns and the agreed upon goals. The patient discusses his or her assets, barriers, and priorities and the nurse shares expert knowledge and may suggest other resources. Knowledge and acceptance of the client's right to alternative solutions and modalities could be incorporated into the plan of care. Nurses should make every effort to acquire appropriate foods, people, artifacts, and so on, as well as to secure space and time for such practices. Nursing practice should always convey a message of respect to the client and their cultural practices and belief system.

Key Terms

- **Acculturation:** The process of the adaptation or accommodation of an individual immigrant or immigrant group to a new culture.
- **Culturally competent health care:** The ability to deliver health care with knowledge of and sensitivity to cultural factors that influence the health and illness behaviors of an individual client, family, or community.
- **Culture:** The values, beliefs, customs, social structures, and patterns of human activity and the symbolic structures that provide meaning and significance to human behavior.
- **Ethnicity:** Designation of a population subgroup sharing a common social and cultural heritage.
- **Ethnocentrism:** A world view based to a great extent on the socialization of individuals within their own culture, to the extent that such individuals believe that all others see the world as they do.
- **Race:** A social classification that denotes a biologic or genetically transmitted set of distinguishable physical characteristics.
- **Stereotyping:** Consigning cultural attributes to a group of people based on assumptions, opinions, or attitudes.

Reflective Practice Questions

1. How do you feel when caring for clients whose cultural backgrounds differ from your own?
2. What are your values and beliefs regarding health and illness in relation to care of the elderly?
3. What are your biases and attitudes toward immigrant clients with various cultural backgrounds?
4. How can you determine whether you are offering culturally competent care in a holistic manner?

References

Achterberg, J. (1990). *Woman as healer.* Boston: Shambhala.

Adler, N. E., & Newman, K. (2002a). Inequality in education, income, and occupation exacerbates the gaps between the health "haves" and "have-nots." *Health Affairs, 21*(2), 60–76.

Adler, N. E., & Newman, K. (2002b). Socioeconomic disparities in health: Pathways and policies. *Health Affairs, 34*(1), 6–14.

Anderson, W. T. (1995). *The truth about the truth.* New York: G. P. Putnam's Sons.

Beach, M. C., Price, E. G., Gary, T. L., Gozu, A., Robinson, K. A., Palacio, A., et al. (2005). Cultural competence: A systematic review of health care provider educational interventions. *Medical Care, 43*(4), 356–373.

Bernal, H. (1996). Delivering culturally competent care. In P. D. Barry (Ed.), *Psychosocial nursing: Care of physically ill patients and their families* (pp. 78–99). Philadelphia: J.B. Lippincott.

Betancourt, J. R. (2006). Cultural competency: Providing quality care to diverse populations. *The Consultant Pharmacist, 21*(12), 988–995.

Bhui, K., Warfa, N., Edonya, P., McKenzie, K., & Bhugra, D. (2007). Cultural competence in mental health care: A review of model evaluations. *BMC Health Services Research, 7,* 15.

Burroughs, V. J., Maxey, R. W., & Levy, R. A. (2002). Racial and ethnic differences in response to medicines: Towards individualized pharmaceutical treatment. *Journal of the National Medical Association, 94*(10), S1–S25.

Campinha-Bacote, J. (2001). A model and instrument for addressing cultural competence in health care. *Journal of Nursing Education, 38,* 204–207.

Centers for Disease Control and Prevention. (2002). *Health status and determinants of health in the United States 2002.* Retrieved June 21, 2008, from http://www.cdc.gov/nchs

Collins, F. (2003). Genomics and health disparities: Disparities in health in America: Working toward social justice. Houston, TX: Summer Workshop at University of Texas MD Anderson Cancer Center.

Cross, T., Bazron, B., Dennis, K., & Isaacs, M. (1989). *Toward a culturally competent system of care* (Vol. 1). Washington, DC: CASSP Technical Assistance Center, Georgetown University Child Development Center.

Degazon, C. (1996). Cultural diversity and community health nursing practice. In M. Stanhope & J. Lancaster (Eds.), *Community health nursing: Promoting health of aggregates, families and individuals* (4th ed., pp. 117–134). St. Louis: Mosby.

Douglas, M. (2002). Developing frameworks for providing culturally competent health care. *Journal of Transcultural Nursing, 13,* 177.

Dreher, M., & MacNaughton, N. (2002). Cultural competence in nursing: Foundation or fallacy? *Nursing Outlook, 50*(5), 181–186.

Engebretson, J. (1996). Considerations in diagnosing in the spiritual domain. *Nursing Diagnosis, 7,* 100–107.

Giger, J., & Davidhizar, R. (1999). *Transcultural nursing: Assessment and intervention* (3rd ed.). St. Louis: Mosby.

Gregg, G. R., & Saha, S. (2006). Losing culture on the way to competence: The use and misuse of culture in medical education. *Academic Medicine, 41,* 1–8.

Hawaii Department of Health. (n.d.). Retrieved June 25, 2008, from http://hawaii.gov/health/statistics/hhs/hhs_05/index.html

Intercultural Cancer Council. (n.d.). *Native Hawaiian and Pacific Islanders and cancer.* Retrieved August 1, 2008, from http://iccnetwork.org/cancerfacts/ICC-CFS5.pdf

Kipnis, K. (1998, November 18). *Quality care and the wounds of diversity.* Paper presented at the meeting of the American Society for Bioethics and Humanities, Houston, TX.

Kluckhohn, F. R. (1976). Dominant and variant value orientations. In P. J. Brink (Ed.), *Transcultural nursing: A book of readings* (pp. 63–81). Englewood Cliffs, NJ: Prentice Hall.

Leininger, M. (2001). *Culture care diversity and universality: A theory of nursing.* Sudbury, MA: Jones and Bartlett.

Lipson, J. G., & Desantis, L. A. (2007). Current approaches to integrating elements of cultural competence in nursing education. *Journal of Transcultural Nursing, 18*(1), 10S–20S.

Macinko, J. A., & Starfield, B. (2002). Annotated bibliography on equity in health, 1980–2001. *International Journal for Equity in Health, 1.* Retrieved June 25, 2008, from http://www.equityhealthj.com/content/1/1/1/

Marmor, T., Barer, M., & Evans, R. (Eds.). (1994). *Why are some people healthy and others not?: The determinants of health of populations.* New York: Aldine de Gruyter.

Oetting, E. R., & Beauvais, F. (1990–1991). Orthogonal cultural identification theory: The cultural identification of minority adolescents. *International Journal of Addiction, 5A, 6A,* 655–685.

Office of Minority Health, U.S. Department of Health and Human Services. (2002). *A practical guide for implementing the recommended national standards for culturally and linguistically appropriate services in health care 2002.* Retrieved August 1, 2008, from http://www.omhrc.gov/assets/pdf/checked/CLAS_a2z.pdf

Postman, N. (1993). *Technopoly.* New York: Vintage.

Purnell, L., & Paulanka, B. (1998). *Transcultural health care: A culturally competent approach.* Philadelphia: F. A. Davis.

Sackett, D. L., Straus, S. E., Richardson, W. S., Rosenberg, S., & Haynes, R. B. (2000). *Evidence-based medicine: How to practice and teach EBM* (2nd ed.). Edinburgh: Churchill Livingstone.

Spector, R. E. (2000). *Cultural diversity in health and illness* (5th ed.). Upper Saddle River, NJ: Prentice Hall.

Underwood, S. M. (2000). Minorities, women, and clinical cancer research: The charge, promise and challenge. *Annals of Epidemiology, 10*(S8), S3–S12.

U.S. Census Bureau. (2000). *2000 census brief.* Retrieved June 21, 2008, from http://www.census.gov/population/www/cen2000/briefs.html

Ethical Decision Making and Moral Choices

Kevin Valadares

LEARNING OUTCOMES

After reading this chapter you will be able to:

- Discuss the definition of personhood and how this definition forms the groundwork of ethical decisions.
- Analyze the purpose of the American Nurses Association *Code of Ethics for Nurses*.
- Understand how the patient bill of rights and advanced directives guide professional codes of ethics.
- Discuss the use of narrative ethics within nursing practice.
- Compare and contrast organizational ethics and patient-centered ethics.
- State the role, function, and underlying goals of ethics committees.
- Explain various ethical conflicts and clarify your values on these issues.

The Importance of Personhood

Nurses and other healthcare professionals function as advocates for patients concerning ethical decisions related to their care. As such, the relationships that form between clients and nurses are bonded in a spirit of trust and respect for the individual as a person. The purpose of this chapter is to provide a

Code of ethics: Standards and behaviors of a profession or organization directed towards its constituents.

Organizational ethics: Ethical analyses and actions taken by healthcare organizations.

Personhood: Various religious and philosophical traditions have definitions of what constitutes a person. These need to be recognized and applied as necessary within a defined healthcare context.

discourse on the ethical context of health care, including the **code of ethics**, patient bill of rights, advance directives, ethical principles and directives in nursing, and **organizational ethics**. The next section of the chapter considers the importance of **personhood** specifically for nurses and within the context of their professional roles as caregivers.

From a religious perspective, the biblical view of the person is based on the teaching that every person is created in the image and likeness of God (known as *Imago Dei*), and therefore, is invaluable and worthy of respect as a member of the human family (Catechism of the Catholic Church, 1994). This definition claims that personhood begins at fertilization and ends with one's death (Ashley and O'Rourke, 1997).

This differs from both the Jewish and Islamic traditions, where life is said to be fully present only from birth. Additionally, the question of personhood does not arise until quickening, thought to be at 40 days (Biale, 1989).

A philosophically geared definition of personhood is found in the teachings of Immanuel Kant (Gaylin, 1984). According to Kant, a person is a rational agent who alone is capable of exercising freedom as autonomy (Kant, 1990). Autonomy, seen as self-determination, confers dignity to persons. From Kant's view, persons have absolute value and must never be used as a means to an end.

Concurring with Kant's definition of personhood, ethicist H. Tristram Engelhardt Jr. distinguishes between persons and humans (Engelhardt, 1996). He applies a strict definition of personhood only to those moral agents who are rational and self-conscious. To speak of a person as a moral agent is to say that the person has a certain degree of autonomy and self-determination, and is empowered to act according to his or her conscience, in freedom, and with knowledge. Therefore infants and young children, the comatose, and the profoundly retarded do not qualify for personhood. However, because they are able to engage in a minimum of social interaction, he does classify them as humans, which he defines in a strictly biological sense.

Although other derivations of personhood exist, primarily from a sectarian framework, the nurse's moral stance on issues is shaped by his or her definition of personhood. This definition forms the groundwork for all ethical decisions made within a healthcare context. Personhood is expressed in numerous ways when nurses function within their professional roles. For example, respecting personhood falls into line with the notion that people should treat others in the same manner in which they desire to be treated. Put in another way, persons should be treated as ends in themselves, not as a means to an end.

Respecting all persons means the nurse should honor human dignity in every encounter with a client and with other healthcare professionals. For the bedside nurse, this can be expressed in small gestures such as closing curtains for privacy, as well as in more obvious gestures such as advocating for patient choice through the establishment of conditions necessary to provide informed consent.

However, the market-driven nature of our current healthcare system strains the concept of personhood in community through the acceptance of economically driven levels of service. The essence of markets is to produce both winners and losers and move products and services to optimal efficiency. This infers an industry-based commodification of persons, supposing exploitation and dehumanization, particularly of those who are marginalized. Moreover, as William-Jones (1999) infers, market-driven initiatives in health care may suggest a materialistic conception of the person, which views the person as a material possession.

The relationship that nurses have with clients is created and sustained in a spirit of trust and respect. For the nurse caregiver, this implies that the client must first be understood as a person through whatever framework of personhood the nurse adheres to.

Codes of Ethics

Most professions, whether its members function within healthcare settings or not, have a code of ethics that illustrates its standards and behaviors as a form of instructions for its members and expectations for its constituents. A code of ethics makes explicit the primary values and obligations of a given profession with a goal of assisting professionals with an ethical component involving conflicts among responsibilities (American Nurses Association, 2003; see Appendix A). Practically, it is the written element for the profession that provides a self-declaration of how the profession and its members should function in their duties and responsibilities and what the public should expect as a competent level of service.

The American Nurses Association's (ANA's) *Code of Ethics for Nurses* was first created as the "Nightingale Pledge" in 1893 and was derived from the physician-driven Hippocratic Oath. From its inception, the *Code of Ethics* has always been concerned with four principles: 1) doing no harm to clients, 2) benefiting others, 3) loyalty to clients, and 4) being truthful in all facets of practice. The current version of the *Code of Ethics* (revised in 2001) focuses on social justice applications for care and emphasizes the connection between the autonomy of the client and the nurse (Hook & White, 2003). (See Figure 15-1.)

The Code of Ethics for Nurses serves the following purposes:
- It is a succinct statement of the ethical obligations and duties of every individual who enters the nursing profession.
- It is the profession's non-negotiable ethical standard.
- It is an expression of nursing's own commitment to its society.

Figure 15-1 The Code of Ethics for Nurses Summarized. *Source:* Hook, K. G., & White, G. B. (2003). *Code of ethics for nurses with interpretive standards. An independent study module.* Retrieved January 7, 2008, from http://nursingworld.org/mods/mod580/cecdeabs.htm.

Patient Bill of Rights

While nurses practice under the guidance of a professional code of ethics, a simultaneous set of directives exists with an understanding and respect for the rights and responsibilities of patients and their families. Nurses and their organizations must practice a healthcare ethic that respects the role of patients in decision making concerning treatment and care choices. This often poses challenges, especially in acute care environments, where patients readily rely on clinicians to offer advice and make healthcare decisions on their behalf.

The rights afforded to patients are couched in the framework of the ethical principle of respect for autonomy. This stands in opposition to the paternalistic culture of health care that was primarily seen through the physician–patient relationship (dominated by physicians) that existed up until the 1980s. Paternalism was ineffective in taking into consideration the viewpoint of patients with respect to their own care. Patients, families, nurses, and other healthcare workers were encouraged to defer to physician decisions and subsequently worked around errors in judgment without directly addressing concerns. A hierarchy related to decision making in health care was the expected norm.

A consumer-driven society necessitates a more fluid patient bill of rights whereby patient autonomy is supported, even if nurses are presented with seemingly contrary clinical decisions by patients. It is then the responsibility of the nurse to work within his or her scope of practice to remain an advocate for patients with their best clinical interests in mind. The ethical principle of autonomy that supports a patient bill of rights also forms the grounding for all practices associated with advance directives.

Advance Directives

The 1990 Patient Self-Determination Act officially requires healthcare institutions to provide patients with information about their state's advance directives policies and procedures at the time of hospital admission or before various outpatient procedures. Almost all states provide for living wills, and most states have at least two statutes, one establishing a living will–type directive, the other establishing a proxy or durable power of attorney for health care. Despite the fact that the general public indicates they desire an advance directive, most Americans lack them (Emmanuel, 1991).

As previously noted with the patient bill of rights, advance directives are rooted in the ethical principle of autonomy. Supporting one's right to choose a course of action that determines both the quantity and quality of life forms the basis for the premise of an advance directive. Professionally, it serves as a guide for clinicians to respect and honor the autonomous decision of the patient when they are in a position to not be able to express their wishes.

The role of nurses concerning the spirit and application of advance directives is one of advocacy. It is this advocacy that fortifies the patient/family–nurse relationship through participating in discussions with surrogates, providing guidance and referral to other resources as necessary, and identifying and addressing problems in the end-of-life decision-making process.

Case Study: Patient Advocacy

Betty Caprice is a 38-year-old woman who lives at home with her parents. When she was admitted to the county hospital for treatment of a bladder infection, she weighed 85 pounds and appeared emaciated. She also had large pressure ulcers on the backs of her legs, indicating that she had not been moved in her bed for quite a long time.

Upon admission, it was discovered that Betty has breast cancer that had spread to her lungs, lymphatic system, and skeletal system. She is in obvious pain. Her mother filled out the admission papers for Betty, listing herself as her daughter's surrogate decision maker. Both she and Betty have been informed of the diagnosis of cancer. When she is alone (away from her mother), Betty says she is in terrible pain and pleads for pain medication. When pain medication is brought to the room, however, Betty's mother tells her daughter, "You're not in pain. You don't need pain medication, do you?" Betty inevitably replies that she does not want the pain medication. This scenario repeats itself two or three times a day. Even if pain medications are started, they are always stopped when Betty, in the presence of her mother, asks for them to be discontinued. Betty and her parents claim that their religion requires them to attempt to heal naturally and that pain medications would interfere with the natural healing process. A psychiatric consult was initiated and the psychiatrist has found that Betty is lucid, oriented as to time and place, understands that she has untreatable cancer, and can discuss her diagnosis, prognosis, and alternatives for care.

What are the ethical issues at this point in Betty's care and what is your role as a nurse caregiver?

> **KEY TERM**
>
> **Principalism:** A methodology used to resolve dilemmas arising in health care by appealing to abstract moral principles.

> **KEY TERM**
>
> **Narrative ethics:** The use of stories to emphasize the importance of context, contingency, and circumstances in recognizing, evaluating, and resolving moral problems applied to health care.

Ethical Principles and Narrative Ethics Within Nursing Practice

The **principalist** approach to applying ethics to health care has dominated the field since the 1970s. This era began with the Belmont Report, which underscored the relevance of key ethical principles, namely: 1) respect for autonomy, 2) proliferation of justice, and 3) exercising beneficence with patients (National Institutes of Health, 1974).

Narrative ethics' primary argument suggests that a core set of principles (commonly referred to as the Georgetown mantra—autonomy, beneficence, justice, non-maleficence) used for ethical decision making are universal in scope and facilitate the objectivity of each clinical dilemma. Beauchamp and Childress (2001) indicate that these principles are drawn from a common morality that binds all persons independent of their situations. The four principles have been grounded in traditional ethical theories and medical codes (including all versions of the *Code of Ethics for Nurses*) throughout history (Beauchamp & Childress).

Another recent approach to understanding ethical dilemmas in health care comes from narratives. Supporters argue that the first-person narrative, or personal story, is a rich medium for qualitative data about the unique lives of individual people. The narrative is not only an important form of communication, but also a means of making life, and specifically the moral life, make sense through the examples put forth by interpreting personal stories.

McCarthy (2003) reiterates that every moral situation is unique and unrepeatable and its meaning cannot be fully captured by appealing to universal principles. For narrativists, understanding an individual's life as an ongoing story and then attempting to interpret it within their healthcare experience enriches and deepens the insight into the moral questions associated with life (McCarthy). With this in mind, when ethically challenging situations arise, it is not the medical chart, the proposed treatment, or even the ethical principles that should govern the care process. Rather, it is the patient's life story that should set the healthcare decisions in motion. In the narrativist mode, clinicians become engaged in a storytelling enterprise as opposed to a treatment process (Brody, 2003).

> **SIDEBAR 15–1**
>
> In narrative ethics, it is the patient's life story that should set the healthcare decisions in motion.

Nurses are most aptly able to assume the narrativist role. The demand for empathetic caregivers does not require one to "step into another's shoes" in order to understand their pain (Brody, 2003). It also does not presuppose that it is ever possible to understand fully another's clinical experience. In some respects, patient will always be an "other" to nurses.

Instead, empathic caregiving demands that nurses bear witness to vulnerability and stand as a "co-human presence" with the patient during their time of care. According to Brody (2003), health professionals cannot offer patients the reassurance that they know and understand them, only the acknowledgement that their story has been listened to and heard. From this viewpoint, no healthcare professional is untouched by a patient's pain and vulnerability (McCarthy, 2003).

Organizational Ethics and the Work Environment for Nurses

Organizational ethics is best described as the integration of values into decision making, policies, and behavior throughout the multidisciplinary environment of a healthcare organization (Magill, 2001). At its heart, it affects the lives of persons, whether it is clients seeking care, employees functioning within the organization, or visitors to the institution.

Organizational ethics is related both to *clinical practices*, in that institutional business decisions affect patient care, and to *business practices*, in that many institutional issues are primarily business concerns involving financial matters, strategic planning, and compliance with regulatory processes. There are three primary concerns related to the impact of organizational ethics on nurses. The first considers nurses as both professionals and employees in a healthcare setting while the second concerns the balance between patient-centered care and organizational practices. Finally, the role of organizational **ethics committees** continues to be a group that nurses can embrace to assist them in unraveling both clinical and non-clinical issues in a healthcare setting.

> **KEY TERM**
>
> **Ethics committee:** Ideally, a multidisciplinary group of healthcare professionals charged with ethics education, policy formation, and review and consultation within an organizational setting.

> **SIDEBAR 15-2**
>
> Organizational ethics is related to both clinical practices and business practices.

Nurses as Professionals and Employees

According to Brandeis (1914), four overarching elements define a profession and those within the profession:

- The necessary preliminary training is intellectual in character, involving knowledge, and to some extent learning, as distinguished from mere skill.
- It is pursued largely for others and not merely for one's self.
- The amount of financial return is not the accepted measure of success.
- It sets and enforces standards.

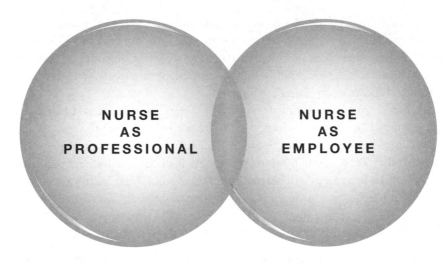

Figure 15–2 Nurses as Professionals and Employees

In applying these elements to nursing as noted in Figure 15-2, it becomes noticeable that some of the ideals have become stretched in directions that challenge the essence of nurses as professionals. For example, in periods where economic labor shortages exist, salaries and financial incentives remain a primary tool of recruitment and retention. Since 2000, the median hospital nursing wage and associated incentives have risen 64 percent to respond to economic shortages and unfilled positions (Simoens, Villeneuve, & Hurst, 2005). Although economic incentives such as bonuses are an effective strategy for recruiting and retaining nurses in the short term, they can stand as an affront to the ideals of nursing, and some indicate that they weaken the healing component of the profession once the glory of the incentive wears off.

Within health care, these elements can be further subdivided into four ethical directives that nurses should integrate into their professional roles (see Figure 15-3).

Confidentiality: Privacy acts such as HIPAA are often associated with confidentiality, and yet the practical reality of implementing a confidential environment poses many challenges. Nurses should respect the persons they are caring for or working with, which sustains the relationship that they possess.

Competence: Credentialing, licensure, and certification attest to basic levels of competence, which are only enhanced by practical experience. This directive is often tested in times of workforce shortages where demand for care exceeds the supply of nurses.

Truthfulness: Disclosing news to patients, families, and co-workers is often challenging. Being truthful in practice again sustains the relationship that exists between patient and clinician.

Relationship-centered: Nurses should recognize the *patient as person*, and this should be the focus of the healthcare relationship.

The notion of nurses as employees, although still retaining the elements of the profession, has undergone a change in the last decade. An adjacent argument that is building momentum when considering nurses as employees concerns the issue of *nurses as customers* within the context of a service industry. The term *customer* is used to embrace a view of the individual that includes more than just a worker performing a necessary job function. A service mentality views the customer as an end-user of an organization's output or service, which includes coworkers who depend on one another to achieve a common good for the organization.

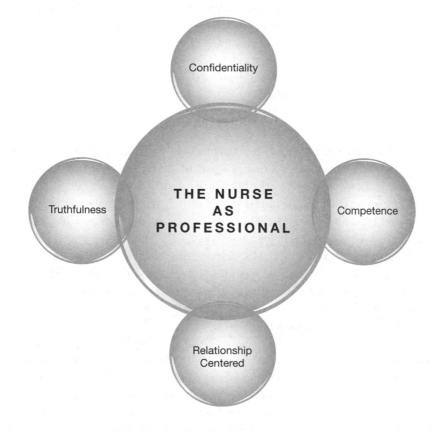

Figure 15–3 The Nurse as Professional

Although customers can encompass healthcare employees, physicians, and the community, it is the client population that is generally recognized as the primary customer. As Spencer and colleagues (2001) conclude, unlike the typical customer, the patient has limited choices and is not always able to exercise choices coherently. Moreover, the vulnerability of a sick patient reduces his or her capacity to affect care delivery, unlike a traditional customer (Spencer).

However, some believe that introducing a customer service mentality into health care is disingenuous to the ethical construct of patient as person and to the clinician as caregiver (Jost, 2007). Retail organizations such as Target stores and hotel chains such as Marriott utilize customer service strategies in part to secure return visits to their business. Within these industries, more satisfied customers often develop a loyalty that translates into repetitive business. Conversely, loyalty within healthcare settings seems at odds with aspects of how nurses practice. Although patients often have a preferred loyalty to physicians and dentists, this does not often translate to nursing. The clinical nurse when functioning as an educator, for example (which is an ongoing role), would often rather not have repeat business because this implies that the goals of previous visits were unattained.

SIDEBAR 15-3

All healthcare organizations are well served by devoting considerable attention to defining who their customers are, particularly if they extend this definition to clinical employees.

Patient-Centered Care vs. Organizational Practices

A second concern within the realm of organizational ethics geared towards nurses stems from an internal conflict that pits patient-centered nursing values against the organization's standard operating procedures. Edmondson (1999) emphasizes how important it is for nurses to feel secure that they have the autonomy to make clinical and ethical decisions concerning the needs of patient care. She refers to this security as psychological safety.

The essence of psychological safety is based on the premise that when employees believe that their suggestions for change will be appreciated, they express themselves freely without fear of embarrassment, rejections, or punishment. They will be able to test assumptions, debate new concepts, and discuss contradictory issues (Chang & Lee, 2001).

As Edmondson (1999) asserts, the key factor ensuring psychological safety lies at each level of the organization's work groups, namely, with first-line supervisors and team leaders. To probe her claim, she conducted a study comparing eight nursing teams from two urban teaching hospitals in order to learn which ones learned and performed better and why. She correlated the medical error rate of the teams in their treatment of patients, anticipating the findings to demonstrate that happier, more stable teams with better leadership would commit fewer medical errors. The data supported a different set of conclusions.

The more positively nurses rated their team's relationships and the levels of coaching and goal-setting they received from their managers, the more errors their team reported. The data reflected the group's new comfort level, which resulted in truthful and accurate reporting of errors. The teams of nurses with the highest reported error rates seemed more comfortable with one another as well as with their managers, who were adept at creating a psychologically safe atmosphere. Teams reporting high error rates were led by managers who showed respect for their subordinates and who valued a collaborative, problem-solving work style. Teams with low reported rates, on the other hand, worked under authoritarian managers and frequently resorted to blaming others for their miscues. She concluded that teams with greater psychological safety not only reported errors and learned more, but also performed more effectively (Edmondson, 1999).

The application of autonomous thought and action to an organizational setting also follows societal influences. Autonomous thought and action are a prevalent Western societal construct whereby the nature of autocratic decision making is questioned. Taylor's (1947) scientific management theories and hierarchical philosophies that governed relationships between management and workers evolved into an empowerment movement emphasizing the contributing ideas of the employee along with reward mechanisms for carrying out ideas to fruition.

Practically, the scope of organizational decision making has become more inclusive. Employee forums and suggestions are part of organizational improvement strategies, and communities are encouraged to express needs that the organization could facilitate. Mission statements include language emphasizing employee uniqueness, all the while attempting to remain focused on core values. The concept of the organization exerting an overbearing position is less apparent as decision making reflects defined stakeholder needs and is reflectively sought through needs assessments.

Conversely, it would be erroneous to suggest that nurse autonomy is the norm in organizational decision making. To a great extent, large-scale decision making is still relegated to those individuals in a position of hierarchical or functional power. However, as the benefits of autonomous decision making concerning patient care have become more clearly aligned with the goal of enhanced clinical outcomes, organizational cultures have adopted similar strategies to improve short- and long-term operations.

Catholic Health Care Organizations has responded to autonomous decision making through its emphasis on the discernment of workers' rights. The 1998 working paper *A Fair and Just Workplace: Principles and Practices for Catholic Health Care* is the result of a candid and constructive dialogue among leaders of Catholic Health Care, the AFL-CIO, and the U.S. Conference of Catholic Bishops (USCCB, 1998). The thesis of the paper speaks to the dignity of work and the rights of workers and identifies new models of relationships between management and labor and between religiously sponsored health ministry and organized labor, all within the spirit of autonomy set in community.

Consider the managerial role that nurses in the emergency department (ED) are often faced with. With EDs governed by the Emergency Medical Treatment and Labor Act (EMTALA), certain non-clinical patient information (e.g., insurance coverage) becomes irrelevant in the decision-making process. In this setting, the nurse is first placed in a position of deciding the priority of patient care in the triage area. Inherently though, just decisions regarding the priority status of patients may come into conflict with an organization's financial mandates.

Another example of the conflict that may exist between the nurse and organization in the realm of patient care concerns individual objections of conscience. The question becomes: Does the autonomous right of the nurse (in exercising his or her beliefs) overrule the practices of the organization or setting?

This has most readily been an issue in both end-of-life and beginning-of-life issues (e.g., dispensing "morning after" pills,) and calls to mind the notion of whether our society would prefer nurses who exercise their personal beliefs concerning a healthcare issue or who simply provide the best care possible while maintaining a neutral stand on an ethical dilemma. It is partly because of these issues that larger healthcare organizations have created separate ethics committees to educate and offer recommendations to clinicians on ethical dilemmas stemming from patient care.

Ethics Committees

An important element that strengthens the ethics within an organization is the creation of an institutional ethics committee. Ethics committees have played clinically relevant roles in organizational settings since the 1960s. Most ethics committees are composed of a variety of clinical and non-clinical employees, although nurses were typically excluded from early participation with committees based on the belief that their role was that of a follower as opposed to a leader (Aulisio, 2004). Thankfully, this imbalance has changed so that today, in most organizations, nurses take leadership roles in all facets of the committee, including functioning as its chairperson.

Ethics committees' functions vary, but usually include three standard components (Aulisio, 2004):

1. General education on the ethical application of patient care. This is geared to all organization employees.
2. Creating policies on ethical questions to serve as a model of practice for the organization.

SIDEBAR 15-4   THE UNDERLYING GOALS OF ETHICS COMMITTEES

- To promote the rights of patients
- To promote shared decision making between patients (or their surrogates if cognitively incapacitated) and their clinicians
- To promote fair policies and procedures that maximize the likelihood of achieving good, patient-centered outcomes
- To enhance the ethical tenor of healthcare professionals and healthcare institutions

3. Offering case consultations, prospectively or retrospectively, on clinical scenarios (usually taken from practice) that are presented to them by fellow clinicians.

Many argue that the consultative practice model is the primary purpose and most effective asset of an ethics committee. Ethics consultations reject the notion of a sole clinician (usually a physician) overseeing all the non-clinical issues that arise in client care. Moreover, it emphasizes that a collaborative philosophy among nurses, social workers, business professionals, and physicians is best suited to offer recommendations to the medical team, the family, and the client.

The infusion of technological interventions into the fabric of client care has certainly complicated the ethical dilemmas that clinicians face. Nurses in particular, who arguably form the strongest bond with client and family, become immersed in the intersection between life-saving techniques that benefit care and those that burden the process.

One of the more recent consultative practices that ethics committees have been engaged with concern operational conflicts that are primarily restricted to employee issues. Some organizations have created sub-committees that solely deal with ethical issues from an organizational perspective, as opposed to those involving direct patient care. A relevant case study illustrates this practice.

Case Study: Management Conflict

Sarah was promoted to nurse manager because of her excellence in delivering patient care and recognized leadership ability. She was an excellent charge nurse, outstanding patient advocate, preceptor, and chair of the practice council. Sarah had been a medical-surgical nurse for over 10 years and enjoyed the variety of clients under her care. She only recently completed her BSN degree and earned her certification in medical-surgical nursing.

When Sarah was in her position for less than 3 months, her immediate supervisor moved to another state because of his wife's promotion. This individual had been a mentor, confidant, and recognized leader in the organization. Sarah tried to make the best of the situation and follow the direction of her new supervisor.

However, from the beginning, she found this individual to be very focused on the negative. As an optimistic person, Sarah found this approach counter to her basic instincts about people. Every time she tried to discuss this difference in approach, her director would say she was naive and that the staff was taking advantage of her good nature. The director used several of her recent project failures to justify her position. However, Sarah understood that these disappointments had been the result of staff illness and institutional reorganization. The crisis point was reached when the director told her to terminate employment of the two staff members who were the most vocal in their dissatisfaction with the reorganization. These individuals were excellent clinical nurses, well-liked by staff, and each had over 12 years of seniority in the organization. Sarah knew that the director did not like these nurses for reasons unrelated to reorganization and their performance. After her third sleepless night, Sarah came to you to ask for guidance.

What advice do you give?

Summary

Nurses and other healthcare professionals have a long history of establishing a relationship of trust and advocacy with clients. Nurses play a key role in functioning as a trusted source of information for clients concerning ethical decisions related to their care. The ANA *Code of Ethics* (2003) provides an ethical infrastructure that outlines the duties and responsibilities for nurses and expectations for the public. Further guidance regarding professional codes of ethics is provided in the patient bill of rights and the 1990 Patient Self-Determination Act. The practicing nurse must continually evaluate the congruency with organizational ethics and the patient-centered ethical directives in the work environment. The ethics committees of organizations are composed of multidisciplinary team members who serve as a model of ethical practice for the organization. The current age of technology and societal changes present complicated ethical dilemmas for nurses, clients and their families, and healthcare organizations. The nurse's moral stance on issues is shaped by his or her definition of personhood, and this definition forms the groundwork for all ethical decisions made within the healthcare context.

Web Links

American Society for Bioethics and Humanities: http://www.asbh.org
ANA Code of Ethics: http://nursingworld.org/mods/mod580/cecde03.htm
ANA Center for Ethics and Human Rights: http://www.nursingworld.org/ethics/
The Belmont Report: Ethical Principles and Guidelines for the Protection of Human Subjects of Research: http://ohsr.od.nih.gov/guidelines/belmont.html
Nursing Ethics Network: http://jmrileyrn.tripod.com/nen/nen.html

Key Terms

■ **Code of ethics:** Standards and behaviors of a profession or organization directed towards its constituents.

■ **Ethics committee:** Ideally, a multidisciplinary group of healthcare professionals charged with ethics education, policy formation, and review and consultation within an organizational setting.

■ **Narrative ethics:** The use of stories to emphasize the importance of context, contingency, and circumstances in recognizing, evaluating, and resolving moral problems applied to health care.

■ **Organizational ethics:** Ethical analyses and actions taken by healthcare organizations.

■ **Personhood:** Various religious and philosophical traditions have definitions of what constitutes a person. These need to be recognized and applied as necessary within a defined healthcare context.

■ **Principalism:** A methodology used to resolve dilemmas arising in health care by appealing to abstract moral principles.

Reflective Practice Questions

1. What is your definition of personhood and where does it come from? Is it based on a religious tradition? How does your definition influence the manner in which you view ethical issues in health care?

2. John has a rare liver disease in which death is imminent unless a liver transplant is done within the next month. The cost of this procedure is $250,000. A matching donor is available. John's insurance will cover up to $200,000. Should your hospital be responsible for the remainder of the expense? Why or why not?

3. Are there instances when nurses should forgo respecting patient confidentiality?

4. If your beliefs as a nurse conflict with that of the organization in which you are working, what is your best course of action?

References

American Nurses Association. (2003). *ANA code of ethics for nurses with interpretive statements*. Retrieved January 7, 2008, from http://nursingworld.org/mods/mod580/cecde03.htm

Ashley, B. M. & O'Rourke, K. D. (1997). Health care ethics: A theological analysis (4th ed.). Washington, D.C.: Georgetown University Press.

Aulisio, M. (2004). Ethics committees and ethics consultation. In S. Post (Ed.), *Encyclopedia of bioethics* (3rd ed., pp. 841–847). New York: Thompson-Gale.

Beauchamp, T. L., & Childress, J. F. (2001). *Principles of biomedical ethics* (4th ed.) New York: Oxford University Press.

Biale, R. (1989). Abortion in Jewish law. *Tikkun 4*(4), 26–28.

Brandeis, L. D. (1914). *Business: A profession.* Boston: Small Maynard.

Brody, H. (2003). *Stories of sickness* (2nd ed.). New York: Oxford University Press.

Catechism of the Catholic Church (English translation). (1994). United States Catholic Conference, Inc., Libreria Editrice Vaticanna. The scriptural reference originates from Genesis 1:26–31.

Chang, H. T., & Lee, A. T. (2001). The relationship between psychological safety, organization context support and team learning behavior in Taiwan. *Global Journal of Engineering Education, 5*(2), 186.

Edmondson, A. C. (1999). Psychological safety and learning behavior in work teams. *Administrative Science Quarterly, 44*(4), 350–383.

Emmanuel, L. L. (1991). Advance directives for medical care; reply. *New England Journal of Medicine, 325,* 1256.

Engelhardt, H. T. (1996). *The foundations of bioethics* (2nd ed.). New York: Oxford University Press.

Gaylin, W. (1984). In defense of the dignity of being human. *Hastings Center Report, 14*(4), 18.

Hook, K. G., & White, G. B. (2003). *Code of ethics for nurses with interpretive statements. An independent study model.* Retrieved January 7, 2008, from http://nursingworld.org/mods/mod580/cecdeabs.htm

Jost, T. (2007). *Health care at risk: A critique of the consumer-driven movement.* Durham, NC: Duke University Press.

Kant, I. (1990). *Foundations of the metaphysics of morals* (2nd ed., L. W. Beck, trans.). New York: MacMillan.

Magill, G. (2001). Organizational ethics in Catholic health care: Honoring stewardship and the work environment. *Christian Bioethics, 7*(1), 67–93.

McCarthy, J. (2003). Principalism or narrative ethics: Must we choose between them? *Journal of Medical Ethics, 29*(2), 65–71.

National Institutes of Health. (1974). *The Belmont report: Ethical principles and guidelines for the protection of human subjects of research.* Retrieved January 7, 2008, from http://ohsr.od.nih.gov/guidelines/belmont.html

Simoens, S., Villeneuve, M., & Hurst, J. (2005). *Tackling nurse shortages in OECD countries. OECD Health Working Papers 19.* Retrieved January 8, 2008, from http://www.oecd.org/dataoecd/11/10/34571365.pdf

Spencer, E. M., Mills, A. E., Rorty, M. V., & Werhane, P. H. (2000). *Organization ethics in health care.* New York: Oxford University Press.

Taylor, F. W. (1947). *Principles of scientific management.* New York: Norton.

U.S. Conference of Catholic Bishops. (1998). *A fair and just workplace: Principles and practices for Catholic health care.* Retrieved January 8, 2008, from http://www.usccb.org/sdwp/national/workplace.shtml

William-Jones, B. (1999). Concepts of personhood and the commodification of the body. *Health Law Review, 7*(3), 11–13.

Legal Issues in Nursing

Eileen K. Fry-Bowers

LEARNING OUTCOMES

After reading this chapter you will be able to:

- Identify and understand the four basic sources of law that govern nursing practice.
- Describe the role and function of a state's nurse practice act.
- Define "standard of care."
- List and describe the four elements of a professional malpractice claim that the plaintiff must prove in order to prevail.
- Discuss the nurse's role and responsibility in obtaining informed consent.
- Consider steps a registered nurse can take to protect him- or herself from disciplinary action and civil or criminal liability.

INTRODUCTION

Consider that:

- There are more than 2.9 million registered nurses in the United States, making nursing the nation's largest healthcare profession (Health Resources and Services Administration [HRSA], 2007).

- More than half (52 percent) of all health profession students in the United States are nursing students (HRSA, 1992).
- Nurses make up the largest single component of any hospital staff, are the primary providers of hospital patient care, and deliver most of the nation's long-term care (HRSA, 2007).

In 1980, 66 percent of working registered nurses were employed by hospitals. By 2004, only 56.2 percent of nurses were employed in the hospital setting as job opportunities for nurses expanded to include settings such as private practices, health maintenance organizations, public health agencies, primary care clinics, home health care, nursing homes, outpatient surgery centers, nursing-school-operated nursing centers, insurance and managed care companies, schools, mental health agencies, hospices, the military, industry, nursing education, and healthcare research (HRSA, 2007). In addition, although nurses work collaboratively with medicine and other fields, the public increasingly recognizes that nurses possess specific skills and may function independent of, not auxiliary to, medicine. Nursing roles range from direct patient care and case management to establishing nursing practice standards, developing quality assurance procedures, and directing complex nursing care systems (American Association of Colleges of Nursing [AACN], 2007). With more than four times as many RNs in the United States as physicians, nurses are relied upon for delivery of an array of healthcare services, including primary and preventive care by advanced nurse practitioners, and services by certified nurse midwives and nurse anesthetists (AACN, 2007).

KEY TERM

Professional malpractice: A type of negligence that results when a professional person fails to perform his or her professional duties in a reasonable manner.

Given the evolution in scope and practice of nursing, the public expects nurses to enter practice prepared to become expert clinicians and, accordingly, holds nurses to increasingly higher levels of accountability with concomitant risk of liability. In fact, more and more nurses are being named as defendants in **professional malpractice** lawsuits (Croke, 2003). Therefore, nurses entering into practice in *any* environment must become aware of the structure and function of their state board of nursing and how their state nursing practice act governs and limits their professional behaviors. Nurses also must appreciate the risks associated with professional malpractice and understand how laws and regulations, such as federal or state privacy law, affect their daily practice. Moreover, nurses must appreciate the basic rights of patients and their personal professional role in safeguarding those rights. A thorough foundation in these matters equips nurses to understand connections among federal and state laws, institutional policies and procedures, professional codes of ethics, and their own professional practice (Priest et al., 2007).

Sources of Law

Understanding the interconnection among federal and state laws, institutional policies, codes of ethics, and professional nursing practice begins with identifying the sources of law that govern behavior and that are enforced by the courts. *Law* may be defined as "any system of regulations to govern the conduct of the people of a community, society or nation, in response to the need for regularity, consistency and justice based upon collective human experience" (Hill & Hill, 2007). There are four basic sources of law, all of which govern the practice of nursing: 1) federal and state constitutional law, 2) laws passed by the federal and state legislatures, 3) the common law, and 4) administrative law.

The primary source of all law in the United States is the federal Constitution. This document sets forth the powers and limitations of the federal government. The first 10 amendments to the Constitution, known as the Bill of Rights, address such familiar concepts as freedom of speech, press, and religion; the right to assembly; and the right not to be deprived of life, liberty, or property without due process of law, among others (U.S. Info, 2007). Each state has a constitution as well, which is also a source of important rights. However, if there is any conflict between the provisions of a state constitution and the federal Constitution, federal law takes precedence; this is known as federal supremacy.

Although the Constitution does not explicitly provide for a right to privacy, the U.S. Supreme Court has nevertheless held that the Constitution does indeed offer such protection. This has profound implications for the practice of nursing because a right to privacy guides courts in deciding significant healthcare issues such as a patient's right to reproductive autonomy, right to refuse medical treatment, and right to die. (See, e.g., *Skinner v. Oklahoma*, 316 U.S. 535 (1942); *Griswold v. Connecticut*, 381 U.S. 479 (1965); *Eisenstadt v. Baird*, 405 U.S. 438 (1972); *Roe v. Wade*, 410 U.S. 113 (1973); *Planned Parenthood v. Casey*, 505 U.S. 833 (1992); *Gonzales v. Carhart*, 127 S. Ct. 1610 (2007); *Jacobson v. Massachusetts*, 197 U.S. 11 (1905); *Washington v. Harper*, 494 U.S. 210 (1990); *Cruzan v. Director, Missouri Department of Mental Health*, 497 U.S. 261 (1990); *Washington v. Glucksberg*, 521 U.S. 702 (1997); and *Vacco v. Quill*, 521 U.S. 793 (1997)).

Congress and state legislatures serve as a second source of law. Laws written by state legislatures, generally effective once signed by the state's governor, and laws drafted by Congress, effective once signed by the President, are called statutes. For example, each state's nurse practice act (NPA) is a state statute that specifically defines the legal limits for the practice of nursing within that state. In addition, all states enact **civil laws** that dictate socially reasonable conduct, as well as criminal laws that protect the public from harmful behaviors.

> **KEY TERM**
>
> **Civil law:** Law that dictates behavior between parties.

The **common law**, or case law, develops as a result of judicial decisions made in settling disputes or "cases," and serves as a third and very important source of law. Courts allow for the resolution of disputes by providing a forum in which the facts can be heard and the law applied. Generally, the facts of the case are presented at a trial court and are heard by a judge or jury. In making her decision regarding any issue, a judge interprets relevant statutes, considers legislative intent, and compares the facts to similar prior cases. The decision rendered may then serve as "precedent," and establishes principles or rules that courts may adopt when deciding subsequent cases with similar issues or facts (Liang, 2002).

Lastly, after the state legislature or Congress passes a law, implementation of the law passes to administrative agencies under the state or federal executive branch, which then make rules and regulations for enforcement of the statute. As a result, these agencies have significant power akin to that of legislative bodies. In addition, they possess what are known as "quasi-judicial" powers. When there is a conflict regarding application and interpretation of the regulations, the administrative agency has the power to adjudicate the dispute through an administrative law process, with final determination subject to review by a court. Courts generally give great deference to decisions made through this process. Examples of administrative boards affecting nursing practice include the Centers for Medicare and Medicaid Services in the Department of Health and Human Services, the National Labor Relations Board in the Department of Labor, the Federal Trade Commission, the Food and Drug Administration, and state boards of health, insurance, medicine, and, of course, nursing (Killion, 2006).

In addition to understanding the sources of law, nurses must distinguish between types of law, and in particular, civil law and criminal law. Civil law can be viewed as the law that dictates behavior between private parties. These disputes take the form of a "lawsuit" and a party's legal claim against another is called a "cause of action." Tort law and contract law are examples of civil law. **Tort law** establishes rules for socially reasonable conduct and imposes liability on a party, a "wrong-doer," for unreasonable conduct. In general, the conduct may be defined as intentional or unintentional, and different rules of law apply to each. Contract law governs agreements and the enforcement of those agreements between parties. Generally, civil cases are determined by the "preponderance of the evidence," meaning that it is more likely than not that one party is responsible for the harm to the other party (Liang, 2002).

Conversely, criminal law serves to protect the public from harm by punishing persons who break societal rules. Rather than a dispute between parties, the state brings the criminal action against the accused. The state must prove its case "beyond a reasonable doubt," a more rigorous standard than that required in a civil action. Thus, a person may be acquitted of criminal wrong-doing but may be held civilly liable.

Judicial System

As noted in the previous section, courts throughout the United States make law through an adjudicative process whereby the court reviews the facts of the case presented through evidence, applies appropriate statutes and precedent, and then renders a decision. Just as each state and territory of the United States has its own set of laws, each possesses a separate court system. In addition, the United States has a court system for deciding disputes involving federal law (known as federal question jurisdiction) or conflicts between citizens of different states meeting a minimum monetary standard (known as diversity jurisdiction).

The courts in each of these systems are organized in a tiered structure. At the lowest level is the trial court, which is generally responsible for discovering the facts and applying the law to a wide variety of subject matters. If a party is dissatisfied with the outcome of a case at the trial level, they may usually appeal the decision, as a matter of right, to the next level of court. This appellate court generally reviews only issues of law related to the dispute and does not revisit the facts of a matter. The appellate court may agree with the trial court's determination and affirm the decision of the lower court or it may disagree and reverse that decision; or the court may agree with some parts of the decision and disagree with other parts, and thus, affirm in part and reverse in part the trial court's decision (Liang, 2002).

If disappointed at the appellate level, the litigant may appeal to the next level of court, generally, the state's highest court (names vary) or the U.S. Supreme Court, depending upon in which system, federal or state, the dispute was adjudicated. Courts at this highest level generally have discretion whether or not to hear an appeal. If the court refuses to hear an appeal, the decision of the appellate court stands.

As noted, Congress and state legislatures delegate significant rule making and enforcement authority to administrative agencies. These agencies may also resolve disputes much in the same manner as a state or federal court, but these hearings do not require a jury, and the evidentiary rules may differ. If a party is dissatisfied with the outcome of this administrative hearing, he or she must first exhaust the administrative agency's appellate process before any appeal may be made to a court of law (Killion, 2006). In general, courts require that the appellant show that the decision of the agency was "arbitrary and capricious" for reversal of an administrative ruling.

Legal Issues in Nursing Practice

Safe and appropriate nursing practice requires more than knowledge of patient conditions and treatment modalities. Nurses must also clearly appreciate the legal issues which govern and impact their practice.

KEY TERM

Licensure: The process by which a state or governmental agency grants permission to an individual to engage in a given profession for compensation.

KEY TERM

Nurse practice act: A state statute that defines the legal limits for the practice of nursing within that state and explicitly identifies the requirements for licensure.

Regulation of Nursing Practice

As previously noted, each state, as well as the District of Columbia and all territories of the United States, have statutes that specifically define the legal limits for the practice of nursing within that state, and explicitly identify requirements for **licensure**; this statute is generally referred to as a **nurse practice act (NPA)** (Fedora, 2001). These legal requirements protect the health, safety, and welfare of the general public and the integrity of the nursing profession. North Carolina passed the first nurse practice act, called the Nurse Registration Act, in 1903. Prior to that time, nursing practice was unregulated and any person could define and practice nursing in any manner (Smith, 2007). Although this first act failed to define nursing practice, minimal educational requirements for nursing, or required registration with the state, many states recognized the need to establish rules and regulations to govern the practice of nursing and followed suit. New York, in 1938, was the first state to pass an act mandating educational prerequisites and licensure by examination for anyone seeking to practice nursing in that state and identify themselves as an "RN" or "registered nurse" (Brent, 2000). In 1955, the American Nurses Association (ANA) published a definition of nursing that served as the foundation for the many state practice acts to follow (since updated and refined on several occasions to reflect changes and expansion of nursing roles). By the 1970s, all states mandated licensure of professional (RN) and practical nursing (LVN or LPN) (Smith, 2007). See Box 16-1 for examples of title protection for registered nurses.

Most state NPAs explicitly provide for the creation of some form of a state board of nursing. The structure and composition of these administrative agencies differ from state to state, as do their roles and authority. In general, however, state boards of nursing are charged with the primary duty of protecting the public's health by ensuring the safe practice of nursing through oversight activities (National Council of State Boards of Nursing [NCSBN], 2007c). Box 16-2 lists the general duties of state boards of nursing.

For the majority of nursing students and practicing nurses, the most direct role that the state board of nursing plays is that of granting licensure, or granting someone the right to use the title registered nurse (RN). Licensure is the process

BOX 16-1   EXAMPLES OF STATUTORY TITLE PROTECTION FOR REGISTERED NURSES

Arizona

A Person who holds a valid and current license to practice professional nursing in this state may use the title "registered nurse" "graduate nurse" or "professional nurse" and the abbreviation "R.N." No other person shall assume or claim any such titles or use such abbreviation or any other words, letters, signs or figures to indicate that the person using it is a registered, graduate or professional nurse. Nurse Practice Act: Section 32-1636

California

It is unlawful for any person or persons not licensed or certified as provided in this chapter to use the title "registered nurse," the letters "R.N.," or the words "graduate nurse," "trained nurse," or "nurse anesthetist."

It is unlawful for any person or persons not licensed or certified as provided in this chapter to impersonate a professional nurse or pretend to be licensed to practice professional nursing as provided in this chapter. Nurse Practice Act: section 2796

Florida

No person shall practice or advertise as, or assume the title of, registered nurse, licensed practical nurse, or advanced registered nurse practitioner or use the abbreviation "R.N.," "L.P.N.," or "A.R.N.P." or take any other action that would lead the public to believe that person was certified as such or is performing nursing services pursuant to the exception set forth in Section 464.022(8), unless that person is licensed or certified to practice as such. Nurse Practice Act: Section 464.015 (6)
Each of the following acts constitutes a misdemeanor of the first degree, punishable as provided in Section 775.082 or Section 775.083:

   (a) Using the name of title "Registered Nurse," "Licensed Practical Nurse," "Advanced Registered Nurse Practitioner," or any other name or title which implies that a person was licensed or certified as same unless such person is duly licensed or certified. Section 464.016 (2)(a)

Kansas

Title and abbreviation. Any person who holds a license to practice as a registered professional nurse in this state shall have the right to use the title, "registered nurse," and the abbreviation, "R.N." No other person shall assume the title or use the abbreviation or any other words, letters, signs or figures to indicate that the person is a registered professional nurse. Nurse Practice Act Section: 65-1115(c)(4)(d)

(continues on page 368)

BOX 16-1 EXAMPLES OF STATUTORY TITLE PROTECTION FOR REGISTERED NURSES
(continued from page 367)

New York
1. Anyone not authorized to use a professional title regulated by this title, and who uses such professional title, shall be guilty of a class A misdemeanor.
2. Anyone who knowingly aids or abets three or more persons not authorized to use a professional title regulated by this title, to use such professional title, or knowingly employs three or more persons not authorized to use a professional title regulated by this title, who use such professional title in the course of such employment, shall be guilty of a class E felony. Nurse Practice Act: Section 6513

Washington
(1) It is unlawful for a person to practice or to offer to practice as a registered nurse in this state unless that person has been licensed under this chapter. A person who holds a license or practice as a registered nurse in this state may use the titles "registered nurse" and "nurse" and the abbreviation "R.N." No other person may assume those titles or use the abbreviation or any other words, letters, signs or figures to indicate that the person using them is a registered nurse.
(2) The same as above for Advanced Registered Nurse Practitioner.
(3) The same as above for an Licensed Practical Nurse.
Nurse Practice Act: Section 18.79.030 and 1994 sps c 9 s 403

Source: Nurse Practice Act: Section 18.79.030 and 1994 sps c 9 s 403.

BOX 16-2 GENERAL DUTIES OF STATE BOARDS OF NURSING

Acting under the direction of the state Nurse Practice Act, the State Boards of Nursing generally:
1) Establish rules and regulations that define and govern safe nursing practice;
2) Set standard nursing educational requirements including developing curriculum requirements, establishing faculty-student ratios for clinical practice, and approving nursing educational programs;
3) Define the criteria and process for licensure, and issuing licenses to practice practical, professional, and advanced nursing;
4) Monitor licensee's compliance with state requirements and taking disciplinary action against licensees who demonstrate unsafe nursing practice or who fail to comply with licensure requirements (Nursing, 2007).

Source: Nursing, 2007.

by which a state governmental agency grants permission to an individual to engage in a given profession for compensation. More specifically, the agency has determined that "the applicant has attained the essential degree of competency necessary to perform a unique scope of practice" (NCSBN, para 1, 2007b).

Licensure should be distinguished from certification, which is another type of credential that affords title protection and recognition of accomplishment, but does not include a legal scope of practice. Generally, certification defines the process by which a non-governmental agency, such as a nursing specialty organization, recognizes individuals who have met certain requirements. Often, state boards of nursing use such professional certification as a requirement toward granting authority for advanced practice registered nurses. (A complete discussion of licensure requirements for advanced practice nursing can be found in Chapter 4.) Readers are encouraged to review the requirements of each state where they wish to practice as well as consult with professional practice specialty associations for specific information.

All state boards of nursing as well as those of the District of Columbia and U.S. territories require candidates for nursing licensure to pass an examination "that measures the competencies needed to perform safely and effectively as a newly licensed, entry level registered nurse" (NCSBN, para 1, 2007d).

Although most nursing students equate passing "boards" with licensure, it is important to note that the licensure examinations are used to *assist* the boards in making licensure decisions and that passage of the licensure examination alone *does not* guarantee licensure. Registered nursing candidates must also comply with all other state, district, or territorial requirements such as meeting background requirements or satisfactory completion of additional educational requirements, which may vary state to state.

In recent years the National Council of State Boards of Nursing (NCSBN), the agency that administers the National Council Licensure Examination for Registered Nurses (NCLEX-RN), has developed a new regulatory model for the profession of nursing, a **mutual recognition of licensure model**, known colloquially as the **nursing interstate compact**, which allows a nurse to maintain one **license** in his or her state of residency and to practice and be "recognized" in another state, physically and/or electronically, subject to each state's practice law and regulation. Any state wishing to enter into a mutual recognition agreement with another state or states must enact legislation or regulations for implementation of the compact (NCSBN, 2007a). A complete listing of the states that have entered into the nurse licensure compact

KEY TERM

Mutual recognition model: Allows a nurse to maintain a license in his or her state of residency and to practice and be recognized in another state, subject to each state's practice law and regulation; also known as the nursing interstate compact.

KEY TERM

Nursing interstate compact: See *mutual recognition model.*

KEY TERM

License: Permission to engage in an activity; a professional license allows the holder to engage in a specific activity for compensation.

TABLE 16-1 STATES PARTICIPATING IN NURSING LICENSE COMPACTS, AS OF JULY 2008

State	Date of Implementation
Arizona	July 1, 2002
Arkansas	July 1, 2000
Colorado	October 1, 2007
Delaware	July 1, 2000
Idaho	July 1, 2001
Iowa	July 1, 2000
Kentucky	June 1, 2007
Maine	July 1, 2001
Maryland	July 1, 1999
Mississippi	July 1, 2001
Nebraska	January 1, 2001
New Hampshire	January 1, 2006
New Mexico	January 1, 2004
North Carolina	July 1, 2000
North Dakota	January 1, 2004
Rhode Island	July 1, 2008
South Carolina	February 1, 2006
South Dakota	January 1, 2001
Tennessee	July 1, 2003
Texas	January 1, 2000
Utah	January 1, 2000
Virginia	January 1, 2005
Wisconsin	January 1, 2000

Source: National Council of State Boards of Nursing (2008). *Nurse Licensure Compact Administrators: Participating States in the NLC,* available at https://www.ncsbn.org/158. htm.

can be found in Table 16-1 and at https://www.ncsbn.org/158.htm. Contemporary Practice Highlight 16-1 further addresses the significance of the nursing mutual recognition model.

No one person has the unequivocal right to practice nursing. A nursing license is a privilege granted by a board of nursing based upon the licensee meeting all requirements for initial licensure or renewal of licensure. A board of nursing can refuse initial licensure and can reprimand, suspend, or revoke the license of a nurse under specific circumstances as outlined in the state's NPA (Wright, 2005). Once granted, however, a nursing license represents a property interest that is

---

CONTEMPORARY PRACTICE HIGHLIGHT 16-1

THE NURSING MUTUAL RECOGNITION MODEL

The evolution of professional nursing roles to include practice in e-health or tele-health, interstate transport nursing, and mobile or travel nursing necessitates a practical strategy to meet the licensure challenges presented by the increased mobility of the nursing population. One such strategy has been the implementation of a mutual recognition of licensure model.

The nursing mutual recognition model, known as the nursing interstate compact, allows a nurse to be licensed in his or her state of residence, but practice in a remote state that is another member of the compact. It is the responsibility of the nurse to know and abide by the remote state's nurse practice act and other applicable regulations, even if different from those of their home state.

An example of a common mutual recognition model is the driver's license. A person with a California driver's license may drive in Arizona but must abide by the driving laws of Arizona. Failure to do so can result in a traffic citation.

Between 1998 and 2007, 22 states enacted compact legislation, with enactment by an additional state (Rhode Island) set for July 2008. Although nearly half of the nation's states participate in the compact model, there has been little formal evaluation of it, and significant controversy regarding the model exists. Consider the following arguments:

Arguments in Favor of Nursing Compact Legislation

- The practice of e-health, tele-health, and transport nursing requires the practice of nursing across state borders. Obtaining and maintaining multiple licenses is burdensome. Compact legislation allows nurses to avoid duplicative licensure and associated fees.
- Because licensure is dependent on the nurse's state of residence, the compact facilitates physical mobility, enabling nurses to take on travel or short-term assignments in other party states.
- The compact prevents implementation of state nurse licensure solutions that fail to provide reciprocal agreements or allow for appropriate information sharing and authority to discipline.
- Information sharing between states regarding nurses will be promoted through the compact. Compact states can have licensure and disciplinary information on each nurse, resulting in great protection of the public.

continues

CONTEMPORARY PRACTICE HIGHLIGHT 16-1 (continued)

Arguments Against Nursing Compact Legislation

- The state of practice, rather than the state of residence, should dictate licensure because the purpose of licensure is to grant a nurse authority to practice while protecting the health and safety of the citizens of the state in which the license is held.
- There are many inconsistencies between states in relation to licensure requirements, such as mandatory continuing education, criminal background checks, and disciplinary causes of action, which leads to the possibility of nurses working side by side with different requirements for practice.
- Many states rely upon licensure fees to sustain their operating expenses. Eliminating the need for duplicative licensure results in decreased revenue to the affected state.
- Because nurses working in a remote state are not required to register with that state's board of nursing, the state will not be aware of the actual number of nurses working in the state, making workforce predictions difficult.
- Variability in state nurse practice acts, as well as civil and criminal laws, raises significant questions related to liability, enforcement, and administrative processes. Nurses may find themselves subject to multiple investigations and disciplinary proceedings arising from the same incident, or be required to defend themselves against civil litigation in a state other than their home state.

Contact your state board of nursing for its specific position statement on this issue. Contact information can be found through the National Council of State Boards of Nursing, https://www.ncsbn.org/515.htm.

Sources: American Nurses Association. (2007). Association of Women's Health, Obstetric and Neonatal Nurses. (1999). *AWHONN position statements: Interstate compact for mutual recognition of state licensure.* Retrieved October 15, 2007, from http://www.awhonn.org/awhonn/content.do?name=05_HealthPolicyLegislation/5H_PositionStatements.htm; National Council of State Boards of Nursing. (2002). *NCSBN position statement: Alternative regulatory licensure models.* Retrieved October 15, 2007, from https://www.ncsbn.org/1270.htm.

protected by the U.S. Constitution and the laws and regulations of each state. Every state has a specific process for filing, investigating, and resolving complaints against nurses but, in each circumstance, a nurse has certain rights. In any licensure matter, a nurse has a right to be informed of the allegations made against them, the right to present their account of the incident, and a right to fair and just legal procedures when action is taken against their license. Moreover, the nurse has the right to consult with legal counsel (and should exercise this right). In addition, the nurse must remember that any disciplinary hearing is, by its very nature, adversarial, because of the board's authority to take action; thus, anything said to a board investigator can be used against the nurse during subsequent proceedings (another important reason to consult legal counsel). The right to use the initials *RN* comes at significant personal cost, effort, and sacrifice, and with great responsibility. Each nurse is accountable for his or her own nursing practice. Box 16-3 provides additional information on how to protect your RN license.

Standards of Nursing Care

In general, much like any statute, the specific content of a state's nurse practice act is broad. These acts and other related regulations are designed to provide general guidelines for nurses, but they do not dictate how to perform procedures associated with the daily functions of a nurse. So then, what does govern how a nurse performs these activities? How do nurses know that their practice is appropriate? In general, nurses must consult the policies and procedures of their employer, which will usually explicitly detail the extent of their nursing responsibilities. An institution may restrict practice to a narrower responsibility than that authorized by the state's nurse practice act, but it may never allow a nurse to take on greater responsibilities. But how does an institution determine its policies and procedures, and will those standards legally protect a nurse in the event of a disciplinary hearing or a lawsuit?

A **standard of care** can be defined as that "degree of care, expertise, and judgment exercised by a reasonable nurse under the same or similar circumstances." This does not mean care must be optimal, or of extraordinary skill, nor does

> **KEY TERM**
>
> **Standard of care:** The degree of care, expertise, and judgment exercised by a reasonable person under the same or similar circumstances.

BOX 16-3 PROTECT YOUR "R.N." LICENSE

1) Review the Nursing Practice Act and all associated rules and regulations of the state(s) where you practice.
2) Obtain personal professional liability insurance with a licensure defense protection benefit which will cover legal costs in the event of disciplinary action.
3) Be familiar with the American Nurses Association Foundation of Nursing Package that includes: *Code of Ethics for Nurses with Interpretive Statements, Nursing Scope and Standards of Practice, and Nursing's Social Policy Statement, 2nd Edition*; and
4) Join a national, state, or specialty nursing association and stay abreast of issues applicable to nursing practice by reading journals, standards, literature, and practice statements.

Source: Smith, 2007; Wright, 2005.

it mean that a nurse may not make an error in nursing judgment. It does require, however, that any error made be *reasonable* under the circumstances (Dempski, 2006).

Sources of standards of care include professional nursing organizations (see Box 16-4 for Web links to professional nursing organizations and standards of care), nursing literature such as peer-reviewed nursing journals, federal or state statutes or regulations (e.g., nurse–patient ratios for federal- or state-funded institutions, the state NPA), the Joint Commission, court decisions that may set new standards (which set precedent), and professional experts (e.g., published authors, nursing professors) (Dempski, 2006).

Hospitals and healthcare-related entities frequently look to these nursing standards of care when determining policies and procedures for their institutions. It is essential, however, that nurses recognize that standards of care are dynamic and change with advancements in health care. Nurses will be held accountable for standards existing at the time of any incident, and not standards they may have learned in school. Thus, it is in any nurse's best interest to stay abreast of changes in practice—this includes ensuring that one's employer's policies and procedures are reflective of changed standards. *A nurse may not be protected in a legal dispute if he or she adhered to standards, albeit "hospital policy," that are outdated.* Box 16-5 provides suggestions on how to keep your practice current as a registered

---

BOX 16-4   WEBLINKS: PROFESSIONAL NURSING ORGANIZATIONS AND STANDARDS OF CARE

Many professional specialty nursing organizations publish evidence-based standards of care. These include, but are not limited to:

1) American Association of Critical-care Nurses (AACN), http://www.aacn.org/
2) American Association of Women's Health, Obstetric and Neonatal Nurses (AWHONN), http://www.awhonn.org/awhonn/
3) American Nurses Association (ANA), http://www.nursingworld.org/
4) Association of PeriOperative Registered Nurses (AORN), http://www.aorn.org/
5) National Association of School Nurses, http://www.nasn.org/
6) Oncology Nursing Society, http://www.ons.org/
7) Society of Pediatric Nurses, https://www.pedsnurses.org/

A comprehensive list of nursing specialty organizations can be found through the Nursing Organization Alliance, http://www.nursing-alliance.org/member.cfm.

FIGURE 16-5   KEEPING YOUR PRACTICE CURRENT

1) Join a nursing organization (see Box 16-4).
2) Subscribe to general professional and specialty nursing journals (often a benefit of membership in a nursing organization).
3) Review nursing articles available via the Internet. One source is the *NursingCenter* at http://www.nursingcenter.com, which provides access to clinical articles from 50 leading nursing journals.
4) Sign-up for email alerts from nursing organizations and state boards of nursing.

---

nurse. (Note: Specialists are held to the standard of other similarly situated specialists. A nurse holding advanced certification or licensure will be held to the standard required of those having such additional training. For example, a Certified Registered Nurse Anesthetist [CRNA] or Pediatric Nurse Practitioner [PNP] would be held to the knowledge level of another similarly situated CRNA or PNP, rather than another RN working in the same setting.)

Civil Liability

Any injured party (plaintiff) can initiate a civil action against a "wrong-doer" (defendant) for unreasonable conduct. If the plaintiff can prove by a preponderance of the evidence that the defendant's action or inaction caused or contributed to the plaintiff's injuries, the defendant will be required to monetarily compensate the plaintiff. These civil actions are based on tort law and are usually classified according to whether the defendant's actions were intentional or unintentional. Even if a defendant's actions were unintentional, they can still be required to compensate the injured party.

Negligence

Negligence is unintentional conduct that falls below a standard of care established for the protection of others against unreasonable risk of harm (Schwartz, 2000). Professional malpractice is a specific type of negligence that results when a professional person fails to perform their professional duties in a reasonable manner. Judges and juries rely on appropriate standards of care to determine the reasonableness of the professional's conduct. Standards of care, however, represent only one aspect of a malpractice claim; the plaintiff must prove several additional factors. Specifically, in a cause of action for

KEY TERM

Negligence: Unintentional conduct that falls below a standard of care established for the protection of others against unreasonable risk of harm.

negligence, and thus, professional malpractice, the plaintiff must prove the following four elements (see Box 16-6).

DUTY The first element of any malpractice claim is **duty**. In a case against a nurse, the plaintiff must prove that the nurse owed a legal duty to the plaintiff (usually the patient and, under some circumstances, the plaintiff's family) that required the nurse to deliver the appropriate standard of care. This duty generally arises with the commencement of the nurse–patient relationship—if there is such a relationship, there is a duty, on the part of the nurse, to act (or not act, as the case may be). In the hospital setting, once nurses are assigned to care for a patient during their shift, this nurse–patient relationship commences and a duty arises. However, a duty can also be established when a nurse is "covering" a patient during a colleague's brief break or even when an unassigned patient on the nurse's unit needs assistance. In the clinic setting, a duty may arise through a simple telephone conversation between nurse and patient. Moreover, if a nurse witnesses a patient receiving inappropriate or inferior care from another nurse or other healthcare professional, including a physician, the law generally imposes a duty on that nurse to intervene on behalf of the patient.

A nurse generally does not have a duty to render assistance at the scene of a car accident but, if the nurse does render assistance, the nurse must not give negligent care (Brooke, 2003). See Contemporary Practice Highlight 16-2 for a discussion about **Good Samaritan laws** that addresses liability related to providing care in emergency situations. In summary, courts generally agree that if a patient presents for care, and care is given or should have been given, legal duty is established.

BREACH OF DUTY Once a plaintiff establishes that the nurse owed a duty of care to the patient, the plaintiff must

> **KEY TERM**
>
> **Duty:** An obligation to act or refrain from acting.

> **KEY TERM**
>
> **Good Samaritan law:** A law enacted by a state that protects healthcare providers and other rescuers from liability if they render aid in an emergency, provided that they use reasonable and prudent judgment under the circumstances based on their education, training, and skill level.

BOX 16-6 FOUR ELEMENTS OF NEGLIGENCE

1) The defendant owed a duty to the plaintiff to use reasonable care;
2) The defendant failed to conform to this standard of care (known as breach of duty);
3) There is a reasonably close causal relationship between the defendant's conduct and the plaintiff's injuries (a two part test); and
4) The plaintiff suffered actual loss or damages (Schwartz, 2000).

CONTEMPORARY PRACTICE HIGHLIGHT 16-2

UNDERSTANDING GOOD SAMARITAN LAWS

Almost all states have "Good Samaritan" statutes that protect from liability those people, including trained healthcare workers, who stop to assist and provide care during an emergency. By providing this protection, states hope to encourage nurses, doctors, paramedics, and other citizens to help victims in an emergency.

Although stopping at the scene of accident may be the appropriate action based upon your own morals and ethics, it is important that you understand your responsibilities under your state nurse practice act and your state's Good Samaritan law. Although most states do not require people to give aid in such cases, two states, Minnesota and Vermont, require such assistance.

Once you render care, you establish a nurse–patient relationship. As a result, you must deliver the same standard of care that a reasonable and prudent nurse would deliver under similar circumstances. Furthermore, you cannot leave the victim until you are able to transfer care to another competent provider of the same or greater skill level.

So how does a reasonably prudent nurse respond in such an emergency? A nurse should provide only that care that is consistent with his or her level of education, training, and expertise.

In general, in most states nurses will be protected from liability if they:

- Assess a patient's status, including level of responsiveness, airway, breathing, and circulation.
- Activate the emergency response system by calling or directing someone to call 911.
- Administer rescue breathing and/or chest compressions if indicated.
- Control bleeding.
- Administer emergency medications such as a glucagon kit or anaphylaxis kit (e.g., EpiPen).
- Use an automated external defibrillator if required.

The protections provided by Good Samaritan laws are limited to emergency situations away from the employment setting and they will not protect a nurse from liability resulting from grossly negligent action.

Of important note, victims rarely sue a person who tries to assist in an emergency. If you render assistance in an emergency, you will be protected if you act reasonably and give the best care possible under the circumstances.

Source: Brooke, P. S. (2003). How good a Samaritan should you be? *Nursing, 33*(6), 46–47.

---

show that the nurse showed a **breach of duty** by failing to perform according to the standard of care for that particular circumstance; specifically, that the defendant nurse failed to do what a reasonable and prudent nurse would have done or not done under the same or similar circumstances. Most often, this standard of care is established through expert testimony and the presentation of additional evidence such as a hospital manual of nursing policies and procedures.

KEY TERM

Breach of duty: Failure to perform according to a specific standard of care once a duty is established.

CAUSATION The plaintiff must do much more than prove that the defendant nurse breached a duty owed to the patient; the plaintiff must demonstrate that the nurse caused the patient's **damages**. **Causation** is a difficult concept to grasp and a detailed discussion is beyond the scope of this chapter. Simply stated, the plaintiff must also show that the nurse's actions were 1) the "cause in fact" (known as the actual or "but for" cause) of the plaintiff's injuries and that 2) the consequences to the patient resulting from the nurse's actions were foreseeable (known as proximate cause).

> **KEY TERM**
>
> **Damages:** Injuries incurred as a result of someone's negligence.

> **KEY TERM**
>
> **Causation:** A determination that if not for the conduct of the defendant, the plaintiff would not have been injured and that the consequences of such conduct were foreseeable.

Cause in fact or actual cause means that *but for* the conduct of the nurse, the patient would not have been injured. Note, however, that more than one person can be held legally responsible for an injury to a patient. In a lawsuit against a nurse, a patient need only show that the nurse's action or inaction contributed substantially to the patient's injury. Once the plaintiff demonstrates cause in fact, he or she must then show it was foreseeable that the patient could have been harmed by the nurse's action or inaction. For example, if a nurse administers a drug to a patient with known sedative effects and then fails to ensure that the patient's bedrails are in the upright position and the patient falls out of bed, the plaintiff may reasonably argue the nurse should have foreseen that the patient was at an increased risk of injury as a result of the medication administered and that the nurse should have taken precaution against such injury. All healthcare providers have a responsibility to foresee harm to those for whom they care and take steps to eliminate if possible, or at least mitigate, that harm.

DAMAGES Finally, the plaintiff must show that he or she indeed suffered injury or "damages" as a result of the nurse's negligent action. Courts award money damages in an attempt to return patients as nearly as possible to their preinjury condition or state. Even if the plaintiff demonstrates duty, breach of duty, and both components of causation, but the patient suffered no injury, there can be no monetary recovery. Money damages are classified as general, special, or punitive and are meant to compensate the patient for pain and suffering, disfigurement and disability, past and future medical expenses, past lost wages and future earning capacity, and so forth.

Respondeat Superior

Respondeat superior, Latin for "let the master answer," is a key legal doctrine which holds that an employer is responsible for the actions of its employee that occur within the scope of the employment relationship (Schwartz, 2000). Thus, although a nurse retains individual responsibility for his or her negligence, he or she shares the liability with their employer. The law recognizes that an employer should bear responsibility for the actions of its employees so as to encourage care in hiring and adequate supervision of employees. In addition, employers are usually in a better position to insure against risks and bear the monetary burden of claims. The doctrine of *respondeat superior* does not apply if nurses act outside the scope of their employment

KEY TERM

Respondeat superior: A legal doctrine which holds that the employer is responsible for the actions of its employees that occur within the scope of the employment relationship.

(or scope of practice), such as performing a procedure that only a physician may do in that institution. Moreover, if a hospital is held liable for the negligence of a nurse, the hospital may have the option of subsequently suing the nurse to recover the damages it paid (known as indemnification). (Note: The doctrine of *respondeat superior* does not apply to work performed by an independent contractor. A nurse hired as a private duty nurse is usually an independent contractor.)

Defenses to Negligence

Once a lawsuit is filed against a nurse, the nurse can raise defenses to the malpractice claim. As noted earlier, a plaintiff must prove all of the elements of negligence in a nursing malpractice claim in order to win a monetary award of damages; thus, asserting that the plaintiff failed to prove just one of the four elements of the claim is a valid defense. Secondly, many states have enacted statutes of limitations that limit the time in which a plaintiff can bring a claim against a defendant. These laws and the cases they address vary from state to state, but if a plaintiff does not bring the cause of action within the time prescribed, their action is barred. Another valid defense that can limit a plaintiff's claim against a nurse is the plaintiff's own actions. The law will not reward a plaintiff who contributed to his or her own injury by failing to act in a reasonable and prudent manner. Examples of such plaintiff behavior are failure to follow instructions and failure to provide truthful information—if these actions contributed to the patient's injury, the court may reduce or even bar any damage award (Schwartz, 2000).

Intentional Torts in Nursing

A nurse's legal liability to a patient can extend beyond negligence to other claims in tort law, known as the intentional torts. Unlike negligence, intentional torts are planned acts that cause harm to another, although this harm may not have been expected by the person who acted. In nursing, any willful act that violates the rights of a patient is an intentional tort. Box 16-7 provides examples of intentional torts. Just as in a negligence/malpractice action, a nurse can be sued for money damages to compensate the patient for the harms caused (Trandel-Korenchuk & Trandel-Korenchuk, 1997).

BOX 16-7   EXAMPLES OF INTENTIONAL TORTS

Assault—Attempting to or threatening to touch a person without his or her consent.
Example—A nurse threatening to give a patient an injection if he or she does not comply with cares.

Battery—Touching a person without his or her consent.
Example—A nurse performing any treatment on a patient without the express or implied consent of the patient or his or her legal guardian.

False Imprisonment—Confining a person without his or her consent.
Example—Unwarranted use of restraints or other restrictions, including pharmacologic, on a patient.

Criminal Liability

As discussed, holding a license as a registered nurse is a privilege, and with that privilege comes significant responsibility. Nurses must recognize that, in addition to civil liability, they may be subject to criminal liability for inappropriate actions taken, in addition to the administrative disciplinary actions regarding licensure as noted above. Often intentional torts, such as those listed in Box 16-7, constitute criminal acts for which a nurse may be disciplined administratively and punished criminally. In addition, inappropriate administration and/or recording of controlled substances violate state and federal drug laws.

Decreasing Elements of Risk

Dealing with any action, whether it is a disciplinary, malpractice or other tort, or criminal action, can be professionally, financially, and psychologically devastating to a nurse. Thus, proactive risk reduction is essential. Box 16-8 provides information about how nurses can reduce their own risk of lawsuit.

Medication errors, which include administering the incorrect medication, incorrect dose, or incorrect route, as well as improper administration, are probably the most common source of nursing negligence (Cavico & Cavico, 1995). Box 16-9 lists common nursing actions leading to malpractice claims. In addition, increased use of unlicensed personnel to complete "nursing tasks" may place a nurse at risk for malpractice and/or disciplinary action for improper **delegation**, which is the delegation of a licensed activity, as defined by the state's nurse practice, to an unlicensed person.

KEY TERM

Delegation: Handing over of a licensed activity, as defined by the state's nurse practice act, to an unlicensed person.

BOX 16-8   REDUCE YOUR RISK OF LAWSUIT

1) Maintain knowledge of state nurse practice act.
2) Comply with and keep current with changes in standards of care, employer's policies, and procedures.
3) Practice appropriate standard of nursing care (e.g., always adhere to "five rights" when administering medications; practice proper hand washing).
4) Communicate clearly and consistently with patient, patient's family, and professional colleagues.
5) Document nursing care accurately, thoroughly, and consistently.
6) Practice adequate supervision of unlicensed personnel.

BOX 16-9   COMMON NURSING ACTIONS LEADING TO MALPRACTICE CLAIMS

In addition to medication errors, common nursing actions leading to malpractice claims include:
1) Failure to follow standards of care
2) Failure to use equipment in a responsible manner
3) Failure to communicate
4) Failure to document
5) Failure to assess and monitor
6) Failure to act as patient advocate

Source: (Croke, 2003)

Recognizing potential risk is the nurse's first step in protecting his or her license and avoiding liability. Second, the nurse should adhere to the principles outlined in Box 16-8 in the performance of his or her professional nursing role. Finally, yet most importantly, a nurse must *always* listen to the concerns of the patient and/or the patient's family *and respond* in a timely and effective manner.

Although a complete discussion of professional liability insurance is beyond the scope of this chapter, all nurses should carefully review their need to obtain such insurance. Factors to consider include the nurse's employment situation and potential risk of lawsuits (e.g., Does the nurse work in a high-risk environment such as labor and delivery?), and personal financial situation (e.g., Could the nurse afford legal representation in the event of a lawsuit or disciplinary action?).

Legal Issues in the Nurse–Patient Relationship

A nurse's duty to his or her patient supersedes all other nursing activities. The prior discussion regarding professional liability makes clear that patients have a right to receive care of a certain standard and quality. In addition, as noted at the beginning of this chapter, the U.S. Supreme Court has carved out additional patient rights. Moreover, subsequent statutes, such as the Patient Self-Determination Act (PSDA), passed as part of the Omnibus Budget Reconciliation Act of 1990, effective December 1, 1991, and the Health Insurance Portability and Accountability Act (HIPAA), enacted by the U.S. Congress in 1996, have provided patients with the legal means to gain control over their health care, including treatment, decision making, and security of health-related information.

The PSDA applies to all healthcare institutions receiving Medicaid funds and requires them to provide individuals receiving medical care written information about their rights under state law to make decisions about medical care, including the right to accept or refuse medical or surgical treatment. Institutions must also provide individuals with information about their right to formulate advance directives such as living wills and durable powers of attorney for health care (42 U.S.C. §§ 1395cc (a)(1) et. seq.). Patients must be made aware of their right to make decisions about these issues upon admission (in the case of hospitals or skilled nursing facilities), enrollment (in the case of health maintenance organizations), on first receipt of care (in the case of hospices), or before the patient comes under an agency's care (in the case of home health personal care agencies) (American Nurses Association, 1991). Title II of HIPAA contains the Privacy Rule, effective in 2003, and establishes regulations for the use and disclosure of protected health information, including information about the health status, provision of health care, or payment for health care that can be linked to a person, and any part of a person's medical record (45 C.F.R. 164.501).

Finally, prominent health-related agencies and organizations have promulgated various versions of a Patients' Bill of Rights to guide healthcare professionals and institutions in their policies of care regarding patients. (See Box 16-10 for Web links that highlight examples of Patients' Bill of Rights.) Since 1998, Congress has attempted to pass legislation known as the Patients' Bill of Rights. In its various forms, such legislation addresses a patient's right to have adverse insurance coverage decisions by employer-sponsored health plans reconsidered and in some cases reversed through a system of internal and external review. As of July 2008, passage has been unsuccessful.

All of these documents and statements stem from a common belief in the patient's right to **self-determination**. Moreover, they serve to address the public's growing mistrust of the healthcare industry, concerns over medical error,

KEY TERM

Self-determination: The right of every individual to control his or her own person, free from interference from others.

BOX 16-10   WEB LINKS: EXAMPLES OF PATIENTS" BILL OF RIGHTS

President's Advisory Commission on Consumer Protection and Quality in the Health Care Industry, Consumer Bill of Rights and Responsibilities, 1997, http://www.hcqualitycommission.gov/cborr/.

American Hospital Association, A Patient's Bill of Rights, 1992, http://www.patienttalk.info/AHA-Patient_Bill_of_Rights.htm.

American Nurses Association, Position Statements: Ethics and Human Rights, multiple statements, http://www.nursingworld.org/readroom/position/ethics/.

American Cancer Society, The Patient's Bill of Rights, http://www.cancer.org/docroot/MIT/content/MIT_3_2_Patients_Bill_Of_Rights.asp.

American Heart Association, Patient's Bill of Rights, http://www.americanheart.org/downloadable/heart/1016226554419patient%20bill%20of%20rights.pdf.

---

and perceptions of a preference for profits over patients. Nurses must familiarize themselves with these statements, and in particular, the American Nurses Association's *Code of Ethics for Nurses with Interpretative Statements*, which holds that nurses have moral and professional obligations to recognize the inherent rights of patients (ANA, 2001).

There is a great and longstanding regard for the principle of respect for autonomy and self-determination in modern Western society, as evidenced by the following quotes from well-known legal cases:

> . . . No right is held more sacred, or is more carefully guarded, by the common law, than the right of every individual to the possession and control of his own person, free from all restraint or interference of others, unless by clear and unquestionable authority of law. . . . (*Union Pacific R. Co. v. Botsford*, 141 U.S. 250 (1891))

> . . . Every human being of adult years and sound mind has a right to determine what shall be done with his own body; and a surgeon who performs an operation without his patient's consent commits assault, for which he is liable in damages. . . . (*Schloendorff v. Society of New York Hospital*, 105 N.W. 92 (1914))

These basic beliefs guide the behavior of healthcare providers in regard to a patient's right to information and right to refuse treatment.

Informed Consent

A patient's right to autonomy and self-determination is most relevant to the issue of **consent**. Under modern rules, any healthcare provider has a duty to inform a patient of all relevant facts regarding a treatment or procedure prior to his or her consent to it. Although physicians, advanced practice nurses, and physician's assistants are often responsible for obtaining informed consent prior to performing procedures, the bedside nurse is also responsible for explaining all nursing procedures to the patient prior to performing them. In such cases, and under most circumstances, a patient's physical acquiescence to bedside care generally constitutes consent.

What constitutes informed consent varies according to jurisdiction, but courts apply one of three standards:

1. *Physician-based standard:* Under this standard, a physician (or nurse practitioner or physician's assistant) has a duty to disclose any information that a reasonable physician in the same or similar circumstances would disclose to the patient for consent purposes.
2. *Patient-based standard:* Under this standard, a physician (or nurse practitioner or physician's assistant) must disclose any information that a reasonable patient would consider material (affect the patient's decision) in making a decision regarding his or her treatment or care.
3. *Hybrid standard:* This standard incorporates both of the above standards and generally requires that disclosure of information meet the physician-based standard and must be sufficient to provide a reasonable person with a general understanding of the procedure or course of treatment (Coulson, 2002).

Regardless of standard, obtaining an informed consent generally requires that the care provider performing the treatment or procedure discuss the following information with the patient:

- Patient diagnosis
- Nature and purpose of proposed course of therapy or procedure
- Expected outcomes from therapy or procedure
- Expected benefits from therapy or procedure
- Name of person performing or responsible for therapy or procedure
- Complications, risks, and side effects of therapy or procedure
- Reasonable alternatives
- Possible prognosis if therapy or procedure is not done (Coulson, 2002; Mackay, 2001).

However, simply providing this information to a patient does not mean that the care provider obtained the informed consent of the patient. Information is but one of three elements necessary for meeting the legal requirements of an informed consent. In order for a patient's consent to a treatment or procedure to be valid, the consent must be *voluntary* and the patient must be *competent* to give his or her consent (Schwartz, 2000).

For a consent to be voluntary, the patient must not be coerced or under any influence, including that of medication that may alter their thought processes, such as a narcotic or sedative agent. Voluntary consent can be expressed verbally, such as stating "yes," or in writing, such as by signature on a consent form. Such affirmation is known as express consent. Consent can also be implied by a patient's actions, such as complying with examination; this constitutes implied consent. Silence, however, cannot be construed as consent if a reasonable person would speak before receiving treatment.

Only a competent patient can give informed consent. Most adults (minors will be discussed next) who can understand relevant information concerning their medical care, demonstrate sufficient understanding of the salient issues, and communicate their choice regarding their care are deemed to be competent. Generally, a nurse is in a very good position to assess the competency of a patient due to frequent interactions with that patient throughout a given nursing shift. Often, it is the nurse who initially detects defects in the patient's attention span, memory, or basic understanding of the situation, each of which can interfere with his or her ability to give informed consent. Any concern regarding patient competence should be immediately shared with the patient's physician or care provider performing the treatment or procedure.

It is the responsibility of the person performing the medical treatment or surgical procedure to obtain informed consent. The care provider performing the treatment or procedure should never delegate obtaining informed consent to the bedside nurse. In other words, that care provider, physician, nurse practitioner, or physician's assistant must be the one to provide the patient with the necessary information to obtain consent, such as the complications, risks, or side effects of the therapy or procedure, as discussed earlier. A nurse may be called upon to witness the consent, which means that the nurse observed the patient signing the consent form, thus giving consent to undergo the procedure. Witnessing a consent is not the same thing as obtaining consent. A nurse may also answer a patient's questions as they pertain to relevant nursing care, but must refer questions regarding medical care to the physician. Documentation of questions asked and information provided is essential. Finally, each nurse must be knowledgeable about consent policies and procedures at his or her institution, as well as be familiar with specific state requirements or issues unique to his or her area of practice (e.g., emergency department, labor and delivery, school-based clinic, etc.). (See Box 16-11.)

REFLECTIVE CASE STUDY 16-1: CONSENT

Mrs. Johnson is a 93-year-old woman with a history of congestive heart failure and chronic renal insufficiency. Her present medications include inderal, lisinopril, digoxin, lasix, warfarin, and a multivitamin. She has been a widow for approximately 40 years. She has 3 living children, 9 grandchildren, and 10 great-grandchildren, most of whom she sees regularly. She lives independently in a "seniors" apartment complex, and, until recently, has participated in many of the complex's activities, including working in the community commissary several mornings a week. She uses a walker in public but manages to move about her apartment unaided. She requires assistance when grocery shopping. Her family members accompany her to medical appointments.

Several days ago, she fell following a trip to the grocery store. She was transported by emergency medical services to the local emergency department. She was diagnosed with left femoral neck fracture with displacement of the femoral head. The orthopedic surgeon has recommended hip replacement surgery. Her family is in support of this procedure.

You are the bedside nurse caring for Mrs. Johnson. In fact, you have cared for Mrs. Johnson for the past 2 days. You have found her to be quiet and cooperative and have noted none of the cantankerous behavior that her family states is characteristic of her. It is 7:30 am, you have received report from the off-going nurse, and have begun your assessment. You note that Mrs. Johnson seems a bit delayed in her responses to your questions. No other changes are noted.

At 7:45 am Dr. Bones, the orthopedic surgeon, enters the patient's room to discuss her upcoming surgery and obtain surgical consent. You remain at the bedside listening to Dr. Bones's comprehensive explanation of the procedure. Throughout his explanation, Mrs. Johnson looks at him and nods her head approvingly. Dr. Bones finally asks Mrs. Johnson if she has any questions, to which she replies, "No sir." Dr. Bones turns to you and states that he will complete the informed consent paperwork and asks you to have Mrs. Johnson sign it.

Shortly thereafter, you bring the consent form to Mrs. Johnson and ask her to sign it. She looks at you and states, "Now Mary, I told you I cannot sign that permission slip. You didn't finish your chores. Now go," and she waves you away. Mary is not your name. Mary is the name of Mrs. Johnson's daughter.

What are the implications of Mrs. Johnson's response? Did Dr. Bones obtain an informed consent from Mrs. Johnson? What should you do?

Special Concerns with Informed Consent

In some circumstances, the usual rules regarding obtaining consent do not apply. Conversely, at other times, additional safeguards are warranted. Nurses working

---

BOX 16–11   YOUR NURSING RESPONSIBILITY IN INFORMED CONSENT

The nurse's primary role in the informed consent process is as patient advocate:
1) Determine your patient's level of understanding and approval of the procedure to be done or care to be given.
2) Identify any patient fears and/or misconceptions and notify care provider.
3) Provide information regarding nursing care associated with the procedure or treatment.
4) Contact the appropriate care provider if you doubt the patient's understanding of the procedure or treatment or his or her decision-making ability.
5) Document questions asked and information provided.
6) Notify your supervisor or follow institution policy if you continue to believe your patient's consent is not voluntary or competent.

The nurse's secondary role in the informed consent process is to act as witness:
1) Witness that the patient has been given information.
2) Witness that the signature on the consent form is, in fact, that of the patient (legal guardian or healthcare proxy agent).

Finally, ensure that the process and signed document conforms to your facility's informed consent policy.

Source: Dunn, 2000.

---

with vulnerable populations, such as minors or the elderly, and those who work in emergency department settings, must know when deviation from the usual rules is required. They must implement the appropriate informed consent rules when necessary.

Minors

In general, minors, individuals under the age of 18, are incapable of providing a valid legal consent, and a parent or court-appointed guardian must provide consent for medical or surgical treatment of the minor. Several statutory exceptions exist. Many states allow minors to consent to treatment for sexually transmitted diseases, including human immunodeficiency virus (HIV); care for the prevention or treatment of pregnancy (including contraception and, in a decreasing minority of states, abortion); treatment for physical abuse; and treatment or counseling for substance abuse. In addition, a minor who can demonstrate to a court that they possess "sufficient understanding and appreciation of the nature and consequences of treatment despite their chronological age" may be judged to be a "mature minor" and capable of consenting to treatment (Rozovsky, 1990, §

5.2.2, p 265). An emancipated minor is one who is financially independent and living apart from his or her parents or guardian, is married, or who is in the U.S. military. Emancipated minors have the same legal capacity as an adult and may consent to treatment. Nurses must be aware of the statutory requirements for the treatment of minors in their respective state of licensure and practice.

Other Consent Issues

A patient who has been adjudicated by a court as mentally incompetent, is intoxicated with alcohol or drugs, is in shock, or is unconscious is not capable of consent. A judicially declared mentally incompetent patient will have a court-appointed guardian who has the legal authority to consent to treatment. It is important to note that there may be restrictions as to what the guardian may authorize. Nurses should consult their institution policies regarding questions or concerns involving the care of the mentally incompetent patient. Often, a legal or ethics consult is needed to address treatment for these patients.

In the case of an emergency, healthcare providers may act in the absence of express consent and provide care to a patient if:

- The patient is unable to give consent due to intoxication, mental incompetence, or the patient is incoherent or unconscious.
- There is risk of serious bodily harm if treatment is delayed.
- A reasonable person would consent to treatment under the circumstances.
- This patient would consent to the treatment under the circumstances (or the healthcare provider has no reason to know that the person would refuse treatment, e.g., knowing that the patient is a Jehovah's Witness or Christian Scientist) (Schwartz, 2000).

Two additional doctrines act as exceptions to informed consent: therapeutic privilege and patient waiver. Under therapeutic privilege, the physician determines that certain information may be detrimental to the patient's physical or emotional well-being and that disclosure should not be made. Clearly, this is risky practice and requires detailed documentation of the circumstances surrounding the decision, including the information disclosed, the information withheld, and the reasons, including medical rationale, for withholding the information (Coulson, 2002). Under patient waiver, patients may decide that they do not wish to know or discuss the various aspects of their care and simply place their care in the hands of their trusted physician. Again, detailed documentation is essential and healthcare providers must remember that the patient can revoke the waiver (Coulson).

Failure to Obtain Consent

Failure to obtain informed consent can have significant consequences for the healthcare team. Providers can be sued for battery, the unauthorized touching of another, or more commonly, for negligence. Because obtaining informed consent is recognized as a professional standard of care, negligence is an appropriate basis for liability. If a nurse knows or should have known that informed consent was not obtained and failed to make the physician or nursing supervisor aware, the nurse may also be liable.

Right to Refuse Medical Treatment

Just as the respect for a patient's right to self-determination dictates that a care provider must obtain informed consent prior to treatments or procedures, it also recognizes that a competent patient can refuse any proposed treatments or procedures, including those that may be life-sustaining or -saving, or motivated by religious belief. As noted, the U.S. Supreme Court recognizes that individuals have a constitutionally protected interest in refusing unwanted medical treatment (*Cruzan v. Director, Medical Department of Health*), although many legal questions remain unanswered. The law remains unclear in cases involving incompetent, terminally ill patients, as well as the role of family members in termination of care. Cases involving refusal or termination of care in minors are complex and a detailed discussion is beyond the scope of this chapter. However, consider the following: If a parent or parents may make such a decision to refuse care for an infant or a young child, can they make that same decision for a school-age child or an adolescent child? At what point should the older child's feelings be considered? What about a cognitively impaired school-age child or adolescent, or an intellectually or emotionally precocious younger child? What if the parents disagree regarding treatment with each other or with the medical staff? Should a court-appointed guardian be allowed to make this decision? What about the feelings, opinions, and beliefs of siblings, grandparents, and other close family members? And, at what point does refusal or termination of the care of a minor constitute child neglect, maltreatment, or abuse?

As with consent, refusal of treatment must be predicated upon information. If a patient refuses care, from a simple dressing change to an invasive procedure, the nurse has a legal duty to the patient to ensure that the patient has the necessary information to make an informed refusal. For example, if a patient refuses to roll over to allow a nurse to perform skin assessment, and the patient is subsequently injured, the nurse may be liable to the patient if he or she did not explain the consequences of failing to assess the patient's skin (Eskreis, 1998).

In addition, nurses must recall their legal responsibilities under the Patient Self-Determination Act (discussed earlier in the chapter) and the various Patients' Bill of Rights in their state, at their institution, or promulgated by their nursing organization. Each of these documents serves as a standard of care to guide nurses in their interaction with patients making healthcare decisions. Institutional legal and ethical consults are often necessary to address questions and concerns regarding refusal of treatment by a patient or his or her family. Healthcare providers should never attempt to circumvent the difficulties of dealing with patient refusal by waiting until an emergency arises and then providing the treatment in question. Proceeding with care under the guise of an emergency violates the patient's autonomy and subjects healthcare providers to legal liability. The prudent, ethical nurse refrains from imposing his or her own beliefs or value system upon a patient or a patient's family.

Privacy

On any given shift, nurses have access to some of the most personal private information about a patient and his or her family. A right to privacy is grounded in Western culture and protected by the U.S. Constitution, various state constitutions, and explicit federal and state statutes (e.g., HIPAA). In addition, the ANA *Code for Nurses* prohibits disclosure of confidential patient information, as do the ethical codes of many other professional organizations. The Joint Commission (formerly JCAHO) mandates that institutions maintain and adhere to policies and standards to protect patient information. Nurses must remember that a right to privacy protects more than the patient's medical record; it protects them from unauthorized photographs and news stories, as well as unauthorized observation by others, even if those others are hospital personnel or healthcare students.

Breach of confidentiality exposes the nurse and his or her employer to lawsuits and federal and/or state legal action. In addition, the nurse can be subjected to disciplinary action by his or her state board of nursing and will likely lose employment because breach of confidentiality can be cause for discharge (Blair, 2003). However, there are several explicit exceptions that allow disclosure of confidential information. See Box 16-12 for examples of exceptions that may allow disclosure of confidential information.

BOX 16-12 EXCEPTIONS WHICH MAY ALLOW DISCLOSURE OF CONFIDENTIAL INFORMATION

1) The patient gives verbal or written permission to release information;
2) Other healthcare workers who have a legitimate reason to know information (e.g., report to charge nurse);
3) Statutory or legal duty to report (e.g., communicable diseases, child abuse, gunshot wounds, etc.);
4) There is a duty to warn (e.g., serious threat to an identifiable victim).

Note that even in the circumstances outlined in Figure 16-12, the disclosure of confidential information may be limited; thus, a prudent nurse will be familiar with his or her institution's confidentiality and privacy policies as well as pertinent laws and regulations affecting their area of practice.

Legal Issues in Nursing Practice, Policy, and Legislation

This chapter has briefly reviewed some of the ways that nursing education, professional practice, policies, laws, and regulations intersect. The healthcare industry and its various professions are highly regulated given their impact on the public. It is in the best interest of those working in healthcare-related roles, and in particular, nurses, to keep abreast of pertinent issues including legislative and community activities that will impact professional practice. In addition, as front line patient advocates, nurses are in an optimal position and, arguably, ethically obligated to speak out about access to care, quality of patient care, adequate hospital staffing levels and safe workplaces, and the many other issues impacting the health of the public. Speaking out takes many forms, from informed voting in local, state, and federal elections to actively advocating specific reforms through letter writing to running for elected office. Chapter 17 further addresses the nurse's role in policy making and political activism.

Each nurse should become familiar with the legislative process and with their elected federal, state, and local representatives. An excellent resource regarding this process is the *AACN Public Policy Handbook* available from the American Association of Critical-Care Nurses. Many other nursing and healthcare professional organizations produce similar materials providing nurses with an in-depth review of the legislative process. Most professional nursing organizations have public policy divisions that follow and advocate for legislative and policy reforms affecting nursing, health care, and public welfare, and provide their membership with information regarding these efforts—another excellent reason to join.

Nurses should also consider community service as a means of advocacy. Nurses are well-respected, highly regarded, accessible members of their communities and they possess knowledge and skills to assist people and communities to make the right choices for themselves. Participating in local or regional community activities gives nurses an opportunity to impact others on a scale not available via other means. Imagine the impact a pediatric nurse has speaking at a local PTA meeting regarding bicycle helmet safety or the effect an intensive care nurse has addressing a community group about organ donation. Nurses can stimulate significant change and influence public opinion through community education and outreach.

Summary

This chapter provided an overview of the legal issues nurses confront in their professional practice. A nurse is never "just a nurse." Those who have earned the legal right to use the initials *RN* after their name have a legal obligation to know about the structure and function of their state board of nursing and how their state nursing practice act governs and limits their professional behaviors. They must recognize that their care must conform to certain standards and they must appreciate how laws and regulations, such as federal or state privacy law, affect their daily practice. Nurses must always advocate for and work to protect the basic rights of their patients.

Key Terms

Breach of duty: Failure to perform according to a specific standard of care once a duty is established.

Causation: A determination that if not for the conduct of the defendant, the plaintiff would not have been injured and that the consequences of such conduct were foreseeable.

Civil law: Law that dictates behavior between parties.

Common law: Law that develops as a result of judicial decision; also known as case law.

Consent: A patient's acquiescence to care; it must be informed, voluntary, and competently made in order to be valid.

Damages: Injuries incurred as a result of someone's negligence.

Delegation: Handing over of a licensed activity, as defined by the state's nurse practice act, to an unlicensed person.

■ **Duty:** An obligation to act or refrain from acting.

Good Samaritan law: A law enacted by a state that protects healthcare providers and other rescuers from liability if they render aid in an emergency, provided that they use reasonable and prudent judgment under the circumstances based on their education, training, and skill level.

License: Permission to engage in an activity; a professional license allows the holder to engage in a specific activity for compensation.

Licensure: The process by which a state or governmental agency grants permission to an individual to engage in a given profession for compensation.

Mutual recognition model: Allows a nurse to maintain a license in his or her state of residency and to practice and be recognized in another state, subject to each state's practice law and regulation; also known as the nursing interstate compact.

Negligence: Unintentional conduct that falls below a standard of care established for the protection of others against unreasonable risk of harm.

■ **Nurse practice act:** A state statute that defines the legal limits for the practice of nursing within that state and explicitly identifies the requirements for licensure.

■ **Nursing interstate compact:** See *mutual recognition model*.

■ **Professional malpractice:** A type of negligence that results when a professional person fails to perform his or her professional duties in a reasonable manner.

Respondeat superior: A legal doctrine which holds that the employer is responsible for the actions of its employees that occur within the scope of the employment relationship.

■ **Self-determination:** The right of every individual to control his or her own person free from interference from others.

■ **Standard of care:** The degree of care, expertise, and judgment exercised by a reasonable person under the same or similar circumstances.

■ **Tort law:** Law that establishes rules for socially reasonable conduct.

Reflective Practice Questions

1. You are a staff nurse working on an acute care medical-surgical nursing unit. You have recently read several peer-reviewed journal articles addressing a new technique that helps reduce the risk of decubitus ulcer occurrence in your patient population. This technique has been shown to reduce the incidence of ulcer formation by a significant amount. Your unit has not implemented this technique. What are the implications of continuing to treat patients according to current hospital protocols? What is your responsibility as a unit staff nurse?

2. According to your state nursing practice act, which of the following procedures can you delegate to an assistant who is not a registered nurse?

   a. Assessment of a patient upon admission to an acute care unit
   b. Administration of oral medications per physician order
   c. Obtaining regularly scheduled vital signs, which include heart rate, respiratory rate, blood pressure, and temperature
   d. Assessment of a telemetry patient's electrocardiogram tracing
   e. Administration of a Demerol intramuscular injection
   f. Performing chest compressions during resuscitation
   g. Transcribing physician's orders
   h. Administration of intravenous antibiotics
   i. Performing discharge teaching
   j. Assessing a patient following an intervention

   What if the assistant is a licensed vocational or practical nurse, or emergency medical technician employed by your facility? Does your answer change? What if your practice environment is a military hospital and your assistants are corpsmen or medics?

3. You are a staff nurse working on an acute care medical-surgical nursing unit. Yesterday, you provided care for Mrs. Baker, an 85-year-old woman who recently underwent a surgical procedure. On review of your notes from the day prior, you realize that you did not document the appearance of her wound or the dressing change you performed. What is the appropriate action to take?

4. You are a registered nurse working in your local public health clinic. A 14-year-old girl presents for treatment of a sexually transmitted disease. During your initial assessment, she confides that her boyfriend is a 19-year-old neighbor with whom she has been sexually active for the past 6 months.

She is concerned that her parents will be notified that she is seeking treatment at the clinic. What is your response? What must you consider?

References

American Association of Colleges of Nursing. (2007). *Nursing fact sheet*. Retrieved May 1, 2007, from http://www.aacn.nche.edu/Media/FactSheets/nursfact.htm

American Nurses Association, 2007; Association of Women's Health, Obstetric and Neonatal Nurses. (1999). *AWHONN position statements: Interstate compact for mutual recognition of state licensure*. Retrieved October 15, 2007, from http://www.awhonn.org/awhonn/content.do?name=05_HealthPolicyLegislation/5H_PositionStatements.htm;

American Nurses Association. (1991). *ANA position statements: Ethics and human rights position statements*. Retrieved July 25, 2008, from http://www.nursingworld.org/MainMenuCategories/HealthcareandPolicyIssues/ANAPositionStatements/ EthicsandHumanRights.aspx

American Nurses Association. (2001). *ANA code of ethics for nurses with interpretive statements*. American Nurses.

Association of Women's Health, Obstetric and Neonatal Nurses. (1999). *AWHONN position statements: Interstate compact for mutual recognition of state licensure*. Retrieved October 15, 2007, from http://www.awhonn.org/awhonn/content.do?name=05_HealthPolicyLegislation/5H_PositionStatements.htm

Blair, P. (2003). Make room for patient privacy. *Nursing Management, 34*(6), 28–29.

Brent, N. (2000). *Nurses and the law: A guide to principles and applications* (2nd ed.). Philadelphia: Saunders.

Brooke, P. S. (2003). How good a Samaritan should you be? *Nursing2003, 33*(6), 46–47.

Cavico, F. J., & Cavico, N. M. (1995). The nursing profession in the 1990's: Negligence and malpractice liability. *Cleveland State Law Review, 43*, 556–626.

Coulson, K. G. (2002). Informed consent: Issues for providers. *Hematology/Oncology Clinics of North America, 16*(6), 1365–1380.

Croke, E. M. (2003). Nurses, negligence and malpractice. *American Journal of Nursing, 103*(9), 54–63.

Dempski, K. M. (2006). Standards of care. In S. W. Killion (ed.), *Quick look nursing: Legal and ethical issues* (pp. 10–11). Sudbury, MA: Jones and Bartlett.

Dunn, D. (2000). Exploring the gray areas of informed consent. *Nursing Management, 31*(7), 20–25.

Eskreis, T. (1998). Seven common legal pitfalls in nursing. *American Journal of Nursing, 98*(4), 34–40.

Fedora, P. A. (2001). Defining nursing practice. In M. E. O'Keefe (ed.), *Nursing practice and the law* (p. 99). Philadelphia: F.A. Davis.

Health Resources and Services Administration. (1992). *Health personnel in the United States, 1991: Eighth report to Congress*. Washington, DC: U.S. Department of Health and Human Services.

Health Resources and Services Administration. (2007). *The registered nurse population: Findings from the March 2004 National Sample Survey of Registered Nurses*. Washington, DC: U.S. Department of Health and Human Services.

Hill, G., & Hill, K. (2007). *Law.com Dictionary*. Retrieved May 1, 2007, from http://dictionary.law.com/default2.asp

Killion, S. W. (2006). The legal environment—Part I. In S. W. Killion (ed.), *Quick look nursing: Legal and ethical issues* (pp. 2–3). Sudbury, MA: Jones and Bartlett.

Liang, B. A. (2002). An overview of United States law. *Hematology/Oncology Clinics of North America, 16*(6), 1315–1330.

Mackay, T. (2001). Informed consent. In M. E. O'Keefe (ed.), *Nursing practice and the law: Avoiding malpractice and other risks* (pp. 199–213). Philadelphia: F.A. Davis.

National Council of State Boards of Nursing. (2002). *NCSBN position statement: Alternative regulatory licensure models*. Retrieved October 15, 2007, from https://www.ncsbn.org/1270.htm

National Council of State Boards of Nursing. (2007a). *Nurse licensure compact*. Retrieved July 2007, from https://www.ncsbn.org/nlc.htm

National Council of State Boards of Nursing. (2007b). *Practice and discipline: Nurse licensure and certification*. Retrieved June 1, 2007, from https://www.ncsbn.org/168.htm

National Council of State Boards of Nursing. (2007c). *What boards do*. Retrieved June 1, 2007, from https://www.ncsbn.org/126.htm

National Council of State Boards of Nursing. (2007d). *What is NCLEX?* Retrieved June 1, 2007, from https://www.ncsbn.org/1200.htm

Priest, C., Kooken, W. C., Ealey, K. L., Holmes, S. R., & Hufeld, P. (2007). Improving baccalaurete nursing students' understanding of fundamental legal issues through interdisciplinary collaboration. *Journal of Nursing Law, 11*(1), 35–42.

Rozovsky, F. (1990). *Consent to treatment: A practical guide*. Boston: Little, Brown.

Schwartz, V. E. (2000). *Prosser, Wade & Schwartz's torts, cases and materials* (10th ed.). New York: Foundation Press.

Smith, M. H. (2007). *Legal basics for professional nursing: Nurse practice acts*. Retrieved June 1, 2007, from http://nursingworld.org/mods/mod995/canlegalnrsfull.htm

Trandel-Korenchuk, D. M., & Trandel-Korenchuk, K. M. (1997). *Nursing and the law* (5th ed.). Gaithersburg, MD: Aspen.

U.S. Info. (2007). *The bill of rights*. Retrieved September 2, 2008, from http://usinfo.state.gov/infousa/government/overview/billeng.html

Wright, L. D. (2005). Bill of rights for nurses in licensure matters. *Journal of Nursing Law, 10*(3),177–180.

Policy and Political Activism

Joanne R. Warner and Sharon Kimball

LEARNING OUTCOMES

After reading this chapter you will be able to:

- Define politics and policy.
- Understand political activism as a valid and significant nursing action.
- Explain the components of political competence for nurses.
- Describe the perspective that positions nurses for successful political activism.
- Link historical examples of political activism to today's context.
- Discuss strategies for getting involved in the political arena.

"I have come to the conclusion that politics are too serious a matter to be left to the politicians."

—Charles De Gaulle, French general and politician (1890–1970)

Introduction

Have you ever wondered why things are the way they are? Have you ever felt "something needs to be done about that"? Have you ever thought "we could do better"? Do you have a vision for what could be? What issues are you

KEY TERM

Politics: Influencing the allocation of scarce resources (Mason, Leavitt, and Chafee, 2007).

KEY TERM

Policy: A plan to guide action or decisions.

passionate about? How would you advance your issue? How would you go about making that change in your community or where you work?

As a nurse, it is your professional responsibility to look around your workplace or your community and ask these hard questions. It is also your professional responsibility to act. Action will require venturing into the world of **politics** and **policy**. It will take your commitment to becoming politically competent.

Is health care political? Yes. Health and health care are inextricably intertwined with social, economic, and political systems. Health care is political because it involves limited resources, important needs, and varied ideas on how to match resources with needs. Health is political because health care is expensive. Someone, somewhere must decide about the allocation of resources that go to health and health care. Nurses need to be involved in those political decisions. Nurses need to be vocal about the policies and politics that affect their practice.

Is nursing political? Of course. There are many legislative and regulatory issues in nursing. Workplace environment, the nursing shortage, migration of nurses, patient rights, patient safety, medical error prevention, violence prevention, licensure, and scope of practice are just a few examples of the critical issues facing nursing. Health care is changing rapidly. As nurses interact with patients and their families, they are often the first providers to see clearly when and how the healthcare system is failing to meet patient needs. Nurses have a choice: to continue trying to make do while feeling victimized by changes over which they feel they have no control (Mick, 2004) or to take action and find opportunities to improve the healthcare system, maintain a strong profession, and bring nursing values into politics and policy formation.

Nurses may forget that, as the largest group of healthcare providers, they could generate enough power to successfully reform the healthcare system based on numbers alone. According to the 2004 National Sample Survey of Registered Nurses, there are 2.9 million registered nurses in the United States (U.S. Department of Health and Human Services, n.d.). This reality continues to offer the nursing profession a formidable power base that is largely untapped in the day-to-day world of politics and legislation (Abood, 2007). Nursing has not developed into a cohesive, powerful professional force that could be a partial counterweight to the dominance of medicine in the policy arena (Mick, 2004). However, involvement of only a fraction of the nation's 2.9 million registered nurses in even the smallest way could become a force for change for the nursing profession and for the healthcare system and the patients it serves (Artz, 2006).

Why is nursing *not* a political force? Why are we sometimes ignored by political leaders and the media? Many nurses are still uncomfortable with the responsibility of asserting their political influence. Many nurses have never considered it their place to challenge the structure of the system in which they work, or seen themselves as experts on healthcare issues (Thomas, Billington, & Getliffe, 2004).

When they choose to take on the role of political or policy activist, nurses often have to move out of the comfort zone of their practice arena and into less familiar arenas where the laws and regulations impacting patient care and nursing practice are developed, and the battles for scarce resources are negotiated and decided. **Political activism** adds a dimension to professional practice that offers the reward of having more control over patient care, outcomes, and nursing practice (Abood, 2007).

Defining Politics and Policy

What is politics? Mason, Leavitt, and Chafee (2007) describe politics as the "process of influencing the allocation of scarce resources" (p. 4). Rains and Barton-Kreise (2001) argue that understanding and engaging actively with the political processes and policies that shape their workplace can help nurses deliver better patient care. Politics also refers to the methods and tactics used to make and apply policy.

A policy is a plan to guide decisions and actions. The term may apply to a government, a private sector organization, a group, or an individual. Examples of policies include presidential executive orders, corporate privacy policies, or workplace policies and procedures. Mason, Leavitt, and Chaffee (2007) differentiate among public policy, social policy, health policy, institutional policy, and organizational policy. **Public policy** is defined as policy formed by governmental bodies (e.g., legislation passed by Congress) and the regulations written from that policy. **Social policy** is policy decisions that promote the welfare of the public. **Health policy** is the decisions made to promote the health of individual citizens. **Institutional policies** govern workplaces (i.e., what the institution's goals are and how it will operate). **Organizational policies** are positions taken by organizations. Each type of policy can affect nurses and their practice.

Health policy is a set course of action (or inaction) undertaken by governments or healthcare organizations to obtain a desired health outcome (Cherry & Trotter Betts, 2005). Public health–related policies come from local, state, or federal legislation; regulations; and/or court rulings that govern the provision of healthcare services. In addition to public policies,

KEY TERM

Political activism: Direct and collective participation in strategies toward specific societal goals; for nursing, this action is based on explicit professional values and focuses on enhancing health.

KEY TERM

Public policy: Policy formed by governmental bodies (i.e., local, state, and federal legislation) and the regulations written from that policy.

KEY TERM

Social policy: Policy decisions that are made to promote the welfare of the public.

KEY TERM

Health policy: Policy decisions that are made to promote the health of individuals.

KEY TERM

Institutional policy: Policy that governs a workplace and describes an institution's goals and how it will operate.

KEY TERM

Organizational policy: Policy that articulates positions taken by an organization.

there are institutional or business policies related to health care. These policies are developed in the private sector by agencies, such as hospitals or accrediting organizations.

Policy may also refer to the process of making important organizational decisions, including the identification of different alternatives such as programs or spending priorities, and choosing among them on the basis of the impact they will have. In political science the policy cycle is a tool used for the analysis of the development of a policy item. One standardized version (Milstead, 2004) includes the stages listed in Box 17-1, and looks a bit like the nursing process. Reflective Case Study 17-1 provides you with an opportunity to consider a health promotion issue and apply the concepts of the policy cycle.

REFLECTIVE CASE STUDY 17-1
DEVELOPING A HEALTH PROMOTION POLICY

Sally is employed on an inpatient acute rehabilitation unit in a large referral hospital. She graduated from her baccalaureate program 2 years ago, and enjoys the interdisciplinary team approach to quality care. Sally is respected as a competent caregiver and an informal leader on the unit. She has never considered herself political.

Through her involvement with her children's preschool, she has become involved in children's safety issues, such as correct helmet fitting and proper car seat installation. She has become quite passionate about these issues because she cares for victims of motor vehicle accidents. She completed a class in proper car seat installation and began exploring the policies in place on the maternity unit of her hospital. She found there was no policy or procedure that included teaching new parents how to properly install and use an infant car seat upon discharge.

1. What is the policy issue?
2. What assessment data does she need to collect to completely understand the issue?
3. How many different ways can this issue be framed? What policy options emerge from each of the different ways to frame the issue?
4. With whom should she network? Who would be potential allies? Who would be potential opponents?
5. Who is the policy-making body that could address this issue?
6. What would the professional risks and rewards be for her if she pursued this?

In order to shape policy and become involved in politics, nurses need to develop political competence. **Political competence** is the skills, perspectives, and values needed for effective political involvement within nursing's professional role. Political competence is needed within nursing to accomplish

---

BOX 17-1   POLICY-MAKING CYCLE

- Setting the agenda and framing the problem
- Forming the policy options
- Making it happen legislatively through decision-making processes
- Implementing the policy
- Evaluating the policy outcomes (decide to continue or terminate?)

Source: Milstead, 2004.

---

many purposes: 1) to reduce or bolster the effect of socioeconomic and environmental influences on health, 2) to give culturally appropriate care, 3) to create with others a humane healthcare system, and 4) to give voice to nursing's values and perspective within policy conversations (Warner, 2003).

You can influence policy. You are the nursing expert. You are the healthcare systems expert. You are a constituent. You are a voter. Nurses have a great understanding of the strengths and weaknesses of the healthcare system, and can use this knowledge to influence politics and policy. What nurses in many instances lack is the belief in their political competence.

Why Political Competence Is Needed In Nursing

Becoming and maintaining oneself as an expert nurse is a rigorous and ongoing process of acquiring knowledge, refining skills, and assimilating into a professional role. In the lengthy list of required abilities, why is political competence needed in nursing? In Box 17-2, Warner (2003) summarizes five reasons for nurses to demonstrate political competence. Each of these reasons is explained below.

BOX 17-2   WHY DO NURSES NEED POLITICAL COMPETENCE?

- Nature of factors affecting health
- Issues of culture and power
- Need for quality improvement and accountability
- Involvement in interdisciplinary practice partnerships
- Need for nursing's voice and values in political decision making

---

Source: Warner, 2003.

Increasingly, the broad nature of societal factors existing outside the health-care system, such as psychosocial factors, political-economic conditions, cultural issues, gender roles, and the state of the environment, is understood to influence the health status of populations (Reutter & Williamson, 2000; Whitehead, 2003). Healthcare providers are challenged to use this broad understanding and intervene with societal factors that threaten or promote health (Reuter & Duncan, 2002). Fagin (2000) praises nursing's holistic focus to providing care and also describes nursing's approach to viewing health and illness, as well as the interaction between health and social problems to be a particular strength of the discipline. Political competence is needed for reform and action that influence these broad variables.

Secondly, a diverse global society requires a culturally competent workforce. "The power and politics embedded in each culture strongly influence many factors that are importantly related to health, such as family social structure, religious traditions and accepted norms/behaviors" (Warner, 2003, p. 136). Political competence is required to intervene within the culturally defined power dynamics in a diverse society.

Third, nurses are accountable for the design and quality improvement of the healthcare system. The most current American Association of Colleges of Nursing (AACN) baccalaureate essentials (1998) underscore the need for knowledge in policy by noting, "health care policy shapes health care systems and helps determine accessibility, accountability, and affordability" (p. 16). Nurses therefore need to understand the political dynamics at play in the healthcare system and have the requisite political skills to contribute to an improved and more accountable system. Interventions at the policy level require partnership, and the skill of graceful interdisciplinary collaboration is one aspect of political competence.

Finally, without nurse activism and political involvement, nursing values and perspective would be lost in the political debate. Mason, Leavitt, and Chaffee (2007) note that nursing's voice brings the values of caring, collaboration, and collectivity to policy conversations. Gebbie, Wakefield, and Kerfoot (2000) explain that nurses bring the clarity of real clinical stories and human implications to abstract policy topics, plus another important perspective: "Nurses' strong beliefs in the capacity and importance of people to care for themselves distinguish nurses from other health professions that share many of the same skills. This belief becomes an orientation toward policy action to enable people to help themselves" (p. 311).

Political competence is a requisite nursing skill for all of these reasons. Political competence will equip nurses to fulfill many aspects of their professional role, including but not limited to the following from the baccalaureate essentials (AACN, 1998):

- Assume accountability for practice
- Form partnerships and serve within interdisciplinary teams
- Communicate and negotiate
- Advocate for patients
- Participate in political and regulatory processes and in shaping the health-care system

Political skills will assist nurses "in improving the health care system, maintaining a strong profession, and bringing nursing values convincingly into policy formation" (Warner, 2003, p. 137).

What Is Political Competence?

Feldman and Lewenson (2000) call for a shift in nursing activism from something abstract, faceless, and self-effacing to a visible leadership on important health and social issues. To accomplish that shift, we need to understand what political competence looks like in a nurse. What behaviors characterize those nurses whose political and social activism wins elections, advocates for successful legislation, and ensures that resources are allocated toward health and healing? Box 17-3 provides a listing of politically competent behaviors for nurses. The following paragraphs provide a synthesis of these politically competent behaviors. Contemporary Practice Highlights 17-1 and 17-2 provide examples of "real-life" political activism that illustrate the use of politically competent behaviors by professional nurses.

Politically competent nurses bring their professional credibility, values, expertise, and background to the table. Annually, nurses rank very high as trusted professionals, above others in health care, so it is nursing's responsibility and opportunity to bring the knowledge and perspective of the profession to policy and political debates. Their nursing credential is worn visibly and proudly, and their experience is often communicated through clinical stories that put a human

---

BOX 17-3   POLITICALLY COMPETENT BEHAVIORS FOR NURSES

- Use nursing knowledge and expertise
- Network and establish relationships
- Commit to collaboration and collective action
- Use the power of persuasion
- Adopt long-term strategic views of issues

Source: Feldman & Lewenson, 2000; Warner, 2003.

CONTEMPORARY PRACTICE HIGHLIGHT 17-1

POLITICAL ACTIVISM AND THE ARCHIMEDES MOVEMENT

The We Can Do Better Web site asks "If anything were possible, how would we design a new health system? If we weren't constrained by the system we have today—the one we all know isn't working—what would a new, better system look like?" In 2006, Dr. John Kitzhaber, former governor of the State of Oregon, emergency room physician, and director for the Center for Evidence-Based Policy at Oregon Health & Science University in Portland, launched the Archimedes Movement to answer those questions. The goal of the movement is to build a grassroots process of civic engagement over the growing concern about our healthcare system. The goal was both creating the vision and realizing the dream through collective action. Nurses have been involved throughout as citizens and as professionals in the Nurses Working Group.

A vision statement was developed through focus groups across Oregon. It reads as follows: "To optimize the health of Oregonians by creating a sustainable system which uses the public resources spent on health care to ensure that everyone has access to a defined set of essential, effective health services." Sounds very compatible with nursing's focus on access, quality, and caring!

Strategies used to realize this vision included a blog, neighborhood meetings to increase awareness and movement membership, drafting of a bill introduced into the Oregon Senate during the 2007 legislative session, and the lobbying and negotiating of the session. The Nurses Working Group met twice with Governor Kitzhaber to provide input on Senate Bill 27 and express the values and perspectives of nursing. The conversations were lively sessions of receptive listening and exchange. SB 27 did not pass, though the activities of the Archimedes Movement continue to work toward reforming the health system and ensuring greater coverage for all Oregonians. Nurses are visible participants in this revolutionary grassroots process.

face on a policy issue. Politically competent nurses know and use nursing expertise and experience to make a difference through policy and political action.

Networking is a significant behavior for politically effective nurses. Networking purposely links the right people and possible ideas at the right time. Nurses have the skills to establish and cultivate relationships. Nurses need to understand that whether someone is an opponent or an ally might change given the political topic, so no one should be considered a perpetual enemy. Related to networking is the commitment of politically competent nurses to collective strength and working collaboratively and in coalition. Our individual effectiveness is made bigger through collective action, such as through professional organizations, agency coalitions, or interdisciplinary unity around a topic.

CONTEMPORARY PRACTICE HIGHLIGHT 17-2

POLITICAL COMPETENCE: SB4 AND NURSING LEADERSHIP AND POLITICAL ACTION

Dr. Kris Campbell serves as the executive director of the Oregon Center for Nursing. She has impeccable credentials in both the academy and the military. She has three degrees in nursing, culminating in a PhD from Oregon Health & Science University, as well as a master's in Strategic Studies from the Army War College. She is a retired Brigadier General from the U.S. Army Reserve, and was the first nurse in the Army Reserve to serve as the Assistant Surgeon General. She was the first nurse and first female to command a medical facility in hazardous duty, specifically Combat Support Hospital in Bosnia. She tells the following story of recent political accomplishments for nursing under her leadership:

> The Oregon Center for Nursing, in partnership with the Oregon Nursing Leadership Council and the Northwest Health Foundation, sponsored legislation in 2007 to support nursing in Oregon. SB4 passed, with modifications, and established funding for the Oregon Center for Nursing, a nursing workforce center established to help solve the nursing shortage in Oregon. SB4 also established the Oregon Center for Nursing as advisory to the Oregon Workforce Investment Board and the Joint Board of Education so that nursing leadership has a voice in workforce and education decisions that affect nursing in Oregon. There were also two retention elements to the bill: one which allows all nurses who work for the state, including faculty, who are retired to continue working without losing retirement pay (PERS relief), and the other created an exception to the requirement for state nurses to work 17.5 hrs to be eligible for group health insurance. The latter exception is also a recruitment incentive.
>
> SB4 was successful because the nursing community in Oregon came together with a collective voice to support nursing. Oregon's nursing leaders developed a strategic plan to solve the nursing shortage in 2001. The statewide collaborative effort by nurse leaders to execute the strategic plan has produced excellent results, such as a 76% increase in nursing school graduates, a new collaborative nursing program to transform nursing education (Oregon Consortium for Nursing Education), a process and program for centralized placement of nursing students in clinical sites (StudentMAX) and the success of the Oregon Center for Nursing, to name a few. These successes demonstrated nursing's credibility in producing outcomes. Nursing leaders also demonstrated a united voice in that representatives from education, practice, workforce and community partners were present at each hearing. The importance of showing up and speaking up made a difference. There were challenges throughout the session, but the focus on funding nursing . . . be it in one's school, facility or community . . . helped keep the focus on what all nurses could all agree to, which was that nurses make a difference to the outcomes of patients, and that funding was needed to support nursing.

Applause to Kris Campbell as one of today's politically competent and active nurses working to improve nursing and health care for society.

The power to persuade and sell an idea is a significant mark of political competence. Nurses are particularly equipped with the power of persuasion—as demonstrated with humor in this quote, "If you can convince someone to drink Metamucil you can convince them to vote" (Warner, 2003, p. 139). Persuasion can take many forms, including speaking in large forums, small hallway conversations, or the written word—all with the goal of health reform or patient advocacy.

Politically competent nurses take a strategic view of issues that includes the complex context as well as consideration of diverse stakeholders and their agendas. They look beyond the immediate and, using a chess analogy, are considering three or four future moves and the long-range vision. Nurses often use this strategic perspective as they incorporate clinical reasoning and multiple environmental factors into decision making. Because the long-range view is often needed for social change, politically competent nurses have the ability to persevere and not define themselves by victories and defeats. Passion and "fire in the belly" for health advocacy sustains politically active nurses for the long haul.

The behaviors that describe politically competent nurses are from the classic set of nursing abilities used to provide clinical care. A slight refocusing of the lens allows these behaviors to be viewed as the pursuit of policies and political decisions supporting health. Nurses could understand their political activism as caring on a grand scale and at the highest collective level.

Incorporating Policy and Politics into Daily Practice

So, how does a nurse become comfortable participating in politics and policy setting? Becoming politically involved and gaining the skills to become politically competent can seem quite daunting. The first requirement is the belief that you have the power to change things. Without that empowered view of your professional role, nurses can be silent and impotent workers in a frustrating system.

What overall perspective is needed for nurses to incorporate policy and politics into their professional role and daily practice? The answer comes in contrasting the scientific and political arenas, and clarity about the expectations within each. Most nurses are educated and socialized to appreciate science and to trust answers that come from use of the scientific method. Within this scientific framework, "truth" is discovered through research and those findings can be repeated. A nurse's world is constructed with reliable and valid principles or facts.

A politician's world is constructed with negotiated truth. Negotiated truth involves what people believe to be true. If there are two "truths," the person who is better at persuading will prevail. Legislation that is passed, or elections that are won, result from skilled communication and the give-and-take of negotiation. Perception is more important than validity; persuasion is more important than reliability. This simplistic view of the nurse's and politician's worlds ignores the merit of policy research and data-driven projects, but is used to make a point to contrast the scientific and political arenas.

To avoid frustration or failure, nurses need to clarify whether the work they are doing that day or at that moment is of scientific or political nature. Once clarified, nurses can honor and follow the unspoken rules of that arena. For example, clinical practice is based on scientific principles and evidence derived from solid research. No negotiation is needed to follow a best practice; sound theory and knowledge developed through research provides guidance to care. However, if nurses are pursuing a policy to fund prenatal care, as an example, persuasion, skilled communication, and negotiation are needed to convince decision makers who are allocating funds. Nurses must speak up, write letters, testify, advocate, and convince decision makers of the "truth" they know.

Without this clarification, nurses are at risk for approaching the political arena with rules from the scientific area. Without understanding what is needed in the political arena, nurses are at risk for thinking that the scientific merit of an issue is inherently right, will not require persuasion or advocacy, and will prevail. Nurses need to understand which arena they are in and what rules to play by.

When nurses can appreciate the differences in the political and scientific arenas, they can use the skills appropriate for that arena. If nurses can successfully match their abilities to the style and requirements of the political arena, they can find the political arena a creative expression of advocacy and social change. Ironically, the ability to differentiate between the two arenas is the precursor to seeing the political in our everyday professional experiences, and moving to a more integrated view of our professional role. Seeing political opportunities in our everyday clinical practice is the key to gaining more control of our profession.

Nursing and Politics in History

Beginning with Florence Nightingale, there have been outstanding examples of individual nurses who have asked the question, "Why are things the way they are?" They have used their passion, perseverance, and understanding of politics and policy to change the nursing profession and improve health care and public health. Nurse activists of previous centuries, including Florence Nightingale, Lillian Wald, and Margaret Sanger, pushed for and achieved tremendous healthcare improvements in their lifetimes.

Today's nurses can examine their legacy to understand how behaviors embodied in becoming politically competent, such as professional credibility, networking, the power to persuade, and a strategic view of the issues, were needed even in the 19th century. Several examples will illuminate each aspect of political competence.

Professional Credibility

Sojourner Truth (1797–1883) was born into slavery. She provided nursing care to Union soldiers and civilians during the Civil War. Because of her professional credibility, in 1865 she was appointed to work with a physician at Freedmen's Hospital in Washington. She was 68 years old. For more than 2 years, she nursed African American soldiers and taught newly recruited nurses. She also organized a group of women to clean the hospital and brought order to the chaotic conditions.

Lillian Wald (1867–1940) attended New York Hospital's school of nursing. She found herself drawn to nursing the inhabitants of New York's lower east side tenements. Her professional credibility opened the door and enabled her to tell the stories of the people living in the tenements to those who held the power to allocate funds. Her political skills were instrumental as she pioneered public health nursing, founded the National Organization for Public Health Nursing, and founded the Henry Street Settlement. Today, the Henry Street Settlement continues to provide social services and arts programming to more than 100,000 New Yorkers each year (Henry Street Settlement, n.d.).

Networking and Collective Strength

Florence Nightingale (1820–1910) was a consummate politician and visionary. She understood the importance of networking. While in the Crimea, she shrewdly invited government officials to see the deplorable hospital conditions firsthand. Those men would later become her collaborators for reform. She wrote thousands of letters, often writing two letters to the same person on the same topic. One of the letters would be designated as public. The second letter would be the private version and would include instructions on who to show the first letter to or how to use the first letter to benefit a cause. She repeatedly discovered and enlisted people with the skills to define problems and formulate solutions.

Networking was also stressed in her nursing schools. All graduates of the Nightingale School were encouraged to see themselves as part of a whole and they were encouraged to keep in touch with each other.

Mary Eliza Mahoney (1845–1926) was the first African American professional nurse in the American Nurses Association (ANA). Realizing the importance of networking, she supported the formation of the National Association of Colored Graduate Nurses (NACGN). She demonstrated to have her alma mater, the New England Hospital, admit more women of color. She was a strong supporter of women's suffrage and was one of the first women in Boston to register to vote, at the age of 76.

The Power to Persuade

During the Civil War, Clara Barton (1821–1912) served as an independent nurse. She lobbied the U.S. Army, at first without success, to bring her own medical supplies to the battlefields. Later, while visiting Europe, Barton worked with a relief organization known as the International Committee of the Red Cross during the Franco-Prussian War. After returning home to the United States, she began to lobby for a U.S. branch of this international organization. Her powers of persuasion helped to found the American Red Cross Society in 1881, and Barton served as its first president.

Susie Walking Bear Yellowtail (1903–1981) worked with the Indian Health Service from 1929 to 1931 to end abuses in the Indian healthcare system, such as the sterilization of Native American women without their consent (American Nurses Association, n.d.). She effectively communicated Native American culture and perspectives to non-Native Americans throughout the country during her career.

Margaret Sanger (1879–1966) was a pioneering force in the field of contraception and helped create the International Planned Parenthood Federation. She concluded that control over childbearing was the key to female emancipation. She wrote newspaper articles on feminine hygiene, put out a militant journal entitled *Woman Rebel*, and in 1914 published a pamphlet, *Family Limitation*, in which she coined the term *birth control* and called for legalization of contraception. She distributed information on birth control when it was illegal. She understood the power of information and civil disobedience to persuade others.

Strategic View of Issues

Lavinia Dock (1858–1956) trained as a nurse at New York City's Bellevue Hospital. She was concerned with the interconnected problems of female education and the advancement of women. She believed that the position of women in society and the status of the nursing profession were inextricably linked. Dock was a common sight on picket lines and at suffrage parades and rallies. She marched in support of the shirtwaist strike, a massive demonstration of New York garment workers (mostly female) that resulted in improved conditions in factories. She spoke to the ANA convention in 1913 urging nurses to support the union movement. She also publicly supported Margaret Sanger's crusades to bring birth control information to all women.

Each nurse is created by the particular social, economic, and political realities of the time that they live in, and each nurse must be held accountable for the future of nursing. Passive acceptance of the status quo will not elevate the status of nursing or enhance the quality of nursing care. Nurses today can look to the nurses in the past for inspiration, and must make a commitment to becoming politically competent and taking action to influence the realities of nursing today.

Making a Difference Through Political Activism

So, how do you wade in? How do you begin to have influence over the myriad of policies, laws, and regulations imposed by government agencies and private sector institutions? How do you hone those newly recognized political competencies? There are multiple ways to become actively involved, ranging from the simple to compensated full-time roles. Examples are discussed in the following sections.

Vote

The first and strongest step you must take, and this is not negotiable, you must *vote*. If you are not yet registered, go to http://www.declareyourself.com for state-by-state information on voter laws and how to register to vote. Without the vote, nurses are not empowered to choose, support, and vote into office a candidate who can support nursing and patient-friendly healthcare legislation. Voting is free and is a democratic right.

Become Familiar with the Nurse Practice Act

Obtain a copy of and become familiar with the ANA's *Scope and Standards of Nursing Practice* and your state's nurse practice act. You must be knowledgeable about state and federal regulations related to your practice, including nurse licensure requirements. Your right to practice and how you practice is outlined in the nurse practice act, which is ultimately governed by the state legislature. It is also important for nurses to keep themselves updated on any changes in their board of nursing's rules, regulations, and practice acts. You can do this by reading the board's newsletters or its Web site. If you do not know your board's Web site address, you can access it from the National Council of State Boards of Nursing website at http://www.ncsbn.org. You can also attend meetings at your state board of nursing.

Join Your Professional Organization

Another step to take is to join your professional or specialty organization. Joining a professional nursing organization is an important way to enhance individual advocacy efforts. Professional nursing organizations are great resources for ideas and venues for networking and sharing concerns. Professional nursing organizations are able to monitor legislation and offer ways for their members to learn about health policy. They also serve as a resource for information from a nursing perspective related to policy issues and policy makers.

Go to the Internet and look at your state nursing organization's Web site. You will find information about legislative bills and proposed regulations that can affect nursing practice or the health of our patients. State nursing organizations and specialty nursing organizations also list ways for nurses to get involved, or you can sign up to receive email updates and action alerts.

Some state nursing and specialty nursing organizations sponsor annual state legislative days, offer policy internships or fellowships, and conduct policy workshops, all designed to give nurses the opportunity to learn more about current healthcare issues and the legislative process.

Review How a Bill Becomes a Law

Most high school government classes cover the steps involved in bringing an idea through the legislative process to become a law or regulation. Nurses need to understand these steps so they can intervene with appropriate timing and actions. One recommended site to review this content is http://www.votesmart.org.

Contact Your Legislators

Legislators often know little about nursing and health care. That's why we need to tell them what we expect from them. Be assured that doctors, hospitals, and other special interest groups are doing just that. Common advocacy activities include letter writing, emails, phone calls, and in-person visits to state and federal senators and representatives. So how do you get started?

First, know the names and contact information of your local council members, state representatives, and federal senators and congresspersons. You can find your House and Senate district numbers on your voter registration card. (You have registered to vote, haven't you?) If you are unsure of the names of your state senator and representative, call your county or state election commission and give them the district numbers, or look them up on the Internet. You can also visit the legislative Web sites at http://www.senate.gov or http://www.house.gov. You may be able to sign up for email information and updates from your legislators' Web sites as well.

Every year numerous bills are introduced into the legislature that could impact your practice and patient care. *You* are the expert on nursing and patient care and your legislators value your knowledge and experience. Many legislative bodies have instituted phone message systems where you can call and leave a message for your representative. Often these calls are toll-free. You can also contact your representative by email.

While your legislators are in their home district make an appointment to meet with them. Take other nurses with you to talk about nursing issues. Invite your senator and representative to come and spend some time at your workplace. That is the ultimate way to teach them about what you do. Then when you call to ask them to vote for or against a bill that affects health care or specifically nursing practice, they will know you are their constituent.

When dealing directly with policy makers, you must be informed. Be concise and be clear about what you want. Writing a well-crafted letter, sending e-mails, leaving a written summary of your issue with staff, and sending thank-you notes are all ways to get one's legislators to consider one as an expert in healthcare and nursing issues. Remember that professional credibility and persuasion are important political skills. They can contact you when they need information related to nursing and health care.

Building Relationships and Networking

It is important to get to know the players. All too often people forget that relationship building with many diverse groups and individuals is the most effective way to gain information, to be invited to participate, and to build personal and organizational intellectual capital. Find a political mentor in your workplace or professional organization. Build community alliances. Human rights groups, crisis centers, parents, educators, social workers, and law enforcement officials can be good allies. They will welcome the expertise of a nurse and you will be able to show your cause is important to a wide range of people. Join with other nurses who share your interests and explore ways you can work together in the political process.

Engage in Workplace Activism

What about activism in your workplace? Joining an existing or new committee in local healthcare facilities can give nurses a powerful voice, especially if the committee has decision-making power, such as a quality improvement, ethics, or policy committee.

On an institutional level, policies and procedures provide basic guidelines for practice, and through participation on committees, nurses can provide input regarding important decisions that will shape nursing practice in that institution.

Put your ideas in writing. Having a written proposal shows you have researched a problem and thought about solutions. Supervisors and managers are more likely to take your suggestions seriously if you have put obvious work into them.

Stay Informed

Turn on your radar and see what nursing and healthcare issues come across the screen. Read your local newspaper, national newsmagazines, professional journals, and newsletters from organizations to which you belong. Search the Internet and check out nursing and healthcare-related Web sites. Most professional and patient advocacy groups have Web sites with excellent links to other Web sites and resources. Sign up to receive online action alerts from organizations.

Learn to Be a Lobbyist

Lobbying means educating and persuading. Nurses make particularly effective lobbyists in issues that relate to health. We bring dedication and energy to our nursing practice—qualities that are easily transferred to lobbying policy makers. Lobbying is not a difficult task, and you can exert more influence than you probably realize. Knowledge is power.

As a nurse, you bring formidable knowledge and conviction to the lobbying process. You have a strong advantage in discussing legislative issues that pertain to your specialty area and health care in general. Secondly, you have your legislator's ear because you are a valued member of his or her constituency. Put that relationship to work. Most legislators care very much about the opinions and positions of the people they represent. However, they are not mind readers. You must let your legislators know how you feel about key nursing practice or healthcare issues. Call, write, email, or visit your legislators. Tell them what action you would like them to take. Be clear, direct, and focused, and keep your message simple.

A personal visit allows you to connect names to faces. Visiting your legislator's office, either in the capital or in his or her home district, is a worthwhile effort to make. If your legislator is not available ask to meet his or her legislative aide.

Aides and other office staff serve as gatekeepers, and legislators listen to their opinions. Treat your legislator's staff respectfully and well. They can make a huge difference in whether your concerns get presented and acted upon. Remember to keep your professional organization informed about any contacts you make. This will help them plan further lobbying efforts, building on the relationships that other members develop with their lawmakers. Box 17-4 provides guidelines on how to effectively lobby your legislator.

Volunteer

Many political candidates maintain Web sites where you can volunteer to work on their campaigns. The Web sites often have a link that enables you to check off the activities you are willing to do. For instance, you can do as little as volunteer to place a sign in your yard or a bumper sticker on your car. You could sign up to be an Internet leader and send e-mail messages to friends. You could host a reception and help with fund-raising activities. Coffees, luncheons, barbecues, walkathons, and kick-off events can also be used to promote a candidate. And volunteers are always needed at the campaign office to help with phone calls and paperwork.

BOX 17-4   HOW TO LOBBY YOUR LEGISLATOR

1. Call in advance for an appointment
2. Be prepared
    a. Be aware of your own prejudices and biases
    b. If you are representing an organization, be well versed on their positions
3. Know your legislator
    a. Try to understand the basis for his/her position
    b. Know his/her record on related legislation
    c. Know his/her constituency pressures
4. Know your issue
    a. Use your own words
    b. Admit when you don't know something and get back to them
    c. Know the status of pertinent legislation
5. Be brief and courteous
6. Identify yourself and establish your own credentials and expertise
7. Give them succinct, easy-to-read literature
8. Express your appreciation for your legislator's interest and support
9. Leave your business card or contact information
10. Follow up with a telephone call or letter within a week

Source: League of Women Voters, 1996.

Donate to a Cause or Political Campaign

Time, people, and money are the resources that fuel most political activities. When we cannot afford time or recruit a group of people, we can contribute money toward a cause or candidate that supports our beliefs. Our donations support media purchases, travel, salaries, and the other costs of getting work done. Financial support of any amount is valued in electoral or issue campaigns.

Run for Office

Nurses make excellent elected officials. Our interpersonal and analytical skills equip us to connect with the constituency and understand complex issues. Ethical behaviors that guide our practice are refreshing standards in office. Possible roles can range from county health boards and professional organizations to state and national legislative bodies.

Summary

Political activism provides the vehicle for social change. It can take one from "something needs to be done" to "look what we have accomplished together." This chapter discussed the skills, perspectives, and values that comprise political competence and why political competence is needed in nursing. Strategies were presented to help nurses craft their own unique expression of political competence. Nurses have or can develop the skills needed for effective political action. Political discussions need and benefit from nursing's values. When we don't fulfill this professional responsibility we lose the opportunity to improve health through policy, to control our practice, and to find the enjoyment of making a difference. How you choose to express your political competence is less important than the fact that you do it.

Key Terms

- **Health policy:** Policy decisions that are made to promote the health of individuals.
- **Institutional policy:** Policy that governs a workplace and describes an institution's goals and how it will operate.
- **Organizational policy:** Policy that articulates positions taken by an organization.
- **Policy:** A plan to guide action or decisions.
- **Political activism:** Direct and collective participation in strategies toward specific societal goals; for nursing, this action is based on explicit professional values and focuses on enhancing health.
- **Political competence:** The skills, perspectives, and values needed for effective political involvement.
- **Politics:** Influencing the allocation of scarce resources (Mason, Leavitt, and Chafee, 2007).
- **Public policy:** Policy formed by governmental bodies (i.e., local, state, and federal legislation) and the regulations written from that policy.
- **Social policy:** Policy decisions that are made to promote the welfare of the public.

Reflective Practice Questions

1. Who do you know who models political competence in a professional environment? Have you seen political competence modeled in nursing practice?
2. What mentors do you have who are assisting you to develop your own political competence? If you don't have a mentor, can you identify someone who would be willing to help you develop your political skills?
3. What propels you toward political action? What inspires you to effect change?
4. How can you promote health and improve quality of life through political activism?
5. Do you believe you can make a difference? What steps will you take to realize your potential for making a difference?
6. When you identify an issue that requires action, how would you go about joining with others to effect change?

References

Abood, S. (2007). Influencing health care in the legislative arena. *Journal of Issues in Nursing, 12*(1). Retrieved July 25, 2008, from http://www.nursingworld.org/ MainMenu Categories/ANAMarketplace/ANAPeriodicals/OJIN/TableofContents/Volume122007/ No1Jan07/tpc32_216091.aspx

American Association of Colleges of Nursing. (1998). *The essentials of baccalaureate education for professional nursing practice.* Washington, DC: Author.

American Nurses Association. (n.d.). *Hall of fame inductees.* Retrieved July 25, 2008, from http://www.nursingworld.org/FunctionalMenuCategories/AboutANA/WhereWe ComeFrom_1/HallofFame/20002004Inductees.aspx

Artz, M. (2006). The politics of caring: Ask not what nursing can do for you. *American Journal of Nursing, 106*(9), 91.

Cherry, B. & Trotter Betts, V. (2005).Health policy and politics: Get involved! In B. Cherry & S. Jacobs (eds.), *Contemporary nursing: Issues, trends & management* (pp. 211–233). St. Louis, MO: Elsevier Inc.

Fagin, C. M. (2000). Foreword. In H. R. Feldman & S. B. Lewenson (eds.), *Nurses in the political arena: The public face of nursing* (pp. ix–xi). New York: Springer.

Feldman, H. R., & Lewenson, S. B. (2000). *Nurses in the political arena: The public face of nursing.* New York: Springer.

Gebbie, K. M., Wakefield, M., & Kerfoot, K. (2000). Nursing and health policy. *Journal of Nursing Scholarship, 32*(3), 309–315.

Henry Street Settlement. (n.d.). Retrieved August 1, 2007, from http://www.henrystreet. org

League of Women Voters. (1996). *How to lobby your legislator.* Retrieved August 1, 2007, from http://www.lwv.org/pubs/how_lobby_your_leg.html

Mason, D. J., Leavitt, J. K., & Chaffee, M. W. (2007). *Policy and politics in nursing and health care* (5th ed.). St. Louis: Saunders.

Mick, S. (2004). The physician surplus and the decline of professional dominance. *Journal of Health Politics, Policy and Law, 20*(4–5), 643–659.

Milstead, J. A. (2004). *Health policy and politics: A nurse's guide* (2nd ed.). Boston: Jones & Bartlett.

Rains, J., and Barton-Kreise, P. (2001). Developing political competence: A comparative study across disciplines. *Public Health Nursing, 18* (4), July–August 2001, pp. 219–224.

Reutter, L., & Duncan, S. (2002). Preparing nurses to promote health-enhancing public policies. *Policy, Politics & Nursing Practice, 3*(4), 294–305.

Reutter, L., & Williamson, D. L. (2000). Advocating healthy public policy: Implications for baccalaureate nursing education. *Journal of Nursing Education, 39*(1), 21–26.

Thomas, S., Billington, A., & Getliffe, K. (2004). Improving continence services—a case study in policy influence. *Journal of Nursing Management, 12*, 252–257.

U.S. Department of Health and Human Services. (2004). *Preliminary findings: 2004 national sample survey of registered nurses.* Retrieved July 25, 2008, from ftp://ftp.hrsa. gov/bhpr/nursing/rnpopulation/theregisterednursepopulation.pdf

Warner, J. R. (2003). A phenomenological approach to political competence: Stories of nurse activists. *Politics, Policy and Nursing Practice, 4*(2), 135–143.

Whitehead, D. (2003). Incorporating socio-political health promotion activities in clinical practice. *Journal of Clinical Nursing, 12*(5), 668–677.

Urban Healthcare Issues

Nena R. Harris and Mary R. Nichols

LEARNING OUTCOMES

After reading this chapter you will be able to:

- Discuss a brief history of population-based nursing.
- Discuss the impact of the environment on the health of individuals and communities.
- Identify selected healthcare issues that place urban residents at risk for poor health outcomes.
- Discuss the role of the nurse in improving health outcomes in urban areas.
- Apply the nursing process to interventions aimed at improving the health of individuals and communities.

Introduction

The Industrial Revolution began at the end of the 18th century and started the process of urbanization in cities across the United States as people left rural areas and moved to cities to take advantage of the many new opportunities. The Industrial Revolution created jobs that were not available in rural towns as advancements were made in agriculture, coal mining, textiles, steam power, and transportation. With the migration of people to urban cities, the influence of the environment on health and well-being began to become apparent. The quality of air and water, food choices, employment choices, family structure and support, housing quality, and access to healthcare services are all factors impacting the health of urban residents (Galea, Freudenberg, & Vlahov, 2005).

The U.S. Census Bureau (2006) has based the most recent classifications of urban and rural cities on the 2000 census. An **urban area** is defined as one that has a population of at least 1,000 persons per square mile or surrounding areas with at least 500 persons per square mile. Any areas outside of these two classifications are considered rural. According to 2000 census data, the five largest urban cities in America are New York, Los Angeles, Chicago, Houston, and Philadelphia. Table 18-1 shows the population of the top 10 urban cities in the United States as well as their population per square mile.

This chapter will introduce you to some of the health issues that are common in urban cities. First, a brief history and background of public health nurses as promoters of health in urban cities will be discussed. Next, an overview of selected

TABLE 18-1 POPULATION OF THE TOP 10 URBAN CITIES IN AMERICA

City	Population in 2000	Population per Square Mile
New York, NY	8,008,278	26,403
Los Angeles, CA	3,694,820	7,877
Chicago, IL	2,896,016	12,750
Houston, TX	1,953,631	3,372
Philadelphia, PA	1,517,550	11,233
Phoenix, AZ	1,321,045	2,782
San Diego, CA	1,223,400	3,772
Dallas, TX	1,188,580	3,470
San Antonio, TX	1,144,646	2,808
Detriot, MI	951,270	6,855

Source: U.S. Census Bureau. (2004). *United States summary: 2000 population and housing counts (Part 1).* Retrieved May 20, 2007, from http://www.census.gov/prod/cen2000/phc3-us-pt1.pdf.

risk factors that contribute to poor health outcomes in urban cities will be presented. Finally, this chapter will end with an application of the nursing process in a discussion of the role of nurses in improving the health of urban residents.

Public Health Nursing: A History of Prevention and Health Promotion

Public health nurses have long played a role in recognizing the impact that the urban environment has had on the health of residents and addressing the health problems that often accompany urbanization. Early public health nurses focused on improving unsanitary conditions caused by inadequate water treatment systems further burdened by overcrowding.

Florence Nightingale was perhaps one of the earliest public health nurses. Known as the founder of modern nursing, Nightingale is known for her early work in England improving the conditions of her patients during the Crimean War (Chinn & Kramer, 2004). Although not officially labeled a public health nurse, Nightingale's observations—published in *Notes on Nursing* in 1680—reflected an understanding of the importance of assessing one's environment as a possible factor contributing to the health of the individual as well as the population. Her work is a representation of the understanding of health in the early 19th century. This time period is known as the Sanitation Era, during which contaminated water, sewage, and poor ventilation were thought to be the main determinants of health (MacDonald, 2004). Nightingale recognized the impact that poor sanitation had on the health of individuals and took the steps necessary to alleviate the environmental threats to her patients' health; preventing illness was accomplished through careful personal hygiene, air quality, and water purification (Chinn & Kramer; MacDonald).

Later in the 19th century, theories about the causes of illness shifted from poor sanitation to the presence of infectious microorganisms (MacDonald, 2004). During this time, public health efforts were aimed at the development of vaccinations and antibiotics that would prevent and treat a variety of acute infectious diseases such as polio, pertussis, and diphtheria; advancements in health care have since made infectious illnesses that once plagued urban cities a rare occurrence (Stern & Markel, 2004; Tomes, 2000). Unfortunately, not all infectious diseases have been eradicated by vaccines or immunizations; and many still affect those living in urban cities (Stern & Markel). Examples of these are tuberculosis and many sexually transmitted diseases (Tomes). It was during this time that **public health nursing** became an official field within modern nursing in the United States, with Lillian Wald being credited as the founder (Jewish Women's Archive [JWA], 2007; MacDonald). She used the term *public health nurse* to describe those nurses who conducted their

> **KEY TERM**
>
> **Public health nursing:** The field of nursing that specializes in improving the health care of the community or individuals in the community setting.

CONTEMPORARY PRACTICE HIGHLIGHT 18-1

HIV/AIDS

Human immunodeficiency virus (HIV) is the virus that causes acquired immune deficiency syndrome (AIDS). It is most commonly transmitted by sexual contact and use of needles that are contaminated by blood. HIV affects the immune system, attacking white blood cells and making it a challenge for infected individuals to fight off disease. AIDS is the final stage of infection and is characterized by a severely weakened immune system. In this stage of the infection, T cells are low in number and infections begin to invade the body.

HIV was first recognized in the United States in homosexual men in the early 1980s. Since this time, however, rates of HIV infection have increased disproportionately among minority men and women. Today, HIV/AIDS is a leading cause of death for both African American men and women; for African American women ages 25–34 years, HIV/AIDS is the number one cause of death (Anderson & Smith, 2005). Although African Americans make up only 13 percent of the U.S. population, they accounted for almost half of new diagnoses of HIV/AIDS in 2005 (Centers for Disease Control and Prevention [CDC], 2007a). According to the CDC, reasons for this disparity include poverty, beliefs in the African American community that lead to non-disclosure of homosexual activity and lack of testing for HIV, increased rates of other sexually transmitted diseases, and injection drug use. Currently, HIV/AIDS is the sixth leading cause of death for all racial groups for individuals ages 25–44 years (Miniño, Heron, & Smith, 2006).

Historically, HIV has been significantly more prevalent in urban cities; rates of infection increase as city population increases. Tables 18-2 and 18-3 illustrate the relationship between city population and AIDS cases and the racial disparities for AIDS.

TABLE 18-2 CURRENT RATES AND CUMULATIVE NUMBER OF AIDS CASES BY POPULATION SIZE, 2005

City Population	AIDS Cases per 100,000	Cumulative Number of Cases
Non-metropolitan (<50,000)	6.4	48,708
50,000 to 500,000	9.3	83,372
>500,000	21.1	777,929

Source: Centers for Disease Control and Prevention (2007b). *HIV/AIDS surveillance in urban and nonurban areas.* National Center for HIV/AIDS, Viral Hepatitis, STD, and TB Prevention. Retrieved September 15, 2007, from http://www.cdc.gov/hiv/topics/surveillance/resources/slides/urban-nonurban/

(continues)

CONTEMPORARY PRACTICE HIGHLIGHT 18-1 (continued)

TABLE 18-3   RACIAL DISPARITIES IN HIV/AIDS CASES BY POPULATION SIZE, 2005

City Population	African American Residents with AIDS	White Residents with AIDS
Non-metropolitan (<50,000)	1,265	1,066
50,000 to 500,000	1,939	1,674
>500,000	16,558	9,195

Source: Centers for Disease Control and Prevention. (2007b). *HIV/AIDS surveillance in urban and non-urban areas.* National Center for HIV/AIDS, Viral Hepatitis, STD, and TB Prevention Retrieved September 15, 2007, from http://www.cdc.gov/hiv/topics/surveillance/resources/slides/urban-nonurban/

care of patients outside of the hospital and within the communities where their patients lived.

Wald is recognized for her role in establishing the Visiting Nurses Service and the Henry Street Settlement in New York City (American Nurses Association [ANA], 2007; JWA, 2007). The Henry Street Settlement, which served as a central station for nurses to see patients and conduct home visits, was founded in 1893. Less than 10 years after its establishment, 18 additional nursing centers were created in order to serve other communities in and around Manhattan and the Bronx. The district centers served more than 4,500 patients a year in 1903; by 1915, settlement nurses treated more than 26,575 patients and conducted more than 227,000 home visits. The history of the Henry Street Settlement is recorded in *The House on Henry Street*, published by Wald in 1915 (JWA, 2007).

Wald began her work in the lower east side settlements of New York City teaching hygiene to its residents (JWA, 2007). However, later in her nursing career, Wald's work began to shift from a focus on the health of individuals to advocating for the residents as a community. She helped to establish a neighborhood playground for children in the settlement who had no source of safe outdoor recreation; this playground became the first municipal playground in New York City (JWA). She also advocated for the hiring of school nurses in New York's public schools, fought for the establishment of a school lunch program (JWA), and worked to improve child labor laws (ANA, 2007). Furthermore, Wald fought for the rights of women in the workplace and was a supporter of New York's women's voting rights (JWA). Not only was Wald influential in addressing the healthcare and sociopolitical needs of New York City's residents, she also helped to educate and train future public health nurses and later became the first president of the National Organization of Public Health Nurses. This professional organization was established to provide practice standards and an advocating body for the growing number of public health nurses (JWA).

The progression from a focus on sanitation and hygiene to a more comprehensive view of the environment reflected society's developing understanding of the factors that influence health. By the middle of the 20th century, causes of death and morbidity shifted from acute infectious diseases to chronic illnesses such as cardiovascular disease, cancer, and diabetes (MacDonald, 2004; Tomes, 2000). The causes of these chronic illnesses were more complex and could not be isolated to a single cause. Chronic diseases are linked to a combination of biological/genetic, psychological, emotional, lifestyle/behavioral, sociopolitical, and environmental factors; the combination of these factors and the relative contribution of each factor vary from one person to the next (MacDonald). Despite the fact that infectious diseases can be linked to a specific contagion, all of these factors contribute to both acute and chronic diseases. In the same way that these factors determine the presence of chronic illness, they also determine the exposure and vulnerability of a person or population to an infectious microorganism as well as subsequent survival (MacDonald). How some of these factors play a role in selected health risks will be discussed in more detail later in this chapter.

When preventing illness and promoting the health of urban residents, it is important to maintain a comprehensive perspective that includes all of the potential factors that may contribute to the health of the individual and population. The next section will present several specific factors that are characteristic of urban cities that will help to inform the nurse caring for patients in an urban setting.

The Urban Environment: An Overview of Selected Risk Factors

The urban environment offers opportunities for increased job availability as well as challenges in public health issues. Risk factors that accompany urban environments are discussed including poverty, pollution, infant mortality, crime, gun safety, and violence.

Poverty

Despite the increased opportunities for employment that exist in urban cities, poverty resulting from underemployment or unemployment plagues urban cities and is more concentrated in inner-city urban neighborhoods (Curley, 2005). As a

> **CONTEMPORARY PRACTICE HIGHLIGHT 18-2**
>
> **LEADING HEALTH INDICATORS**
>
> The Office of Disease Prevention and Health Promotion has identified 10 health indicators that represent areas of public health concern in the United States. These Leading Health Indicators are:
>
> - Physical activity
> - Overweight and obesity
> - Tobacco use
> - Substance abuse
> - Responsible sexual behavior
> - Mental health
> - Injury and violence
> - Environmental quality
> - Immunization
> - Access to health care
>
>   Visit the Web sites for the National Center for Health Statistics and Healthy People 2010 for more information on these and other issues in urban cities at http://www.cdc.gov/nchs/datawh/nchsdefs/healthypeople2010.htm.

result, homelessness and other problems related to poverty affect many families. The definition of poverty used by the U.S. Census Bureau (2007) accounts for the income of a household and number of family members living in the household. A person or family is living in poverty when they earn an income less than the set threshold. Recent reports indicate growing economic inequality; those who live in poverty have become more poor in recent years (Aron-Dine, 2007; Center on Budget and Policy Priorities, 2004). The percentage of poor people living in poverty, as well as the severity of poverty, was greater in 2003 than in any other year since 1975 (Center on Budget and Policy Priorities). Despite a recent lack of growth in the median income, the incomes of those earning at the high end of the spectrum rose significantly, contributing more to economic inequality (Aron-Dine, 2007; Center on Budget and Policy Priorities). Table 18-4 provides examples of the 2006 **poverty threshold**s for families of varying types.

Growing economic inequality is especially evident in urban cities, where poverty is concentrated in inner-city neighborhoods (Curley, 2005; Earls, 2000; Wilson, 2003). One of the theories that helps to explain the concentration of poverty in urban cities is based on the movement of manufacturing

KEY TERM

Poverty threshold: An income amount set by the government that accounts for household size and earnings. A family whose income falls below this threshold is considered to be living in poverty.

TABLE 18-4	POVERTY THRESHOLDS FOR 2006 FOR VARIOUS FAMILY TYPE
Family Type	2006 Poverty Threshold
Over 65 years old, living alone	$ 9,669
Over 65 years old, married couple	$ 12,186
Single mother with 2 children	$ 16,242
Single mother with 4 children	$ 23,691
Married couple with 2 children	$ 20,444
Married couple with 4 children	$ 26,938

Source: U.S. Census Bureau, Housing and Household Economic Statistics Division. (2007). *Poverty definitions.* Retrieved August 1, 2007, from http://www.census.gov/hhes/www/poverty/definitions.html

KEY TERM

Decentralization: A process occurring in urban cities in which employment opportunities and social capital move into suburban areas. This process is suggested to be one of the causes of urban poverty.

and industrial jobs—once prevalent in urban cities—to suburban or rural areas. This process, known as **decentralization**, resulted in an increase in service-oriented jobs in urban cities; jobs such as those in health care, education, and information technology require skills and training that individuals formerly employed in low-wage, entry-level jobs did not have (Curley; Rankin & Quane, 2000; Wilson). Those with low-paying jobs often do not have the resources to commute to entry-level jobs that have been moved to suburban or rural areas, resulting in a lack of jobs for those with low skills in urban cities.

Due to decentralization, segregation of urban neighborhoods has also increased (based primarily on education and income), resulting in fewer and fewer resources in low-income neighborhoods (Wilson, 2003). Furthermore, the migration of middle- and working-class families out of inner-city neighborhoods into suburban areas further contributed to urban poverty by removing vital social networks and stability that once buffered many of the ill effects of poverty (Rankin & Quane, 2000). This absence of social capital and role modeling led to the deterioration of neighborhood organizations that reinforced social mores that valued education, gainful employment, and family cohesiveness (Curley, 2005; Rankin & Quane; Wilson).

Unemployed individuals and those employed in low-wage jobs have similar chances of being unemployed in the future (Stewart, 2007); simply being employed does not protect one from future unemployment and poverty if the job is one with low earnings. In fact, low-wage jobs may lead one down the path of future unemployment, especially if the low-wage job was preceded by a period of unemployment (Stewart).

It is important to note that urban cities offer many benefits in regards to health care, education, and social and psychological well-being (Galea et al., 2005; Vlahov, Galea, & Freudenberg, 2005; Wilson, 2003). It is for this reason that many rural residents are prompted to relocate to urban cities. Unfortunately, relocation from rural to urban cities does not always facilitate mobility out of poverty for unemployed or low-wage workers coming from rural areas; mobility out of poverty is low for those who are unemployed or low-wage workers even for rural-to-urban migrants and especially for African Americans (Mauldin & Mimura, 2001; Mimura & Mauldin, 2005). The presence of concentrated poverty in urban cities has created a dichotomy of haves and have-nots, in which case the urban poor are excluded from many of the benefits of urban life (Mercado, Havemann, Sami, & Ueda, 2007). Concentrated poverty is associated with poor health, high crime, and violence (Earls, 2000), as well as drug activity and use (Fishbein et al., 2006; Freisthler, Lascala, Gruenewald, & Treno, 2005; Khan, Murray, & Barnes, 2002). Health care for the poor is limited due to lack of insurance coverage, which has decreased in recent years due to the decline in employer-based coverage and the rising costs of insurance premiums (Center on Budget and Policy Priorities, 2004). Fear of crime severely diminishes the mental well-being and quality of life for impoverished urban residents (Earls, 2000), as does drug use. Nurses working with urban residents must be aware of the factors that contribute to poverty for many of its residents and its associated health-related outcomes.

The Urban Structural Environment

Substandard housing is a major problem in U.S. urban cities, which are often characterized by aging, deteriorating buildings and other poor environmental conditions (Jackson, 1998). Low-income and minority families are disproportionately the victims of inadequate and substandard housing that exposes them to such conditions as high lead levels, poor heating or cooling, roach and rodent infestation, and unsafe electrical wiring (Bashir, 2002; Kjellstrom et al., 2007). Not only does housing in urban cities affect the health status of urban residents, but the higher prevalence of convenience stores, fast food restaurants, and liquor stores in urban cities and neighborhoods makes unhealthy choices easily accessible and healthy ones more difficult to maintain (Bashir). Dependence on public transportation and motor vehicle transportation has contributed to increasing rates of obesity due to lack of physical activity and the convenience of obtaining unhealthy meals via the drive-throughs of fast food restaurants

Air pollution (mostly from automobiles, buses, and other types of urban transportation) is a primary cause of increased asthma and other respiratory illnesses

CONTEMPORARY PRACTICE HIGHLIGHT 18-3

LEAD POISONING

Efforts at decreasing incidence of lead exposure and poisoning, mainly in children, over the last 30 years have been largely successful. A variety of organizations joined together to decrease the amount of lead poisoning that plagued urban neighborhoods. Some of these organizations included the Environmental Protection Agency, the Department of Housing and Urban Development, the Food and Drug Administration, and the Consumer Product Safety Commission. Together, the efforts of these organizations have led to the removal of lead from gasoline, paint, food cans, and toys (Jackson, 1998). Furthermore, the medical community played a large role in the early screening of children and in educating parents about the dangers of lead poisoning (Jackson), which include developmental, neurological, and intellectual deficits (Bashir, 2002). However, more than 1 million children continue to be affected each year. These children are disproportionately residents of urban neighborhoods and aging, substandard housing. Continued efforts are needed in order to continue to prevent lead poisoning, screen for exposure, and educate parents on protecting their children from the dangers of lead.

in urban cities (Akinbami, 2006; Frumkin, 2002). Traffic emissions have resulted in increases in air pollution and contribute to up to 60,000 respiratory-related deaths per year in the United States (Galea et al., 2005). Adverse respiratory-related outcomes include poor lung function, hospitalizations, increased medication use, school/work absenteeism, and death (Frumkin). Asthma, the most prevalent respiratory illness, disproportionately affects urban residents (Jackson, 1998); triggers for asthma and other respiratory illnesses that are prevalent in urban cities include traffic emissions, cigarette smoke, mold, and droppings from cockroaches and rodents found in substandard housing (Bashir, 2002; Peters, Levy, Rogers, Burge, & Spengler, 2007). It is estimated that 6.5 million children in the United States suffer from asthma (National Center for Health Statistics, 2007). Asthma also affects poor children and black children disproportionately; the disparity between white and African American children has increased in recent years (Akinbami, 2006) and may be a reflection of the increasing concentration of poverty and racial segregation evident in inner-city urban neighborhoods (Bashir). Almost 16 million adults currently suffer from asthma (National Center for Health Statistics). Although many urban residents are affected in some way, those with pre-existing cardiopulmonary disease, the elderly, and the young are most vulnerable to the effects of air pollution present in urban cities (Frumkin).

In addition to air pollution, the quantity of automobiles and other forms of transportation have contributed to the incidence of motor vehicle accidents (MVAs) in urban cities (Frumkin, 2002). The quantity of people relying on transportation and the increased need for commuting to work signify an increased exposure to potential MVAs for urban residents. Increased suburban living with travel into the city for employment increases the risks for MVAs while inner city residents reliant on public transportation are at risk for pedestrian accidents (Frumkin). Although the most densely populated urban cities—when compared to less densely populated cities—seem to have created systems that result in lower rates of MVA and pedestrian deaths, the relative number of all vehicle-related deaths in urban cities remains costly (Frumkin). Automobile-related accidents are the number one cause of death in people ages 1–24 years (Frumkin; Miniño et al., 2006).

Tuberculosis

Tuberculosis (TB) is a respiratory illness caused by the airborne transmission of the bacteria *Mycobacterium tuberculosis* (National Institute of Allergy and Infectious Diseases [NIAID], 2006). The incidence of TB is higher in urban areas primarily due to the ease of transmission among people living in crowded environments (Galea et al., 2005). Specifically, TB is easily transmitted in places such as prisons, homeless shelters, and long-term care facilities for the elderly. Furthermore, individuals living in these environments often have compromised immune systems due to poor nutrition as well as alcohol and drug abuse (NIAID). On average, there is an increase in TB cases as the population increases; this is a reflection of a mechanism of transmission that is facilitated by increases in population (see Table 18-5).

Maternal and Child Health

Maternal and child health indicators are a reflection of the quality and efficacy of care provided to childbearing women and their children (Save the Children, 2007).

TABLE 18-5 COMPARISON OF TB CASES

Cities with ≥1 Million Residents[+]	TB Cases per 100,000[*]	Cities with ≤600,000 Residents[+]	TB Cases per 100,000[*]
New York, NY	11.3	Nashville, TN	7.5
Los Angeles, CA	9.8	Portland, OR	3.5
Chicago, IL	6.4	Oklahoma City, OK	5.0
Houston, TX	9.1	Las Vega, NV	5.0
Philadelphia, PA	4.2	Tucson, AZ	3.6

+ Based on 2000 Census Data

* Centers for Disease Control and Prevention, 2005

Often, indicators such as infant mortality, maternal morbidity, and maternal mortality are used in comparing healthcare systems around the world. Prenatal care, aimed at reducing maternal and infant morbidity and mortality, is the provision of services during pregnancy aimed at screening for, monitoring, and treating potential complications in the mother and baby (National Center for Health Statistics, 2006). Ideally, prenatal care should begin in the first trimester of pregnancy and continue until the birth of the baby. Unfortunately, the United States has been unable to prevent many of the maternal and fetal complications of pregnancy when compared to other developed countries, despite the steadily increasing healthcare dollars invested in obstetrical care in this country. One of the reasons for this trend is the constellation of social, psychological, and environmental factors that influence the health of mothers and babies in addition to physical factors (CDC, 2007c). In urban areas, some of these additional factors may play a different role in the everyday lives of women than in rural areas. These might include previously discussed factors such as poverty, challenges in accessing healthcare services, fear of crime, discrimination, drug use, and employment in low-skilled, physically demanding jobs (Earls, 2000; Freisthler et al., 2005; Mercado et al., 2007). All of these factors play a role in the pregnancy-related health outcomes of infants and mothers.

Maternal morbidity is defined as the presence of any pregnancy-related complication or disorder that potentially threatens the health of the mother and the fetus she is carrying (CDC, 2007c). Such disorders can occur during or after pregnancy and include ectopic pregnancy, gestational diabetes, gestational hypertension and pre-eclampsia, pregnancy-related cardiomyopathies, breast and uterine infections, postpartum hemorrhage, and depression. The most severe pregnancy-related complication is maternal death. According to a report from the National Center for Health Statistics (Hoyert, 2007), the **maternal mortality rate** in 1915 was 608 deaths per 100,000 live births; in 2003, the rate was 12 deaths per 100,000 live births. After a drastic decline in recent decades, reported maternal deaths are on the rise, likely due in part to changes in reporting classifications (National Center for Health Statistics, 2006). True estimates of maternal mortality and other maternal/child health indicators fluctuate due to differences in reporting systems and identification of the events represented by these indicators.

Infant mortality is defined as the death of a child one year or younger. The **infant mortality rate (IMR)** is calculated for the number of infant deaths per 100,000 live births. The United States, despite being one of the most medically advanced countries in the world, has an infant mortality rate much higher than other developed countries. Table 18-6 displays the 2002 IMRs for selected developed and developing countries. The United States is currently ranked 26th in the world for its IMR (Save the Children, 2007).

KEY TERM

Maternal mortality rate: The number of maternal deaths per 100,000 live births. Maternal deaths are those that occur during pregnancy or within 42 days after the pregnancy has ended.

KEY TERM

Infant mortality rate (IMR): The number of infant deaths per 100,000 live births. Infant deaths are those that occur during the child's first year of life.

TABLE 18-6   INFANT MORTALITY RATES OF SELECTED DEVELOPED AND DEVELOPING COUNTRIES, 2002

Country	Infant Mortality Rate (per 100,000 live births)
Developed countries	9
Developing countries	58
Japan	3
France	4
Germany	4
Netherlands	4
Singapore	4
Australia	5
Canada	5
Czech Republic	5
Spain	5
Greece	6
United States	7
Cuba	7
South Korea	7
Russia	20
Mexico	25
North Korea	27
Ghana	54
Haiti	78
Ethiopia	104
Liberia	134
Afghanistan	145

Source: Save the Children, 2007.

Some of the leading causes of infant mortality include congenital malformations, deformations, and chromosomal abnormalities; conditions related to preterm birth (less than 37 weeks gestation) and low birth weight (less than 2,500 grams); sudden infant death syndrome; effects of maternal complications during pregnancy; respiratory distress; and effects of complications of the placenta, umbilical cord, and membranes (Miniño et al., 2006).

Rates of preterm birth and low birth weight are similar in the largest U.S. cities and the most rural cities (i.e., those not in close proximity to a metropolitan area; Hillemeier, Weisman, Chase, & Dyer, 2007); however, urban cities are characterized by significant variations in infant health indicators across racial groups. Congenital malformations and chromosomal abnormalities were the leading cause of infant mortality in 2002, the latest year the data are currently available (NCHS). Together, preterm birth and low birth weight comprise the second leading cause of all infant mortality; for infants born to African American mothers, preterm birth and low birth weight are the leading causes of infant mortality (Miniño et al., 2006). Preliminary reports of 2004 data indicate that the IMR for all African American infants was nearly 2.5 times the IMR for white infants (13.65 vs. 5.65, respectively; Miniño et al.). Furthermore, the racial disparity in infant mortality is, in part, a reflection of the higher rates of preterm birth and low birth weight among African American infants. This disparity persists in infants born to college-educated African American women when compared to those born to white women with similar socioeconomic status, indicating the presence of other complex factors (e.g., racial segregation) that may interact and play a role in infant mortality. According to 2003 data, the IMR for infants born to African American mothers with 13 or more years of education was 11.2; the rate for infants born to white mothers with the same educational background was 4.3 (National Center for Health Statistics, 2006).

The third leading cause of infant mortality is sudden infant death syndrome (SIDS), despite significant decreases in SIDS since the late 1980s (Miniño et al., 2006). During this time, the American Association of Pediatrics issued a statement detailing the risks of placing infants to sleep on their stomachs and recommended that infants be placed on their backs to sleep (National Institute of Child Health and Human Development [NICHHD], 2006). According to the NICHHD, the back-to-sleep campaign has contributed to a decrease of over 50 percent of deaths from SIDS by changing the behaviors of parents; however, other causes of SIDS—such as environmental smoke and pollution prevalent in urban environments—have proven more difficult to change and continue to contribute to the deaths of infants.

Crime and Safety

Criminal activity has long characterized urban cities and is cited by many as a reason to avoid urban cities and reside in suburban or rural areas. Criminal activity invokes fear in urban residents, contributing to social isolation, anxiety, and stress, all of which have a negative effect on physical and mental health (Earls, 2000). Trends in criminal activity statistics indicate that as the population increases, so does crime. According to the Bureau of Justice Statistics (2007), large cities with more than 1 million residents have the highest crime rates; those with fewer than 250,000 residents have the lowest rates among urban cities. From 1976 to 2005, more than 50 percent of all homicides have been committed in large cities (those with more than 100,000 residents). Nearly 25 percent of homicides were committed in large cities with over 1 million residents . Furthermore, the types of crimes committed vary by geographic location. The largest cities tend to have higher numbers of drug- and gang-related homicides, whereas family- and work-related homicides characterize smaller cities (those with less than 100,000 residents; see Table 18-7). In 2005, rural areas had a higher relative number of intimate homicides than small cities

TABLE 18-7 PERCENTAGE OF HOMICIDES COMMITTED, BY URBANICITY, 1976–2005

Type of Homicide	Large Cities	Suburban Areas	Small Cities	Rural Areas
All homicides	57.3%	21.0%	11.5%	10.2%
Gang-related	69.3%	16.9%	13.1%	0.7%
Drug-related	67.4%	18.1%	9.9%	4.5%
Gun	59.3%	19.8%	10.6%	10.4%
Intimate partner	40.7%	28.0%	14.5%	16.8%
Family member	38.7%	29.1%	13.2%	19.0%
Workplace	31.4%	37.2%	13.4%	17.9%

Source: Bureau of Justice Statistics. (2007, July 11). *Homicide trends in the U.S.: Trends by city size.* U.S. Department of Justice, Office of Justice Programs. Retrieved August 5, 2007, from http://www.ojp.usdoj.gov/bjs/homicide/city.htm

Gun Safety

Gun possession may be a response to the dangers perceived by residents of urban, low-income neighborhoods (Vacha & McLaughlin, 2004). Members of households in urban cities are more likely to witness criminal acts such as homicide, gang activity, theft, home invasion, and selling of drugs. As a result, residents of urban cities—especially those in low-income neighborhoods—are more likely to fear victimization and possess a firearm in an effort to protect themselves and their families. Those who keep guns for protection (as opposed to hunting or other sporting hobbies) are more likely to keep the gun loaded and readily available for use in the event of threat of victimization. Exposure to loaded, unsecured guns leads to more accidental injuries and deaths from guns, especially among young children (Vacha & McLaughlin). Among adults, rates of intentional firearm deaths are similar in urban and rural cities. However, there is a variation in the type of firearm deaths between urban and rural cities; intentional homicides are more characteristic of urban cities, whereas suicides are more common in rural areas (Branas, Nance, Elliott, Richmond, & Schwab, 2004).

Gang Violence

As shown in Table 18-7, gang violence is a major source of crime in large cities (Bureau of Justice Statistics, 2007); in addition to homicides, gangs contribute to drug-related offenses as well as other crimes such as illegal gun possessions, vandalism, thefts, and non-fatal assaults (Vigil, 2003). A gang is defined as a group of individuals who come together for the purpose of identity, cohesion, and sense of belonging. Gangs can range in type from innocent social gatherings to those that participate in delinquency and violent behaviors (Ruble & Turner, 2000). Urban gang members, when compared to rural gang members, are more concerned about their personal safety. Urban youth in general report having more friends in gangs than rural youth, indicating a potential normalization of gang activity in urban neighborhoods (Evans, Fitzgerald, Weigel, & Chvilicek, 1999). Gang membership is influenced by concentrated poverty; hopelessness, fueled by poverty and exposure to crime, is associated with future involvement in criminal activity in adolescents (Bolland, 2003).

Families living in poor high-crime neighborhoods tend to become isolated out of fear of victimization. Parents may become either overprotective of their children as a result of this fear or, due to severe poverty, be unable to provide adequate supervision in order to deter future delinquent behavior (Tolan, Gorman-Smith, & Henry, 2003). Children, especially young boys, growing up in overprotective environments may seek out compensatory socialization as they become adolescents. Those growing up in unmonitored environments may have formed early peer groups in which delinquent behaviors are typical. In both scenarios, the formation of unhealthy ties to peers may result in increasingly delinquent gang activity and crime (Tolan et al., 2003).

Violence Against Women

Abuse during adulthood may be classified using one of several labels that describe violence during this time, including *domestic violence, spousal abuse, battering, intimate partner violence, marital rape,* and *date rape* (Manfrin-Ledet & Porche, 2003). Physical abuse is defined as the use of force with the intention of causing bodily harm; this definition encompasses such acts as punching, hitting, shaking, biting, choking, scratching, slapping, and use of restraints (CDC, 2006a). According to the Centers for Disease Control and Prevention (CDC, 2006b), acts of sexual violence include nonconsensual attempted or completed contact, intentional contact, penetration, and noncontact abuse (e.g., voyeurism, pornography, threats of abuse). Acts in which an individual is unable to consent (i.e., due to the influence of alcohol or drugs, age, or disability) or unable to refuse (i.e., due to use of weapon, physical violence, or other threats of harm) are also considered sexual violence (CDC, 2006b). The Rape, Abuse, and Incest National Network (RAINN, 2006) reports that one in six women have been sexually assaulted. Experiencing childhood and/or adult trauma in the form of physical and/or sexual abuse often sets the stage for a life that is characterized by substance abuse and participation in other behaviors that leave a woman at high risk for contracting HIV and other sexually transmitted diseases (Miller, 1999).

Resources for victims of abuse are generally more present in urban cities than in rural ones (Eastman & Bunch, 2007; Grossman, Hinkey, Kawalski, & Margrave, 2005). Battered women's shelters, legal advocacy groups, and social service resources are usually common in urban cities, whereas these services might not be typical of some rural towns. Factors influencing the challenges of offering and accessing these services in rural areas may include attitudes of acceptance of violence against women, geographical isolation, and lack of public transportation (Eastman & Bunch). In a study comparing rural and urban service provider perceptions of consumer needs, resource availability, funding, and other factors impacting public access to domestic violence services, Eastman and Bunch found that rural service providers described family expectations, cultural norms, and personal belief systems as having a greater impact on the likelihood of seeking services than did urban service providers.

Even for perpetrators of violence against women, services are more readily available in urban cities. Logan, Walker, and Leukefeld (2001) found that rural males in their sample had significantly more prior and slightly fewer subsequent domestic violence convictions than urban males (34 percent and 16 percent for rural males; 31 percent and 19 percent for urban males), and implied that this difference reflects possible differences in the justice systems of rural and urban cities. Rural justice systems may have more challenges deterring domestic violence due to tolerance of these behaviors. Furthermore, Logan et al. found that urban males were significantly more likely to have participated in anger management counseling than their rural counterparts (33 percent vs. 16 percent, respectively), indicating a possible discrepancy in these services between urban and rural cities.

Although there is generally increased availability of domestic violence services in urban cities, this may not necessarily translate to better access or use of services for urban residents; reasons for not accessing available resources may persist regardless of the lack of or presence of various agencies established to assist victims of domestic violence. Barriers to accessing abuse resources can exist for women regardless of residency and may include fear of abuse escalation due to lack of confidentiality or an attempt to leave the relationship, lack of awareness or low self-esteem, lack of access to public transportation, mistrust in healthcare providers' ability to provide appropriate referrals, fear of losing custody of children, and fear of judgment (Petersen, Moracco, Goldstein, & Clark, 2003). Barriers to accessing domestic violence services for low-income and minority women—especially African American women—in urban cities may be similar to those experienced by women in rural areas and differ from higher income women in urban cities (Grossman et al., 2005).

Access to Healthcare Services

In light of the various factors that may harm health in the urban environment, it is important to recognize the presence of factors that may enhance health (Vlahov et al., 2005). One of the benefits of life in urban cities is the availability of more healthcare services for those who can access them. In general, death rates per 100,000 of the population in urban, metropolitan cities are lower than in rural, non-metropolitan areas; this geographical trend remains across gender and racial groups (National Center for Health Statistics, 2006; Vlahov et al.). The prevalence of healthcare facilities and healthcare providers in urban cities is higher than in rural areas. The presence of governmental agencies and social organizations that respond to the needs of residents is also a benefit of urban living (Vlahov et al.). Resources for assistance with basic necessities, as well as social networks centered around ethnic, cultural, religious, educational, and professional interests, are more prevalent in urban cities and may contribute to the health of urban residents.

The Role of the Nurse in Improving Health Outcomes in Urban Settings

The nursing process provides a framework from which nurses can make clinical decisions that will contribute to the overall well-being of individuals and communities (Smith & Bazini-Barakat, 2003). For public health nurses, clinical scenarios may consist of interactions with an individual person or family, a community, or policy makers. The steps of the nursing process—assessment, diagnosis, planning, implementation, and evaluation—provide the nurse with a systematic process by which the needs of urban residents are identified and actions are planned and carried out. The results of interventions are then evaluated for efficacy, sustainability, and appropriateness for the individual and community. The process may be non-linear as nurses gain more information through ongoing assessment and interventions are revised in consideration of new data (Potter et al., 2004).

As a part of assessment, nurses working in urban cities must be aware of the many issues that play a role in the life of urban residents and communities. Specifically, the nurse must have an intimate knowledge of the community within which she or he works; nurses new to a community must put forth additional effort to obtain this information in order to effectively serve the community (Tanner, 2006). This involves developing a knowledge base from which the nurse can make sound clinical judgments that will improve the health of individuals and the community. Assessment also includes evaluation of an individual's or community's readiness for actions aimed at improving health. Nurses make clinical judgments within the scope of nursing practice and plan for action on behalf of the individual or community. Planning for interventions can be a lengthy process as the nurse conducts ongoing assessments of patient and community needs, prioritizes appropriate interventions based on the best available evidence, and gathers resources needed for implementation of the decided interventions. Addressing the needs of the individual or family should be an interdisciplinary effort for the nurse in urban settings; community-based interventions will involve interaction with key leaders in the community and the identification of available resources to maximize the success of the intervention (Office of Disease Prevention and Health Promotion, 2001; Tanner). Interventions can be classified as primary, secondary, or tertiary (Smith & Bazini-Barakat, 2003); nurses must make decisions about interventions based upon whether individuals or communities have actual or potential needs, or if they are at risk for certain needs. Lastly, evaluation is an ongoing process that involves determining the attainment of the objectives identified and the success of all interventions. Successful interventions will be those that result in improved health and quality of life for the individual and community (Smith & Bazini-Barakat, 2003).

The information that follows consists of principles that can be used by the nurse to improve health outcomes in an urban setting. The principles, adapted from the Office of Disease Prevention and Health Promotion (2001) and Smith and Bazini-Barakat (2003), are primarily applicable to community-level scenarios, but can be used to guide care for individuals as well. Table 18-8 displays examples of how nurses can apply some of the following principles to interventions for individuals in areas such as acute care settings or private clinics.

| TABLE 18-8 | EXAMPLES OF APPLICATION OF COMMUNITY PRINCIPLES TO THE INDIVIDUAL | |

Phase of Nursing Process	Community Principle	Application to Scenarios Involving Individuals
Assessment	Prioritize community concerns based on available data.	Review patient medical records. Conduct a thorough patient history.
Diagnosis	Identify community needs as actual, potential, or at risk for. Prioritize needs that will be the target of interventions.	Assign nursing diagnoses as appropriate. Prioritize health needs, addressing immediate threats to life first.
Planning	Establish specific and measurable objectives with dates for accomplishment.	Example: Within 1 hour of acetaminophen administration, patient temperature will fall within the range of normal.
	Identify essential action steps for meeting each objective, assigning each step to the most appropriate team member or partnering organization.	Identify all members of the healthcare team needed to meet each objective (e.g., physician, nurse, nurse aide, and ancillary services).
Implementation	Set regular times for contact between all team members and for communication of progress.	Example: RN and nurse aide agree to use patient chart for communication of patient temperatures; MD to be contacted via phone.
Evaluation	Conduct ongoing reassessments throughout the implementation process to ensure that steps for meeting all objectives remain feasible in light of new data.	Example: Lab report indicates dehydration, so IV fluids are started. Temperature assessments continue to monitor effect of IV fluids and acetaminophen.

Assessment:

1. Identify the population (i.e., an individual patient, a family, or the community) that will be the target of your intervention.

2. Conduct an assessment of your population to identify strengths and areas for improvement. For a community, involve key members of the community by conducting focus groups or personal interviews.

3. Prioritize community concerns based on community assessment and available quantitative data as well as qualitative data that consist of the perceptions and opinions of key community members. Quantitative data may consist of census data, school records, hospital records, morbidity and mortality data obtained from federal sources, and incidence and prevalence rates for conditions of interest. Consult resources such as the Healthy People 2010 document, the Centers for Disease Control and Prevention, and the National Center for Health Statistics.

4. Identify the contributing factors to the identified health concerns. Consider individual, psychosocial, environmental, social, economic, and political factors.

Diagnosis:

1. Identify actual conditions, potential conditions, or situations that place individuals or the community at risk for a certain condition.

2. Analyze collected data (quantitative and qualitative) and prioritize those community concerns and needs that will be the target of planned interventions.

3. Assign identified needs to their corresponding conditions, whether actual, potential, or at risk for.

Planning:

1. Establish specific and measurable objectives with dates for accomplishment. For example, a goal to increase healthy food choices in school-age children might be reflected in an objective that states: "By June 2009, 50 percent of fourth through sixth graders will be able to identify the food groups of the food pyramid and recognize correct serving sizes." Consider identifying incremental objectives as well (e.g., By December 2008, 25 percent of fourth through sixth graders will be able to identify . . .).

2. Identify essential action steps for meeting each objective, assigning each step to the most appropriate team member or partnering organization.

3. Identify and locate all resources needed for implementation. For areas where resources are lacking, consider alternative options based on available resources.

4. Clarify the role for all team members and partner organizations in achieving the identified objectives. Make sure all parties are in agreement.

Implementation:

1. Set guidelines for continuing quality assurance before the implementation phase begins. Set regular times for contact among all team members and for communication of progress.
2. All team members and partner organizations carry out their specified roles in achieving the stated objectives.

Evaluation:

1. Using the dates determined for each objective, assess whether each was reached; identify barriers that prevented unfulfilled objectives from being reached.
2. Identify the effectiveness of all interventions implemented.
3. Conduct ongoing reassessments throughout the implementation process to ensure that steps for meeting all objectives remain feasible in light of new data.

Summary

The focus on the impact of environment on the health of individuals has a long history, dating back to Florence Nightingale, Lillian Wald, and other early public health nurses. Health and environment are very complex, interrelated issues that influence both short- and long-term health outcomes and quality of life for citizens nationally and globally. The factors that influence health include a combination of biological/genetic, psychological, emotional, lifestyle/behavioral, sociopolitical, and environmental factors; nurses must consider the role that these factors play in the health of individuals. Risk factors in the environment such as poverty can dramatically alter the health status of individuals and families. Poverty in urban cities is thought to be the result of decentralization, increased racial segregation, unemployment, and increasing economic disparities. Risk factors that play a specific role in the health of urban residents include poverty, substandard housing, air pollution, crime and violence, and access to healthcare services.

Urban cities are characterized by health-related issues that may contribute to health as well as harm health. Those suffering from poverty in urban cities encounter challenges in accessing many of the benefits of urban living, making them more vulnerable to poor health outcomes. Nursing professionals must continue to assess risk factors in the client's environment. Nurses can act as change agents and advocate for policies that improve access to care and decrease public health risk factors.

Key Terms

- **Decentralization:** A process occurring in urban cities in which employment opportunities and social capital move into suburban areas. This process is suggested to be one of the causes of urban poverty.
- **Infant mortality rate (IMR):** The number of infant deaths per 100,000 live births. Infant deaths are those that occur during the child's first year of life.
- **Maternal mortality rate:** The number of maternal deaths per 100,000 live births. Maternal deaths are those that occur during pregnancy or within 42 days after the pregnancy has ended.
- **Poverty threshold:** An income amount set by the government that accounts for household size and earnings. A family whose income falls below this threshold is considered to be living in poverty.
- **Public health nursing:** The field of nursing that specializes in improving the health care of the community or individuals in the community setting.
- **Urban area:** An area that has a population of at least 1,000 persons per square mile or surrounding areas with at least 500 persons per square mile. Any areas outside of these two classifications are considered rural.

Reflective Practice Questions

1. You are a nurse working in an urban health department conducting home visits for mothers and their newborn infants living in a low-income neighborhood. Your patient today is Nicole, a teenage mother who lives with her mother, grandmother, and two younger siblings in a three-bedroom home. Nicole was given education about SIDS prevention during her postpartum stay at the hospital. However, upon arrival, you notice that the baby, who is 1 week old, is sleeping on his stomach on Nicole's bed. Nicole notices your observation and proceeds to tell you about the pressure she received from her mother and grandmother to place the baby on his stomach after trying, unsuccessfully, to get him to sleep on his back. His crying was beginning to keep everyone awake and this was the only thing that helped. Both Nicole's mother and grandmother told her repeatedly that they put their babies to sleep on their stomachs and everything turned out fine. In fact, they believed that this practice helped their babies sleep better at night. What steps would you take to educate Nicole and her family on the risks of stomach sleeping and the benefits of placing babies on their backs to sleep? Outline your steps as they follow the nursing process.

2. You are working in a community health center and facilitating a support group for people with diabetes. Today, you are discussing the benefits of exercise in controlling blood glucose levels and maintaining a healthy weight. The community center is in a high-crime, low-income

neighborhood with no parks, sidewalks, or exercise facilities. Group members express fear about exercising in their neighborhood. You decide to convene a group of community members in order to assess the problem in the community and come up with potential solutions. What actions would you take to conduct a full assessment of recreation barriers and resources in the community? What are some possible solutions?

3. What are some potential factors present in the urban environment that contribute to each of the Healthy People 2010 Leading Health Indicators discussed in this chapter?

References

Akinbami, L. J. (2006). *The state of childhood asthma, United States, 1980–2005.* Centers for Disease Control and Prevention. Retrieved September 15, 2007, from http://www.cdc. gov/nchs/data/ad/ad381.pdf

American Nurses Association. (2007). *ANA hall of fame 1976–1982 inductees: Lillian Wald.* Retrieved August 1, 2007, from http://nursingworld.org/FunctionalMenuCategories/ AboutANA/WhereWeComeFrom_1/HallofFame/19761982/waldld5595.aspx

Anderson, R. N., & Smith, B. L. (2005, March 7). *Deaths: Leading causes for 2002.* Centers for Disease Control and Prevention. Retrieved September 9, 2008, from http://www. cdc.gov/nchs/data/nvsr/nvsr53/nvsr53_17.pdf

Aron-Dine, A. (2007). *New data show income concentration jumped again in 2005: Income share of top 1% returned to it 2000 level, the highest since 1929.* Center on Budget and Policy Priorities. Retrieved July 26, 2008, from http://www.cbpp.org/1-23-07inc.htm

Bashir, S. A. (2002). Home is where the harm is: Inadequate housing as a public health crisis. *American Journal of Public Health, 92*(5), 733–738.

Bolland, J. M. (2003). Hopelessness and risk behaviour among adolescents living in high-poverty inner-city neighbourhoods. *Journal of Adolescence, 26*(2), 145.

Branas, C. C., Nance, M. L., Elliott, M. R., Richmond, T. S., & Schwab, C. W. (2004). Urban-rural shifts in intentional firearm death: Different causes, same results. *American Journal of Public Health, 94*(10), 1750–1755.

Bureau of Justice Statistics. (2007, July 11). *Homicide trends in the U.S.: Trends by city size.* U.S. Department of Justice, Office of Justice Programs. Retrieved August 5, 2007, from http://www.ojp.usdoj.gov/bjs/homicide/city.htm

Center on Budget and Policy Priorities. (2004). *Census data show poverty increased, income stagnated, and the number of uninsured rose to a record level in 2003.* Retrieved July 26, 2008, from http://www.cbpp.org/8-26-04pov.htm

Centers for Disease Control and Prevention. (2005). *Tuberculosis cases and case rates per 100,000 population: Metropolitan statistical areas with ≥500,000 population, 2005 and 2004 (Table 46).* Retrieved May 20, 2007, from http://www.cdc.gov/tb/surv/surv2005/ PDF/table46.pdf

Centers for Disease Control and Prevention. (2006a). *Intimate partner violence surveillance: Uniform definitions.* Retrieved April 10, 2007, from http://www.cdc.gov/ncipc/pub-res/ ipv_surveillance/05_UNIFORM_DEFINITIONS.htm

Centers for Disease Control and Prevention. (2006b). *Sexual violence surveillance: Uniform definitions for sexual violence.* Retrieved April 10, 2007, from http://www.cdc.gov/ncipc/ pub-res/sv_surveillance/04_uniform_definitions.htm

Centers for Disease Control and Prevention. (2007a). *HIV/AIDS.* National Center for HIV/ AIDS, Viral Hepatitis, STD, and TB Prevention. Retrieved July 26, 2008, from http:// www.cdc.gov/hiv/ and http://www.cdc.gov/nchhstp/

Centers for Disease Control and Prevention. (2007b). *HIV/AIDS surveillance in urban and nonurban areas.* National Center for HIV/AIDS, Viral Hepatitis, STD, and TB Prevention. Retrieved July 26. 2008, from http://www.cdc.gov/hiv/topics/surveillance/ resources/slides/urban-nonurban/

Centers for Disease Control and Prevention. (2007c). *Maternal and infant health.* Retrieved August 2, 2007, from http://www.cdc.gov/reproductivehealth/MaternalInfantHealth/ index.htm

Chinn, P. L., & Kramer, M. K. (2004). Nursing's knowledge development pathways. In (Chinn & Kramer, Eds.), *Integrated knowledge development in nursing* (6th ed., pp. 19–54). St. Louis: Mosby.

Curley, A. M. (2005). Theories of urban poverty and implications for public housing policy. *Journal of Sociology and Social Welfare, 32*(2), 97–119.

Earls, F. (2000). Urban poverty: Scientific and ethical considerations. *The Annals of the American Academy of Political and Social Science, 572*(1), 53–65.

Eastman, B. J., & Bunch, S. G. (2007). Providing services to survivors of domestic violence: A comparison of rural and urban service provider perceptions. *Journal of Interpersonal Violence, 22*(4), 465–473.

Evans, W. P., Fitzgerald, C., Weigel, D. A. N., & Chvilicek, S. (1999). Are rural gang members similar to their urban peers? Implications for rural communities. *Youth Society, 30*(3), 267–282.

Fishbein, D. H., Herman-Stahl, M., Eldreth, D., Paschall, M. J., Hyde, C., Hubal, R., et al. (2006). Mediators of the stress–substance-use relationship in urban male adolescents. *Prevention Science, 7*(2), 113–126.

Freisthler, B., Lascala, E. A., Gruenewald, P. J., & Treno, A. J. (2005). An examination of drug activity: Effects of neighborhood social organization on the development of drug distribution systems. *Substance Use & Misuse, 40,* 671–686.

Frumkin, H. (2002). Urban sprawl and public health. *Public Health Reports, 117,* 201–217.

Galea, S., Freudenberg, N., & Vlahov, D. (2005). Cities and population health. *Social Science & Medicine, 60,* 1017–1033.

Grossman, S. F., Hinkey, S., Kawalski, A., & Margrave, C. (2005). Rural versus urban victims of violence: The interplay of race and region. *Journal of Family Violence, 20*(2), 71–81.

Hillemeier, M. M., Weisman, C. S., Chase, G. A., & Dyer, A.-M. (2007). Individual and community predictors of preterm birth and low birthweight along the rural-urban continuum in central Pennsylvania. *Journal of Rural Health, 23*(1), 42–48.

Hoyert, D. L. (2007). *Maternal mortality and related concepts.* National Center for Health Statistics, Vital Health Statistics. Retrieved July 30, 2007, from http://www.cdc.gov/ nchs/data/series/sr_03/sr03_033.pdf

Jackson, R. J. (1998). Habitat and health: The role of environmental factors in the health of urban populations. *Journal of Urban Health: Bulletin of the New York Academy of Medicine, 75*(2), 258–262.

Jewish Women's Archive. (2007). *Lillian Wald.* Retrieved August 1, 2007, from http:// www.jwa.org/exhibits/wov/wald/lwbio.html

Khan, S., Murray, R. P., & Barnes, G. E. (2002). A structural equation model of the effect of poverty and unemployment on alcohol abuse. *Addictive Behaviors, 27*(3), 405.

Kjellstrom, T., Friel, S., Dixon, J., Corvalan, C., Rehfuess, E., Campbell-Lendrum, D., et al. (2007). Urban environmental health hazards and health equity. *Journal of Urban Health: Bulletin of the New York Academy of Medicine, 84*(1), i86–i97.

Logan, T. K., Walker, R., & Leukefeld, C. G. (2001). Rural, urban influenced, and urban differences among domestic violence arrestees. *Journal of Interpersonal Violence, 16*(3), 266–283.

MacDonald, M. A. (2004). From miasma to fractals: The epidemiology revolution and public health nursing. *Public Health Nursing, 21*, 380–391.

Manfrin-Ledet, L., & Porche, D. J. (2003). The state of science: Violence and HIV infection in women. *JANAC: Journal of the Association of Nurses in AIDS Care, 14*(6), 56–68.

Mauldin, T., & Mimura, Y. (2001). Exits from poverty among rural and urban Black, Hispanic, and White young adults. *The Review of Black Political Economy*, 9–23.

Mercado, S., Havemann, K., Sami, M., & Ueda, H. (2007). Urban poverty: An urgent public heath issue. *Journal of Urban Health: Bulletin of the New York Academy of Medicine, 84*(1), i7–i15.

Miller, M. (1999). A model to explain the relationship between sexual abuse and HIV risk among women. *AIDS Care, 11*(1), 3–20.

Mimura, Y., & Mauldin, T. A. (2005). American young adults' rural-to-urban migration and timing of exits from poverty spells. *Journal of Family and Economic Issues, 26*(1), 55–76.

Miniño, A. M., Heron, M. P., & Smith, B. L. (2006, June 28). *Deaths: Preliminary data for 2004.* Centers for Disease Control and Prevention. Retrieved August 10, 2007, from http://www.cdc.gov/nchs/data/nvsr/nvsr54/nvsr54_19.pdf

National Center for Health Statistics. (2002). *Supplemental Analyses of Recent Trends in Infant Mortality.* Retrieved September 9, 2008, from http://www.cdc.gov/nchs/products/pubs/pubd/hestats/infantmort/infantmort.htm

National Center for Health Statistics. (2006). *Health, United States, 2006, with chartbook on trends in the health of Americans.* Centers for Disease Control and Prevention. Retrieved July 27, 2008, from http://www.cdc.gov/nchs/data/hus/hus06.pdf

National Center for Health Statistics. (2007). *Home page.* Retrieved September 15, 2007, from www.cdc.gov/nchs

National Institute of Allergy and Infectious Diseases. (2006). *Tuberculosis fact sheet.* Retrieved May 17, 2007, from http://www.niaid.nih.gov/factsheets/tb.htm

National Institute of Child Health and Human Development (NICHHD). (2006). *SIDS: "Back to sleep" campaign.* National Institutes of Health. Retrieved September 15, 2007, from http://www.nichd.nih.gov/sids/

Office of Disease Prevention and Health Promotion. (2001). *Healthy people in healthy communities: A community guide using Healthy People 2010.* Department of Health and Human Services. Retrieved September 5, 2007, from http://www.healthypeople.gov/Publications/HealthyCommunities2001/healthycom01hk.pdf

Peters, J. L., Levy, J. I., Rogers, C. A., Burge, H. A., & Spengler, J. D. (2007). Determinants of allergen concentrations in apartments of asthmatic children living in public housing. *Journal of Urban Health: Bulletin of the New York Academy of Medicine, 84*(2), 185–197.

Petersen, R., Moracco, K. E., Goldstein, K. M., & Clark, K. A. (2003). Women's perspectives on intimate partner violence services: The hope in Pandora's box. *Journal of the American Medical Women's Association, 58*, 185–190.

Potter, P., Boxerman, S., Wolf, L., Marshall, J., Grayson, D., Sledge, J., et al. (2004). Mapping the nursing process: A new approach for understanding the work of nursing. *Journal of Nursing Administration, 34*(2), 101–109.

Rankin, B. H., & Quane, J. M. (2000). Neighborhood poverty and the social isolation of inner-city African American families. *Social Forces, 79*(1), 139–164.

Rape, Abuse and Incest National Network. (2006). *Statistics.* Retrieved July 27, 2008, from http://www.rainn.org/statistics

Ruble, N. M., & Turner, W. L. (2000). A systematic analysis of the dynamics and organization of urban street gangs. *The American Journal of Family Therapy, 28*, 117–132.

Save the Children. (2007). *State of the world's mothers, 2007: Saving the lives of children under 5.* Retrieved August 15, 2007, from http://www.savethechildren.org/jump.jsp?path=/publications/mothers/2007/SOWM-2007-final.pdf

Smith, K., & Bazini-Barakat, N. (2003). A public health nursing practice model: Melding public health principles with the nursing process. *Public Health Nursing, 20*(1), 42–48.

Stern, A. M., & Markel, H. (2004). International efforts to control infectious diseases, 1851 to the present. *Journal of the American Medical Association, 292*, 1474–1479.

Stewart, M. B. (2007). The interrelated dynamics of unemployment and low-wage employment. *Journal of Applied Econometrics, 22*, 511–531.

Tanner, C. A. (2006). Thinking like a nurse: A research-based model of clinical judgment in nursing. *Journal of Nursing Education, 45*(6), 204–211.

Tolan, P. H., Gorman-Smith, D., & Henry, D. B. (2003). The developmental ecology of urban males' youth violence. *Developmental Psychology, 39*(2), 274–291.

Tomes, N. (2000). Public health then and now: The making of a germ panic, then and now. *American Journal of Public Health, 90*(2), 191–198.

U.S. Census Bureau. (2004). *United States summary: 2000 population and housing counts (Part 1).* Retrieved May 20, 2007, from http://www.census.gov/prod/cen2000/phc3-us-pt1.pdf

U.S. Census Bureau. (2006). *Census 2000 urban and rural classifications.* Retrieved May 15, 2007, from http://www.census.gov/geo/www/ua/ua_2k.html

U.S. Census Bureau. (2007). *Poverty definitions.* Housing and Household Economic Statistics Division. Retrieved August 1, 2007, from http://www.census.gov/hhes/www/poverty/definitions.html

Vacha, E. F., & McLaughlin, T. F. (2004). Risky firearms behavior in low-income families of elementary school children: The impact of poverty, fear of crime, and crime victimization on keeping and storing firearms. *Journal of Family Violence, 19*(3), 175–184.

Vigil, J. D. (2003). Urban violence and street gangs. *Annual Review of Anthropology, 32*, 225–242.

Vlahov, D., Galea, S., & Freudenberg, N. (2005). Toward an urban health advantage. *Journal of Public Health Management and Practice, 11*(3), 256–258.

Wilson, W. J. (2003). Race, class and urban poverty: A rejoinder. *Ethnic and Racial Studies, 26*(6), 1096–1114.

chapter

19

Nursing and Rural Healthcare Issues

Wanda Bonnel, Amanda Alonzo, Patricia E. Conejo, and Sylvia Heinze

LEARNING OUTCOMES

After reading this chapter you will be able to:

- Describe common rural health and nursing practice issues including access to care and care resources in the rural setting.
- Consider broad health promotion needs and approaches for working with rural patients.
- Examine diverse health professionals' challenges and roles in delivering rural health care.
- Identify strategies for collaborating and maximizing the use of technology within broader health provider networks for the purpose of delivering quality rural health care.
- Discuss approaches to integrate evidence-based practice and quality improvement in rural health care and nursing practice.
- Plan education and career development for the care of rural patients and nursing practice in rural settings.

Introduction

Many nurses will either practice in rural settings or care for patients who reside in rural communities. Although there are similarities across all

447

healthcare settings, unique factors impact the healthcare needs of rural patients. All nurses need to be familiar with issues that impact the care they provide to rural patients. And those nurses who are considering practicing in rural communities need to be familiar with the issues associated with rural health care.

A recent Institute of Medicine report (Board on Healthcare Services, Institute of Medicine, 2005) highlighted the challenges of providing health care in rural settings. Although rural populations have healthcare needs similar to urban populations, there are fewer healthcare agencies and resources available to them. For example, there are significant and growing problems with alcohol and drug dependence in many rural settings; however, there are also fewer mental health professionals available to provide assistance. Greater geographical distances often separate patients, providers, and specialists; this makes healthcare transportation a particular challenge in the rural setting, which can impact healthcare outcomes. The percentage of traumatic injuries is commonly higher in rural settings with poorer healthcare outcomes often related to the lack of emergency response training and transportation issues (National Rural Health Association, 2006).

Diverse rural populations with a variety of needs can stress limited rural healthcare resources. In addition to healthcare specialist shortages, rural communities often cope with shortages of primary care providers including physicians, nurses, dentists, and allied health personnel. Care for populations with specialized healthcare needs such as those patients with cancer or HIV can be even more problematic given the limited resources available in rural communities.

Particularly in the rural setting, a care focus on populations, as well as individuals, is required to maximize resources. Because healthcare resources tend to be less available, identifying and maximizing the resources that are available in the community setting is critical. The nurse's skill at partnering with families and local resources to develop and deliver creative health programming becomes very important. For example, health promotion activities such as weight management and smoking cessation may be important population programs delivered in connection with local churches or community organizations. Optimizing technology partnerships such as telemedicine with local and urban healthcare networks provides another opportunity to maximize resources. Nurses also have roles in helping clients gain self-advocacy skills and helping individuals be better prepared to monitor their own care and their families' care as well.

By recognizing and building on the strengths of the rural community, nurses have many opportunities to impact population health. As in all settings, goals in caring for rural patients and populations include effective, efficient, quality care. This chapter provides an overview of rural healthcare issues that nurses need to be familiar with to meet the goal of providing quality health care to rural populations.

Rural Descriptions

The U.S. Census broadly defines a rural community as an area not designated as urban and having less than 2,500 inhabitants. Twenty percent of the citizens in the United States can be considered to be living in a rural area, and in 30 states at least 25 percent of the citizens are considered to be in rural areas. Rural hospitals make up 44 percent of the total number of U.S. hospitals and include 21 percent of all hospital beds (Board on Healthcare Services, 2005).

Although rural healthcare resources may vary from county to county, overall, fewer healthcare providers and facilities for health care are available in rural areas. Rural populations are officially considered **medically underserved populations (MUPs)**, meaning they lack needed healthcare providers and face economic, cultural, or linguistic barriers to health care. MUP designations are made based on computations specific to community poverty level, elderly population, infant mortality rate, and number of physicians in a geographic area (Hartley & Gale, 2003). Rural areas that do not qualify as a MUP, but generally have limited healthcare providers, are officially called **health professional shortage areas (HPSAs)**. These include shortages of healthcare providers such as those who deliver primary, dental, or mental health care. Often these designations are used in the allocation of federal grant resources to help rural communities enhance access to primary health care. A sample rural community is described in Box 19-1.

Health disparities in rural versus urban settings are related to a variety of factors including economic, social, and cultural differences as well as educational differences. Rural counties often have higher minority populations who work at relatively low-paid agricultural or farm jobs and experience economic disadvantages that impact the quality of living and ability to afford health care. Safety net programs are required to provide adequate primary care services to these populations, especially in the areas of obstetric and pediatric care services (Board on Healthcare Services, 2005). A sample of reported health disparities in rural settings is provided in Box 19-2.

> **KEY TERM**
>
> **Medically underserved populations (MUPs):** This designation is assigned to healthcare service areas that face economic, cultural, or linguistic barriers to health care and is based on computations specific to community poverty level, elderly population, infant mortality rate, and ratio of primary care physicians per 1,000 population (Health Resources Service Administration, 2006).

> **KEY TERM**
>
> **Health professional shortage area (HPSA):** This designation identifies defined communities that have shortages of healthcare providers such as primary care, dental, or mental health care (Health Resources Service Administration, 2006).

> **KEY TERM**
>
> **Health disparities:** Differences in conditions that exist among specific population groups in the United States, including incidence, prevalence, mortality, and burden of diseases.

Healthcare Roles in Rural Settings

Having a diverse and adequate supply of health care providers is a challenge in many rural communities. This section describes the healthcare roles most commonly found in rural settings.

BOX 19-1   RURAL HEALTH SETTING EXEMPLAR—RURAL KANSAS

Kansas is a predominately rural state. On the far western edge of the state several counties have a frontier-type population based with 2-3 people per square mile. In many rural Kansas counties the elderly comprise 25-30% of the entire population. Some Kansas counties have had double-digit growth in minority populations during the last decade due to the introduction of the beef processing industry in the larger, rural communities. As of 2006, 78 of 105 counties in Kansas were designated as Primary Care Health Professionals Shortage Areas (HPSAs). The large state universities work with Area Health Education Centers (AHECs) in these underserved areas to help provide education and resources to local multidisciplinary providers for promoting health and improving patient care. These state demographic characteristics have significant implications for nursing practice and healthcare delivery in the state of Kansas. The Web site for the Office of Local and Rural Health within the Kansas Department of Health and Environment provides additional information regarding the delivery of health care in rural Kansas.

Source: http://www.kdheks.gov/olrh/index.html

BOX 19-2   CHARACTERISTICS AND HEALTH DISPARITIES IN RURAL SETTINGS

The National Rural Health Association summarizes that while there is great variability in rural communities, the following characteristics and health disparities commonly exist in rural settings.
- Lack of health insurance coverage
- Higher incidence of poverty
- Higher incidence of hypertension and stroke
- Delayed time to cancer diagnosis
- Increased chronic disease complications such as diabetes
- Increased injury rates from motor vehicle accidents
- Higher rates of alcohol and tobacco use by teenagers
- Fewer healthcare resources including dental and mental health services

Source: National Rural Health Association, http://199.237.254.34/about/sub/different.html

---

Nursing

Nurses are currently in short supply in all regions of the country, but the shortage of nurses and other healthcare providers is even worse in rural areas, presenting unique challenges. In acute care hospitals, even though a shortage of nurses exists, the census of most units does not provide enough work for nursing staff to be dedicated to a certain unit and patient population; nurses are required to "float" and provide staffing where they are needed. This means that those nurses must maintain broad, generalized nursing skills and competencies, varying from those required to care for the hospital's only pediatric patient to the critically ill young adult as well as the older adult receiving palliative care.

The rural nurse must also excel in triage and decision making. In the emergency room, on any given day, the nurse may encounter and provide care to an infant with colic, an adult with pneumonia, a woman experiencing an obstetrical emergency, and a patient who has been critically injured in a motor vehicle accident, all without the benefit of a comprehensive healthcare team consisting of specialists trained to diagnose and treat the patients' emerging health crises. The nurse must be able to make immediate and potentially life-saving decisions about when to transfer a patient via air to regional healthcare centers better equipped to meet the patient's healthcare needs—a decision that has significant financial implications, as well as patient care implications.

In the rural hospital, nurses often serve as coordinators of care, linking and coordinating services and working with other care providers to minimize the patients' length of stay. The nurse communicates with physicians, case managers, physical therapists, pharmacists, and other facility contacts as needed. When transferring patients to other facilities, the nurse may be responsible for contacting the facility, arranging transport (via private vehicle, ambulance, or helicopter), and communicating with the physician, patient, family, and the accepting facility. At times, nurses may be required to accompany patients when they are transferred via ambulance.

Nurses are often the coordinators of care in the rural community setting itself. It is frequently the nurse's responsibility to screen for clients with health risk factors, identify problems, and help locate specific resources including both informal and formal healthcare services. Nurses work closely with patients and informal caregivers to identify care needs and consider what health or service options are available to help the patients and families obtain the needed services. Nurses working in the broader community, such as in primary care clinics, community health, or public health nurse roles are required to balance numerous, simultaneous demands. Providing and clarifying health information for rural patients on diverse issues is a significant nursing responsibility; for example, rural healthcare nurses may be expected to provide information to patients regarding available community resources such as car seat safety inspection, how to obtain discounted prescriptions or free immunizations, as well as referrals to other healthcare and social agencies.

Primary Care Providers

Rural primary care providers are most likely to be general practice physicians, nurse practitioners (NP), and physician's assistants (PA). Midlevel providers are often called on to extend physician resources. Networking with specialists, these individuals are typically the backbone of the rural healthcare system. These rural primary care providers face challenges similar to those in urban settings, but bring unique perspectives to coping with legal, reimbursement, and regulatory issues. These issues include reimbursement issues such as those related to system costs and fewer numbers of patients; regulatory issues, which are often designed for larger provider systems and those having regulatory officers; and legal issues such as those related to "duty to treat" and transferring patients to other healthcare facilities. Rural primary care providers often have limited peer networks or even inadequate support resources in their work settings to help them deal with these issues and challenges. Graduate health professions' programs often provide little education on rural issues to help prepare practitioners to successfully address them (Lindeke, Grabau, & Jukkala, 2004). Additionally, the lack of specialty physicians in rural areas often results in general practice physicians, with the assistance of NPs and PAs, providing specialty services in areas such as obstetrics and gynecology, pediatrics, general surgery, intensive care, and emergency medicine.

Emergency Care Providers

First responder emergency medical service (EMS) providers play key roles in rural care that are different from those in urban settings. In the rural setting, it is common for EMS personnel to be volunteer firefighters or other local community volunteers who receive basic required training, but not advanced life support training. When emergency calls are received, agency service providers should be staffed by the appropriately designated level of care provider. If appropriate staff are not available, however, the basic technician may need to call upon the assistance of the nearest ambulance service equipped with full-time paid and adequately trained staff, thus causing a delay in patient assistance.

Case Manager Roles and Resources

Case management is commonly considered a system of assessment, coordination, and monitoring designed to help clients connect with appropriate health and social services, both formal and informal. Formal case manager roles vary in structure, but in rural care settings the nurse is most likely to serve as an informal case manager, helping families screen for problems and identify local resources to address those problems.

Rural case managers need adequate access to supportive resources for patient and family referrals. Appropriate social services and coordinated health care are particularly critical with the limited healthcare services and providers available in rural communities. Core services that make up a formal service network and commonly provide patient and family support in larger communities are noted in Box 19-3. Although many states have home and community-based service programs to assist patients, these services may be less available to rural residents.

BOX 19-3   CORE HOME-BASED COMMUNITY SERVICES NEEDED FOR RURAL POPULATIONS

- Transportation
- Nutritional support services
- Homemaker support services
- Personal care services
- Home health nursing services
- Chore services

Further information on community based services can be gained at the following: http://www.aoa.gov/eldfam/Service_Options/Service_Options.asp

In rural settings, nurses can assess the community for these core services, determine the gaps in services, and then consider who might fill the gaps to provide these services if they are not available. Agencies such as AARP, National Association of Area Agencies on Aging, and local health departments often provide good starting points for identifying community resources. Parish nurse programs also can make important contributions to local service continuums. People often have a trusting relationship with parish nurses from their faith communities, so the parish nurses can be excellent resources for promoting health and providing support services related to chronic health problems (Catanzaro, Meador, Koenig, Kuchibhatla, & Clipp, 2007). Highlights of the parish nursing role can be found in Contemporary Practice Highlight 19-1.

CONTEMPORARY PRACTICE HIGHLIGHT 19-1

PARISH NURSING

Parish nurses work within the faith community of rural churches to:
- Educate, counsel, and advocate for health promotion
- Advise community members on health problem referrals
- Develop support groups for health-related concerns

Characteristics of parish nurses:
- Registered nurses experienced in hospital- or community-based settings
- Completion of basic preparation courses in parish nursing
- Embrace the four main concepts of parish nursing:
  - Spiritual formation
  - Professionalism
  - Health and wholeness as God's intent
  - Respect of culture and diversity in the community

For more information on parish nursing, see http://www.parishnurses.org.

Other Care Providers

Recruiting and retaining all levels of qualified healthcare professionals can present major challenges in rural settings. Direct care workers such as nursing assistants, support technicians, and home health aides are often in short supply in the rural setting. To help remedy this shortage, some communities use an educational ladder approach to promote recruitment for healthcare careers, providing mobility options for healthcare workers to increase their knowledge and levels of formal healthcare training to better serve their own communities.

Volunteers also play an important role in rural health care. Rural healthcare and social support volunteers may come from social, faith, and work communities. A challenge can be that few people may be available to volunteer, and their roles may tend to overlap among the various community networks. Lack of available transportation systems, child care, and other infrastructure issues may also impact these volunteers' efforts. It is essential that nurses working in rural communities learn to effectively recruit and partner with volunteers so as to maximize resources and not overburden the available, but potentially scant, number of volunteers.

Patients and families are also important partners on the rural healthcare team. Family caregivers often have multiple roles with numerous responsibilities varying from assisting with such daily tasks as meal preparation and personal hygiene care to performing complex clinical skills such as completing dressing changes and administering medications. Such responsibilities require extensive patient and family education from the nurse; thus, the nurse must be a skilled patient care educator. In addition, with extended periods of caregiving, the caregivers' physical and mental health can be adversely affected, with feelings of burden and depression being common. A burned-out caregiver leads to not one patient but two (Montgomery & Williams, 2001). The nurse must be adept at screening for caregiver problems and providing tools and resources that can help caregivers more effectively manage their responsibilities without burning out.

Common Rural Health Problems and Health Disparities

Common rural health problems mirror those of larger populations and relate to the specific rural community. Although there is great variability in rural populations, in general, rural communities have a higher percentage of their population not covered by health insurance, more poverty, higher incidences of hypertension and stroke, longer delays in cancer diagnosis, increased chronic disease complications such as diabetes, and increased injury rates from motor vehicle accidents. Heart disease, alcohol abuse, and trauma are common in rural settings (National Rural Health Association, 2006). Challenges exist in managing common health problems because rural populations tend to be older, the economy is agriculturally driven, and economic factors affect healthcare coverage.

Rural dwellers are often self-employed and may be uninsured or under-insured for healthcare costs. For example, self-employed farmers with their money invested in land, equipment, and operational expenses such as animals and veterinary care may not budget money to buy health insurance coverage. Although perceived as "rich" by those outside of the agricultural economy, they may have limited disposable income and may need to work another job for insurance benefits or gain insurance through a spouse's employment. Other rural workers, who are not farmers but live in the rural setting, work at low-paying jobs with limited benefits (National Rural Health Association, 2006).

As noted, rural healthcare services are vastly different from those in urban settings. Those healthcare problems requiring treatment from specialists may have increased impact because of fewer healthcare resources. Specialty services are typically limited in the rural setting because the population is geographically diverse and a specialty service would have only a few clients and not be financially viable. Even patients with obstetric care needs beyond the basic pregnancy care provided from primary care providers may need to drive to an urban center for services. Specialty cardiology services are another example of services that are limited in rural areas (Pierce, 2007).

Health Promotion Issues

Data suggest that rural community residents have greater health risk behaviors including smoking more, exercising less, having less nutritional diets, and being more likely to be obese than urban residents. This suggests there may be a need for more culturally sensitive health promotion approaches in the rural setting (Hartley, 2004). Nurses in all rural settings take on broad roles in health promotion and public health. Health promotion programs that engage and work collaboratively with community members promote a focus on the health of the larger population. In rural settings there may be fewer opportunities for education about the prevention of health problems. As in urban areas, some individuals would not consider certain behaviors such as smoking and heavy drinking as a health risk and would often not consider getting outside assistance. National guidelines such as Healthy People 2010 (U.S. Department of Health and Human Services, 2000) provide the nurse and other care providers with direction for community health interventions. An example of a community-wide rural substance abuse program is provided in Box 19-4.

Rural nurses teach in diverse settings and play a very significant role in providing patient education for health promotion and disease prevention. Educational topics nurses might provide in a given setting can vary daily, from older adults' diabetic foot care to smoking cessation. Rural nurses may educate about blood pressure at a local church event, give a talk on sexually transmitted diseases at the local high school, or explain a new diagnosis of congestive heart failure to a

---

**BOX 19-4 SUBSTANCE ABUSE: RURAL MENTAL HEALTH
PROGRAM EXEMPLAR IN SOUTHEAST ALASKA**

Since rural populations often have limited providers and resources for dealing with substance abuse, a consortium approach (including use of professional staff and village provider teams and technology) was used in southeast Alaska to help provide mental health services to residents of the region. Use of indigenous village counselors ensured that the care was culturally appropriate, promoted greater longevity of the counselors and improved employment in the depressed area. Telepsychiatry and telehealth from larger cooperative sites were used as well. Services for assessment, early intervention, education, counseling for emergency and crisis intervention, aftercare/continuing care, relapse prevention, and community development were employed. For more information on Rural Health Promotion Programs, see: http://srphnt08.srph.tamhsc.edu/centers/rhp2010/Volume1.pdf.

---

patient at a private care clinic. In addition they provide education at health fairs sponsored by the community where they live and even at the grocery store when someone will stop them to ask for advice. Coffee shops, gas stations, or beauty shops may offer the best places for health posters and brochures.

Nurses can optimize opportunities to provide healthcare education in primary care settings as well. The challenge to rural nurses is to be knowledgeable about a wide array of topics and be able to communicate with diverse populations. Rural populations and common health concerns are listed in Box 19-5 and discussed in the following sections.

Common Health Problems for Agricultural Workers

An agriculturally driven economy lends itself to certain occupational and environmental hazards that are unique to the rural setting. Safety issues and other potential problems are pervasive for farm workers. There are no regulatory organizations such as the Occupational Safety and Health Administration (OSHA) in family farm operations. The harvest season brings a higher incidence of accidents. Farmers may work around equipment after they are tired from working a shift at another full-time job. Many times teenagers work on farms or as "summer help" at local industries. These teens may not be adequately trained for these tasks, resulting in injuries or illness. Skin cancer is another common problem with farmers and field workers. Nurses have important opportunities to teach prevention of accidents and injuries and promote appropriate screening for skin cancer.

Deaths from unintentional injuries, such as motor vehicle accidents, are also higher in rural areas. According to the National Rural Health Association

BOX 19-5   RURAL POPULATIONS AND COMMON HEALTH CONCERNS

Agricultural workers
- Rural occupational health and safety needs

Rural teens
- Safety needs
- Limited recreational activities
- Potential problems with drinking and drugs

Diverse patients
- At-risk groups needing safety nets such as obstetrical and pediatric care services
- Rural culture and potential distrust of outsiders

Further information can be gained from the National Rural Health Association (2006). http://www.nrharural.org/advocacy/sub/policybriefs/HlthDisparity.pdf

(2006), one-third of all motor vehicle accidents occur in the rural setting, with two-thirds of all deaths from motor vehicle accidents occurring on rural roads. Nurses can play a role in educating teens and employers on potential risks they may encounter as well as general safety guidelines. Web resources for promoting health and rural safety are provided in Box 19-6.

Common Health Problems for Rural Teens

Teenagers are an at-risk population in general, but certain factors may put them at increased risk in the rural setting. Because of limited recreational activities in rural areas, teens are at particular risk for alcohol abuse, drug use, and other

BOX 19-6   WEBLINKS FOR PROMOTING RURAL HEALTH AND SAFETY

- Safety for Agricultural Educators
  http://www.nycamh.com/resources/sage/entry_list.asp
- Rural Women's Health, Frequently Asked Questions
  http://www.raconline.org/info_guides/public_health/womenshealth.php
- Emergency Preparedness in Rural Areas for Large Disasters
  http://srphnt08.srph.tamhsc.edu/centers/osp/USACenter/library.htm#RER
- Rural Healthy People 2010, Volume 1
  http://www.srph.tamhsc.edu/centers/rhp2010/Volume1.pdf

safety issues such as drunk driving or car racing. Rural nurses can address these issues with teens as part of school health promotion activities and athletic physical exams in primary care, and with parents in settings such as high school orientation programs. Rural nurses may also need to work with school officials to gain population access and lead discussions on common problems such as sexually transmitted diseases.

Rural teens may have additional challenges in obtaining access to health care. For example, the rural teenager who desires birth control may not have ready transportation to the health department clinic. Privacy may also be an issue if she gets to the health department and finds that her neighbor is the nurse staffing the clinic. Further research and strategies are needed to promote positive teen health behaviors in rural communities.

Clients with Diverse Cultural Backgrounds

Different cultural backgrounds affect the communication of health information between providers and patients. Different cultural meanings and even different languages between patients and providers can lead to health treatment misunderstandings. Issues may exist when educating to promote adherence to health prescriptions, especially if patients don't have the money or other resources to manage their healthcare problems. Sometimes rural adults have a very self-sufficient mentality that may lead to suspicion of outsiders or even an antagonistic relationship with healthcare providers. There may also be different ways of defining health and needed healthcare actions in rural populations (Hartley, 2004). Additionally, the use of folk remedies is frequent; patient assessments should include questions about their use. It is not clear whether the use of folk remedies is more a cultural phenomenon or a healthcare access factor (Easom & Quinn, 2006).

Seasonal migrant workers may be another at-risk population within the rural setting. There are approximately 3 million migrant workers in the United States at risk for a variety of health issues. Many workers do not seek out health services until a major issue has developed because of a fear of negative consequences such as loss of employment eligibility or even deportation. Back problems and other musculoskeletal injuries, depression, sexually transmitted diseases, and acute issues such as dehydration are all common problems in migrant workers. Areas of focus for rural nurses include teaching about the need to seek early health care and assisting workers to find resources for affordable health care (Connor, Rainer, Simcox, & Thomisee, 2007).

Health Literacy in the Rural Setting

Health literacy has been described as the degree to which individuals have the capacity to obtain, process, and understand basic health information and services

needed to make appropriate health decisions. Higher prevalence of poor health literacy has been linked to lower levels of
education and higher poverty rates, both of which are found
in many rural communities (Rural Assistance Center, 2007).

> **KEY TERM**
>
> **Health literacy:** An individual's capacity to obtain, process, and understand the basic health information needed to make appropriate health decisions.

With fewer healthcare providers and resources available,
health literacy issues may present even larger problems in the
rural setting. Patients with low health literacy are at greater
risk of misunderstanding their diagnoses, their directions for self-medication,
and their self-care instructions. All these issues impact patient quality of life and
add expense to the healthcare system.

The importance of the nurse assessing each patient regarding his or her specific
learning needs, learning styles, and readiness to learn is noted. Although illnesses
are similar, patients are not. Nurses should also address any patient misconceptions about health problems. Diverse teaching strategies including individual
education, group education, and a variety of teaching methods can help meet
the needs of diverse learners in rural settings. Good patient follow-up and educational reminders such as handouts with key teaching points provide opportunity
for reinforcing teaching. Broad educational approaches related to chronic diseases include classes such as stress management with relaxation training and even
pet therapy. Materials to enhance local agency resources can be obtained from
organizations such as the Centers for Disease Control and Prevention (CDC) and
national health associations for health promotion and chronic disease management. Sharing accurate information and promoting good healthcare communication are important issues that rural nurses have the potential to impact. Examples
of resources for rural nurses are provided in Box 19-7.

BOX 19-7   WEB LINK RESOURCES FOR RURAL NURSES

National Rural Health Association
 http://www.nrharural.org/
Online Journal of Rural Nursing and Health Care
 http://www.rno.org/journal/issues/Vol-6/issue-2/TOC.htm
Rural Nurse Organization
 http://www.rno.org/
Rural Health Clinic Services
 http://www.cms.hhs.gov/MLNProducts/downloads/rhcfactsheet.pdf
**National Nursing Centers Consortium (nurse-managed health
centers serving vulnerable people across the country)**
 http://nncc.us/

Care Resources and Access to Care

Rural hospitals are typically much smaller than urban ones. Hospitals in rural areas range in size from less than 25 beds to 100+ beds. Of the approximately 2,100 rural community hospitals, 12 percent have less than 25 beds, 34 percent have 25–49 beds, and 31 percent have 50–99 beds. In comparison, only 26 percent of urban hospitals have less than 100 beds, and of those, 59 percent have 50–99 beds (Committee on the Future of Rural Health Care, 2005). Typically, primary care providers treat patients in small community clinics or hospitals. Local churches may also be used as sites for healthcare screening and low acuity treatment.

Rural hospitals must optimize resources to be successful. Services such as pharmacy or the laboratory may be staffed for limited hours or even be absent from the setting. Nursing supervisors often take on additional roles in obtaining necessary medications and treatments for newly admitted patients. Respiratory therapy, nutritional support, and many other specialty services may be non-existent or provided by mobile staff who visit the agency on a scheduled basis. Patients treated by these visiting specialists in both the acute care and community settings have complex medication regimes that rural nurses must manage.

The small rural hospital, in order to meet accreditation standards, must have staff trained in a variety of areas because often they need to float or cover different unit types. Even those staff who provide palliative care for hospice patients, for example, also need to have advanced cardiac life support (ACLS) training and be prepared to provide life-sustaining care in the emergency department. Although rural hospitals may also depend on agency staff to meet staffing shortfalls, agency nurses may find it difficult to meet the demands of providing both acute and chronic care for various patients along the birth to death continuum. Rural nurse partners can help agency nurse partners feel welcome in unique rural settings.

Lack of Local Specialty Services

To gain access to specialty health services, rural patients and families typically need to drive to large urban areas that may seem strange and forbidding. Patients with cancer, for example, may have to drive over 100 miles one way to an oncology clinic. Patients with renal failure might choose not to have dialysis rather than drive to the city. In some cases people, quite literally, would choose to die rather than leave their rural comfort zone. For transportation to these distant healthcare sites, privately owned vehicles are often the only option. Family or friends often have to miss work to take loved ones to healthcare appointments because there are no buses and very limited, if any, other types of transportation. Critical communication services such as phone and Internet may not be consistently available and complicate care arrangements as well.

Patients with more specialized health problems such as cancer or HIV are particularly at a disadvantage in terms of services. Although they may rely on distant communities for access to adequate health care, there are still issues concerning the lack of local community education and educational resources to promote understanding of illnesses. Patients have reported value in being part of support groups and speaker bureaus for HIV; they have also noted concerns about their diagnosis stigmatizing their families in intimate rural communities (Gaskins & Lyons, 2007).

Critical Access Facilities

Many hospitals in rural areas are designated **critical access facilities**. These facilities have a limited number of beds (15–25) available for admitting patients, and their services provide a type of healthcare safety net function. To gain critical access designation they must provide emergency services and meet specified population and geographic criteria. Critical access facilities gain Medicare reimbursement for actual costs, enabling them to be financially viable (Williams, 2007). Besides providing a healthcare safety net, critical access facilities can benefit the community in other ways as well. For example, a hospital can provide economic benefits for a rural community by serving a role as a major employer in the region (Ormond, Wallin, & Goldenson, 2000).

> **KEY TERM**
>
> **Critical access facility:** A small rural hospital that is the sole community hospital provider and is reimbursed by the Centers for Medicare and Medicaid Services for actual costs.

Swing Beds

In addition to receiving in-patient care in the hospital, some patients remain hospitalized under the distinction of **swing beds** for more long-term care. These patients may have been admitted to the hospital from home, but they are not well enough to return home and do not want to go to a nursing home to receive additional treatment. Many times patients in swing beds are returning to the community hospital from a metropolitan hospital following an invasive surgery such as heart bypass or a recent stroke or an extensive wound. They still require specific therapies that cannot be provided at home.

> **KEY TERM**
>
> **Swing beds:** Excess hospital beds that are designated for patients needing long-term skilled nursing care.

Long-Term Care Resources

Most rural settings have easier access to a long-term care nursing facility than to hospitals, and data suggest that these facilities are well used in the rural setting (Gamm & Hutchison, 2004). Long-term care settings are different from urban facilities in that they do not typically provide extended services such as specialty units for clients with dementia, adult day care programs, or respite services for family caregivers. Additionally, resources such as home care and assisted living are often not available in rural settings. Recruitment and sometimes retention for these facilities can be challenging.

Collaboration Among Community Providers

To stay financially viable and treat the needs of a diverse rural population, rural healthcare and service agencies may best meet patient care needs via collaborative efforts. This includes local and regional collaborations with nontraditional health agencies as well as other clinical providers.

Maximizing Traditional Healthcare Resources

Statewide incentive programs are often developed to attract physicians and their families to rural areas. When there are inadequate numbers of healthcare providers, regional services provide interim medical coverage to some rural communities that contract with these programs. This can be an incentive to retired physicians and even new physicians who are seeking extra income. Some companies provide services to fly in surgeons with more experienced specialty skills to assist local surgeons. Clark and Leipert (2007) discussed the advantages and disadvantages of mobile and outreach service teams, noting not only the benefits, but also the challenges with insider versus outsider status that may exist in rural communities.

Collaboration between rural community health centers and hospitals can be a useful approach to extending scarce resources. Sample collaborative activities include sharing electronic patient medical record systems, electronic information systems, training and technical support for clinical providers, and health promotion and disease prevention community projects. These collaborations can also include partnered health education, combined recruitment, training, human resources, and sharing case managers and service resources. Partnerships may enable agencies to make joint efforts in qualifying for and gaining grant funds and other resources (National Rural Health Association, 2007). The National Rural Health Association (NRHA) is a non-profit organization that provides leadership on rural healthcare issues. A summary of the NRHA's leadership activities is provided in Box 19-8.

Good documentation becomes particularly important when collaboration for quality patient care is required. Keeping multiple providers, consultants, and those transferring between rural and urban care centers informed is a key safety issue, requiring clear documentation. When there are multiple team members, the benefit of using templates and checklists for communication throughout a patient's care is obvious. Electronic health records that provide quick access to comprehensive patient information are needed. These resources are discussed further in the technology section later in this chapter.

BOX 19-8   NATIONAL RURAL HEALTH ASSOCIATION (NRHA)

- Non-profit organization that provides leadership on rural healthcare issues
- Mission is to improve the health and well-being to rural Americans and to provide leadership on rural health issues
- Areas of focus include: NRHA Quality Initiatives, EMS agenda for the future, and sponsor of Rural Medical Educators and NRHA Student Group
- Advocates legislative and regulatory policies and positions before Congress and the White House
- Members actively participate to bring about appropriate rural health policy and legislation
- Volunteer membership

For more information on the National Rural Health Association, see: http://www.nrharural.org

---

Maximizing Non-traditional Healthcare Resources

Rural partnerships might also include less traditional partners such as schools, **cooperative extension offices**, health departments, mental health centers, and senior citizen agencies. Additionally, local chapters of agencies such as the American Heart Association, American Lung Association, and American Red Cross may be available. Rural cooperative extension offices, funded by the U.S. Department of Agriculture, provide leadership in programming and address issues of concern specific to families, youth, and rural communities. Affiliated groups, such as 4-H clubs, are frequently involved in health-related community service projects. Some community colleges in rural areas offer healthcare screening and education through wellness centers operated and staffed by nursing faculty and students. Collaboration among these groups, other community agencies, and local churches can provide for the more efficient use of scarce resources to improve the health of rural residents.

KEY TERM

Cooperative extension office: Funded by the U.S. Department of Agriculture, these offices provide leadership in programming, addressing issues of concern specific to families, youth, and rural communities.

Maximizing Educational Opportunities and Technology for Rural Health Care

Developing and maximizing a rural nursing workforce can be challenging. There are fewer healthcare providers in rural settings and the skills of those available need to be maximized. Especially with the rapid pace of change, rural nurses work hard to access educational resources and keep up with changing healthcare practices. Educating new professionals, orienting new nurses, and promoting staff development can all present special challenges in rural settings. **Area health education centers (AHECs)**, community colleges, and distance education partnerships can all play important roles in this effort. Technology and rural/urban partnerships are central forces in rural health care as well.

AHECs and community colleges promote health profession education in many rural states. AHECs are federally funded partnerships between health science center universities and local health agencies. AHEC partners, with particular knowledge and expertise in the interests and needs of rural students and graduates, assist rural healthcare agencies with the facilitation of rural relationships, strategic planning, and program marketing. The continuing education offered to healthcare providers in the field enhances the level of care provided, particularly in counties where few healthcare agencies and health profession schools exist, ultimately improving patient care in underserved areas.

Community colleges play a central role in nursing education in rural states. Often these schools are the only regional access to professional clinical education such as practical nursing and associate degree nursing programs. In addition to basic healthcare educational programs, community colleges can provide a foundation for educational career ladders that partner with distant colleges and universities. Issues that impact rural community colleges can include a shortage of available clinical sites, a limited range of clinical experiences, and a shortage of nursing faculty. Extensive travel may be involved for rural nursing students to obtain clinical experiences with a variety of patients.

Because advanced clinical education programs typically are not available in rural communities, technology provides a way to extend health profession education. The concepts of "growing your own" and educational career ladders often incorporate distance education strategies that provide opportunity for students unable to travel to college campuses to continue their education. Web-based transition programs such as RN to BSN programs allow diverse students to access advanced education from home communities. A diverse group of healthcare providers can be gained who are more likely to stay in their rural communities and potentially improve the distribution of health profession workers to underserved areas. There are several online graduate nursing programs that provide opportunities to specialize in rural nursing leadership.

Integrating the use of technology into health care can change the quality of practice in rural settings. Patient simulators are a good example of opportunities for technology partnerships in the rural setting. Simulators have implications for both staff development and professional education. Simulators, available in multiple forms, are tools in healthcare education that mimic patient encounters and provide practice application of theoretical concepts and skills.

In particular, new high-fidelity patient simulators (HFPS) provide students and clinicians opportunities for skill practice in a safe setting. Simulators provide an opportunity to offer a diverse range of clinical experiences to students and the current nursing workforce. Rural nursing staff can demonstrate critical assessment skills, maintain practice on unusual cases, and gain continuing education without extensive travel.

Technology partnerships are particularly important in the rural setting, providing convenience in connecting with larger urban centers and specialists. **Telehealth** and **telemedicine** use telecommunications technology to deliver, manage, and coordinate care and provide rural practitioners with the opportunity to work with practitioners in urban specialty centers. Virtual health professional teams can be developed that connect rural primary care clinics with urban specialists via telemedicine. Healthcare providers can monitor patients and/or consult with rural care providers from a distance, collaboratively diagnosing patients, designing treatment plans, and monitoring patient outcomes. Real-time, two-way visual and audio connectivity between patient and provider are made possible using assistants and specially made equipment at the rural site. With appropriate resources, settings such as primary care, long-term care, hospitals, and even patient homes can be sites for telemedicine.

> **KEY TERM**
>
> **Telehealth:** Healthcare services delivered, managed, and coordinated by nurses and other healthcare providers using electronic information and telecommunications technologies.

> **KEY TERM**
>
> **Telemedicine:** A component of telehealth focusing on medicine's approach to deliver, manage, and coordinate care via telecommunications technologies.

Furthermore, telehealth technology can allow patient assessment data such as heart and lung sounds to be transmitted electronically to specialty providers. Digital images such as x-rays or pictures of skin lesions can be transmitted. Given the appropriate technology, healthcare providers can connect with patients and families in their homes for routine check-ins and electronic reminders. Competencies needed in telehealth nursing include both technical and interpersonal skills, practice knowledge, and administrative skills including documentation and resource management (American Academy of Ambulatory Care Nursing, 2007).

Additional technologies that assist clinicians in promoting the public's health include the web, personal digital assistants (PDAs), and electronic records. These technologies promote systematic approaches to information retrieval as well as patient-related care. Use of web-based libraries and resources of all types promote efficient access to clinical resources. The concept of fingertip knowledge is expanded as evidence-based protocols are accessed for practice. Particularly in rural settings, with the need for a broad range of information for dealing with diverse situations, these electronic resources help practitioners provide quality care. As in urban settings, use of PDAs assists in systematic documentation and makes Web resources easily available for fingertip knowledge. These resources can help rural nurses implement evidence-based practice.

Use of electronic records promotes safety in patient care as well as providing data for quality assurance. Electronic records provide a systematic approach to record-keeping and easy data retrieval for patient care. Uses include not only provider documentation, but also prescribing, insurance claims processing, data exchange, and communicating information to promote efficient patient transfers. Outcomes evaluation and continuous quality improvement are facilitated with electronic records.

The Web serves as a resource in patient education and caregiving as well. Appropriate online support groups and educational resources can be recommended to patients and families such as those with breast cancer, cystic fibrosis, Parkinson's disease, or caregivers of family members with Alzheimer's disease.

A current national focus is on the development of best structures and networks for electronic system communications (Board on Healthcare Services, 2005). In the rural setting, technology-savvy resource people are needed to promote efficient technology use. In particular, nurses are needed who can help determine best practices in the use of technology for patient care, ensuring that patients receive high-touch care along with the use of advanced technology.

Technology can positively influence healthcare practice in rural settings. Student and staff development is enhanced. In addition, efficiency and safety within health care are two advantages to having access to appropriate technology that is used in efficient ways. Technology has relevance for all practitioners and plays an important role in facilitating evidence-based practice and continuous quality improvement. Contemporary Practice Highlight 19-2 describes a current initiative that promotes the use of technology to improve patient safety.

CONTEMPORARY PRACTICE HIGHLIGHT 19-2

TECHNOLOGY

Broad attention is currently being given to the need for appropriate technology to promote safe quality care for patients. Effective electronic record systems are one approach to communicating and transferring information across healthcare systems. Although there are federal initiatives promoting technology for a connected and seamless healthcare system, implementing technology systems can challenge and burden rural health care. Nurses have a role in both making electronic record needs known within their systems and providing ideas for point-of-care approaches. Nationally, nurses are involved in the Technology Informatics Guiding Educational Reform (TIGER) initiative. The purpose of the TIGER initiative is to increase the technology capabilities of nurses and identify best practices to facilitate effective information management. One of the TIGER goals is to establish guidelines for organizations to follow as they integrate informatics into practice and academic settings.

Source: Report from the Technology Informatics Guiding Educational Reform (TIGER) Initiative (Health Information Technology). https://www.tigersummit.com.

Evidence-Based Practice and Quality Improvement in Rural Nursing

Quality improvement projects require leadership and time resources. In the rural setting many nurses are non-baccalaureate prepared and may have a limited theory or research background for quality improvement projects. Nurses who have the educational preparation, skills, and dedicated time required to direct data collection and quality assurance studies specific to the increasingly complex needs of diverse patients in a technology-driven, chaotic healthcare system are needed. The common rural issue of too few people to fulfill multiple roles can challenge quality improvement efforts. Although quality assurance positions are emerging in the rural hospital, with limited staff it is often the nurse manager who attempts to forward quality assurance efforts along with a myriad of other responsibilities. Nurse leaders are needed to help organizations become more quality focused with a learning community approach that addresses ongoing professional development and culture change.

The improved healthcare outcomes linked to evidence-based practice are critical for rural settings. Because time and resource barriers may present challenges to evidence-based practice, project partnering is often a necessity for rural healthcare providers. Leaders in rural nursing organizations can promote partnerships and help promote quality initiatives. For example, a nursing specialist in pressure ulcer prevention and treatment may not be available in the rural setting, but national organizations such as the American Association of Clinical Nurse Specialists can provide resources or suggest nurse consultants.

Evidence-based protocol development can be more efficiently done within a network of rural providers. National organizations and federal agencies such as the CDC, American Diabetic Association, American Heart Association, and others can serve as resources for helping nursing staff obtain and organize best practice evidence. Additionally, the rural context needs to be considered in evidence-based practice, asking, for example, if there are differences in how protocols need to be implemented in rural versus urban settings. There are a variety of interest groups, ranging from hospitals and specialty groups to governmental agencies, all intent on identifying how evidence-based practice can promote quality care, patient safety, and system efficiency, and decrease costs.

Implications for Rural Nursing Practice and Education

The rural nurse has an opportunity to create a role to match the needs of a particular rural community. Strategies such as preparing, organizing, and collaborating can help guide readiness for practice in the rural setting. Sample practice tips for rural nursing are highlighted in Box 19-9.

BOX 19-9   PRACTICE TIPS FOR RURAL NURSING

The following guidelines will help you prepare for nursing practice in a rural health care setting:

- Acquire a broad, generalist nursing education and expertise
- Use a population focus in health promotion, building on available resources and working with people in their communities to promote health
- Work with primary care settings to identify educational resources and promote best practices for problems such as farm safety, child/teen safety, and coping with chronic illnesses
- Develop community-wide interventions using resources such as schools and churches and other relevant networks
- Develop an understanding of coordinator and case manager roles, gaining familiarity with local and regional resources for client support
- Emphasize the positive, work with and build on available informal and formal community networks and resources
- Promote and encourage use of collaborations and technology to promote expanded resources for health care
- Be active in national nursing organizations that provide collegial support as well as resources for practice
- Be familiar with continuous quality improvement approaches and resources for evidence-based practice

---

Preparing for a rural nursing practice includes obtaining a good generalist education that prepares one to provide care to a broad range of patients. This includes being able to identify and access resources and provider networks to assist in caring for those patients with less common health problems. This also includes being knowledgeable of common challenges in addressing rural health promotion and safety issues, and effectively working with people in their communities to promote health. The rural health nurse needs to understand how to consider and apply "best" nursing approaches broadly in community health systems, gaining guidance from resources such as Healthy People 2010 (U.S. Department of Health and Human Services, 2000).

Organizing for a rural nursing practice includes knowing formal and informal resources available in the community that can extend health capacity and caregiving capabilities. This includes assessing the strengths and weaknesses of these community resources. Organizing or taking leadership in community health-building efforts can promote ongoing projects with schools, churches, and community groups. Because volunteer efforts often play a central role in extending healthcare resources, the rural health nurse must be able to optimize volunteer opportunities, understand the principles of volunteerism, and work effectively with community volunteers.

Collaborating within local and regional networks promotes partnerships for increasing quality and efficiency of services. Examples of such collaboration can include building bridges with technology between care partners, participating with national organizations on evidence-based practice committees, and helping local healthcare organizations select and participate in meaningful quality improvement projects. Being active in nursing organizations also provides collegial support as well as resources for practice; this can help build bridges for support via regional and national organizations.

Nurses can do a self-assessment to make sure they have the competencies needed by rural nurses. Hurme (2007) organized 25 different competencies to include the major categories of clinical and technical skills, critical thinking, interpersonal communication, and management/organizational skills. Competencies needed by the rural nurse are noted in Box 19-10.

Summary

Designing a nursing role in rural health involves a good generalist preparation, working with the community for health promotion, being aware of resources, knowledgeably using technology tools, and having a willingness to work collaboratively with partners in care to ensure best-care practices. This includes partnerships at local, regional, and national levels. Concepts of preparing, organizing, and collaborating can guide the nurse in determining his or her readiness for practicing in rural community settings. Rural nursing provides the opportunity to practice the best of population-based care, acute care, and chronic care management skills.

BOX 19-10   COMPETENCIES FOR RURAL NURSES

- Maintains broad clinical and technical skills
- Employs critical thinking and problem solving in caregiving
- Participates as a collaborative healthcare team member
- Utilizes informatics in meeting diverse patient care needs and promoting efficient healthcare systems
- Utilizes good interpersonal communication and teaching/learning strategies with culturally diverse patients and families
- Promotes community-wide efforts for maintaining a healthy community
- Utilizes clinical best practices and pursues quality assurance efforts

Expanded competencies from IOM Health Professions Competencies, Health Professions Education: A Bridge to Quality, http://www.nap.edu/catalog.php?record_id=10681

Key Terms

- **Area health education centers (AHECs):** Federally funded partnerships between health science center universities and local community clinical and educational resources that work together to improve education to local multidisciplinary providers and ultimately improve patient care in underserved areas.
- **Cooperative extension office:** Funded by the U.S. Department of Agriculture, these offices provide leadership in programming, addressing issues of concern specific to families, youth, and rural communities.
- **Critical access facility:** A small rural hospital that is the sole community hospital provider and is reimbursed by the Centers for Medicare and Medicaid Services for actual costs.
- **Health disparities:** Differences in conditions that exist among specific population groups in the United States, including incidence, prevalence, mortality, and burden of diseases.
- **Health literacy:** An individual's capacity to obtain, process, and understand the basic health information needed to make appropriate health decisions.
- **Health professional shortage area (HPSA):** This designation identifies defined communities that have shortages of healthcare providers such as primary care, dental, or mental health care (Health Resources Service Administration, 2006).
- **Medically underserved populations (MUPs):** This designation is assigned to healthcare service areas that face economic, cultural, or linguistic barriers to health care and is based on computations specific to community poverty level, elderly population, infant mortality rate, and ratio of primary care physicians per 1,000 population (Health Resources Service Administration, 2006).
- **Swing beds:** Excess hospital beds that are designated for patients needing long-term skilled nursing care.
- **Telehealth:** Healthcare services delivered, managed, and coordinated by nurses and other healthcare providers using electronic information and telecommunications technologies.
- **Telemedicine:** A component of telehealth focusing on medicine's approach to deliver, manage, and coordinate care via telecommunications technologies.

Reflective Practice Questions

1. What are your experiences working with patients from a rural setting? What aspects of this chapter support your understanding of rural healthcare issues? What surprises were there as you read about healthcare issues of rural patients?

2. What do you think are some of the similarities and differences in caring for patients in rural and urban settings? If you interviewed a patient from a rural setting and one from an urban setting with the same diagnosis, such as breast cancer, what similar concerns would you expect? What different concerns?

3. What role should nurses in rural areas play in creating healthcare partnerships with non-traditional healthcare resources such as 4-H clubs or Boy Scout organizations?

4. What do you see as the most important benefits of technology in rural health care? What skills would you personally need to develop in your nursing practice to effectively work in telehealth? How can you learn more about this healthcare approach?

5. Visit the National Rural Health Association (http://www.ruralhealthweb. org/) and explore some of the links within it. If you were a nurse practicing in a rural area, what resources could you derive from this site that would help you provide better care and teaching to your patients?

References

American Academy of Ambulatory Care Nursing. (2007, Jan/Feb). Telehealth nursing practice. *American Academy of Ambulatory Care Nursing Viewpoint*. Retrieved October 12, 2007, from http://findarticles.com/p/articles/mi_qa4022/is_200701/ai_n18705860

Catanzaro, A., Meador, K., Koenig, H., Kuchibhatla, M., & Clipp, E. (2007). Congregational health ministries: A national study of pastors' views. *Public Health Nursing, 24*(1), 6–17.

Clark, K. J., & Leipert, B. D. (2007). Strengthening and sustaining social supports for rural elders. *Online Journal of Rural Nursing and Health Care, 7*(1), 13–26. Retrieved October 12, 2007, from http://www.rno.org/journal/index.php/online-journal/article/view-File/6/177

Committee on the Future of Rural Health Care. (2005). *Quality through collaboration: The future of rural health care.* Washington, DC: The National Academies Press.

Connor, A., Rainer, L. P., Simcox, J. B., & Thomisee, K. (2007). Increasing the delivery of health care services to migrant farm worker families through a community partnership model. *Public Health Nursing, 24*(4), 355–360.

Easom, L., & Quinn, M. (2006). Rural elderly caregivers: Exploring folk home remedy use and health promotion activities. *Online Journal of Rural Nursing and Health Care, 6*(1), 32–46. Retrieved October 12, 2007, from http://www.rno.org/journal/index.php/online-journal/article/viewFile/30/159

Gamm, L. D., & Hutchison, L. L. (2004). *Rural healthy people 2010: A companion document to healthy people 2010* (Vol. 3). College Station, TX: The Texas A&M University System Health Science Center, School of Rural Public Health, Southwest Rural Health Research Center. Retrieved October 12, 2007, from http://srphnt08.srph.tamhsc.edu/centers/rhp2010/Volume1.pdf

Gaskins, S., & Lyons, M. (2000). Self-care practices of rural people with HIV disease. *Online Journal of Rural Nursing and Health Care, 1*(1), 18–27. Retrieved October 12, 2007, from http://www.rno.org/journal/index.php/online-journal/article/viewFile/64/63

Hartley, D. (2004). Rural health disparities, population health, and rural culture. *American Journal of Public Health, 94*(10), 1675–1678. Retrieved October 12, 2007, from http://www.pubmedcentral.nih.gov/articlerender.fcgi?artid=1448513

Hartley, D., & Gale, J. (2003). *Tools for monitoring the health care safety net, rural health care safety nets.* Retrieved October 12, 2007, from http://www.ahcpr.gov/data/safetynet/hartley.htm

Health Resources and Services Administration. (2006). *Shortage designation.* Retrieved October 12, 2007, from http://bhpr.hrsa.gov/shortage/

Hurme, F. E. (2007). *Competencies for rural nursing practice.* Doctoral dissertation, Louisiana State University, Baton Rouge, LA. Retrieved October 12, 2007, from http://etd.lsu.edu/docs/available/etd-04052007-112941/

Lindeke, L. L., Grabau, A. M., & Jukkala, A. J. (2004). Rural NP perceptions of barriers to practice. *Nurse Practitioner, 29*(8), 50–51. Retrieved October 12, 2007, from http://findarticles.com/p/articles/mi_qa3958/is_200408/ai_n9454132/

Montgomery, R., & Williams, K. (2001). Implications of differential impacts of care-giving for future research on Alzheimer care. *Aging and Mental Health, 5*(2 Supp), S23–S34.

National Rural Health Association. (2007). *National rural health association mission* Retrieved July 26, 2008, from http://www.ruralhealthweb.org/go/top/about-the-nrha/our-mission

Ormond, B., Wallin, S., & Goldenson, S. (2000). *Supporting the rural health care safety net.* Retrieved July 26, 2008, from http://www.urban.org/publications/309437.html

Pierce, C. (2007). Distance and access to health care for rural women with heart failure. *Online Journal of Rural Nursing and Health Care, 7*(1), 27–34.

Rural Assistance Center. (2007). *Rural health literacy frequently asked questions.* Retrieved October 12, 2007, from http://www.raconline.org/info_guides/healthliteracy/health literacyfaq.php

Technology Informatics Guiding Education Reform (TIGER). (2008). About TIGER. Retrieved February 20, 2008, from https://www.tigersummit.com/.

U.S. Department of Health and Human Services. (2000). *Healthy people 2010: Understanding and improving health* (2nd ed.). Washington, DC: U.S. Government Printing Office. Retrieved October 11, 2007, from http://www.healthypeople.gov/Document/tableofcontents.htm

Williams, S. (2007). Urban care in rural settings. *Nursing Spectrum (New England edition), 11*(14), 8–9.

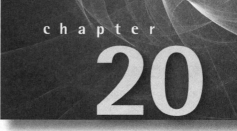

20

Informatics and Healthcare Technology

Elizabeth M. LaRue, Susan K. Newbold, Gilan EL Saadawi,
and Karen L. Courtney

LEARNING OUTCOMES

After reading this chapter you will be able to:

- Define informatics and healthcare technology.
- Identify changes in the practice of health care due to technology infiltration.
- Discuss ethical concerns with technology in the healthcare arena.
- Explain security issues related to the use of healthcare technology.
- Describe how automated tools can help promote quality patient outcomes.
- Describe the role of the nurse in implementing information technology that promotes evidence-based practice.
- Discuss three issues related to the implementation of information technology in health care.
- Predict future uses of technology in health care.

Introduction

Nursing practice has been and will continue to be significantly altered by the use of **informatics** and **healthcare technology**. Ranging from something as simple as the use of an electronic thermometer to the

Healthcare technology: Technology used to deliver care in the prevention, diagnosis, and treatment of health problems.

Informatics: The study of the structure and properties of information.

sophistication of leading-edge intensive care unit hemodynamic monitors and fully computerized clinical management information systems, informatics and healthcare technology have revolutionized the delivery of health care and created a level of complexity never before experienced by healthcare providers. Telehealth, e-ICUs, and networked clinical information management systems that provide immediate access to patient medical records are just a few examples of the increasingly common technology being used in healthcare organizations. The explosion of technology in health care has created the need for nurses and other healthcare providers to be savvy users of technology, with an understanding of the legal, ethical, and financial issues associated with the use of technology.

This chapter provides an overview of informatics and healthcare technology and describes how the use of technology affects nursing practice and patient care outcomes. Informatics and healthcare technology will be defined and the legal, ethical, and financial considerations associated with the use of technology also will be addressed. Changes in health care and the way technology has influenced those changes also will be presented.

Nursing informatics (NI): A specialty that integrates nursing science, computer science, and information science to manage and communicate data, information, knowledge, and wisdom in nursing practice.

Nursing Informatics

Nursing informatics (NI) is a specialty that integrates nursing science, computer science, and information science to manage and communicate data, information, knowledge, and wisdom in nursing practice. NI supports consumers, patients, nurses, and other providers in their decision making in all roles and settings. This support is accomplished through the use of information structures, information processes, and information technology (American Nurses Association [ANA], 2008). Nursing informatics is part of the larger field of healthcare informatics.

The first master's degree in nursing informatics was offered by the University of Maryland, Baltimore School of Nursing in 1989. Nursing informatics was recognized as a specialty field for registered nurses by the American Nurses Association (ANA) in 1992. In 1995 the American Nurses Credentialing Center offered the first certification examination for informatics nurses. There are approximately 8,000–10,000 nurses currently working in the field of informatics in the United States, and there is a growing need for more nurses specializing in informatics. There are not enough informatics nurse specialists to analyze, develop, test and maintain, implement, and evaluate systems that support patient care and aid the profession of nursing.

Nursing Informatics: Not Just for the Specialists

Informatics concepts cannot be left to the informatics nurse specialists, but must be adopted by all nurses. The work of Staggers, Gassert, and Curran (2002) delineates informatics competencies for the beginning nurse, the experienced nurse, the informatics specialist, and the informatics innovator. The competencies include computer skills and informatics skills that can be used by faculty to create curricula or by an employer to determine skills needed by the nursing workforce.

In 2005 the TIGER Initiative (Technology Informatics Guiding Education Reform) was created to "enable practicing nurses and nursing students to fully engage in the unfolding digital era of health care. The purpose of the initiative is to identify information/knowledge management best practices and effective technology capabilities for nurses" (TIGER, 2008). The vision for the future of nursing is to bridge the quality chasm with information technology, enabling nurses to use informatics in practice and education to provide safer, higher-quality patient care. More information about the TIGER initiative can be found at the following Web site: http://www.tigersummit.com.

Nurses as Knowledge Workers

Knowledge is information that is synthesized so that relationships are identified and formalized. Nurses are knowledge workers, taking information from many sources and combining it in meaningful ways. As knowledge workers, nurses make numerous decisions that affect the life and well-being of individuals, families, and communities (ANA, 2008). Decisions are best when supported with data, often housed in electronic sources. Nursing informatics can help nurses synthesize knowledge, manage information, and make decisions that promote quality patient care outcomes.

One of the tenets of nursing informatics is the focus on efficient and effective delivery of complete and accurate information in order to achieve quality outcomes (ANA, 2008). Table 20-1 contains measurement criteria, as cited in the *Scope and Standards of Nursing Informatics Practice* (ANA, 2008) as being a standard for the informatics nurse, although these standards can apply to all nurses. It is clear that every nurse needs to have an understanding of the continuum from data to information to knowledge to wisdom in order to make decisions about patient care needs. Such an understanding promotes utilization of research evidence and results in the implementation of evidence-based practices.

Use of Informatics and Outcomes in Evidence-Based Practice (EBP)

Evidence-based practice (EBP) is the conscientious use of current best evidence in making decisions about patient care. It is a problem-solving approach to clinical

TABLE 20-1	SCOPE AND STANDARDS OF PRACTICE FOR NURSING INFORMATICS (ANA, 2008)

The informatics nurse formulates expected patient outcomes by:

- Involving the patient and family members, nurses, healthcare providers, and other stakeholders.

- Considering cost-benefit ratios, environmental factors, potential risks, evidence-based findings, and expert knowledge

- Defining outcomes within the context of patient values, ethical considerations, the environment, and the organization

- Identifying a time line for achieving the established outcomes

- Developing outcomes that will provide stakeholders with a clear plan of action

- Modifying anticipated outcomes as appropriate based upon evaluation data and changes in patient's situation

- Documenting goals for achieving outcomes that are measurable

- Determining that outcomes are established by considering scientific evidence and utilizing evidence-based practices

- Achieving outcomes using economically responsible methods that optimize the potential for quality, efficiency, and effectiveness

- Supporting the integration of clinical guidelines with information systems, informatics informed solutions, and knowledge bases to achieve outcomes

Source: Adapted from American Nurses' Association, 2008. *Nursing Informatics: Scope and Standards of Practice.*

practice that integrates a systematic search and critical appraisal of the most relevant evidence related to a specific clinical question, with one's own clinical expertise and the patient's preferences, while also valuing the humanistic component of providing care (Melnyk and Fineout-Overhold, 2005).

Various informatics tools and techniques can be utilized to bring the best available evidence about nursing and health care to the point of care in order to support the patient's health and decision making. These tools help in the conversion of data to information. At the most simple level, automation can help ascertain the accuracy of the data. Edit checks can validate whether the data entered is within the appropriate range; for example, a temperature could not be entered as 112° Fahrenheit. Tools such as spreadsheets or graphics can display vital signs over time in a way that is more meaningful than numbers alone. At a more complex level, data from hundreds of cases may be used to predict risk; for example, nurses can use an automated method to quickly and accurately identify patients at risk for rapid deterioration in medical status.

In health care, large amounts of data have been collected in electronic formats but it is hard to derive information from this data. Data mining is the technique of sorting through large amounts of data and selecting relevant information. Data mining is one step in the process of knowledge discovery in large databases. According to Abbott (2000), knowledge discovery in large databases is the melding of human expertise with statistical and machine learning techniques to identify features, patterns, and underlying rules in large collections of healthcare data. This fusion of approaches leads to the detection of nonintuitive, previously undiscovered relationships in the data.

Barriers to Utilization of Research Evidence

Understanding informatics concepts can provide the nurse with tools to overcome perceived barriers to research utilization. Hutchinson and Johnson (2006) cited barriers to nurses' utilization of research evidence. Nurses perceive they do not have time to search for evidence. They lack confidence in their critical appraisal skills and believe they lack authority to make decisions based on evidence. The organization's infrastructure and lack of support may be additional barriers in some organizations. Nurses may not have access to information from the point of care and there may be a lack of evidence on the topic in question. Generally there may be a lack of understanding of what evidence-based content is and how to integrate it within clinical systems.

Fundamentally, the nurse may not be well-versed in information seeking. Pravikoff, Tanner, and Pierce (2005) revealed in a study of over 3,000 staff nurses that although 64.5 percent of nurses report needing information weekly or several times weekly, only 26.7 percent have received training in using tools to access evidence. Only 11 percent cite searching for information from evidence weekly or more often, and nearly half (48.5 percent) are not familiar with the term *evidence-based practice*. See Chapter 11 for further discussion of evidence-based practice.

Current Issues in Informatics

There are many issues related to the use of informatics in health care. These include technology barriers, developing **standardized languages**, ethical concerns (privacy, security, and confidentiality), and the social and economical impact of technology.

> **KEY TERM**
>
> **Standardized language:** A collection of terms with definitions that are used in informational system databases.

Technology as a Barrier

The technology itself can be a barrier to its adoption. The lack of interoperable systems is one of the main technical hindrances to the implementation of electronic records. Today, the available systems have many technological variations in how they operate and communicate. There are many proprietary systems and multiple standards, which have led to a fragmented infrastructure that lacks the ability to exchange information across software applications.

Standardized Language

The ANA (2008) defines a standardized language as "a collection of terms with definitions for use in informational systems databases. They enable comparisons to be made because the same term is used to denote the same condition." When a standardized language is used with an electronic documentation system it provides a way to enter and access data in a systematic way. Having specific and consistent descriptions of nursing care allows for data abstraction for research purposes and makes the contributions to outcomes made by nursing care more measurable. The relationships between standardized language and evidence-based practice include linking of clinical practice guidelines to appropriate patients during the patient–provider encounter and matching potential research subjects to research protocols for which they are potentially eligible (Saba & McCormick, 2006). These relationships provide a foundation with which to build nursing practice and nursing science.

Nursing needs standardized terminology to summarize medical information and to document clinical details (problems, interventions, and outcomes) over time. Nursing has set some standards for nursing terminology but these nursing classifications are not included in all clinical information systems. Nursing, in general, has not seen the need to demand the use of these nursing classifications. For a list of the nursing classifications recognized by the ANA, see Table 20-2.

Ethical Issues: Privacy, Security, and Confidentiality

KEY TERM

Privacy: Expected behavior that regulates the professional relationship between patients and their healthcare providers.

KEY TERM

Security: Involves protecting data and information systems, including ensuring the integrity of the information and protecting against accidental or purposeful misuse of the data and loss due to physical damage.

Safeguards to patients' privacy, security, and confidentiality are key to the successful adoption of the electronic health record (EHR). **Privacy** is the individuals' right to keep certain information to themselves and not disclose it. Maintaining a patient's right to privacy has always been a concern of healthcare providers and institutions, but the increasing use of information technology and technology networks in all healthcare systems has complicated and extended the scope of this concern. **Security** involves protecting information and systems, including ensuring the integrity and availability of the information. It includes the physical means and procedures that protect data and information against accidental or purposeful misuse and other disasters. **Confidentiality** is the practice of permitting only certain authorized individuals

TABLE 20-2	NURSING CLASSIFICATIONS RECOGNIZED BY THE AMERICAN NURSES ASSOCIATION

North American Nursing Diagnosis Association (NANDA)
Nursing Interventions Classifications (NIC)
Nursing Outcomes Classification (NOC)
Home Health Care Classification (HHCC)
Omaha System
Patient Care Data Set (PCDS)
AORN Perioperative Nursing Dataset (PNDS)
Systematized Nomenclature of Medicine—Clinical Terms (SNOMED CT)
International Classification for Nursing (ICNP)
ABC Codes
Nursing Minimum Data Set (NMDS)
Nursing Management Minimum Data Set (NMMDS)

Source: American Nurses Association (2008). Recognized languages for nursing (revised April 2008). Retrieved July 29, 2008, from http://www.nursingworld.org/MainMenuCategories/ThePracticeofProfessionalNursing/DocInfo/NIDSEC/RecognizedLanguagesfornursing.aspx.

to access information, with the understanding that they will disclose it only to other authorized individuals as appropriate. Confidentiality is a legal protection and the assurance of an individual's right to privacy to the fullest extent allowable by state law; however, information is not confidential unless there exists a treatment relationship between the patient and care provider (Shortliffe & Cimino, 2006).

> **KEY TERM**
>
> **Confidentiality:** Legal protection ensuring individuals their right to privacy to the fullest extent allowable by law.

Privacy and confidentiality are inherently expected by the *International Code of Ethics for Nursing* (International Council of Nurses [ICN], 2008). The Code makes it clear that every nurse has the duty to respect human rights, including the rights to life, to dignity, and to be treated with respect. The ICN *International Code of Ethics for Nursing* guides nurses in everyday choices and supports nurses' refusal to participate in activities that conflict with caring and healing.

In addition to the ethical considerations that must always be considered in a nurse/patient professional relationship, federal and state governments have enacted a number of laws in an attempt to create standards for ensuring the right to privacy and confidentiality of personal information while still creating electronic systems that will enhance and improve all levels of healthcare systems. For example, the Privacy Act of 1974 (Department of Justice, 2003) mandates a written consent before the disclosure or use of any personal information. The Privacy Act also states that if the institution maintains a record of any individual, this individual has the right to review and copy any portion of this record and has the right to make any amendments or changes (Hodge, Gostin, & Jacobson, 1999). Individual institutions have developed policies and security systems that ensure these rights within their own system, but once any information is transmitted across various forms of media networks, the mechanisms for ensuring this privacy become extremely complex.

The U.S. Department of Health and Human Services (HHS) has created security standards for electronic health data, mandated under the **Health Insurance Portability and Accountability Act of 1996 (HIPAA)**, also known as the Kennedy-Kassebaum Act (HHS, 2007). The main aims of HIPAA are to improve the efficiency of healthcare delivery and to standardize electronic data interchange while enforcing standards to protect patients' confidentiality. It specifies that individuals have the right to control their data and to be informed of their privacy rights. The law covers all medical records or any individually identifiable health information and mandates that healthcare providers give clear written explanations of how their information is going to be used. It also gives individuals the right to see and copy their records and request amendments. Individuals also have the right to file a formal complaint if they feel that their privacy was violated. This act has had a great impact on healthcare delivery systems; it has initiated the development of unique identifiers for both patients and employees, secure user authentication software, and major advances in security systems and firewalls.

To reinforce ethical behavior, institutions usually provide employee education emphasizing the importance of protecting patient privacy and the confidentiality of patient information. Violation of patient confidentiality usually invokes disciplinary action and quite possibly termination of the employee. Moreover, to deter the breach of confidentiality, obstacles have been placed within the technology itself to create access barriers and track user access. One method of reinforcing ethical behavior and confidentiality is the audit trail in which the identity, time, and context of all users accessing a computer system is automatically recorded. Other measures of monitoring ethics and confidentiality are enforcing strong user authentication, installing firewalls and rights management software where the content is segmented and encrypted, and granting users access based on their right to know (Rindfleisch, 1997).

Social Impact

Information technology (IT) is transforming the social, cultural, and economic landscape of health care. Several common themes permeate the literature regarding IT's social impact, including the creation of the digital divide, the impact of information technology on economics and the work environment, and the effects of globalization enabled by the Internet. Some have noted that to understand fully the social impact of IT one should include an examination of the economic, political, cultural, legal, environmental, ergonomic, health, and psychological effects of IT on human life.

Although the number of Americans who have access to the Internet is growing, some of the most vulnerable healthcare populations remain disenfranchised from accessing or gaining benefit from healthcare information found on the Internet. This concept has been termed the *digital divide*. The "digital divide" is not confined to individual patients however; in many cases smaller health care practices and organizations cannot afford to financially support the infrastructure and maintenance required to computerize patient health care records, deliver telehealth, or monitor patient care.

Economic Impact

The economic realities of delivering health care are being transformed by the implementation of health information technology. According to the Agency for Healthcare Research and Quality (AHRQ) 2006 report, *Costs and Benefits of Health Information Technology (HIT)*, "HIT has the potential to enable a dramatic transformation in the delivery of health care, making it safer, more effective, and more efficient (p.v)." The report continues, adding that, "The quantifiable benefits of HIT are projected to outweigh the investments' cost. However, the predicted time needed to break even varied from three to as many as 13 years (p.v)." Costs involved in implementing HIT include the initial capital investment for installing hardware and software, staff training on the use of the system, and the costs assoiciated with a temporary decrease in productivity while the system is being implemented. Ongoing maintenance of the system is another cost.

Healthcare Technology

A technology can be anything that aids in accomplishing a task. Most of the time technologies are idealized as a tangible mechanism such as a monitor, an invasive device, or even a blood pressure cuff; however, technology can take other forms as well, such as a radioactive dye, an enzyme, or heat. Healthcare technology can be defined as technology that is used to deliver care in the prevention, diagnosis, and treatment of health problems.

Healthcare technology has evolved to the point that in the 21st century we think of it primarily as computer software applications and computer hardware that interact to become a medical device to improve health care. The infusion of technology into health care means there is not a practicing nurse who does not use daily at least one form of health technology in her or his profession. This has resulted in an expansion in nurses' expected skill sets to include knowledge of technology and to demonstrate adeptness in its use and capabilities. This knowledge has provided nurses the opportunity to test, develop, and implement technologies for their practice and general health care. As new technologies emerge and existing technologies change over time, this requires nurses to maintain an ongoing commitment to learning.

The role that nurses play and their level of involvement within the technology team are vital factors for the successful implementation and utilization of any technology. Implementing the use of new technology requires changing attitudes, cultures, and the practice of providing health care (Oroviogoicoechea, Elliott, & Watson, 2008). When future users participate in the design and development or selection of information technologies the likelihood of successful implementation and use of these systems increases (Barki & Hartwick, 1994; Demiris, 2006; Foster & Franz, 1999).

Nurses may be involved in all phases of choosing a new technology, including design, development, or selection of the technology. Nursing involvement in technology design or development frequently means nurses help technology designers understand the clinical workflow of a setting and help with prototype testing of user interfaces and functions (Lee, 2007). Nurses' understanding of the clinical workflow within the work setting is also invaluable to technology implementation teams when they are selecting an existing commercial technology rather than developing their own. As team members, nurses can help identify priority functions as well as identify potential clinical practice problems with a technology design. If the clinical workflow is not considered in technology design or selection, nurses and other healthcare providers often resort to workarounds, which can eliminate the safety features or benefits of a technology (Vogelsmeier, Halbesleben, & Scott-Cawiezell, 2008).

As part of the implementation team, nurses are involved in identifying resources and needs (such as additional staff, hardware, or training), designing and delivering effective training, and potentially serving as "power users" or "unit champions" (Lee, 2007). Nurses help to provide the necessary customization for the clinical setting for general implementation plans. Nurse administrators also must recognize the organizational issues that require administrative resource support in addition to identifying the nurses who will be the power users and the unit champions who will help facilitate the technology use in their clinical practice setting (Moen, 2003). Because of the practice implications, nurses need to be involved in the design or selection of technologies and the implementation of technologies within their clinical work setting.

Changes in Workflow and Practice

Information technology can be used to create dynamic, data-using applications that go beyond simply developing electronic versions of existing paper forms.

These types of data-using applications can also change nursing practice and workflow. For instance, creating an electronic version of a paper form can make data retrieval easier and help to reduce errors from poor handwriting or missing forms. Because of nurses' understanding of the paper documentation of care and its use in their practice and health care, it is mandatory that they work with the IT people in converting the process of paper documentation to an electronic format. Although some means of paper documenation can easily be formatted to become an electronic form, the access, utilization, and storage of the form all become new issues. Contemporary Practice Highlight 20-1 provides an example of how workflow and practice can be changed by the introduction of a new means of documenting care.

Another example of changing practice can occur when **computerized physician order entry (CPOE)** systems are implemented and physician medication orders are transmitted directly from the physician to the pharmacy, bypassing the nurse who would have reviewed the order prior to it being sent to the pharmacy (Koppel et al., 2005). This new information system reduces the time it takes for medication orders to reach the pharmacy and decreases handwriting or transcribing errors. However, this type of change also removes an additional nursing review of the medication order, which could lead to delays in medication administration or increased medication errors if the nurse is unaware of the new order.

Similarly, proponents have lauded the ability of the EHR to make a patient's chart readily accessible to multiple members of the healthcare team at any point;

> **KEY TERM**
>
> **Computerized physician order entry (CPOE):** A computer system used by physicians to place orders.

CONTEMPORARY PRACTICE HIGHLIGHT 20-1

TRANSFORMING NURSING PRACTICE WITH TECHNOLOGY

The implementation of a point-of-care documentation system for an intravenous (IV) nurse team provides one example of how information technology can transform nursing practice (Bosma, Balen, Davidson, & Jewesson, 2003). This system used a handheld computer with a relational database to capture IV-team nursing interventions at the bedside (Bosma et al., 2003). In addition to accurately capturing the data for patient consultations during a 7-month period, the system identified more than 200 follow-up opportunities, which resulted in IV team–initiated consultations (Bosma et al.). These IV team–initiated consultations were a new practice for the team that occurred because they had new information generated by the data captured in the database.

Information systems have the capability to transform raw data into information that can enhance the nursing process. One example of this transformation is displaying data graphically over time (trend lines). This type of information display can yield patient trend information and help nurses understand patient information more quickly.

however, the number of available computer workstations and their locations also need to be addressed. If the number of workstations is inadequate, delays in charting and receiving orders ensue and omissions in the record may increase. Likewise, the location of electronic access can change practice patterns. Bedside terminals or handheld computers can increase access to the patient's health record but also can inhibit patient–provider communication if the nurse or other healthcare provider focuses on the technology rather than the patient (Frankel et al., 2005; Rouf, Whittle, Lu, & Schwartz, 2007).

Implementation of any type of information technology system can affect practice and workflow in general as well as in technology-specific ways. In one study that examined the effects of implementation of electronic patient records and handheld computers in nursing homes, administrators noted that the increased facility-wide information access and the ability to examine documentation easily was resulting in further changes in workflow processes and training (Alexander, Rantz, Flesner, Diekemper, & Siem, 2007). Of particular note, the administrators estimated that workload tripled during the conversion to the electronic record, and documentation time following the conversion was still higher than prior to the system implementation (Alexander et al., 2007).

Incorporating information technology into the workplace also generates new information needs and training on the part of the healthcare provider. Thirty-two percent of all healthcare providers who participated in a telemedicine survey (Demiris, Edison, & Schopp, 2004) stated that they did not know whether practicing telemedicine over the telehealth network could increase the risk of security and privacy violations. Similarly, 25 percent of nurse PDA (personal digital assistant) users were uncertain if HIPAA would apply to PDA use in general (Courtney, Pack, & Porter, 2005). Nearly three-fourths of the nurse PDA users (72.5 percent) were unsure or felt that HIPAA did not apply to their use of the handheld computers (Courtney et al., 2005), when in reality it does apply. Both nurses and administrators will need to be aware of the additional educational needs of nurses in the context of new information technologies.

Interdisciplinary Teams: Diversity in the Workforce

Nurses work in an increasingly diverse workforce environment. Professionals from the fields of information science and engineering, among others, have joined the workforce in health care. These professionals bring a diverse set of skills beyond those of the healthcare providers. With different perspectives and knowledge bases the individual team members focus on the goal of implementing technology to deliver quality patient care; this single goal serves to bond the different disciplines into a team. A collaborative team requires utilization of knowledge from each unit layer in the institution's work force, from financial personnel to facility electricians and beyond.

When implementing any type of technology, a project team of individuals with a variety of skill sets needs to be formed (Thielst, 2007). As an example, when implementing an EHR a collaborative team of people is needed including select administrative personnel, facilities management, select nurses and physicians, computer scientists, librarians, informaticians, and staff. The number of people on the team will evolve over the project's duration, as the specialized knowledge of each member is required. For instance, when one healthcare medical center began implementing an electronic medical record (EMR), they reported that 60 members of the project team responsible for the implementation were selected in-house and about 60 external temporary hires, or consultants, were needed to complement the skill set of the internal team members (Gensinger, 2006). Even with the established team, an extra 35 consultants were hired later during the critical implementation phase to assist with installing the technology. The project manager realized that the existing team did not have enough people and/or enough people with the necessary skill sets to ensure that the project team would successfully meet the project completion deadline. Thus, they employed more people with the required skills to ensure the project would be completed on schedule and that it would be functional. As the technology became more ubiquitous and the project reached its end, the temporary hires and consultants were no longer on the project team and the hospital employees went back to their original duties.

Information technology cannot be considered in isolation from the social systems in which it is embedded. "Any new health service might (and probably must) entail innovation in clinical roles, work processes, and culture change as well as the new technologies drawn from the treasure chest" (Coiera, 2004, p. 1198). When these processes are not carefully considered and addressed prior to technology implementation, there can be unintended consequences that negatively affect nursing practice and patient care. The level of collaboration that occurs within the team can directly impact the quality of care a person receives (Fewster-Thuente & Velsor-Friedrich, 2008). Research reports that nearly 70 percent of all adverse events in health care are a result of poor communication (Joint Commission, 2006). Utilization of communication tools, such as e-mail, networked PDAs, or a shared folder on a server, provides ways for sharing information, thus making it less proprietary. To collaborate successfully, people have to communicate and make information available.

The Electronic Health Record

The **electronic health record (EHR)**, also known as the electronic medical record (EMR), is an electronically maintained compilation of a person's lifetime health status and health care. The EHR is not yet widespread in the United States and there is no standardized definition for the EHR.

KEY TERM

Electronic health record (EHR): Patient-specific information made available in an electronic format for clinical purposes.

Although the development of electronic patient records was originally for the use of the financial department of the hospital for billing purposes, physicians and other clinical staff began to access the records for patient information (Haux, 2006). Despite the fact the records contained a patients' health information, the actual patient was usually denied direct access to the electronic files. As the transition to electronic health records continues to progress, individuals are now increasingly being granted access to their health record. With this new privilege, patients now may hold partial responsibility for maintaining the information their record contains. This migrates and blurs the naming of the technology from an EHR or EMR, which is included in a clinical information system (CIS), to what is known as a personal health record (PHR), which may or may not be included in a CIS. Although the terms may be used synonymously, there are distinct differences between them.

Computerized Records: PHRs vs. EHRs

The EHR is connected to the CIS, and the provider can control who has access to the information and who can add information to the record (U.S. Department of Health and Human Services [HHS], 2006). Thus, at this present date, only approved healthcare personnel add information to an EHR. Access to the various data fields contained within an EHR also are restricted, so rarely does a nurse and/or patient see all the available data. Security within an EHR is very tight to ensure no loss of confidentiality or privacy.

In contrast, a PHR is controlled by the patient, and the patient has the discretion to permit numerous people to have reading and data adding privileges. The existence of two separate electronic records creates potential problems related to having multiple health information sources (EHR & PHR) for a patient; for example, knowing which database is the most current, deciding who has access to make additions or corrections to the information, and determining how to make a PHR information available to clinicians. The security of a PHR is also problematic because of the broad audience that can typically access a PHR. Including a secure but unregulated system (where anyone can be granted access) inhibits the inclusion of a PHR into a CIS (HHS, 2006). A workgroup of the National Committee on Vital and Health Statistics has proposed that CISs become interoperable with PHRs so health personnel and patients have access to all the most up-to-date health information on a patient.

Recently, insurance companies and Internet start-up companies have begun providing consumers Web-based EHRs/PHRs for their individual use. All members of the UPMC Health Plan, for example, now have access to an online PHR that connects them to their insurance claims, immunization schedules, drug allergies, and any health assessment information (Taylor, 2007). Use of the PHR is optional, but the insurance company stresses the importance of electronically tracking personal health information to share with one's healthcare providers. They propose that the information from the PHR, when used, can make the provider–patient interactions during healthcare visits more meaningful and ultimately result in better care. Although UPMC Health Plan's service is not connected to a patient's EHR, or connected to a hospital CIS, it is connected to his or her insurance agency's health plan. Although this is a small step, it is one step toward the development of a fully integrated system and is an example of future interoperable uses of EHRs and PHRs.

Clinical Information Systems

Although EHRs and EMRs get a great deal of attention from the media, they are only a part of a larger information technology system, the clinical information system. Clinical information systems (CIS) provide a computerized means by which to support documenting patient care, monitoring patient status, and providing data for the nurse and other healthcare providers to use for decision support. Clinical systems may be designed to support specific healthcare settings such as critical care, community health, and ambulatory care systems. An array of computerized applications also fall under the category of clinical systems— nursing documentation, care planning, computerized provider order entry, barcode medication administration systems, case management, decision making, and discharge planning.

A CIS is a suite of software programs and computer hardware working together to manage health information. These systems can provide forms, notes, work lists, care plans, medication administration records, and many other features. They can consist of ancillary service systems such as picture archiving and communication systems (PACS), laboratory and radiology systems, and biomedical equipment. Each system or device has its unique function tailored to the discipline it is serving. The development and purpose of the CIS is to provide healthcare practitioners with up-to-date patient information and permit patients to access their health information.

Because of improved technology, the CIS has become available on mobile technology. Wireless PDAs, tablets, and laptops can be used to retrieve, store, and input patient data at any time within the secured wireless environment. For instance, in every patient's room at OhioHealth Incorporated's Dublin Methodist Hospital, there is a laptop available for use (Vaughan, 2008). The laptop provides access to the patient's health record and general health information for the patient and care provider. Because of the wireless environment, nurses are able to use a wireless bar-code scanner connected to the CIS. When the nurse scans the patient's ID bracelet and the bar-coded medication, she or he is assured the proper medication is being given at the correct time and the system is dynamically updated at the point of care. This use of the medication system and technology, which is part of the CIS, adds a safety check for the nurse and patient, saves time, and automatically updates the appropriate records in the patient's file at the time of the event.

Administrative, Research and Educational Information Systems

There are a number of other computerized information systems including those with administrative, research, or educational applications that nurses can utilize to support their practice. Administrative applications range from systems designed to support nurse staffing and scheduling, maintain incident reports, manage inventory, monitor infection control rates, and support budgeting and payroll activities. Research applications include using the computer to collect, manage, and analyze large amounts of data, prepare proposals, conduct online surveys, and manipulate data with statistical packages. In the educational arena, there are computerized information resources such as MEDLINE and CINAHL, health reference databases, and the World Wide Web. Another educational application includes learning management tools (course management systems) that are used for the delivery of online course materials, teaching students either on-site or at a distance.

Telehealth and E-Health

Health information technology is rapidly changing point of care. Telehealth is the use of communication technologies to deliver health care at a distance (Demiris, 2004). Examples of telehealth include remote patient monitoring, virtual nursing visits, and remote specialist consultations. Telehealth focuses on connecting healthcare providers to remote patients or other healthcare providers.

Simultaneously with the increased diffusion of telehealth into clinical practice, increased consumer co-management of their health care has led to the development of e-health innovations. E-health refers to "health services and information delivered or enhanced through the Internet and related technologies" and implies the active involvement of the consumer as well as the healthcare provider in health decision making (Eysenbach, 2001, http://www.jmir.org/2001/2/e20). Unlike in traditional telehealth, e-health consumers are not always interacting with healthcare providers, but may be involved in peer-to-peer networks or virtual patient communities.

Using Technology to Provide Patient Care at a Distance

Telehealth in home care or telehome care uses advanced technologies such as videoconferencing, the Internet, and portable monitoring devices to enable a healthcare provider at a clinical site to communicate with patients in their homes. Such an interaction is called a **virtual visit** in contrast to an *actual visit* in which the healthcare provider makes a traditional visit to the patient's home (Demiris et al., 2004). Nurses are trained to conduct virtual visits using videophones or Internet-based videoconferencing and process datasets of vital signs from the remote monitoring of patients. Similar projects are underway using telehealth technology to deliver supportive interventions to home hospice family caregivers (Parker Oliver, Demiris, Day, Courtney, & Porock, 2006) and bringing hospice patients and their caregivers "virtually" to hospice interdisciplinary team meetings for participation (Parker Oliver, Demiris, & Courtney, 2006).

> **KEY TERM**
>
> **Virtual visit:** Using technology to provide a digitized view of a patient and healthcare provider engaged in real-time communication.

Providing e-ICU Nursing Care

Evidence suggests that physicians and nurses who are specially trained in intensive care deliver better patient outcomes in intensive care settings, but clinician shortages and financial concerns often limit specialist staffing. In response to these challenges, hospitals are beginning to use telehealth technology in ICUs to provide e-ICU or virtual ICU care (Rabert & Sebastian, 2006). The virtual ICU is a remote monitoring station staffed with specialist physicians and nurses that is connected to ICUs via telemedicine technology. This allows the remote staff to virtually visit with both patients and hospital staff. Through virtual visits, the remote physicians and nurses can provide expert second opinions and assist the local staff in monitoring the care of critically ill patients. These virtual ICUs change the point of care for the clinicians who work in them because they may be providing care to patients at several different hospitals simultaneously.

Using the Internet

To Support Nursing Practice

Nursing is a profession that requires a commitment to life-long learning. To maintain a nursing license, annual continuing education units (CEUs) are mandated in some states; in other states continuing education is a voluntary activity. Many universities, colleges, hospitals, and businesses have created online learning modules and/or tutorials that practicing nurses can complete to meet their responsibility for continuing professional development.

As our society progresses with using Internet technology, resources will become better and more accessible. However, this does require nurses to have the requisite computer skills needed to access the Internet. One study that evaluated the use of online tutorials for CEUs showed that of 473 nurses who registered for the course only 52 percent completed the tutorials (Sweeney, Saarmann, Flagg, & Seidman, 2008). The researchers concluded that although the online tutorials were good, nurses overestimated their computer skills, and continuing professional development opportunities which teach basic computer and Internet skills are still necessary.

Staying up-to-date with the clinical practice and nursing research literature is easier than ever with online databases, journals, and other resources made available on the Internet. Databases have been created that specialize in evidence-based practice information, quality measures, patient safety, and allied health (Batten, 2006). For example, the National Library of Medicine has released PubMed (http://www.pubmed.gov), a free access database that indexes literature from the life sciences with a focus on biomedicine. Taking time to meet with your hospital or academic health sciences librarian to learn the specific resources available is an important aspect of being an informed, knowledgeable nursing professional.

For Patient Education

Virtual patient visits are made possible through the use of the Internet. The decrease in the cost of technology has helped to expand the popularity of the Internet, resulting in a broader use of its software applications and tools. While providing a backbone for virtual visits, the Internet is also being used to establish electronic support groups for patients, provide patient education, and provide continuing education courses for nurses.

Patient support groups are, like so many social networks that develop on the Internet, a group of individuals that have something in common and begin exchanging information in a chat room or through a blog so frequently that they establish themselves as an information-sharing resource. Patients with chronic illnesses have been one of the biggest and most frequent users of Internet support groups.

Many such Internet patient support groups are actually established and supported by professional healthcare organizations or healthcare agencies to provide access to quality information and expert clinicians who respond to posted questions through a Web-based portal. For example, one large hospital in Boston provided a Web portal for patients to contact their clinicians and access their EMR. Primarily, the patients who accessed the site used the portal to contact registered nurses by e-mail. The nurses provide the patients with information about their health problem, Suggest additional online information resources for them to view, and encourage the patients to seek treatment for their health problem as appropriate (Allen, Lezzoni, Huang, Huang, & Leveille, 2008). Using technology in this manner to provide patient education, it actually extends the outreach capabilities for nursing and leads to better patient care.

For Consumer Use

Many consumers are taking increased responsibility for their health and participate in their care with a healthcare professional. As a result, consumers in large numbers now seek health information to care for themselves and they need it in a format they can understand. In today's healthcare environment consumers are less inclined to call health professionals for information or obtain informational brochures from physicians' offices and health clinics. Instead, the Internet has become a significant source of healthcare information for many.

Considering that an estimated 335 million people in North America access the Internet, this means that approximately 70 percent of the population in North America (Miniwatts Marketing Group, 2007) potentially has access to an informational tool that is perfect for providing health information. It has been found that health information is one of the most common subjects individuals search for on the Internet. According to Fox and Fallows (2003), approximately one-half of adult U.S. Internet users, 93 million people, have searched for health-related information and 7 million people connect to Internet resources for health-related information each day.

One reason for the popularity of the Internet for accessing health information may be because consumers can access information anonymously. This change in how many people obtain health information is transforming the way nurses communicate with patients and provide care. Nurses, along with other healthcare providers, must add to their regular patient education protocol to now inform consumers about evaluating the quality and reliability of health information they obtain from the World Wide Web (Anderson & Klemm, 2008), suggest Web pages for patients to access, and field questions patients derive from the Internet.

To meet this increasing consumer need for information, healthcare providers (including nurses), health insurance companies, hospitals, and researchers, as a small example, have created a variety of health information applications, such as patient portals, podcasts, video cases, and health-specific Web sites. For example, the University of Wisconsin, Madison, has developed and has been testing for numerous years a computer-based system called CHESS (Comprehensive Health Enhancement Support System) that is accessed through the Internet. As a patient portal, CHESS currently provides its users with social support, decision-making and problem-solving tools, customized information, and a central location from which to access answers to their health queries (CHESS, 2008; Gustafson, Hawkins, & Boberg, 2002).

Recent additional Internet technology applications for consumer information support include podcasts and/or videocasts (vcasts) so individuals can access health information at any time and download it to MP3 and video MPEG players. For instance, the American Society of Cataract and Refractive Surgery is an example of one organization that provides MP3s and vcasts from its Web site (American Society of Cataract and Refractive Surgery, 2008). To promote greater dissemination of health information, the Centers for Disease Control and Prevention (CDC) provides podcasts on topics ranging from water safety to living with diabetes (Centers for Disease Control and Prevention, 2007).

Although technology may decrease face-to-face information exchange, it has increased the distribution of health information and made it possible to share the same information in multiple formats. Using podcasts, vcasts, patient portals, and other Internet technologies has increased nurses' outreach and provided an array of information formats to meet patients' needs.

How to Evaluate Information on the Internet

It is obvious that patient participation in decision making and self-care has shifted the patient's position from that of a simple recipient to one of active participant and that technology has been a major impetus for this shift. This has empowered patients and their families to use the Internet and any available resources, collectively known as consumer health information resources, to seek information about their diseases or conditions. The major problem consumers face is being able to evaluate the credibility of the medical information they find on the Internet. Security and confidentiality of online medical records and health information exchanged on the Internet with others is another potential problem.

Research studies have attempted to assess the quality of health information available online through the Internet (Goldsmith, 2000). Although many of these resources are legitimate and provide accurate information about health problems and treatment, just as many resources are no more than someone's personal opinions or a form of advertisement promoting products to unwary consumers. While Web sites and online support groups can provide valuable education and emotional support to consumers, the information found on these sites can be detrimental if it is misleading or out-of-date. Even major Web sites sponsored by medical centers can contradict each other or contain inaccurate information.

These issues have prompted the development of ethical guidelines for e-health (Eysenbach, 2000). Some of these projects are geared towards educating consumers about how to "filter" information (Eysenbach & Diepgen, 1998; Wilson, 2002) and decide which Web sites to trust. Criteria to evaluate Web sites have been established by many organizations like the National Institutes of Health (Kimball & O'Neil, 2002) and the American Medical Association (2008). Another initiative involves encouraging health-information providers to validate and rate their own Web site. This can be achieved by following a user guidance system to determine if the Web site complies with established standards.

One example of a user guidance system is the Health on the Net (HON) Foundation (HON Foundation, 2007), which was originally developed to ensure quality of healthcare information posted on the Internet and to identify ethical guidelines that can be used to guide development of healthcare information Web sites. The HON Foundation has developed a code of conduct listing eight elements that should be present in medical and healthcare Web sites (HON Foundation, 2007). Box 20-3 identifies the HON Code of Conduct.

BOX 20-3   HON CODE OF CONDUCT FOR MEDICAL AND HEALTH CARE WEBSITES

Web sites providing medical and health care information should include attention to the following ethical elements:

Authoritative—authors' qualifications are clearly indicated

Complementarity—the information is intended to be supportive of the doctor-patient relationship

Privacy—the privacy and confidentiality of any information provided by the patient should always be respected

Attribution—all published information should have cited sources with clearly identified dates of when the webpage was last updated

Justifiability—if any claims are made by the website to promote positive treatment benefits the claims must be substantiated by clearly established evidence

Transparency—contact information for the webmaster and others involved in the development and support of the website must be clearly available and accessible to the consumer

Financial disclosure—all funding sources related to the design, development and maintenance of the website should be clearly identified

Advertising policy—any advertising contained on the website will be clearly identified as such and distinguished from the actual information provided by the site

---

Source: Health on the Net Foundation. Retrieved on June 22, 2008 from http://www.hon.ch/HONcode/Conduct.html

---

Other user guidance systems include:

- *DISCERN (DISCERN, n.d.):* A brief questionnaire for users to validate information on treatment choices.
- *Net Scoring (Net Scoring, 2001):* Gives guidance on all health-related information.
- *QUICK (QUICK, n.d.):* Targets children and tries to provide a guide to their search on the Web for health information.
- *MedPICS Certification and Rating of Trustworthy Health Information on the Net (medCERTAIN, 2000):* Funded by the European Union, it actually evaluates the information published and displays a warning when a user accesses a fraudulent Web site, thus acting as a third party that certifies the Web site complies with quality criteria.
- *URAC (URAC, n.d.):* The U.S. medCERTAIN equivalent; an independent, nonprofit organization that started a health Web site accreditation and certification program.

The National Library of Medicine has created a Flash tutorial "Evaluating Internet Health Information" that discusses how to evaluate the quality of information on a Web site (National Library of Medicine, 2006). One additional quick tool that can be used to help people evaluate the quality of the information presented on a Web page is to use the mnemonic "SPAT," which stands for site, publisher, audience and timeliness. The site URL should clearly identify where the information is coming from (e.g., .com, .edu, .org); the publisher of the page should be clearly identified; the intended audience for the Web site should be identified; and the date of when the page was last updated should be clearly posted (LaRue, 2006).

Educating the consumer on how to evaluate the quality of healthcare information on the Internet is a role for the nurse when designing patient education plans. Nurses can teach the patients and their families how to become savvy consumers of information. Nurses can also act as information brokers and interpreters for patients. With the widespread adoption by consumers of the use of technology to obtain healthcare information, it is imperative that the nurse be aware of ethical considerations associated with providing information via the Internet and how to properly evaluate information found online.

The Cost of Technology and Access

Although the adoption of healthcare technology increases the quality of life, it has been repeatedly cited that it is "the major" cause of the increasing cost of health care (McClellan & Newhouse, 1997; Okunade & Murthy, 2002). This has prompted a debate over whether the adoption of technology in health care is cost effective (Bunker, Frazier, & Mosteller, 1994; Cutler & McClellan, 2001; McClellan & Newhouse, 1997).

Technology adoption might be in the form of a new treatment modality or expanding the availability of an existing therapy to treat more people. In most cases, the improvement in patients' care and outcome, due to use of new technology, outweighs the increase in spending. Cutler and McClellan (2001) show this desirable effect in cases of heart disease, the care of low-birth-weight infants, and depression treatment. On the other hand, they also show that this effect is not observed in breast cancer treatment, where the increase in cost due to use of new technology was substantial enough to neutralize the improvement in patients' outcome.

Another often cited benefit of technology adoption is that it enables care providers to perform their jobs more efficiently and in a timely manner. A perfect example would be the introduction of computerized physician order entry (CPOE) systems. Although many studies have proven that CPOE decreases prescription errors (Potts, Barr, Gregory, Wright, & Patel, 2004; Taylor, Loan, Kamara, Blackburn, & Whitney, 2008; Walsh et al., 2008), other studies argue that adoption of CPOE is not always cost effective. In a study by Travers and Downs (2000), the success in adopting technology in two different pediatric practice settings varied due to organizational differences and readiness for change in these practices. The cost of the technology was not the sole factor considered by the practices. Similarly, the preliminary research done by Waterman et al. (2007) suggests that technology adoption may not have a totally positive impact on employees, but may instead lead to significant emotional and job-related stress, including depression and diminished job satisfaction.

The take-home message from all of these studies is that we cannot evaluate the cost of technology independent of the setting in which the technology is used. Users should evaluate their needs and balance the cost effectiveness and the benefits of individual technologies, not just the purchase cost.

Trends in the Use of Informatics and Healthcare Technology

New and emerging technologies, such as smart devices that have decision support tools or artificial intelligence built into the tools, are rapidly being deployed in the healthcare arena. Many technologies are converging and providing new tools to support patients in their homes. As an example, see Contemporary Practice Highlight 20-2 for a description of how technology can help the elderly to remain in their own homes.

Some new technologies may help mitigate the nursing shortage. Womack, Newbold, Staugaitis, and Cunningham (2004) reviewed technology that would help solve nursing workplace issues, including not having enough nurses to manage workloads, reassignment to unfamiliar care areas, time spent on non-direct care activities, balancing the demands of home and work, and improving quality. For example, in the category of balancing the demands of home and work, there are technologies that allow nurses to see their work schedule from home and to bid on additional shifts.

Future computing technology will become smaller, more transparent, wireless, portable, equipped with sensor monitors, and therefore will be ubiquitous. Technology will not only monitor structures, including humans, externally via cables and portable computers, but also will be internal, wireless, and work on operating systems designed to support wireless sensor networks (Tiny OS applications) (Culler, 2006). Sensors, often in the form of a node, will be placed in clothing and

---

CONTEMPORARY PRACTICE HIGHLIGHT 20-2

GERONTECHNOLOGY

The emergence of new automated tools is particularly important for the growing elderly population and helping to support elderly patients in their homes. This convergence of gerontology and IT is the new field of gerontechnology, and it is receiving a lot of attention from engineers, gerontologists, healthcare providers, and major businesses. An example of a smart tool that can be used to assist in the care of the elderly is a medication administration system that can transmit whether an elderly patient has taken his or her medications.

implanted in bodies to monitor stress, heat, and movement, to name only a few of their possible functions (Jong-Wan, Takao, Sawada, & Ishida, 2007). They will have the potential to monitor human diets, behavior and motion, and physiologic functions. In clinical trials small computer chips (RFID tags) containing all the information in a person's health record are being implanted into that person's subcutaneous fat (O'Connor, 2006). These chips, called VeriChips, are as small as a grain of rice and can use **radio-frequency identification (RFID)** technology to transmit the person's data (VeriChip, 2006). This data, incorporated into the right system, can set off alarms to notify or prompt necessary action in response to changes in the patient's data.

Technologies will become increasingly dynamic, less expensive, and more accessible. More communication will take place with mobile devices that can display video. Patients will communicate with their healthcare professionals through e-mail, text messages, and telemedicine and have less face-to-face communication. Consumers will have more responsibility for keeping personal health records and these consumers must be well informed. The Internet will continue to play a growing and more prominent role in providing health information to consumers.

Nurses will need to become increasingly adept at utilizing informatics and healthcare technology in the management and delivery of patient care. The role of hand-held devices as resource tools and decision support tools will continue to evolve. Clinical information systems, as they become more common in all healthcare agencies, will provide a means of electronic connectedness across healthcare providers. These information systems will have significant impact on the work of the nurse and workflow in patient care settings. Security and confidentiality issues will become more complex, as will the ethical issues associated with the use of healthcare technology. All nurses have the professional responsibility to become computer literate, knowledgeable users of technology, and involved in understanding the impact that healthcare technology can have on patient outcomes.

Summary

This chapter defines informatics and healthcare technology and addresses the impact of technology on nursing practice and the outcomes of patient care. The ethical concerns related to technology and ensuring security, privacy, and confidentiality are also addressed. The introduction of electronic health records, clinical information systems, and telehealth and how these means of technology are changing the delivery of health care is discussed, and the nurse's role in implementing healthcare technology is emphasized. In order to practice safely and competently, nurses must be willing to adapt to the technological advances that are rapidly occurring in health care, and at the same time remain sensitive to the importance of emphasizing the caring, humanistic aspects of providing patient care in a high-tech environment.

Key Terms

Computerized physician order entry (CPOE): A computer system used by physicians to place orders.

Confidentiality: Legal protection ensuring individuals their right to privacy to the fullest extent allowable by law.

Electronic health record (EHR): Patient-specific information made available in an electronic format for clinical purposes.

Health Insurance Portability and Accountability Act (HIPAA): A government mandate that aims to improve efficiency in healthcare delivery and standardized electronic data interchange while enforcing standards to protect patients' confidentiality and privacy with their right to control their data.

Healthcare technology: Technology used to deliver care in the prevention, diagnosis, and treatment of health problems.

Informatics: The study of the structure and properties of information.

Nursing informatics (NI): A specialty that integrates nursing science, computer science, and information science to manage and communicate data, information, knowledge, and wisdom in nursing practice.

Privacy: Expected behavior that regulates the professional relationship between patients and their healthcare providers.

Radio-frequency identification (RFID): A smart bar code that provides access to data via use of computer microchips.

Security: Iinvolves protecting data and information systems, including ensuring the integrity of the information and protecting against accidental or purposeful misuse of the data and loss due to physical damage.

Standardized language: A collection of terms with definitions that are used in informational system databases.

Telehealth: Delivery of health care using telecommunication technology.

Virtual visit: Using technology to provide a digitized view of a patient and healthcare provider engaged in real-time communication.

Reflective Practice Questions

1. List four technologies currently employed in health care that you have utilized in your clinical experiences. Describe how they have changed your current nursing practice.

2. Explain two applications of RFID technology in health care. Consider how RFID technology could be used in operating rooms for surveillance of inventory.

3. You are currently working in the critical care unit and want to propose using a point-of-care documentation system. Provide examples of three ways this technology will transform your current nursing practice.

4. You are working in a clinic and a patient brings you a printed document from the Internet on diabetes that has some inaccuracies. In your role as a nurse and healthcare provider, what do you do?

References

Abbott, P. A. (2000). Knowledge discovery in large data sets. In M. J. Ball, K. J. Hannah, S. K. Newbold, & J. V. Douglas (Eds.). *Nursing informatics: Where caring and technology meet (3rd ed.)*. New York: Springer-Verlag.

AHRQ. (2006). Costs and Benefits of Health Information Technology. AHRQ Publication NO. 06-E006. Washington, DC: United States Department of Health and Human Services. Health Insurance Portability and Accountability Act Of 1996, http://www.hhs.gov/ocr/hipaa/

Alexander, G. L., Rantz, M., Flesner, M., Diekemper, M., & Siem, C. (2007). Clinical information systems in nursing homes: An evaluation of initial implementation strategies. *CIN: Computers, Informatics, Nursing, 25*(4), 189–197.

Allen, M., Lezzoni, L., Huang, A., Huang, L., & Leveille, S. (2008). Improving patient-clinician communication about chronic conditions: Description of an Internet-based nurse e-coach intervention. *Nursing Research, 57*(2), 107–112.

American Medical Association. (2008, June 1). *Guidelines for medical and health information sites on the Internet*. Retrieved June 8, 2008, from http://www.ama-assn.org/ama/pub/category/1905.html

American Nurses Association. (2008). *Nursing Informatics: Scope and Standards of Practice*. Silver Spring, MD: American Nurses Publishing.

American Nurses Association. (n.d.). Glossary. www.nursingworld.org/npii/glossary.htm

American Society of Cataract and Refractive Surgery. (2008). *As seen from here*. Retrieved June 11, 2008, from http://www.asseenfromhere.com

Anderson, A., & Klemm, P. (2008). The Internet: Friend or foe when providing patient education? *Clinical Journal of Oncology Nursing, 12*(1), 55–63.

Barki, H., & Hartwick, J. (1994). Measuring user participation, user involvement and user attitude. *MIS Quarterly, 18*(1), 59–82.

Batten, J. (2006). Evidence-based resources for nurses on the Web. *Journal of Hospital Librarianship, 7*(1), 101–115.

Bosma, L., Balen, R. M., Davidson, E., & Jewesson, P. J. (2003). Point of care use of a personal digital assistant for patient consultation management: Experience of an intravenous resource nurse team in a major Canadian teaching hospital. *CIN: Computers, Informatics, Nursing, 21*(4), 179–185.

Bunker, J. P., Frazier, H. S., & Mosteller, F. (1994). Improving health: Measuring effect of medical care. *Millbank Quarterly, 72*(2), 225–258.

Centers for Disease Control and Prevention. (2007). *Podcasts at CDC*. Retrieved June 11, 2008, from http://www2a.cdc.gov/podcasts/

CHESS, University of Wisconsin-Madison. (2008). *What is CHESS?* Retrieved June 11, 2008, from http//chess.wisc.edu/chess/projects/about_chess.aspx

Coiera, E. (2004). Four rules for the reinvention of health care. *BMJ, 328*, 1197–1199.

Courtney, K. L., Pack, B., & Porter, G. (2005). Within their grasp—hand-held computer use among registered nurses. *Business Briefings: U.S. Healthcare Strategies*, 14–15.

Culler, D. E. (2006). Operating system design for wireless sensor networks. *Sensors, 23*(5), 14–20.

Cutler, D., & McClellan, M. (2001). Is technological change in medicine worth it? *Health Affairs, 20*(5), 11.

Demiris, G. (2004). Electronic home healthcare: Concepts and challenges. *International Journal of Electronic Healthcare, 1*(1), 4–16.

Demiris, G. (2006). Examining health care providers' participation in telemedicine system design and implementation. *AMIA Annual Symposium Proceedings*, 906.

Demiris, G., Edison, K., & Schopp, L. H. (2004). Shaping the future: Needs and expectations of telehealth professionals. *Telemedicine Journal and e-Health, 10*(suppl. 2), S-60–S-63.

Department of Justice. (2003). *The Privacy Act of 1974.* Retrieved September 25, 2007, from http://www.usdoj.gov/oip/privstat.htm

DISCERN. (n.d.). *Quality criteria for consumer health informatics.* Retrieved September 14, 2007, from http://www.discern.org.uk

Eysenbach, G. (2000). Towards ethical guidelines for e-health: JMIR theme issue on e-health ethics. *Journal of Medical Internet Research, 2*(1), e7.

Eysenbach, G. (2001). What is e-health? *Journal of Medical Internet Research, 3*(2), e20. Retrieved June 11, 2008, from http://www.jmir.org/2001/2/e20/

Eysenbach, G., & Diepgen, T. L. (1998). Towards quality management of medical information on the internet: Evaluation, labelling, and filtering of information. *BMJ, 317*(7171), 1496–1500.

Fewster-Thuente, L., & Velsor-Friedrich, B. (2008). Interdisciplinary collaboration for healthcare professionals. *Nursing Administration Quarterly, 32*(1), 40–48.

Foster, S. T., & Franz, C. R. (1999). User involvement during information systems development: A comparison of analyst and user perceptions of system acceptance. *Journal of Engineering and Technology Management, 16*, 329–348.

Fox, S., & Fallows, D. (2003). *Internet health resources.* Washington, DC: Pew Internet and American Life Project.

Frankel, R., Altschuler, A., George, S., Kinsman, J., Jimison, H., Robertson, N. R., et al. (2005). Effects of exam-room computing on clinician-patient communication: A longitudinal qualitative study. *Journal of General Internal Medicine, 20*(8), 677–682.

Gensinger, R. (2006). Able to adapt. *Healthcare Informatics: The Business of Healthcare Information Technology, 23*(9), 36.

Goldsmith, J. (2000). How will the Internet change our health system? *Health Affairs, 19*, 148–156.

Gustafson, D. H., Hawkins, R. P., & Boberg, E. W. (2002). CHESS: 10 years of research and development in consumer health informatics for broad populations, including the underserved. *International Journal of Medical Informatics, 65*, 169–177.

Haux, R. (2006). Health information systems—past, present, future. *International Journal of Medical Informatics, 75*, 268–281.

Health on the Net Foundation. (2007, June 18). *Health on the Net Foundation.* Retrieved July 26, 2007, from http://www.hon.ch/HomePage/Home-Page.html

Health on the Net Foundation. (n.d.). *HON code of conduct (HONcode) for medical and health web sites.* Retrieved September 4, 2007, from http://www.hon.ch/HONcode/Conduct.html

Hodge, J. G., Jr., Gostin, L. O., & Jacobson, P. D. (1999). Legal issues concerning electronic health information: Privacy, quality, and liability. *Journal of the American Medical Association, 282*(15), 1466–1471.

Horrigan, J. B. (2006). Online news: For many home broadband users, the Internet is a primary news source. Retrieved October 9, 2008, from http://www.pewinternet.org/search.asp

Hutchinson, A. M. & Johnson, L. (2006). Beyond the BARRIERS Scale: Commonly Reported Barriers to Research Use. *Journal of Nursing Administration, 36*(4), 189-199.

International Council of Nurses. (2008). *ICN code of ethics*. Retrieved September 5, 2007, from http://www.icn.ch/ethics.htm

Joint Commission. (2006). Sentinel event statistics. Retrieved May 8, 2008, from http://www.jointcommission.org

Jong-Wan, K., Takao, H., Sawada, K., & Ishida, M. (2007). Development of radio frequency transmitters including on-chip antenna for intelligent human sensing systems. *IEEJ Transactions on Electrical and Electronic Engineering, 2*(3), 365–371.

Kimball, B., & O'Neil, E. (2002). *Health care's human crisis: The American nursing shortage*. Princeton, NJ: Robert Wood Johnson Foundation.

Koppel, R., Metlay, J. P., Cohen, A., Abaluck, B., Localio, A. R., Kimmell, S. E., et al. (2005). Role of computerized physician order entry systems in facilitating medication errors. *Journal of the American Medical Association, 293*(10), 1197–1203.

LaRue, E. M. (2006). *A study on the adoption of a web page content assessment tool: SPAT*. Pittsburgh, PA: University of Pittsburgh.

Lee, T. T. (2007). Nurses' experiences using a nursing information system: Early stage of technology implementation. *CIN: Computers, Informatics, Nursing, 25*(5), 294–300.

Madden, M. (2006). *Internet penetration and impact*. Pew Internet & American Life Project.

McClellan, M., & Newhouse. J. P. (1997). The marginal cost-effectiveness of medical technology: A panel instrumental-variables approach. *Journal of Economics, 77*, 39–64.

medCERTAIN. (2000). *The future European trustmark for reliable health information*. Retrieved September 9, 2008, from http://www.hi-europe.info/files/2000/medcertain.htm

Melnyk, B. M. & Fineout-Overhold, E. (2005). *Evidence-based practice in Nursing & Healthcare: A guide to best practice*. Philadelphia: Lippincott Williams & Wilkins.

Miniwatts International. (2006, June 30). *Internet world stats: Usage and population statistics*. Retrieved July 26, 2007, from http://www.internetworldstats.com

Moen, A. (2003). *Nursing leadership and the electronic patient record (EPR)—the odd couple?* Paper presented at the NI 2003, 8th International Congress in Nursing Informatics, Rio de Janeiro, Brazil.

National Library of Medicine. (2006, February 15). *Evaluating Internet health information: A tutorial from the National Library of Medicine*. Retrieved July 26, 2007, from http://www.nlm.nih.gov/medlineplus/webeval/webeval.html

Net Scoring. (2001, July 18). *Criteria to assess the quality of health Internet information*. Retrieved September 14, 2007, from http://www.chu-rouen.fr/netscoring/netscoringeng.html

O'Connor, M. C. (2006). Insurer running Verichip trial. *RFID Journal*. Retrieved July 27, 2007, from http://www.RFIDjournal.com/article/articleprint/2496/-1/1/

Okunade, A. A., & Murthy, V. N. R. (2002). Technology as a "major driver" of health care costs: A cointegration of the Newhouse conjecture. *Journal of Health Economics, 21*, 147–159.

Oroviogoicoechea, C., Elliott, B., & Watson, R. (2008). Review: Evaluating information systems in nursing. *Journal of Clinical Nursing, 17*(5), 567–575.

Parker Oliver, D., Demiris, G., & Courtney, K. L. (2006). Patient and family involvement in hospice interdisciplinary team meetings in the United States. *Palliative Medicine, 20*(3), 278.

Parker Oliver, D., Demiris, G., Day, M., Courtney, K. L., & Porock, D. (2006). Tele-hospice support for elder caregivers of hospice patients: Two case studies. *Journal of Palliative Medicine, 9*(2), 264–267.

Potts, A. L., Barr, F. E., Gregory, D. F., Wright, L., & Patel, N. R. (2004). Computerized physician order entry and medication errors in a pediatric critical care unit. *Pediatrics, 113*(1 Pt 1), 59–63.

Pravikoff, D. S., Tanner, A. B., & Pierce, S.T. (2005). Readiness of U.S. nurses for evidence-based practice: Many don't understand or value research and have had little or no training to help them find evidence on which to base their practice. *American Journal of Nursing, 105*(9), 40–51.

QUICK. (n.d.). The QUICK guide to checking information quality. Retrieved September 14, 2007, from http://www.quick.org.uk

Rabert, A. S., & Sebastian, M. M. (2006). The future is now: Implementation of a tele-intensivist program. *Journal of Nurse Administration, 36*(1), 49–54.

Rindfleisch, T. C. (1997). Privacy, information, technology, and health care. *Communication of the ACM, 40*(8).

Rouf, E., Whittle, J., Lu, N., & Schwartz, M. D. (2007). Computers in the exam room: Differences in physician-patient interaction may be due to physician experience. *Journal of General Internal Medicine, 22*(1), 43–48.

Saba, V. K. & McCormick, K. A. (2006). *Essentials of Nursing Informatics* (4th ed.). New York: McGraw-Hill.

Shortliffe, E. H., & Cimino, J. J. (2006). *Biomedical informatics: Computer applications in health care and biomedicine* (3rd ed.). New York: Springer.

Staggers, N., Gassert, C., & Curran, C. (2002). A delphi study to determine informatics competencies for nurses at four levels of practice. *Nursing Research, 51*(6), 383–390.

Sweeney, N. M., Saarmann, L., Flagg, J., & Seidman, R. (2008). The keys to successful online continuing education programs for nurses. *Journal of Continuing Education in Nursing, 39*(1), 34–41.

Taylor, J. A., Loan, L. A., Kamara, J., Blackburn, S., & Whitney, D. (2008). Medication administration variances before and after implementation of computerized physician order entry in a neonatal intensive care unit. *Pediatrics, 121*(1), 123–128.

Taylor, M. (2007). *UPMC Health Plan launches new personal health record.* Retrieved June 11, 2008, from http://www.upmchealthplan.com/media/news/2007_09_04.html

Technology Informatics Guiding Education Reform (TIGER) (2008). About TIGER. Retrieved February 20, 2008, from https://www.tigersummit.com/About_Us.html.

Thielst, C. B. (2007). The future of healthcare technology. *Journal of Healthcare Management, 52*(1), 7–10.

Travers, D. A., & Downs, S. M. (2000). Comparing user acceptance of a computer system in two pediatric offices: A qualitative study. *AMIA Annual Symposium Proceedings,* 853–857.

URAC. (n.d.). *URAC health web site accreditation.* Retrieved September 5, 2007, from http://www.urac.org/consumers/resources/accreditation.aspx

U.S. Department of Health and Human Services. (2006). *Personal health records and personal health records systems: A report and recommendations from the National Committee on Vital and Health Statistics.* Washington, DC: Author.

U.S. Department of Health and Human Services, Office for Civil Rights—HIPAA. (n.d.). *Medical privacy—national standards to protect the privacy of personal health information.* Retrieved September 5, 2007, from http://www.hhs.gov/ocr/hipaa/

Vaughan, D. (2008, March 10). *New Ohio hospital maximizes wireless procedures.* Retrieved June 12, 2008, from http://include.nurse.com/apps/pbcs.dll/article?AID=/20080310/MW02/803100307

VeriChip. (2006). *RFID for people.* Retrieved July 27, 2007, from http://www.verichipcorp.com/content/company/1117572449

Vogelsmeier, A. A., Halbesleben, J. R. B., & Scott-Cawiezell, J. R. (2008). Technology implementation and workarounds in the nursing home. *Journal of the American Medical Informatics Association, 15*(1), 114–119.

Walsh, K. E., Landrigan, C. P., Adams, W. G., Vinci, R. J., Chessare, J. B., Cooper, M. R., et al. (2008). Effect of computer order entry on prevention of serious medication errors in hospitalized children. *Pediatrics, 121*(3), e421–e427.

Waterman, A. D., Garbutt, J., Hazel, E., Dunagan, W. C., Levinson, W., Fraser, V. J., et al. (2007). The emotional impact of medical errors on practicing physicians in the United States and Canada. *Joint Commission Journal on Quality and Patient Safety, 33*(8), 467–476.

Wilson, P. (2002). How to find the good and avoid the bad or ugly: A short guide to tools for rating quality of health information on the Internet. *BMJ, 324,* 598–602.

Womack, D., Newbold, S. K., Staugaitis, H. & Cunningham, B. (2004). *Technology's Role in Addressing Maryland's Nursing Shortage: Innovations & Examples.* Baltimore, MD: Technology Workgroup, Maryland Statewide Commission on the Crisis in Nursing. http://maryland.nursetech.com/F/NT/MD/NursingInnovations2004.pdf

The Transition into Nursing Practice

Ellen Wathen

LEARNING OUTCOMES

After reading this chapter you will be able to:

- Explain the difference between the novice and advanced beginner in professional nursing practice.
- Describe the knowledge, competencies, and skills required for the transition into professional nursing practice.
- Discuss learning experiences and strategies that will enhance the nursing student's transition from the educational environment into the practice environment.
- Describe the maturation process related to decision making and clinical nursing judgments.
- Describe key elements to be considered when selecting a work environment.

Role Transition

Transitioning from the role of a student into the role of a practicing registered nurse is often accompanied by feelings of accomplishment, excitement, uncertainty, anxiety, and yes, even fear. The realization that graduation brings with it the opportunity to secure one's first position in practice as a professional nurse is exciting and empowering; however, with that opportunity comes the full responsibility for managing and providing patient care—without the security of having nursing faculty nearby to validate one's clinical decisions or of providing care to only a few patients as was frequently the case in nursing school. The purpose of this chapter is to explore some of the issues that nursing students will face as they make this important transition into practice and to offer strategies to help ease this potentially challenging time in their new professional careers.

In an effort to prepare nursing students for a successful transition into practice, nursing faculty are beginning to incorporate contemporary learning experiences into nursing curricula that focus on specific competencies required for practice in today's complex healthcare settings. These competencies include a focus on patient-centered care, teamwork and collaboration, evidence-based practice, quality improvement, safety, and informatics (Cronenwett et al., 2007). Each of these competencies will be elaborated upon in this chapter and are further discussed in other chapters within this book. Nursing students share the responsibility with their faculty to seek out learning experiences that will provide experiential opportunities to acquire a foundation in each of these competency areas. The lived experiences that their faculty can share will serve as resources for nursing students as they enter the workforce. As nursing students transition into their roles as registered nurses, these competencies will serve as a blueprint for their success in the nursing profession.

What is expected of nursing students as they begin the transition into their first practice role as a registered nurse? What can be done to make the transition less "bumpy" as they learn how to coordinate the multiple facets of their new role as a nursing professional? And at what point can new graduates expect to feel like they have the knowledge and skills needed to provide basic and competent care to their patients? These are some of the major questions that will be addressed in this chapter.

From Novice to Advanced Beginner

When new nursing graduates enter the workforce, they may feel that they are expected to know "everything" in order to provide nursing care to their patients. This is an unrealistic expectation for a **novice** practitioner; actually, it is an unrealistic expectation for any practitioner because the complexity of nursing practice means that all nurses are continually in a learning role to stay current and competent. Most new graduates will have the benefit of an orientation period in their new position. The usual goals for these orientation periods include reviewing regulatory and institutional policies, nursing policies and responsibilities, patient care equipment and technology, and role expectations. Orientation programs are addressed at further length later in this chapter. Although the nature and length of the orientation period will vary among institutions, new graduates must remember that the orientation period was established to facilitate their role transition and is designed to provide them with the opportunity to work alongside an experienced nurse as they assume their patient care responsibilities. The primary role of this experienced nurse, who may be termed a **preceptor** or **mentor**, is to explain the organization's policies and procedures, assist with assimilation into the culture of the organization, provide guidance in clinical decision making, and, in general, be available to answer questions. It is important for the new graduate to maximize the opportunities the orientation period provides and fully capitalize upon the assistance and learning experiences that are formally provided by the organization during this time frame.

KEY TERM

Preceptor: Someone who orients or provides guidance to a novice or advanced beginner in a given situation or over a fixed period of time (Alspach, 2000).

KEY TERM

Mentor: Someone who develops a professional relationship or bond with a novice or advanced beginner (Alspach, 2000).

Once released from their orientation period, novice nurses will likely encounter new challenges as they begin to independently manage their patient care assignment. They may feel alone as they coordinate their patients' care and engage in the never-ending, critical decision-making processes that characterize nursing practice, even though they are surrounded by experienced nurses and other healthcare professionals. Novice nurses may also feel uncomfortable about asking for help, fearful of being a "bother" to others, or appearing unknowledgeable, dependent, or unskilled and incompetent. Unfortunately, at times more experienced practitioners may either unintentionally or intentionally convey these attitudes to the new graduate. However, the single biggest mistake novice nurses can make in their new role is to not ask questions and enlist assistance with decision making when they are uncertain of how to proceed in a clinical situation. And one of the most serious and unprofessional injustices that experienced nurses can commit is not offering to assist novice nurses, but instead waiting to see if the new graduate will "sink or swim."

Why do new graduates feel insecure within their role as a nurse? Some of these feelings of insecurity are based on their limited patient experience in the clinical setting (Etheridge, 2007). **Graduate nurses** need time and experience to fortify and expand their skill set (McNiesh, 2007). Benner (1984) explained the skills acquisition concept in her outline of the five stages of nursing proficiency in her book, *From Novice to Expert: Excellence and Power in Clinical Nursing Practice* (see Table 21-1). The five stages of skills acquisition are novice, **advanced beginner**, **competent**, **proficient**, and **expert**. Benner applied the Dreyfus model of skills acquisition to nursing. As novice nurses gain experience, they are better able to analyze patient situations and use

KEY TERM

Graduate nurse: A nursing student who has graduated from a nursing program, but not yet taken the NCLEX examination.

Advanced beginner: Someone who has limited experience with a given situation (Benner, 1984).

Competent: Someone with 2–3 years of experience who is consciously aware of a given situation in its individual parts and can develop a long-range action plan (Benner, 1984).

Proficient: Someone with the experience to see a given situation in wholes rather than individual parts, who can analyze the situation and determine whether the typical picture is not materializing, and who can determine what needs to be revised within the plan of care in response (Benner, 1984).

Expert: Someone with the vast experience to intuitively assess a given situation and accurately target the problem area without being distracted by other unrelated symptoms (Benner, 1984).

their past patient encounters to respond with appropriate interventions. The goal is to eventually be able to draw upon their past experiences to analyze patient problems, foresee potential complications, and intervene with preventative care.

Nursing students and new graduates are considered novices because they have very little experience in assuming responsibility for patient care in various clinical situations. Throughout their nursing education, in both the classroom and the clinical setting, students are provided with a set of rules to follow for providing care to their patients in selected situations. Even though these sets of rules assist nursing students in providing patient care, their inexperience leaves these novices with the inability to adapt or modify their provision of care based on variances within the patients' actual conditions.

With time and experience novices become what Benner (1984) refers to as advanced beginners—those nurses who have limited patient experiences, but can recognize the similarities between current patient care situations and past patient care experiences. Most graduate nurses enter the workforce as novices, because they are faced with many patient care situations that they have never before experienced. They find that each patient brings a new and individualized variation to what may have been a seemingly familiar clinical scenario. Newly graduated nurses need to file away experiences that vary from the norm for future referencing as they learn how to adapt in situations based on these past patient encounters.

To summarize, new graduates will inevitably face some challenges as they transition from the role of the student to the role of a registered nurse. However, there are skill sets and strategies that nursing students can develop and use while still in their nursing program to assist in this transition.

Preparing for Transition into Practice

It is important that nursing students possess the attitude that learning is a shared responsibility between students and faculty. Nursing faculty can facilitate students' acquiring knowledge of the discipline, and developing psychomotor skills and professional values. Nursing students can engage in self-assessment of learning needs and communicate those needs to faculty. Being actively engaged and self-directed in the learning process will help nursing students as they prepare for their transition into the role of licensed professional nurses (Knowles,

TABLE 21-1   DREYFUS MODEL APPLIED TO NURSING

Stages	Performance Characteristics
1. **Novice**	No experiences Rules-oriented behaviors
2. **Advanced Beginner**	Prior limited experiences Recognition-based behaviors
3. **Competent**	Two to three years of experience Mastery, organization skills
4. **Proficient** 5. **Expert**	Experience-based abilities Perceptions of the whole Experience-based intuitions Accurately targets problems

Source: Data taken from Patricia Benner's *From Novice to Expert: Excellence and Power in Clinical Nursing Practice* (1984).

1980). This section of the chapter provides an overview of activities that will help nursing students maximize their learning experiences in their final semesters of study with a focus on the demands of contemporary nursing practice.

Skill Set

Upon graduation from nursing school, all new nurses should possess a basic skill set, including cognitive knowledge, psychomotor skills, and professional nursing values and attitudes. The ultimate goal is for newly graduated nurses to critically think and use their acquired knowledge, psychomotor skills, and attitudes to provide competent patient-centered care, cooperate in a spirit of teamwork and collaboration, utilize evidence-based findings, participate in quality improvement practices, instill safety measures, and apply informatics as appropriate (Cronenwett et al., 2007). Quality and Safety Education for Nurses (QSEN) is one resource available to nursing faculty to assist students in the development of this competency skill set. This relatively new initiative, funded by the Robert Wood Johnson Foundation, has developed a comprehensive set of nurse competencies related to quality and patient safety. The goal for QSEN is to provide information for nurses to continuously improve the quality and safety of the patient care environment. Table 21-2 provides a general description of the six competencies (Cronenwett et al., 2007), which were adapted from the Institute of Medicine. A full description of these competencies is available on the QSEN Web site at http://www.qsen.org.

TABLE 21-2 QUALITY AND SAFETY COMPETENCIES

Competencies	Defining Characteristics
1. Patient-Centered Care	Nurses should use the patient's needs, preferences, and values as the central focus when developing the plan of care.
2. Teamwork and Collaboration	Nurses should work as part of a team to effectively execute the patient-driven plan of care.
3. Evidence-Based Practice	Nurses should use evidence-based data in conjunction with patient preferences and values to implement the plan of care.
4. Quality Improvement	Nurses should be involved in the continual monitoring of patient data to determine areas for process improvement.
5. Safety	Nurses should ensure patient safety by providing patient care in accordance with organizational policies.
6. Informatics	Nurses should use technology as available to support the safe implementation of patient care.

Source: Data taken from Cronenwett et al.'s *Quality and Safety Education for Nurses* (2007).

Nursing students begin to build this competency skill set throughout their educational experiences, particularly in the semesters immediately prior to graduation, as they synthesize all they have learned in their program in their final clinical learning experiences. It is during this time that students should make every effort to further strengthen their knowledge base by working collaboratively with faculty to seek out the individual clinical learning experiences they may not previously have had the opportunity to acquire.

Cognitive Knowledge Base

Nursing students are expected to integrate the knowledge they gain in the classroom into the patient care they provide in the clinical setting (QSEN, 2007). In the classroom, nursing students are likely to be provided with content related to illnesses and health problems including associated signs and symptoms, outcomes, and potential complications. Case study exemplars may also be provided for discussion and to stimulate critical thinking. Clinical learning experiences essentially provide opportunities to apply what is learned in the classroom. To increase the focus on developing competency in quality and patient safety, as called for in the QSEN initiative, students must go beyond acquiring this fundamental cognitive knowledge base. For example, preparation for clinical learning experiences can include a review of the current best practices related to quality and safety for their patients' diagnoses and treatment plans (QSEN). This review of best practices can also be used to guide the development of patients' plans of care and shared with other nursing students during pre- or postconferences. Nursing students can also compare and contrast what the literature supports as recommendations for patient care and what they actually find being practiced within the clinical setting. These are just a few examples of how students can best use their clinical experiences to increase their knowledge base and prepare for transition into the "real" world of practice.

Psychomotor Skills

Nursing students learn how to perform many psychomotor skills throughout their schooling; as they master these skills they should always be focused on safety for the patient (QSEN, 2007). It is important for students to assume responsibility for actively seeking out opportunities to enhance the development of their psychomotor skills. In addition to learning the skills required to perform the procedure, these repeated experiences allow students to learn the nuances of patient care that cannot be found in textbooks or institutional policies. Although it is common to hear nursing students make such comments as "I have already inserted a Foley catheter," thus inferring that they don't need another opportunity to do so, it must be understood that a one-time psychomotor skill experience does not facilitate the acquisition of skill competence. Nursing students are better served by having the opportunity to perform the same skills as often as possible in different patient care settings. This repetition will help nursing students to become more comfortable in their skills for these procedures and also gain the necessary confidence to perform new procedures in complex settings, thus easing their transition from student to practitioner upon graduation.

Professional Values and Attitudes

Acquiring and demonstrating the values and attitudes of a professional are critical competencies for the new graduate. Some of these values and attitudes include demonstrating integrity, open communication, and mutual respect of others; engaging in collaboration and teamwork; and understanding and acknowledging one's own strengths and limitations (QSEN, 2007). As one means of easing the transition from student to practicing nurse, nursing students can engage in self-reflection about strengths and weaknesses and then clearly communicate their self-identified learning needs to faculty, as well as seek out and be open to constructive criticism from others.

In addition, the healthcare team is becoming more culturally diverse and consists of professionals with varied levels of experience across numerous age groups. Respect for cultural and generational differences among the healthcare team is of paramount importance in the work environment because misunderstandings among team members can divert needed attention away from patient care and adversely affect patient safety. Developing an understanding and appreciation of these workforce generational and cultural differences now, while still in nursing school, can greatly facilitate how quickly the new graduate becomes an accepted member of the healthcare team in the work environment.

KEY TERM

Critical thinking: A systematic process of assessing, grouping, and evaluating data to determine the best plan of action for each patient care issue (Etheridge, 2007).

Critical Thinking/Problem Solving

The art of **critical thinking** and problem solving is one of the most important skills for nursing students to master. Critical thinking is defined as "thinking about all of the implications of and options for each issue of patient care" (Etheridge, 2007, p. 26). Nursing students have limited time in most clinical settings and frequently do not have the opportunity to see the outcomes of the clinical decisions being made by the experienced nurses with a multi-patient case load. Due to this limited time, nursing students may not fully appreciate the vast amount of knowledge that is necessary to make clinical decisions until they are immersed in the clinical setting after graduation (Beauregard, Davis, & Kutash, 2007; Etheridge, 2007; McNiesh, 2007; Nelson et al., 2006; Starr & Conley, 2006). Nursing students have reported that they thought the physicians would make all the decisions and nurses would follow through with the physicians' orders. Other nursing students have reported that they thought there would be a flowsheet or algorithm to guide their decision-making process (Etheridge).

A small pilot study conducted with graduate nurses found that they were overwhelmed by the amount of critical thinking that was necessary on a daily basis (Etheridge, 2007). These graduate nurses found that over a period of time they developed confidence in their decision-making abilities, accepted responsibility for their decisions, and depended less on other healthcare team members for decision making. These graduate nurses felt they could not truly appreciate the magnitude of the responsibility and the amount of decisions needing to be made until they were in orientation and beyond.

What can nursing students do to prepare themselves for making critical patient care decisions? The first step is to develop a good foundational knowledge base, such as that acquired through the nursing curriculum, as a starting point for the decision-making process. What are more difficult to prepare for, however, are the clinical variations and complications in patients that can impact treatment protocols and nursing care. Asking "why" questions of other more experienced practitioners is vital to the student and novice nurse's understandings of the rationale for clinical decisions made in patient care situations. Asking "why" questions of nursing faculty and experienced nurses in the clinical setting prompts these experienced nurses to "think out loud" and share their expertise about how and why clinical decisions are made.

Again, nursing students should assume responsibility for obtaining as many hands-on clinical experiences as possible, even if they have already had multiple patients with similar admitting diagnoses (Etheridge, 2007). Patients with identical diagnoses will have individualized differences from which students can learn. For example, will a patient undergoing a cholecystectomy with a history of diabetes receive a different postoperative plan of care than a patient without diabetes? How does the history of diabetes affect medication administration issues, postoperative incision care, and postoperative infection rates? What if the patient with diabetes has nausea and vomiting postoperatively? How does this impact their dietary intake and insulin administration?

When nursing faculty quiz students about their thought processes while caring for patients, they are actually trying to help nursing students develop their critical thinking skills (Etheridge, 2007). This quizzing usually takes place while in the patient care setting or in pre- or postconference sessions. When nursing students are preparing for their clinical experiences, they should ask themselves "why" questions. For instance, why are specific tests being ordered, were the test results normal or abnormal, and how do these results impact the patient? Or what medications are ordered, what conditions are the medications used for, and why are these medications ordered for this particular patient? Nursing students can practice asking themselves "why" questions by reviewing the exercises provided within this chapter (Box 21-1). These types of exercises are also an excellent means of preparing for the NCLEX-RN examination. Additional critical thinking exercises will be discussed in the prioritization section of this chapter.

Time Management/Organization

All new nurses need to possess time management and organizational skills. Seldom is the patient's plan of care managed and directed by the nurse without revisions or interruptions. These alterations can be caused by changes in patients' conditions, tests being performed without preset schedules, new patient admissions, patient discharges, emergencies (e.g., code blue, seizures, patient falls), unanticipated delays in supplies and equipment, and interruptions from other healthcare providers, family members, and more. Nursing students not only need to learn how to organize their responsibilities for patient care and manage time effectively, they also need to learn to be flexible and comfortable with adapting

---

BOX 21-1   CRITICAL THINKING EXERCISE

You can develop your critical thinking skills either by yourself or with a group of your peers with this exercise. First, review your patient's clinical data. Then ask yourself and/or your peers the following questions:

- What clinical signs are being exhibited by the patient and is there any reason to be alarmed?
- Which data are considered normal?
- Which data are considered abnormal? Why?
- Which data abnormalities are pertinent for the physician to be notified about immediately? Why? What would happen if this data were not called to the attention of the physician immediately?
- Which abnormalities can you wait to notify the physician about (i.e., physician can review the data on patient rounds during the current shift)? Why?

These crucial "why" questions will assist you with your critical thinking skills and patient care decisions as you "think out loud" and seek answers to the "why" questions. Develop the habit of approaching all of your patient care assignments in this manner.

Source: Etheridge, 2007

---

to unexpected changes in their work plan. Developing these skills while still in nursing school will help students make the transition to caring for multiple patients in practice.

The standard principles of time management can be taught, but the method of implementing these principles into the work environment is individualized rather than uniform. Each nursing student needs to find a method of time management that works for them and consistently seek experiences to develop those skills. Observing how other nursing students and experienced nurses organize their responsibilities can be very helpful, as can asking experienced nurses why they organize their work in certain ways. Discussing various time-management methods with nursing faculty can provide additional insight and another voice of experience.

A time-management system does not need to be complex. For example, it can be as easy as A-B-C. Nursing students can review the responsibilities for the patients in their care, and then categorize these tasks as an A (must be done), a B (should be done), or a C (could be done). The A responsibilities are priority interventions such as suctioning a tracheostomy and ensuring the patient has a clear airway. B responsibilities have a lower priority than the A responsibilities but are still important; for example, taking the patient's vital signs every 4 hours. The C responsibilities are less vital to patient care and can be postponed to a later time on the current or later shifts, such as changing a postoperative dressing on a stable patient. The important point is that the nursing student consciously considers means by which to develop his or her time-management skills and organize the delivery of patient care. More details on time management will be discussed within the delegation and prioritization sections of this chapter.

Delegation

Safe delegation of nursing care to other care providers is a key responsibility of the registered nurse. Nursing students usually deliver the majority of their assigned patients' care during their clinical assignments, and therefore do not have much opportunity to develop their delegation skills. When nursing students graduate and assume their first nursing position, they quickly learn the importance of being able to function as a leader and member of the healthcare team, and the need to be able to effectively delegate tasks to appropriate team members. Otherwise, the responsibility for the total care of their assigned patients can be overwhelming.

Many new graduates find assuming the responsibility for safe delegation to be daunting initially. How do new nurses learn what they can delegate and who they can delegate to? Who is responsible for the delegation of patient care? A first step to learning about the act of delegation for nursing students is to understand the legal responsibilities associated with the process. Observing the amount of delegation occurring in their clinical settings can also be a good initial learning experience for students.

Delegation is defined as "transferring to a competent individual authority to perform a selected nursing task in a selected situation" (National Council of State Boards of Nursing [NCSBN], 1995, p. 1). The five rights of delegation are listed in Box 21-2 (Henderson et al., 2006; NCSBN). These five rights of delegation outline the registered nurse's legal responsibilities associated with delegation.

The delegation of patient care is based on state nurse practice acts and healthcare institutions' job descriptions. An example of one state's nurse practice act

---

BOX 21-2   FIVE RIGHTS OF DELEGATION

- Identify the right task to delegate
- Identify the right circumstances for delegation
- Select the right person for delegation
- Use the right direction and communication when delegating

Source: Henderson et al., 2006

(Indiana's) can be found at the following website: http://www.in.gov/pla/files/ ISBN_2008_EDITION.pdf. Each state's nurse practice act addresses the registered nurse's responsibility for delegation.

The registered nurse who is delegating patient care must know what responsibilities are in the other healthcare provider's job description. For instance, can a nursing assistant insert a urethral catheter or change a dressing over a postoperative incision? If the registered nurse delegates patient care duties to other healthcare workers and those duties are not allowed within their job description, then the registered nurse can be held liable for inappropriate delegation. The healthcare worker to whom duties are being delegated is also responsible for informing others if the duties being delegated are not within his or her job description. If the healthcare worker performs the delegated duties despite being aware that the duties are not within the job description, then the healthcare worker can also be held responsible and liable. The bottom line is that delegation is an important skill for nursing students to learn to use because it will be essential in their professional practice after graduation.

Nursing students can learn how to effectively delegate within a team by practicing a strategy called the Four Ps (Hansten & Washburn, 2001; Nelson et al., 2006). The Four Ps are purpose, picture, plan, and part, and they utilize the elements of delegation and prioritization. In this strategy, nursing students review the *purpose* of the patient's admission to the hospital, the *picture* or goals for this patient during the current shift, the *plan* for meeting these goals, and the *part* each team member will play in meeting these preset goals. This strategy allows nursing students to test their knowledge of what can be delegated and practice effective communication skills with nursing assistants and other healthcare team members.

Prioritization

The ability to prioritize patient care needs is one of the most important skills that nursing students can develop and is a skill they will be expected to demonstrate as new nurses. The challenge for students and novice nurses, of course, is to identify which patient care needs demand immediate attention and which can wait. Nursing students should seek opportunities to observe how experienced nurses prioritize care not only for one patient, but also between patients, asking "why" questions as appropriate. For example, should the nurse suction Patient A's tracheostomy before administering his IV pain medication? Or, is it appropriate for the nurse to suction Patient A's tracheostomy before administering Patient B's IV pain medication? In both cases the nurse should attend to the patient's tracheostomy before administering the pain medication. Why? Maintaining an open airway is always a priority! This is a simplified example of clinical decision making, but it illustrates the point that nurses are called upon frequently to meet important and competing patient demands, and must be able to prioritize the order in which they will address them.

Prioritization begins with "being able to learn how to distinguish the relevant from the irrelevant and the abnormal from the normal" and it takes the novice nurse time to develop this skill (McNiesh, 2007, p. 77). There are exercises, however, that nursing students can incorporate into their study to learn how to prioritize safely and appropriately. Case Study 21-1 and Box 21-3 illustrate one of these exercises. Further highlighting the importance of critical thinking skills in prioritizing patient care, Contemporary Practice Highlight 21-1 provides a scenario that presents some of the simultaneous nursing care decisions that are very typically required in an acute care healthcare setting.

CASE STUDY 21–1
PRIORITIZING PATIENT NEEDS

It is 10:00 am and you are faced with the following tasks with five of your patients:

Patient 1	Wears a bed alarm and is now climbing out of bed with the alarm ringing.
Patient 2	A scheduled antibiotic is due.
Patient 3	Wants ice water because NPO order was just discontinued and is thirsty.
Patient 4	Needs vital signs every 4 hours—due now.
Patient 5	Just returned from an arteriogram and oozing is noted at the arterial puncture site.

Which needs should be handled first? Why? In what order should the remainder of patient needs be addressed? Why? Use the various prioritization methods in Box 21-3 to decide how to prioritize the care of your five patients and answer these questions. Which method worked best for you?

Pick a method to use in the clinical setting on your next patient assignment. Review all the patient's needs and prioritize the order for addressing those needs. Discuss this list with your nursing instructor or within a postconference. Once you determine a method or a variation of one of these methods that works best for you, continue to use it and develop it while in nursing school. This integration of a prioritization system will help you when you graduate and are faced with multiple patients with different levels of needs.

BOX 21-3   THREE METHODS FOR PRIORITIZING PATIENT CARE

Use these three different methods for prioritizing patient care to address the patient care scenario given in Case Study 21-1.

Five "F"s for Prioritizing

The "Five Fs for Prioritizing" developed by Alspach (2000) uses the categorization of job elements. The five categories are fatal, fundamental, frequent, fixed, and facility. **Fatal** elements are of highest priority and failure to complete these elements in a timely manner could result in the patient's death or injury (e.g., respiratory distress related to secretions in tracheotomy). **Fundamental** elements are vital for the nurse's job role (e.g., patient assessment). **Frequent** elements are those that are repeated many times (e.g., vital signs). **Fixed** elements are those that had to be performed within a specific interval (e.g., antibiotic administration). **Facility** elements are those that were mandated by the healthcare institution (e.g., patient care conferences per week). Look at the list of patient needs and attempt to categorize them according to this prioritization system. Did this help?

Marny's Four

Marny's Four uses four categories of needs and desires that are comparable to Maslow's Hierarchy of needs to help guide prioritization of patient needs. Maslow's (1968) model emphasized that the patient's basic needs must be met prior to the higher level needs of esteem and self-actualization. Marny's Four includes: meeting the needs of the patient (e.g., pain, nutrition, and elimination); meeting the needs of the nurse (e.g., physician orders, patient education, and medication administration); meeting the patient's desires (e.g., glass of water, sharing pictures of loved ones); and meeting the desires of the nurse (e.g., straightening up patient rooms, combing patient's hair). Look at the list of patient needs and attempt to categorize them according to this prioritization system. Did this help?

Christine's CURE

Christine's CURE uses a prioritization method that ranks patients' needs from highest to lowest importance. This method emphasizes the fact that all patient needs are important, but nurses need a system to prioritize these needs accurately as they provide care for multiple patients. The CURE method consists of the prioritization categories of critical, urgent, routine responsibilities, and extras needs. The critical needs are of highest priority since these could be life-threatening if left untreated (e.g., patient with sudden weakness on one side of the body with slurred speech). Urgent needs are next in priority since these are usually related to eliminating harm or relieving discomfort for the patient (e.g., confused patient attempting to climb out of bed on own). Routine responsibilities are next in priority and include patient activities that are scheduled throughout the shift (e.g., patient with vital signs ordered every 4 hours). Extras are of the lowest priority since these needs are related to patients' desires (e.g., patient requesting a cup of water). Look at the list of patient needs and attempt to categorize them according to this prioritization system. Did this help?

Source: Nelson et al., 2006

CONTEMPORARY PRACTICE HIGHLIGHT 21-1

EFFECTIVE PRIORITIZATION OF PATIENT CARE

Being able to critically think through clinical problems and effectively prioritize and delegate care is vital to the delivery of safe patient care. Frequently the nurse is faced with a situation in which more than one patient has the same level of priority need. How does the nurse decide which patient's needs should be addressed first?

In this case scenario, the nurse has been given responsibility for the care of the following six patients. Having just received the hand-off report on the patients, the nurse begins to make rounds on the patients to assess and evaluate the patients' status.

Patient 1   The family has called out and said the patient needs his tracheostomy suctioned. He has tried to cough up the mucous but it is too thick.

Patient 2   The blood bank has called and informed you that the blood is ready for the patient. The patient, who has been diagnosed with lung cancer, has a Hgb of 7.0.

Patient 3   The patient, who is 2 days postoperative a colon resection, is requesting pain medication; she states that her pain is at a level of 10. The nurse notes that the patient's pain medication was last administered 4 hours ago.

Patient 4   The family has called out requesting the patient be placed on a bedpan; the patient has been having diarrhea for the last 24 hours.

Patient 5   The patient has some questions regarding the colonoscopy that is scheduled for tomorrow morning.

Patient 6   The patient's wife is on the phone and wants to speak to the nurse .

For this exercise, prioritize these patients' needs into the proper categories using CURE (critical, urgent, routine, and extras; see Christine's CURE in Box 21-3) (Nelson et al., 2006).

OUTCOME

More than one patient has a need at the same level of acuity. Patient 1 has a critical need. Patients 2, 3, and 4 have urgent needs. Patients 5 and 6 have routine needs. They should be addressed as follows:

- The nurse's first priority is suctioning mucous from the tracheostomy because maintaining the airway is most important. The nurse will need to address the patient with respiratory distress first.
- The nurse's second priority is attending to the following patients: Patient 2 who needs a blood transfusion started because his Hgb is 7.0, Patient 3 who is requesting pain medication, and Patient 4 who is requesting the bedpan.
- The nurse's third priority is answering questions for the wife of Patient 6 and answering questions from Patient 5.

Within this example, the nurse had three urgent tasks and two routine tasks in addition to the critical need. So how does the nurse prioritize within the same category? Which one of these should the nurse do before the other(s) within the same category?

(continues)

CONTEMPORARY PRACTICE HIGHLIGHT 21-1 (continued)

After suctioning Patient 1 (critical need), the nurse should do the following:

- First, place Patient 4 on the bedpan if no one else is available to delegate this task to (nursing technician or another nurse). This can be done fairly quickly and the patient's need is urgent due to the diarrhea.
- Next, the nurse would administer the pain medication to Patient 3 because the pain was rated as a 10 and some time has elapsed since the patient's last pain medication. Administration of the pain medication is a task that can be accomplished within a short period of time.
- The nurse would then call the blood bank and request the blood be sent up for Patient 2 after determining the patient's IV site is patent, the blood consent form has been signed, and the physician's order for administering the blood has been reviewed.
- While waiting for the blood to arrive on the unit, the nurse could speak to the wife of Patient 6.
  - While the nurse was taking care of the other critical and urgent needs, he or she could have asked the secretary, another nurse, or a nursing technician to let the wife know that the nurse would be able to speak to her in 15 minutes if she wants to hold or would be glad to call her back in 15 minutes.
- After the blood is started on Patient 2 the nurse could finish patient rounds, speaking to Patient 5 and answering questions about the colonoscopy.
  - Since his procedure is not until the next day, the nurse can wait to address the patient's questions about the procedure while assessing his status.

The bottom line is if two responsibilities are of the same level of importance, then the activity taking the least amount of time to accomplish should be completed first in most cases.

Source: This exercise was adapted from methods in Nelson et al. (2006). Teaching prioritization skills: A preceptor forum. *Journal for Nurses in Staff Development, 22*(4), 172–178.

Patient Safety

Nursing students and novice nurses need to realize the limits of their knowledge base and openly share these limits with their instructors and/or supervisors to ensure patient safety (McNiesh, 2007). The safe delivery of patient care incorporates the mastery of all the nursing skills—knowledge, psychomotor, attitude, critical thinking, time management, delegation, and prioritization. Healthcare institutions are accredited by various organizations to ensure the effective and safe delivery of patient care. Organizations such as the Joint Commission, Centers for Disease Control and Prevention, and State Department of Health provide these healthcare institutions with standards to be met for their accreditation. These standards impact nursing's role in patient care delivery. As one example of how these standards impact the delivery of patient care, one accreditation standard is that upon admission and during every shift patients are to be assessed for their risk for falling. When patients are identified as being at a high risk for falls, measures are implemented to prevent patient falls; these measures must be assessed routinely and documented. It is important for nursing students to be aware of these standards and how they are addressed within the healthcare institution's policies; for new graduates, it is also common that these types of safety measures are addressed in the institution's orientation programs.

Nursing students can increase their knowledge and awareness of such patient safety measures by observing the practice of experienced nurses, participating in the delivery of patient care, identifying the policies and procedures that guided nursing decisions and interventions, and noting any variations from the established policies as well as the reasons for the variations. Discussing these observations and care experiences with experienced nurses, faculty, and other healthcare professionals can foster in students a deeper understanding of patient safety issues in the healthcare setting. Chapter 8 further addresses the culture of safety and how it impacts the delivery of health care. Learning the importance of following institutional policies, identifying safe vs. unsafe care, and recognizing when nurses need to deviate from policies will help nursing students in their transition after graduation (QSEN, 2007).

Interprofessional Communication

Prior to graduation, nursing students have nursing faculty and experienced nurses to assist them with the coordination of patient care and collaboration with other healthcare team members. Nursing students can take advantage of their clinical experiences to learn how to communicate clearly with the patient and other members of the healthcare team, observe how to mediate any controversies, and incorporate the family into the plan of care as appropriate (QSEN, 2007). Observing and participating in patient care conferences also enhance the development of the teamwork and collaboration skills that will be so important to a successful transition into the work environment after graduation.

Maximizing the Benefits of Student Intern/Extern Programs

Students may want to consider seeking out opportunities to gain additional clinical experiences in programs designed to allow them to work under the direct supervision of an experienced nurse. In a 2007 survey, nursing students indicated they felt only somewhat prepared to care for patients after graduation and were naturally concerned about making patient care errors (AMN Healthcare, 2007). Given the complexity of nursing and health care, these findings are hardly surprising. Intern, extern, and residency programs have been developed at many healthcare institutions to meet the experience and learning needs of nursing students. These programs have also been reported to positively affect school performance (Beauregard et al., 2007; Starr & Conley, 2006). Nursing students may find that the additional experiences offered through the intern and extern programs will ease the transition to their new role of graduate nurses because these programs offer an opportunity to perfect and expand their skill set. In addition, many students elect to accept intern/extern positions at institutions where they hope to practice as registered nurses upon graduation, thus providing them with an opportunity to become familiar with the institution's culture and policies.

There are some subtle differences in extern and intern positions. *Extern programs* are usually offered when nursing students have limited clinical experience and wish to gain more hands-on patient encounters under the direct supervision of registered nurses. Externs working alongside registered nurses are able to gain insights into the many roles nurses fulfill during their shifts. Extern programs offer an opportunity for nursing students to develop skill with specific tasks within their limited skill set, become more confident in these skills and their role in patient care delivery, and feel less fearful of making mistakes.

Intern and residency programs may be offered during the last semester of nursing school or as part of the new graduate orientation. These programs offer nursing students or graduate nurses the opportunity to develop their prioritization, time-management, and critical thinking skills as they take a full patient assignment under the direct supervision of registered nurses (Beauregard et al., 2007; Rosenfeld, Smith, Iervolino, & Bowar-Ferres, 2004). The goal of the intern and residency programs is to ease students and graduate nurses into the real world of nursing, with all the complexities and decisions to be made for a full caseload of patients. As a result, these nursing students and graduate nurses may feel more prepared for their role as registered nurses.

Another advantage of participating in intern and extern programs is that many nursing students are hired as graduate nurses based on the relationships they build with the manager and nursing staff within these programs (Beauregard et al., 2007; Rosenfeld et al., 2004; Starr & Conley, 2006). Managers and staff nurses are able to examine the nursing students' potential during their extern and intern programs prior to graduation and determine their preference for hiring them based on their performance. In turn, nursing students can also use the extern and intern programs to determine if the healthcare institution is where they wish to work upon graduation and in what area.

With the extra clinical experiences provided in the extern and intern programs, students may have a smoother transition to the graduate nurse role. Nursing students not only have been able to improve their skill set within these programs, but also have been able to increase their confidence levels related to skills performance (American Association of Colleges of Nursing [AACN], 2002). These programs have also yielded higher retention rates, which may indicate that new nurses experience greater job satisfaction postgraduation due in part to participating in these programs (Beauregard et al., 2007; Halfer & Graf, 2006; Rosenfeld et al., 2004).

Beyond Nursing School

You have accepted your first position as a registered nurse and are scheduled to begin work the week following your graduation. You have maximized your last semesters in nursing school as suggested in this chapter by seeking out learning experiences that have helped you further refine your skill set and your clinical decision-making abilities. In addition, you have been a student nurse extern for the past year at the institution in which you have accepted a registered nurse position. So what else do you need to consider in facilitating your role transition from student to professional nurse? This section of the chapter will provide you with an overview of what to expect in those first months in your new position and how to make the most of the experiences to which you will be exposed.

The Orientation Period

In most institutions, new graduates can expect a detailed orientation when they are first hired. During the interviewing process, it is appropriate to ask about the length and type of orientation period that will be provided. The formalized orientation after graduation acquaints new nurses with their role responsibilities and expectations, emphasizes policies related to the safe delivery of patient care, provides opportunity to demonstrate psychomotor skills and learn new skills as required for the position, and familiarizes them with available resources within the institution. During this formal orientation period, new graduates are also assigned to work alongside experienced nurses who have the responsibility for providing and overseeing patient care experiences that will promote the acquisition of additional knowledge and skills. In addition, these experienced nurses will provide information about the nursing unit layout, location of equipment, unit-based responsibilities, how patient assignments are posted, when meal breaks are taken, how report is given between shifts, and how staff communicates within the shift (i.e., phones, pagers, etc.)—in general, orienting the new nurse to the expectations related to the daily routine of the unit.

Healthcare institutions may provide both agency orientation and nursing department orientation sessions. The agency orientation may include information for all new employees, such as benefits, confidentiality, fire and electrical safety, and emergency preparedness. Nursing department orientation may include information specifically for the job role, such as medication safety and nursing policies, and hands-on practice with patient care equipment. The agency orientation may be 1–2 days in length. Nursing department orientation typically can range anywhere from 4 weeks for non-intensive care units to several months for intensive care units. In some cases the period of orientation may be adjusted depending on how quickly the new nurse acclimates to her or his role responsibilities.

If new graduates have been previously oriented as students to the institution in which they have been hired, they may think some information is repetitious from when they were students. This is somewhat true. In fact, this orientation may make graduate nurses feel like they are still in school. Regulatory agency standards may not be different, but after graduation your responsibility changes in relation to these standards. As a nursing student you were not ultimately responsible for the safety of patients in your care—the registered nurse held that responsibility. Role transition from student to registered nurse brings new responsibilities that put a different perspective on what you need to know about these standards and other institutional policies.

It is important to realize that the information provided during orientation, albeit repetitious in some cases, is being presented for reasons that may not be fully appreciated until the orientation period is completed and the new graduate has assumed total responsibility for patient care. Be sure to keep an open mind and a respectful, professional attitude toward those who are providing the orientation sessions. Make note of information that will be useful to you later and be sure to ask questions as appropriate throughout the orientation period. The time in orientation passes relatively quickly. Commit to using the orientation period as effectively as you can to gain a fuller understanding of your new role and responsibilities as a registered nurse.

Preceptor's Role in Orientation

Many institutions use the preceptor model in their orientation programs to assist in the orientation of new nurses. Preceptors are experienced nurses who are assigned to new graduates for the length of their orientation period. In most cases, the graduate nurse is assigned the identical work schedule as the preceptor. The advantages of using a preceptor model for the orientation of new graduates are the consistent one-on-one supervision, individualization of learner needs, and the opportunity for continual feedback related to performance (Alspach, 2000).

Nursing students may not realize that experienced nurses who serve as preceptors can assist them with transitioning to the nursing role even while they are still students. These experienced nurses are not only trained to precept others, but genuinely like to teach and usually possess caring attitudes (Schumacher, 2007). Students should ask questions of these experienced nurses to glean as much learning as possible from their clinical experiences prior to graduation. Expert nurses who have been in practice for a while can sometimes forget to explain the rationale for their actions and decisions, because they may assume the topic in question is common knowledge. Nursing students can also ask these preceptors to share stories about their own experiences as nursing students and as new graduates. This type of information sharing reinforces the fact that feelings of insecurity as a new nurse are normal.

Mentor's Role in Orientation

Mentors differ from preceptors in that serving as a mentor is not an assigned role, nor does it exist for a specified period of time as does the preceptor role (i.e., the length of new graduate orientation). Mentors are experienced nurses who form a professional relationship with nursing students and new nurses on a voluntary basis (Bally, 2007). Mentors are viewed as role models who provide advice and guidance on patient care issues as well as professional development issues. A mentor-mentee relationship will last as long as it is mutually beneficial to both parties.

Nursing students may want to research which healthcare institutions provide a mentoring program or foster professional mentoring relationships. They should ask for the specifics of the program—how mentors are selected, what training mentors receive, how long the program has been in existence, how many nurses have participated, whether the program has been evaluated by both mentors and mentees, and whether a summary of these evaluations is available for review.

Having a professional mentor can be very helpful to the new graduate during role transition. Above all, a mentor should be someone who is a good listener and conveys interest in the new graduate's professional growth, someone who the new graduate can turn to for guidance with career issues and concerns. For some new graduates, former faculty may continue to serve as mentors; others may find mentors in the institution in which they are employed or through professional organization activities. Seeking a mentor is a proactive strategy for managing the stress of a new role and is one strategy that all new graduates should seriously consider to help them cope with the "reality shock" that has been inevitably associated with becoming a registered nurse.

Reality Shock

Reality shock is a common phenomenon in nursing that many new graduates face as they enter the workforce and assume the complex responsibilities associated with the role (Kramer, 1974). Kramer identified four phases that new graduate nurses experience as employees: honeymoon, shock, recovery, and resolution. The honeymoon phase begins as they enter the workforce after graduation, expending a lot of energy to develop their nursing skills and acquaint themselves with their new co-workers and job role. The shock phase appears several weeks later as the reality of their new responsibilities settles in and creates a sense of feeling overwhelmed and insecure. New graduates may begin to feel angry, want to quit their job, and lose their prior energy level. The recovery phase begins when the graduate nurses realize that they are going to make it. The graduate nurses will show a re-emergence of their preshock personality and sense of humor. The resolution phase is evidenced by new strategies that the graduate nurses decide to use as they begin to adjust and cope with the demands of their new role.

Signs of Reality Shock

Nursing students need to know what the signs of reality shock are so they can prepare themselves for this common occurrence. Typically, the signs exhibited include anger, negativity, low energy levels, and discouragement (Kramer, 1974). Preceptors and mentors can assist new nurses through the shock phase by helping them find a healthy resolution to accepting their new role and all the related responsibilities. Preceptors may ask new graduates what they are thinking and feeling while watching for the signs of reality shock. It is helpful during this time for new graduates to be open and honest about what they are thinking and feeling so their preceptors, mentors, and others can assist them through the phases of reality shock.

What Is Normal?

Caring for human lives is an enormous responsibility that can lead to feeling overwhelmed, frustrated, and fatigued. Words of encouragement and reassurances from preceptors and the other experienced nurses that these feelings are quite normal will help new graduates as they assume their new responsibilities. Time is both a friend and a foe. Nursing students and new graduates typically want to know and be able to do everything the job entails immediately upon graduation. Although it is not comfortable to feel inexperienced in a role that has responsibilities with such high human stakes, it is unrealistic to expect to be able to automatically function as those with more nursing experience. With the passage of time and an ever growing body of experience, the requisite knowledge and skills needed to function as competent nurses will develop and mature. It is quite common for 6–12 months to pass before novice nurses begin to feel more comfortable with their skills and new role. Patience is essential during this time. During this period, the novice nurse should be asking questions and aligning with a mentor or other experienced nurses for guidance and support.

New nurses can effectively cope with reality shock by first recognizing the symptoms and talking to their preceptor, a mentor, their manager, and other experienced nurses. These individuals can assist the graduate nurses in identifying the positive aspects of their new role and setting realistic expectations and goals. At the very beginning of accepting a new position, the new graduate should take steps to identify and incorporate self-care activities into his or her lifestyle, as one means of coping with work-related stressors and avoiding burn-out. These strategies can be as simple as daily exercise, healthy eating, and scheduled leisure activities. Networking with other new graduates under the guidance of an experienced nurse can also assist new graduates in realizing their feelings of reality shock are normal and will subside with time and experience.

Support Systems

Having support systems in place can be an effective strategy for coping with role transition and reality shock. New graduates should seek out the individual(s) that they feel most comfortable sharing their thoughts with or asking questions. Preceptors and mentors can be effective members of the support system; those two roles have been addressed previously in this chapter. Additional members of a new graduate's support system can be faculty, other experienced nurses, clinical educators, nurse managers, peers and discussion groups, and professional organizations.

Faculty

Teacher–student interactions can have positive effects on the student's performance (Chou, Tang, Teng, & Yen, 2003; Ironside, 2003), especially when teachers exhibit a caring attitude and belief in their students (Chou et al.). New nurse graduates have also identified faculty as role models, and indicated in hindsight how beneficial it was for their faculty to challenge them as students in their decision making regarding patient care issues (Etheridge, 2007). Just as faculty can serve as role models during nursing school, they can continue to serve as important support systems and mentors to new graduates. New nurse graduates should not hesitate to seek out their former faculty and nursing programs as one means of support postgraduation. Among other words of advice, faculty can provide expert guidance on professional development opportunities.

Experienced Nurses

Experienced nurses who are not identified as preceptors or mentors can also provide guidance to nursing students preparing to graduate and new nurse graduates as needed. Experienced nurses have a wealth of valuable expertise to share and are frequently very willing to help students and new graduates find opportunities for new clinical learning experiences if they know what experiences are needed. Nursing students can ask these experienced nurses if they remember doing a specific skill the first time and what helped them to feel more comfortable performing or perfecting the skill. This type of question can create an open dialogue between the student and nurse, and lead to more learning opportunities. New nurse graduates should also ask questions of experienced nurses as one means by which to become socialized to their new work environment and colleagues.

Clinical Educators

Many healthcare institutions have clinical educators in specific specialty areas in addition to centralized nursing education departments. These clinical educators are usually charged with providing support and guidance to nurses at the bedside where patient care is delivered. They have the opportunity to take advantage of the teachable moments with nursing students and new nurse graduates as they arise in the patient care setting and can be wonderful resources in terms of support and clinical information for new nurses.

Nurse Managers

Nurse managers are also important members of the new nurse graduate's support system. Graduate nurses will want to seek guidance from their nurse manager about their performance and progress toward mutually agreed-upon goals for orientation and beyond. Developing a positive, mutually respectful professional relationship with the nurse manager is an important factor in smoothing the transition into practice.

New Nurse Graduate Peers and Discussion Groups

One source of support for nursing students who are anticipating graduation can be new nurse graduates who are already in the work world. Nursing students can also obtain information from graduate nurses on what they found to be the most useful components of their schooling. Nurses who have recently graduated can share their experiences of the first year in their new role—what surprised them, what was the most difficult part of their new role, what they liked the most about their new role and why, and what they liked least about their new role and what could make this issue less unappealing.

Nursing students should research healthcare institutions to identify which ones provide new nurse networking or discussion groups. These discussion groups provide a venue for new nurse graduates to discuss the challenges they are experiencing in their new roles. This discussion group can be a mechanism for graduate nurses to hear from their peers and realize that they are not alone in their challenges or feelings of insecurity. A facilitator sets ground rules so that these discussion groups are safe havens for sharing experiences without repercussions (Etheridge, 2007). Some healthcare institutions may incorporate nurse networking within their mentor programs.

Professional Organizations

Numerous professional organizations can provide students and new graduates with support and resources. National and state student nurse associations provide resources for NCLEX-RN examination preparation and study aids, and information on scholarships, financial aid, and the job market. The local chapter of the International Honor Society of Nursing, Sigma Theta Tau, can provide opportunities to meet with other nurses and discuss mutual topics of interest related to improving global nursing issues and provide information on scholarships, research, and education. Graduate nurses can join other organizations that discuss issues related to specific nursing specialties. Overall, the goals of these professional organizations are to discuss current issues of nursing practice, promote nursing fellowship, and develop standards of patient care. Web links for some of these professional organizations and resources are provided in Box 21-4.

BOX 21–4   PROFESSIONAL RESOURCE WEB LINKS

1. Quality znd Safety Education for Nurses or QSEN (http://www.qsen.org) – link to competency definitions and ideas for developing these competencies in the classroom and clinical setting
2. Nurse Zone (http://www.nursezone.com) - link to a student nurse center with information on topics such as financial assistance, student nurse associations, study tips and tools, NCLEX examination prep, finding a job, and networking to multiple organizations
3. National Student Nurses' Association (http://www.nsna.org/) – link to network and support systems
4. Sigma Theta Tau (http://www.nursingsociety.org/index.html) – link to multiple resources, such as education and research, online library, and professional development
5. American Nurses Association (http://www.ana.org) – link to multiple resources, such as nursing issues and programs, publications, and online journal

Source: Henderson et al., 2006

Developing Confidence in Clinical Decision Making as a New Nurse

The ability to apply acquired knowledge to the unique circumstances of each patient is learned through the process of lived experiences. New nurse graduates need to realize that they will continue to consult frequently with their preceptors and other experienced healthcare professionals for advice and guidance even after their orientation phase has ended.

Repeated clinical experiences will assist the new graduate in providing appropriate and safe care, and with mastering the ability to make clinical decisions and adapt when an alternate approach is required. New nurse graduates have reported feeling more confident in their abilities to provide nursing care after 6 months of experience postgraduation (Etheridge, 2007). At the same time, nursing students and new graduates should also realize that it is rare for an experienced nurse to work through a shift without consulting with a colleague regarding the care of a patient. Knowing that such collaboration is common among healthcare workers should be a comfort to nursing students nearing graduation.

Confidence can be defined as "the belief in oneself, in one's judgment and psychomotor skills, and in one's possession of knowledge and ability to think and draw conclusions" (Etheridge, 2007, p. 25). One of the factors that can influence one's self-confidence is the environment in which one is functioning. For example, research has indicated that students experience more academic success when teachers create positive learning experiences and provide words of encouragement to their students (Angulo, 2002; Pitino, 2003). Research also has indicated that when teachers portray a belief in students' success then these students tend to be more successful. In addition, when students have more positive perceptions of their teacher's feelings toward them they tend to have more positive perceptions of themselves and are more successful (Zohar & Dori, 2003). Given that students have repeatedly reported feeling more self-confident in their abilities when working in a supportive environment, it would not be surprising to find that new nurse graduates also respond positively to a supportive work environment and colleagues who encourage them and foster their growth as professionals. New graduates should actively seek out experienced colleagues who are supportive and encouraging, promoting the development of their self-confidence. The combination of acquiring additional patient care experience and working with supportive colleagues will increase the new graduate's sense of self-confidence and the chances of a successful transition to practice.

Learning to take responsibility for one's own knowledge, skills, and actions can be overwhelming for new graduates (Etheridge, 2007; McNiesh, 2007). While in nursing school, nursing students are frequently limited in the patient care they can provide their assigned patients and do not assume total responsibility for coordinating the care of patients. Thus, students do not feel the full impact of their nursing responsibilities until they graduate.

New nurse graduates should assume their new role with the understanding that they have shared responsibility for identifying their learning needs. For example, in orientation they may be asked to complete a skill set checklist to identify what skills they have performed previously and feel competent in, what skills they have limited experience with, and what skills they have never performed. The preceptor supervising their orientation will review this list and verify competence in the performance of all skills. It is important that novice nurses be honest when expressing their comfort level with various patient care experiences so that the preceptor can seek out appropriate opportunities to help them further develop their decision-making skills. As novices, they also need to be open to constructive feedback related to their nursing skills so that they can continue to improve in the role. Participating regularly in continuing education offerings that are made available by the institution or through professional organizations is another strategy that can boost a new graduate's confidence in performance.

Work Environment

In a survey completed by nursing students, the quality of the workplace environment ranked higher than pay or geographic location when citing important elements for employment consideration (AMN Healthcare, 2007). When seeking their first position postgraduation, what should nursing students look for in the work environment? What are some of the key characteristics of a good work environment? For instance, do the nurses have varied levels of experience or are they all new graduates? What is the mix of the other healthcare workers and how do they get along? Do nurses have a voice in their practice or are all the decisions made at the administrative level and passed down to staff?

Multi-generational differences can influence the nature of the work environment, as can the governance structure and the presence of collective bargaining units. Each of these work environment elements is briefly addressed in the sections that follow.

Multi-Generational Workforces

The generational composition of healthcare work environments is increasingly diverse. Being aware of the generational differences and differing core values and beliefs held among healthcare team members is an important element in promoting a cohesive working environment. Typically there are four generations in the current workforce; these generations and some key characteristics for each are listed in Table 21-3 (Sherman, 2006). Life events during the formative years for those born in these generations molded the characteristics they exhibit in the work environment. Veterans lived through the events of World War II and the Great Depression. Baby Boomers were born in the postwar era when extended families became less common. Generation Xers grew up when divorce rates soared and single parent families became more common. Millennials were

TABLE 21-3   FOUR GENERATIONS IN THE WORK ENVIRONMENT

Generation	Characteristics
1. Veterans, Traditionalists or Mature (1925–1945)	Loyal / supportive of organization hierarchy Disciplined work habits
2. Baby Boomers (1946–1964)	Individualistic / Rewriting society's rules Work related to self-worth
3. Generation X (1963–1980)	Self-Reliant Balance work and life responsibilities
4. Millennial (1980–2000)	Technology-driven lives Balance work and life responsibilities

Source: Data taken from Rose Sherman's *Leading a Multigenerational Nursing Workforce: Issues, Challenges, and Strategies* (2006).

raised in the midst of terrorism and increasing violence in the world around them (Sherman, 2006).

Each generation brings positive elements to the working environment. Being aware of and respecting the differences in other generations will enhance the communication and teamwork on the healthcare team. Nurses and other healthcare workers must find a way to make their diversity a positive influence in their working relationships instead of a detriment. Communication and conflict resolution are conducive to promoting a positive work environment for all. Finding value in each other's contributions and demonstrating respect for each other despite these differences can lead to a strong team caring for patients and their families (Etheridge, 2007; QSEN, 2007; Sherman, 2006). As new nurse graduates enter the workforce they must be aware of and sensitive to these differences in values and beliefs, and strive for open communication and mutual respect among all members of the team.

Governance Structures

How are nursing decisions made? Who is fundamental in creating and implementing these changes? Is nursing empowered to be proactive in making policy changes to meet the future needs of patients and staff? Knowing who makes the decisions related to patient care should be an important element of the work environment for many graduate nurses. If they wish to work in a patient care unit where they make the decisions on how the care is provided, then a shared governance structure will be more inviting. If they are satisfied with the administrators of the healthcare institution directing their methods of care delivery, then a centralized governance structure may be more appealing.

Shared Governance

The American Association of Colleges of Nursing (2002) developed a document that identified the characteristics of a professional nursing practice environment. These "hallmark" characteristics included elements that recognize and promote nursing knowledge, skill, and professional development, and an environmental structure that utilizes bedside nurses for clinical decision making.

Models demonstrating staff nurse involvement at the decision-making level in nursing are referred to as shared governance models. The organizational structure of such organizations is relatively flat as compared to the more typical hierarchal design. The patient care unit is the central location where decisions are made, partnering nursing staff with management. Within shared governance structures, nursing staff have the power, autonomy, and accountability to make patient care decisions or changes within their nursing practice (Green & Jordan, 2004; Hess, 2004). Nursing management is charged with providing the nursing staff with the necessary resources to implement these patient care delivery decisions or changes

(Caramanica, 2004). Despite the variations of the shared governance models that exist in multiple healthcare institutions, the core element of autonomy should be evident in nursing practice. Staff nurses must know that they have the power to change nursing actions that impact patient care.

Examples of shared governance include creating nursing councils (or committees) for practice, research, quality, education, and recruitment and retention. Council membership consists of nursing representatives from patient care units who meet on a regular basis to assess the need for changes in practice. These nursing representatives are charged with collecting evidence-based data to support changes and recommend policy changes. Nursing representatives share these decisions with their colleagues within their patient care unit and seek feedback. This communication between the council representatives and the nurses on the patient care units is essential for the success of shared governance.

Another example of shared governance would be the use of collaborative teams for systems improvement. Continual process improvement is part of the healthcare environment, and nursing plays a key role due to nurses' direct patient contact. Nurses see firsthand what the issues are in patient care and can collect the necessary data for evaluation. Nurses are asked to serve on the teams with other healthcare workers and administrative staff to analyze patient care data and provide recommendations on proposed changes in patient care delivery.

For example, nurses on a patient care safety team could identify gaps in the current practice of changing central line catheter dressings (QSEN, 2007), and collect and analyze data supporting the use of occlusive vs. gauze dressings. The nurses could then assist with the policy development, education plan for the nursing staff, and time line for implementing the change in practice.

New nurse graduates have expressed major dissatisfaction when they do not feel they have a voice in their nursing practice (Halfer & Graf, 2006). Whether or not a future employer has a shared governance structure can be a vitally important consideration to new graduates when selecting a position. Asking how policy decisions that affect nursing practice are made in the organization is an acceptable question to ask in the interview process.

Centralized Governance

Models that demonstrate the more typical hierarchical design for decision making are referred to as centralized governance structures. The decisions are made by management with very limited, if any, input from the nursing staff. Policy changes related to patient care decisions are made without the staff nurses' direct involvement. Although healthcare institutions with centralized governance structures can provide acceptable patient care, the nursing staff lacks the empowerment to seek out and implement changes. Nurses would not be members of the policy-making committees within these healthcare institutions (Green & Jordan, 2004; Hess, 2004).

Collective Bargaining

According to the American Nurses Association (ANA) Bill of Rights "nurses have the right to negotiate the conditions of their employment, either as individuals or collectively, in all practice settings" (Wiseman, 2001). The ANA is nursing's professional organization that works to advocate and support the rights of nurses in the workplace. "The ANA advances the nursing profession by fostering high standards of nursing practice, promoting the rights of nurses in the workplace, projecting a positive and realistic view of nursing, and by lobbying the Congress and regulatory agencies on health care issues affecting nurses and the public" (ANA, 2007). Since 1946, the ANA has supported collective bargaining as a means to seek solutions for nursing shortages. More recently a new approach within collective bargaining systems focuses on using shared governance structures as a means to give nurses more voice in their overall practice (Budd, Warino, & Patton, 2004).

Many nurses still think of strikes and picket lines when they are confronted with discussions on collective bargaining. Nurses do not like the union fees or loss of work while on the picket line (Budd et al., 2004). They also worry about the impact of strikes on the delivery of patient care. Nursing students must consider their options regarding whether they want to work within an environment that is unionized. In healthcare institutions where collective bargaining does not exist, nurses should work within their institution's committees (e.g., recruitment and retention, policy and procedure) to make sure elements of the ANA Bill of Rights are incorporated into nursing practice as appropriate (Wiseman, 2001).

From Advanced Beginner to Competent Nurse

Benner (1984) identifies the advanced beginner as one who has limited experiences but can recognize the similarities between current patient situations and past patient experiences. As expressed by preceptors and graduate nurses the element of time is critical to skill set development (Etheridge, 2007; McNiesh, 2007). Nursing students may not be able to fully appreciate this concept until after graduation when they are faced with the realization of a patient care assignment and the amount and complexities of decisions needing to be made and procedures to be performed. New nurse graduates will continue developing their fundamental skill set over the first 12 months in their new job role before feeling more comfortable with their performance in psychomotor and decision-making activities (Etheridge). Nursing students and new nurse graduates need to be reminded over and over again that they cannot rush this period of time; only with time and experience will the skill set develop.

With additional time the novice nurse's skill set becomes more varied and perfected. Benner (1984) identifies the competent nurse as one who has 2–3 years of experience and has developed the art of conscious, deliberate planning for patient care. This transition from advanced beginner to competent nurse is more than just the passage of an established time frame. Within this transition to the competent level the nurse develops the ability to engage in long-range planning. The competent nurse also feels like he or she has mastered skills and is able to cope with the complexities of the patient care unit.

Even after being on the job for years, nurses continue to encounter new clinical situations and technologies that warrant new skills acquisition. Being a competent nurse requires a lifelong commitment to learning and embracing new knowledge.

Summary

This chapter described some of the challenges that nursing students are faced with as they transition from the role of student to the role of registered nurse. It also described strategies for acquiring the necessary experiences that will help new nurses successfully make this transition. Assuming responsibility for their own learning and being proactive in seeking out needed learning experiences are two of the best strategies that nursing students can employ to help prepare themselves for practice in the real world.

Graduating and accepting your first position as a registered nurse is an exciting time in your new career. Use your time wisely before graduating to prepare yourself for this transition, seek out mentors, develop your support systems, and find the right work environment for you. Welcome to the nursing profession!

Key Terms

- **Advanced beginner:** Someone who has limited experience with a given situation (Benner, 1984).
- **Competent:** Someone with 2–3 years of experience who is consciously aware of a given situation in its individual parts and can develop a long-range action plan (Benner, 1984).
- **Critical thinking:** A systematic process of assessing, grouping, and evaluating data to determine the best plan of action for each patient care issue (Etheridge, 2007).
- **Expert:** Someone with the vast experience to intuitively assess a given situation and accurately target the problem area without being distracted by other unrelated symptoms (Benner, 1984).
- **Graduate nurse:** A nursing student who has graduated from a nursing program, but not yet taken the NCLEX examination.
- **Mentor:** Someone who develops a professional relationship or bond with a novice or advanced beginner (Alspach, 2000).
- **Novice:** Someone who has no experience with a given situation (Benner, 1984).
- **Preceptor:** Someone who orients or provides guidance to a novice or advanced beginner in a given situation or over a fixed period of time (Alspach, 2000).
- **Proficient:** Someone with the experience to see a given situation in wholes rather than individual parts, who can analyze the situation and determine whether the typical picture is not materializing, and who can determine what needs to be revised within the plan of care in response (Benner, 1984).

Reflective Practice Questions

1. You are working with a nursing technician who tells you she is allowed to change dressings and apply antibiotic ointment to wounds. You consult the job description for nursing technicians to determine if this task can be delegated. What do you think you will find? Is the nursing technician allowed to change dressings? Is the nursing technician allowed to apply antibiotic ointment? Is this antibiotic ointment considered a medication? Depending on your state laws and institutional guidelines, what is your response to the nursing technician?

2. You are working the evening shift with Pam, who is 50 years old, and Christy, who is 35 years old. You are discussing the self-scheduling system for the staff on your unit. Christy is verbalizing her disgust with her schedule after the manager has adjusted the final schedules. Christy feels she is working more than her share of evening shifts on her day/evening position. Christy thinks she should be able to work fewer evening shifts because she

has a young family at home and is missing out on their growing years. Pam tells Christy that she should be happy to have a job when so many people are facing layoffs or are unemployed. Christy becomes angry and asks your opinion on the issue. Christy wants you to tell her who is right, Pam or Christy. What do you say? What is your best approach in dealing with these sensitive generational issues?

3. You are seeking a job as a registered nurse and have narrowed it down to two hospitals on the west coast. Both hospitals state that they have shared governance structures, and similar wages, professional development programs, and benefits. One hospital is unionized and the other is not. What other questions do you need to have answered before making your final decision between the two hospitals?

4. Consider your own nursing practice development needs as you prepare to graduate. What additional learning experiences will be most helpful to you? How do you plan to acquire these experiences?

References

Alspach, G. (2000). *From staff nurse to preceptor: A preceptor development program. Instructor's manual* (2nd ed.). Aliso Viejo, CA: American Association of Critical Care Nurses.

American Association of Colleges of Nursing. (2002). *Hallmarks of the professional nursing practice environment.* Retrieved July 22, 2007, from http://www.aacn.nche.edu/Publications/positions/hallmarks.htm

American Nurses Association. (2007). *About ANA.* Retrieved November 24, 2007, from http://www.nursingworld.org/FunctionalMenuCategories/AboutANA.aspx

AMN Healthcare. (2007). *AMN Healthcare: 2007 survey of nurse students.* San Diego: Author.

Angulo, N. (2002). The use of feminist pedagogical strategies to promote mathematics achievement by community college minority females. *Dissertation Abstracts International, 63*, 529.

Bally, J. (2007). The role of nursing leadership in creating a mentoring culture in acute care environments. *Nursing Economics, 25*(3), 143–148. Retrieved July 29, 2007, from http://www.medscape.com/viewarticle/559316_print

Beauregard, M., Davis, J., & Kutash, M. (2007). The graduate nurse rotational internship: A successful recruitment and retention strategy in medical-surgical services. *Journal of Nursing Administration, 37*(3), 115–118.

Benner, P. (1984). *From novice to expert: Excellence and power in clinical nursing practice.* Menlo Park, CA: Addison-Wesley.

Budd, K. W., Warino, L. S., & Patton, M. E. (2004). Traditional and non-traditional collective bargaining: Strategies to improve the patient care environment. *Journal of Issues in Nursing, 9*(1). Retrieved July 25, 2008, from http://www.medscape.com/viewarticle/490769

Caramanica, L. (2004). Shared governance: Hartford hospital's experience. *Online Journal of Issues in Nursing, 9*(1). Retrieved April 15, 2007, from http://www.nursingworld.org/MainMenuCategories/ANAMarketplace/ANAPeriodicals/OJIN/TableofContents/Volume92004/Number1January31/HartfordHospitalsExperience.aspx

Chou, S. M., Tang, F. I., Teng, Y. C., & Yen, M. (2003). Faculty's perceptions of humanistic teaching in nursing baccalaureate programs. *Journal of Nursing Research, 11*(1), 57–64.

Cronenwett, L., Sherwood, G., Barnsteiner, J., Disch, J., Johnson, J., Mitchell, P., et al. (2007). Quality and safety education for nurses. *Nursing Outlook, 55*(3), 122–131.

Etheridge, S. (2007). Learning to think like a nurse: Stories from new nurse graduates. *Journal of Continuing Education in Nursing, 38*(1), 24–30.

Green, A., & Jordan, C. (2004). Common denominators: Shared governance and work place advocacy—strategies for nurses to gain control over their practice. *Journal of Issues in Nursing, 9*(1). Retrieved July 25, 2008, from http://www.nursingworld.org/ MainMenuCategories/ANAMarketplace/ANAPeriodicals/OJIN/TableofContents/ Volume92004/Number1January31/SharedGovernanceandWorkPlaceAdvocacy.aspx

Halfer, D., & Graf, E. (2006). Graduate nurse perceptions of the work experience. *Nursing Economics, 24*(3), 150–155.

Hansten, R., & Washburn, M. (2001). Outcomes-based delivery. *American Journal of Nursing, 101*(2), 24A–24D.

Henderson, D., Sealover, P., Sharrer, V., Fusner, S., Jones, S., Sweet, S., et al. (2006). Nursing EDGE: Evaluating delegation guidelines in education. *International Journal of Nursing Education Scholarship, 3*(1), Article 15. Retrieved July 20, 2007, from http:// www.bepress.com/ijnes/vol3/iss1/art15

Hess, R. (2004). From bedside to boardroom—nursing shared governance. *Journal of Issues in Nursing, 9*(1). Retrieved July 25, 2008, from http://www.nursingworld.org/ mods/mod680/govtoc.htm

Indiana State Board of Nursing. (2008). Indiana State Board of Nursing: A compilation of the Indiana Code and Indiana Administrative Code. Retrieved November 23, 2007, from http://www.in.gov/pla/files/ISBN_2008_EDITION.pdf

Ironside, P. M. (2003). Trying something new: Implementing and evaluating narrative pedagogy using a multimethod approach. *Nursing Education Perspectives, 24*(3), 122–128.

Knowles, M. S. (1980). *The modern practice of adult education. Andragogy versus pedagogy.* Englewood Cliffs, NJ: Prentice Hall/Cambridge.

Kramer, M. (1974). *Reality shock: Why nurses leave nursing.* St. Louis: Mosby.

Maslow, A. (1968). *Toward a psychology of being.* Princeton, NJ: Van Nostrand.

McNiesh, S. (2007). Demonstrating holistic clinical judgment: Preceptors' perceptions of new graduate nurses. *Holistic Nursing Practice, 21*(2), 72–78.

National Council of State Boards of Nursing. (1995). Delegation: Concepts and decision-making process. *National Council Position Paper.* Retrieved July 27, 2007, from https:// www.ncsbn.org/323.htm

Nelson, J., Kummeth, P., Crane, L., Mueller, C., Olson, C., Schatz, T., et al. (2006). Teaching prioritization skills: A preceptor forum. *Journal for Nurses in Staff Development, 22*(4), 172–178.

Pitino, D. (2003). Gift giving. *Teaching PreK-8, 33*(8), 12–14.

Quality and Safety Education for Nurses. (2007). *Home page.* Retrieved June 6, 2007, from http://www.qsen.org

Rosenfeld, P., Smith, M., Iervolino, L., & Bowar-Ferres, S. (2004). Nurse residency program: A 5-year evaluation from the participants' perspective. *Journal of Nursing Administration, 34*(4), 188–194.

Schumacher, D. (2007). Caring behaviors of preceptors as perceived by new nursing graduate orientees. *Journal for Nurses in Staff Development, 23*(4), 186–192.

Sherman, R. (2006). Leading a multigenerational nursing workforce: Issues, challenges and strategies. *Online Journal of Issues in Nursing, 11*(2). Retrieved July 14, 2007, from http://www.medscape.com/viewarticle/536480

Starr, K., & Conley, V. (2006). Becoming a registered nurse: The nurse extern experience. *Journal of Continuing Education in Nursing, 37*(2), 86–92.

Wiseman, R, (2001). The ANA develops bill of rights for registered nurses: Know your rights in the workplace. *American Journal of Nursing, 101*(11), 55–56.

Zohar, A., & Dori, Y. J. (2003). Higher order thinking skills and low-achieving students: Are they mutually exclusive? *Journal of Learning Sciences, 12*(2), 145–181.

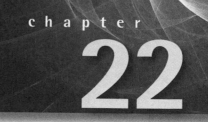

The Future of Nursing in Health Care

Pamela B. Koob and Monique Ridosh

LEARNING OUTCOMES

After reading this chapter you will be able to:

- Describe the changes in the philosophy of science that drive the future of nursing.
- Discuss the changes and challenges impacting the future of nursing in practice.
- Discuss the changes and challenges impacting the future of nursing in education.
- Discuss the changes and challenges impacting the future of nursing in research.
- Discuss the linkage of change events in practice, education, and research.
- Create a strategic plan for your own career pathway in the future.

The healthcare system and the nursing profession are at a critical turning point of transformation. New technologies, different models of care, shifts in the philosophy of science, consumer demand for cost-effective quality care, and an evidence-grounded profession are driving the healthcare system and nursing profession toward transformation. Rituals or the "ways we are used to doing things" are outdated and ineffective. To lead nursing into the future, "each leader must become a revolutionary in residence" (Porter-O'Grady & Malloch, 2007, p. 348).

Pathway for the Future

The purpose of this chapter is to review critical turning points of transformation for nursing and how they link to create a pathway for the future. The chapter will discuss four major arenas that will influence this pathway: 1) nursing philosophy, 2) nursing practice, 3) nursing education, and 4) nursing research. After discussing the complex conditions impacting transformation, the reader will be able to contemplate the linkages of these four elements to direct their own future career pathway. The chapter will also examine challenges that must be addressed to achieve nursing goals and standards of excellence for the future of nursing.

Future Pathway for Nursing Philosophy

While many nursing theorists, philosophers, and futurists provide perspectives to explicate visions of the future of nursing, Sister Callista Roy is one example of a theorist whose recent writings pose a vision to assist nurses planning for the future. Sr. Roy highlights the importance of transformation to integrate person with environment and promote unity in knowledge by collaboration. Emphasis is placed on the human ability to think and feel while sharing accountability for realizing the potential of all other human beings (Roy, 2000a). Sr. Roy envisioned the nurses' role in shaping the preferred future by being knowledgeable of visible and invisible issues of the environment.

Examples of visible issues and trends are emergence of the information age such as the electronic record and changing demographics including aging of the population, increased ethnic diversity, and widening income gap. Nurses need to be aware of common trends such as consumers may be better educated yet not necessarily better informed, and technological advances in pharmacology, genetics, and transplantation will often dramatically change practice. Healthcare reform with an emphasis on quality assurance, performance improvement, and cost of health care are other common visible issues. Invisible issues include personal and professional values and commitments. Sr. Roy defined the person to include "purposefulness of human existence, unity of purpose, activity and creativity, and value and meaning of life" (Roy, 2000b). Nurse leaders need knowledge of future issues and trends to engage in care models targeting the new consumer while maintaining regard for values and committments.

Futurists in nursing knowledge (Coile, 2001; Reed, 1995, 2006; Whall, Sinclair, & Parahoo, 2005) as well as experts in the history of nursing knowledge (Carper, 1978) inform

> **KEY TERM**
>
> **Futurist:** A forecaster of systems influenced by current and past trends and innovations. Predictions are shaped by social, organizational, political, and global perspectives.

the transformation of knowledge. New technology, practice models, and evidence-based nursing contribute to today's philosophical premise of nursing science. Reed (1995, 2006) stated that **neomodernism** is the current **philosophy of science** driving the future of nursing knowledge. Neomodernism links knowledge production and practice to generate scientific theory. It is a scientific philosophy that demands the use of new methods and technologies in nursing practice and research. Neomodernism blurs the dividing line between knowledge production and practice. "In neomodern thought, the nurse practitioner is not merely a knowledge consumer or user, but is a knowledge producer" (Reed, 2006, p. 36). According to neomodernist philosophy, the nurse and patient partner together to produce knowledge. This philosophy promotes the linkage of the nursing roles of practitioner, researcher, and educator to advance nursing knowledge and evidence-based nursing (EBN). Reed (2006) reported that the education system must change to educate nurses for the neomodern practice of EBN. (See Chapter 11 for more on evidence-based nursing.) "Neomodern clinicians need to be educated in how to employ various patterns of knowing—from aesthetic and empirical to technologic and sociopolitical—to generate theories of nursing in practice" (Reed, 2006, p. 37).

> **KEY TERM**
>
> **Neomodernism:** A philosophy of science linking knowledge production and practice to generate scientific theory.

> **KEY TERM**
>
> **Philosophy of science:** Assumptions and foundations of a discipline forming the body of knowledge for practice. Nursing's philosophy of science is based on knowledge acquired through quantitative and qualitative research. Theories generated through scientific inquiry are the basis of nursing's body of knowledge.

Future Pathway for Nursing Practice

The future of nursing practice is being transformed by multiple complex factors including consumer demands, data-driven initiatives for quality and safety, constant change at a rapid pace, and the need for universal access to care. The Institute of Medicine (IOM, 2003) stated that care must be safe, effective, patient-centered, timely, efficient, and equitable. The responsibility of ensuring that these practice initiatives are realized in all types of healthcare settings is critical for nurses. Safety and quality are at the core of every strategic plan for the future. The current and future healthcare environments are driven by the trend toward public reporting and increased scrutiny. Nursing executives and leaders are making quality and safety a top priority. The future of nursing practice is reviewed regarding standards for practice and the guiding principles for future patient care delivery.

The American Nurses Association outlines standards for practice to guide professional development for the future of nursing. Standards include evaluating the quality and effectiveness of care, evaluating one's own practice and adherence to professional standards, maintaining currency in education, contributing to professional development of others, acting ethically, working collaboratively, and utilizing evidence and research for practice.

The American Organization of Nurse Executives (AONE) taskforce established in 2005 described the guiding principles for future patient care delivery. These principles were developed based on the forecast of workforce shortage, the need to define future in order to prepare the workforce, the identification of priority changes, and emphasis on evidence-based practice and research. The AONE principles emphasized the core of nursing is knowledge and caring, and knowledge is both access-based and synthesized. These AONE principles can be applied to changes in healthcare organizations by nurse leaders to emphasize the maintainance of core values, critical thinking, provider and consumer relationships, and advocacy. Information and the toolkit for application of the AONE Guiding Principles are at the link http://www.aone.org/aone/resource/guidingprinciples.html (American Organization of Nurse Executives, 2005).

The following sections discuss some of the key trends influencing the future practice of nursing.

Changing Sociodemographics for Nurses

The demographic profile of the nursing profession as well as the public is rapidly changing. Most nurses are over 40 years of age (approximately 70 percent). The majority of nurses continue to be white; only 12 percent are Latino, African American, or Asian. Over 1 million nurses have an associate degree, 800,000 are diploma or baccalaureate graduates, and 275,000 have master's and/or a doctoral degree. In 1980, 3.7 percent of nurses worked as faculty members; that number has now decreased to 2 percent (Box 22-1). There is a shortage of registered nurses, and it is expected to worsen over the next 5–10 years (American Association of Colleges of Nursing [AACN], 2006).

Rating Tools for Healthcare Providers and Internet Health Information

Insurance providers have initiated a rating tool for clients who have Well-Point and/or Blue Cross/Anthem health insurance to evaluate their providers (Knopper, 2008). Physicians, advanced practice nurses, physician assistants, and nurse midwives are evaluated on a 30-point scale on the four criteria of trust, communication, availability, and environment. The survey provides data on

---

BOX 22-1   BARRIERS IN THE NURSING SHORTAGE

Many individuals seeking to enter the profession cannot be accommodated in nursing programs due to faculty and resource constraints.

The primary barriers to accepting all qualified students at nursing colleges and universities continue to be insufficient faculty, a limited number of clinical placement sites, and a lack of classroom space (AACN, 2008).

the provider-client relationship that indicate whether the respondents felt the providers were supportive, trustworthy, and encouraged informed decision making. It is limited in focus and is exclusive of critical data about quality and safety (Knopper, 2008). Other limitations to online provider surveys include concerns about the potential for fraudulent online submissions, providing access to information for clients who are not technically savvy, and development of valid tools that measure client-provider relationships as well as quality and

safety. Clients can also be overwhelmed by the plethora of reported data. Clients still need to have a nurse they feel they can communicate with and ask questions comparing care options and cost. However, online surveys are part of a growing trend toward online provider and agency rating systems. HealthGrades.com and Hospital Compare (http://www.hospitalcompare.hhs.gov) are other online survey tools available to the information-savvy consumer. The futurist nurse must be prepared to realize that client **satisfaction** and cost are going to drive healthcare decisions more than ever.

In the future, the Internet will be an increased source of health information for clients, and access to the information will be available on more portable minia-ture devices. The futurist nurse should act as an advocate to educate consumers on access to Internet health information. Importantly, nurses should help clients to evaluate the credibility of the data and information they find on the Internet. In this age of technology and knowledge explosion, futurist nurses should encourage clients to evaluate multiple sources of evidence and make informed decisions after deliberation with nurses, family members, and physicians.

Healthcare Infrastructure and Client Care Delivery Systems

Workplace environments may be "outdated, designed to support a now defunct clinical and financial model" (Arnold et al., 2006). Delivering excellence in nursing care is the standard, but this must be molded around environments that are focused on nursing outcome measures. Future models of care incor-porate teamwork, multidisciplinary collaboration, and technology that is min-iature, decreases work flow inefficiencies, and is designed to be nurse-friendly (Box 22-2). Infrastructure is changing to include private rooms for consumers, portable computer stations, and patient supply areas close in proximity to point of care. These changes are based on research to improve processes. Changes in workflow eliminate nonessential work and provide nurses more time for direct care activities (Arnold et al., 2006; American Academy of Nursing [AAN], 2008).

Improved Emergency Response Process

Natural disasters such as Hurricane Katrina and the September 11, 2001, attack have acted as catalysts to improve response to public health threats. The U.S.

BOX 22-2 HEALTHCARE TECHNOLOGY PROCESSES

Technology Drill Down is a process from a project called "Technology targets: A synthesized approach for identifying and fostering technological solutions to workflow inefficiencies on medical/surgical units." Results of this project may include:

- More input into the design of medical devices
- Computerized provider order entry
- 100 percent electronic medical records
- Improved ways of tracking supplies
  Technology must be intuitive to the nursing process; otherwise, nurses will work around it (AAN, 2008).

Department of Health and Human Services & Centers for Disease Control (2008), *Public Health Preparedness: Mobilizing State by State*, highlights improvements that have been made in the United States between 2002 and 2007. All states now have plans to receive and distribute supplies from the Strategic National Stockpile, a national repository of antibiotics and other life-saving medication. Additionally, all states now maintain 24-hour participation in the Health Alert Network, which allows for rapid exchange of public health information. The CDC reported that having professionals prepared for emerging health threats is critical to the safety of the public. The nurse must be educated and prepared to respond to public health and global threats, including pandemics. (See Chapter 12 for more on emergency planning and response.)

Future Pathway for Nursing Education

The ever-changing practice environment has created a cascade of changes in nursing education for faculty and students alike. "Nurse educators must be knowledgeable enough of the practice environment to design new curricula to ensure graduates have the requisite skills in areas that have been designed by the Institute of Medicine (2003) as essential for health care professionals—patient-centered care, evidence-based practice, quality improvement, interdisciplinary practice, and informatics" (Halstead, 2007, p. 117). A top priority among nursing educators, executives, and practitioners is developing the core educator **competencies** among faculty in order to teach the practice competencies to new graduates and the entire nursing workforce. These competencies do not exist uniformly in academia or the current healthcare system (NLN, 2005) (Box 22-3).

KEY TERM

Competencies: Measurable levels of knowledge, skills, and attitudes required to perform in a professional role.

> ### BOX 22-3   GAP IN RESEARCH REGARDING CURRICULUM CHANGE
>
> "The fundamentals of making curriculum decisions in a rapidly changing world with limited time and resources have not been adequately addressed in the literature" (Halstead, 2007, p. 107).

Nurses aware of the current trends and issues of the bedside are called to leadership. Healthcare organizations as well as educational institutions need to prepare successor leadership as nursing management begins retirement phase. Arnold et al. (2006) emphasized that the healthcare system and the public rely on nurses at the bedside and on the treatment frontline to take a leadership role in delivering and managing care. Progressive educational development of these nurses is critical for safety, quality, and leadership-based competencies. "Many believe that there is a leadership crisis in nursing at all levels; immediate action is required to develop leadership capabilities in our organizations and to establish a strong leader workforce for the future" (Arnold et al., 2006, p. 213).

The following sections discuss key trends in the future of nursing education to develop and sustain competencies in educators, new graduates, and experienced nurses.

Establishing Collaborative Relationships

Partnerships among schools of nursing, healthcare organizations, and various stakeholders such as consumers, governing agencies, and funding entities provide opportunities to advance the practice and leadership capabilities of students, faculty, nursing staff, and managers (Box 22-4). This has proven to be one way to approach the nursing leadership challenge at hand (Arnold et al., 2006). As examples, the federal government has partnered with universities to develop nursing expertise to promote the health of veterans, and collaborative relationships are commonly formed in shared governance structures with hospital systems and universities. Partnerships are formed at various levels of organizations and across

> ### BOX 22-4   TRANSFORMING NURSING EDUCATION
>
> "The overriding purpose of nursing education is to prepare individuals to meet the health care needs of the public; therefore, education programs must be well aligned with changes arising from health care reform" (National League for Nursing [NLN], 2005).

types of systems to improve outcomes and support excellence in healthcare and nursing education.

Continuing Education for Professional Development

Clinical environments are increasingly complex. New graduates and experienced nurses require continued skill development in communication, financial management, and outcomes management. Nurses have opportunities to participate in organizational educational programs for professional development. Examples are research conferences offering continuing education credits, in-service programs, or interdisciplinary grand rounds. Nurses must be knowledgeable regarding accreditation criteria such as core measurement data. Nurses can play a role in multidisciplinary programs to design measurement tools regarding satisfaction expectations to target areas of improvement. Hospitals are investing in new graduate nurse traineeships or residency programs to further develop the expertise of new nurses lasting anywhere from 3 months to a year. These programs provide a combination of didactic instruction pertinent to a specialty area and supportive mentorship to increase retention of new nurses. As the demand for quality and safety becomes ever more intense, so too will the demand for a highly skilled faculty and nursing workforce. It is imperative that undergraduate and graduate nursing curricula and continued nursing education programs focus strongly on these skills and competencies for future nurses.

Evolving Nurse Roles

"Nurse practitioners are becoming the comprehensive primary care practitioners of American medicine" (Apold, 2008, p. 107). The United States has seen an increased emphasis on primary care, which nurse practitioners provide a cost-effective alternative for. This trend has been paralleled by an increase in APN and physician assistant (PA) programs, and the tasks involved in primary care have become the basis of their practices (Bourgeault & Mulvale, 2006).

As health care continues to change rapidly, the need for changes in our traditional nursing roles has never been more apparent. Traditional models of health care have focused on curing illness. Today, however, health care must be client-directed, and nurses will be at the forefront of changes that will provide quality, cost-effective care for the betterment of the client, family, and community. The Doctor of Nursing Practice (DNP) may be an opportunity to advance nursing knowledge to improve the health of the nation. *The Essentials of Doctoral Education for Advanced Nursing Practice* (AACN, 2006) outlined the competencies for DNP programs. The DNP curriculum and educational standards and the measurement of client outcomes must be maintained as a **benchmark** of quality for the future of nursing education and practice.

> **KEY TERM**
>
> **Benchmark:** Quality performance measurement data shared among healthcare providers and organizations for quality improvement and safety. The National Committee for Quality Assurance (NCQA) maintains benchmarking data.

Future Pathway for Nursing Research

Evidence-based nursing practice (discussed in more detail in Chapter 11) is developing as a practice standard globally. The gap between published research and translating these findings into practice is recognized as a critical issue for the future of nursing. Using evidence to guide clinical practice is challenging in an environment with competing demands for time, resources, and budgetary or grant funding for research consultation and researcher salaries. A few key future trends influencing the future of nursing research are discussed in the following sections.

Innovative Approaches to the Integration of Practice and Research

Creating structures and support for nurses in hospitals, schools, and community organizations to use evidence in practice will promote excellent client outcomes. Some examples of strategies to implement evidence-based nursing practice are found in organizations that have achieved ANA Magnet recognition status (Box 22-5).

In 1983, the American Academy of Nursing's (AAN's) Taskforce on Nursing Practice in Hospitals conducted a study to determine common variables in hospitals that were influential in recruiting and retaining excellent nurses. Forty-one of the 163 organizations shared characteristics that became "Forces of Magnetism" in these "Magnet" organizations. The American Nurses Credentialing Center (ANCC) developed a **Magnet** designation in 1990. Now this designation has evolved into a recognition

> **KEY TERM**
>
> **Magnet:** A healthcare organizational environment that promotes a culture of professional development and quality patient outcomes within the global healthcare climate (ANCC, 2008).

BOX 22-5   EXAMPLES OF STRATEGIES TO INTEGRATE PRACTICE AND RESEARCH

- Create an evidence-based practice committee. Select champions from this committee who will act as change agents on their practice units.
- Require attendance at a yearly research conference for all nurses.
- Form collaborative research teams consisting of faculty and clinicians.
- Identify senior nurse researchers who will provide mentorship and oversight to the clinical research.
- Require funding for research consultation in hospital operational budgets.
- Establish monthly research grand rounds.
- Encourage nurses to submit a clinically based study for a poster or presentation at a research conference.
- Revise infection control and other policies and procedures to reflect the current literature for evidence. Cite literature references for all policies.

program to acknowledge organizations providing nursing excellence. The program is a mechanism to benchmark excellence for consumers and professionals. The Magnet program is based on research regarding quality indicators and standards of practice. The program can be viewed as a framework for dissemination of best practice strategies to professionals. "Approximately 4.79% of all health care organizations in the United States have achieved ANCC Magnet Recognition® status" (ANCC, 2007).

In 2008, the framework was revised based on statistical analysis of evaluations. The evaluation findings resulted in a reorganization of Forces of Magnetism evidence into groups, leading to a new empirical model for the program. (See Figure 22-1). The five components of the framework model are transformational leadership, structural empowerment, exemplary professional practice, new knowledge including innovation and improvements, and empirical quality results (ANCC, 2008):

- Transformational leadership is essential to the success of today's nurse administrator. A transformational leader will prepare nurses for future challenges. The mindset of this leader must be that of a futurist to prepare the organization to be engaged in the change process. Organizations today are revising their strategic plans and creating new visions to meet the demands

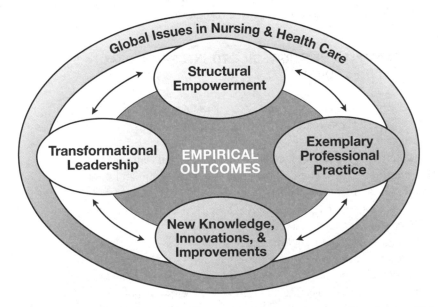

Figure 22-1 2008 Magnet Model. *Source:* © 2008 American Nurses Credentialing Center. All Rights Reserved.

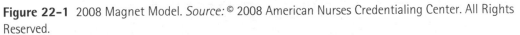

of the future. For example, a change in mission to provide services to consumers regardless of ability to pay may lead an organization to expand outpatient clinical services and strengthen community programs and clinical resource management to link the uninsured with health services that will ease the burden of expensive emergency room utilization for primary care services. The transformational leader would reallocate resources and engage staff to promote health based on priorities of organization.

- The second component of the framework, structural empowerment, refers to the development of new structures and processes that will engage the organization to meet goals and desired outcomes. Innovative programs such as Transforming Care at the Bedside (TCAB), an initiative led by the Robert Wood Johnson Foundation and the Institute for Health Care Improvement, created a framework for change on medical/surgical units in four categories: safe and reliable care, vitality and teamwork, patient-centered care, and value-added care processes.

- Exemplary professional practice, the third component, is considered the "essence" of a Magnet organization. Professional practice is demonstrated by nurses applying new knowledge and evidence in practice. Nurses now are engaged in practice councils and shared governance to act as change agents.

- New knowledge, innovation, and improvements are the fourth component of the model, and they incorporate all prior components of leadership, empowerment, and exemplary practice to produce new models of care. This component is the application of existing and new evidence to contribute to the body of nursing knowledge. Organizations are revising the patient care model so it is grounded in theory, and are applying the model to enhance the nursing process.

- Empirical quality, the fifth component, focuses on outcome measurement. Organizations must be accountable for producing results versus simply changing structure and processes. Qualitative benchmarking will occur in areas of clinical outcomes related to nursing, workforce outcomes, patient and consumer outcomes, and organizational outcomes. The question now is, "What difference have you made?" (ANCC, 2008).

This Magnet model utilizes outcome measurement and documentation. The Magnet vision focuses on the communication of knowledge in the global delivery of nursing care. This is evidenced by the charge to continuously strive for discovery and innovation to lead the future of the nursing profession. As healthcare reform evolves, magnetism contributes to the success of organizations. It provides direction for organizations to survive in the climate of nursing shortage and to maintain excellent patient outcomes. Coile (2001), a healthcare futurist, suggested the Magnet hospital culture favorably impacts recruitment and retention of nurses more significantly than wages.

KEY TERM

Information literacy: The ability to identify the need for information, search appropriate databases for it, evaluate the results, and utilize the information.

Integrating Evidence–Based Practice and Information Literacy

"In the new millennium, healthcare environments will increasingly demand nurses to be flexible, innovative and 'information literate' professionals, able to solve complex patient problems by utilizing the best available evidence" (Shorten, Wallace, & Crookes, 2001, p. 86). Nurses now need competency in **information literacy** as a tool for lifelong learning. They also must have the skills to access and process the vast information provided by the software utilized in bedside hospital computer systems. Nurses practicing today frequently have a mixed skill set because the majority of nurses were initially trained in the traditional classroom where they accessed material in a physical library building. The ability to access current materials online has increased the volume and changed the type of information that needs to be processed.

To be information literate, the nurse must be able to identify the need for information, search appropriate databases, evaluate results, and utilize the information. The patient consumer in today's healthcare environment is information-savvy. The nurse must be prepared to quickly identify keywords of a topic to search and retrieve information that is accurate and reliable for patient education. Selecting appropriate databases is an important first step to finding appropriate information. Some current databases include Medline, Cumulative Index to Nursing and Allied Health (CINAHL), Cochrane Database of Systematic Reviews, and HealthSource, Consumer edition. Searching keywords in various databases will yield different results, and basic search techniques such as using the Boolean operators AND, OR, or NOT can limit search results. Using wildcards expands searches by determining the root of words and adding "*" to ensure that all endings of a word are included in the search. For example, a primary care nurse performs a literature review on childhood obesity for parents using the database Health Source—Consumer edition. Searching with the keywords "child*" and "obesity" yields over 700 articles. Narrowing the search by adding the keywords "diet" and "nutrition" then yields about 50 articles with pertinent consumer information. The final step for the nurse is to evaluate the information based on the reliability of the source and the validity of the content. Following this process to filter articles should yield information and materials that can be utilized to provide current patient education.

Linking Change Events in Practice, Education, and Research

Porter-O'Grady and Malloch (2007) compare the old healthcare paradigm with the new. Hospital-based nursing was the hallmark of nursing in years past. Today, most procedures are done on an outpatient or overnight basis. Care models are designed to bring the center of care to the client's community. Telehealth, school clinics, and mobile vans that travel to schools and nursing homes are commonplace. Hierarchical management is no longer the norm as organizational decision making flows in all directions (Porter-O'Grady & Malloch). Technology, miniaturization, and globalization have altered how we practice and do business. Today nurses at all levels of the organizational structure are involved in decentralized budgeting, shared governance, and strategic planning. The nurse is not an employee, but a career-focused professional. Focus has moved from "sick care" to health care and promotion, prevention, and continuity of care. Cost containment is still important, but "customer" satisfaction and caregiver/agency accountability are vital. Documentation has moved from being written to being electronically recorded.

Thus, nurses are challenged to provide high-quality, cost-effective, and efficient care in a more complex environment with scarcer resources. Creativity is valued. Nurses are in a unique position to redefine the role of nursing to positively influence health care in this country as well as internationally. Nurses today have more opportunities to be a part of improving health care for our country by providing more preventative services. Nursing professionals can make a tremendous difference in preventing and controlling disease as well as improving outcomes for those who have the potential to develop a chronic illness; they can also decrease morbidities in those individuals who already have chronic problems. There has never been a better time for nurses to be creative, visible, and present in our communities. Now is the time for nurses to be active participants in the prevention of healthcare problems as well as making it known publicly who nurses are and what nurses do.

Summary

This chapter has summarized key turning points for the future transformation of nursing philosophy, practice, education, and research. Health care has changed drastically over the past century. Citizens are more involved and participatory in their health care. Advances in technology will continue to be a driving force for change. Consumers are becoming more Internet-savvy. Providers are using the Internet for telemedicine and communication with their patients. Nurses will need to increasingly focus on health promotion and preventive care for the community and the public. Futurist thinking will drive changes in organizational structure to achieve the desired outcomes and demonstrate nursing excellence. Nursing professionals have a major role to play in improving care outcomes through the application of evidence-based care and information literacy. The futurist nurse is one who is grounded in values and commitment and advanced knowledge in evidence-based delivery of care within a complex healthcare system.

Key Terms

- **Benchmark:** Quality performance measurement data shared among healthcare providers and organizations for quality improvement and safety. The National Committee for Quality Assurance (NCQA) maintains benchmarking data.
- **Competencies:** Measurable levels of knowledge, skills, and attitudes required to perform in a professional role.
- **Futurist:** A forecaster of systems influenced by current and past trends and innovations. Predictions are shaped by social, organizational, political, and global perspectives.
- **Information literacy:** The ability to identify the need for information, search appropriate databases for it, evaluate the results, and utilize the information.
- **Magnet:** A healthcare organizational environment that promotes a culture of professional development and quality patient outcomes within the global healthcare climate (ANCC, 2008).
- **Neomodernism:** A philosophy of science linking knowledge production and practice to generate scientific theory.
- **Philosophy of science:** Assumptions and foundations of a discipline forming the body of knowledge for practice. Nursing's philosophy of science is based on knowledge acquired through quantitative and qualitative research. Theories generated through scientific inquiry are the basis of nursing's body of knowledge.
- **Satisfaction:** A measure of the quality of a service or organization based on consumer or employee perceptions. Satisfaction ratings provide outcome measurement, contributing to consumerism and improvement processes to increase productivity and retention.

Reflective Practice Questions

1. How do you see yourself as a contributor to a standard of excellence in the future of nursing?
2. You are on a multidisciplinary team that is developing a patient satisfaction survey for completion at discharge. What questions do you feel reflect the most critical aspects of patient satisfaction that are a direct result of nursing care?
3. In the next 5 years, approximately 340,000 nurses are expected to retire from the profession. Many nurses have already worked 30 to 40 years. What educational and care delivery models will capitalize on the collaboration of experienced nurses with new graduates to enhance nursing excellence? As

a new graduate, what type of mentorship are you seeking? What will you contribute back to your mentor?

4. Which nursing content or courses do you think are less relevant or should be changed in the nursing curriculum? How can nursing educators change what has been traditionally taught and teach it in a truly innovative way? For example, should pharmacology be taught differently since the era of PDAs and electronic PDRs?

5. How will you develop financial management skills and an understanding of the operational budget in your workplace? What approaches to nursing budget development will give nurses the best preparation to balance the quality-cost equation in the future?

6. Taking risks and being able to make mistakes (at least non-life-threatening ones) are essential to innovation and transformation. Reflect on an innovative practice idea that you would like to implement in practice. How would you act as a change agent? What are the best strategies for advancing your idea to the nurses, physicians, and other healthcare professionals on your team? What kind of evidence would you provide that led you to think this might improve outcomes or make a difference? If your idea does not work, how could you use this as a learning tool for future progress?

7. How much more education do you feel you need in nursing? Where do you see yourself in the profession in 5 years? Ten years? Have you thought about getting a master's degree in nursing, or becoming a nurse practitioner, nurse anesthetist, or other advanced practice nurse? Where would you start with your plan and how would you accomplish this?

8. How do we enhance research skills in our current nursing workforce? How should we engage senior nurse researchers in the patient care environment with other nurses and healthcare professionals?

9. How should we more effectively prepare nurses to integrate evidence-based practice and information literacy in practice settings?

References

American Academy of Nursing. (2008). *Study, "Technology targets: A synthesized approach for identifying and fostering technological solutions to workflow inefficiencies on medical/surgical units."* Retrieved September 1, 2008, from http://www.aannet.org/i4a/pages/index.cfm?pageid=3318

American Association of Colleges of Nursing. (2004). *Position statement on the practice doctorate in nursing.* Retrieved April 10, 2008, from http://www.aacn.nche.edu/DNP/DNPPositionStatement.htm

American Association of Colleges of Nursing. (2006). *The essentials of doctoral education for advanced practice nursing*, pp. 1–28. Retrieved April 2, 2008, from www.aacn.nche. edu/DNP/pdf/Essentials.pdf

American Association of Colleges of Nursing. (2008). *Nursing faculty shortage.* Retrieved April 8, 2008, from http://www.aacn.nche.edu/Media/factsheets/nursingfaculty shortage.htm

American Nurses Credentialing Center. (2008). *Announcing a new model for ANCC's Magnet Recognition Program®.* Retrieved August 28, 2008, from http://www.nurse credentialing.org/Magnet/NewMagnetModel.aspx

American Nurses Credentialing Center. (2007). *Growth of the program.* Retrieved April 20, 2008, from http://www.nursecredentialing.org/magnet/growth.html

American Organization of Nurse Executives (2005). AONE Guiding Principles for Future Patient Care Delivery Toolkit. Retrieved September 1, 2008, from http://www.aone. org/aone/resource/guidingprinciples.html

Apold, S. (2008). The doctor of nursing practice: Looking back, moving forward. *The Journal for Nurse Practitioners, 4*(2), 101–109.

Appleby, J. (2007). *Wellpoint Doctors to get Zagat Rating.* Retrieved September 1, 2008, from http://www.usatoday.com/money/industries/health/2007-10-21-wellpoint-zagat_N.htm

Arnold, L., Campbell, A., Dubree, M., Fuchs, M. A., Davis, N., Hertzler, B., et al. (2006). Priorities and challenges of health system nursing executives: Insights for nurse educators. *Journal of Professional Nursing, 22*(4), 213–220.

Baker, L., Wagner, T., Singer, S., & Bundorf, M. (2003). Use of the Internet and email for health care information: Results from a national survey. *Journal of the American Medical Association, 289*(18), 2400–2406.

Bourgeault, I. L., & Mulvale, G. (2006). Collaborative health care teams in Canada and the USA: Confronting the structural embeddedness of medical dominance. *Health Sociology Review, 15*(5), 481–494.

Carper, B. A. (1978). Fundamental patterns of knowing in nursing. *Advances in Nursing Science, 1,* 13–23.

Coile, R. (2001). Magnet hospitals use culture, not wages, to solve nursing shortage. *Journal of Healthcare Management, 46*(4), 224–227.

Halstead, J. (2007). *Nurse educator competencies.* New York: National League for Nursing.

Institute of Medicine. (2003). *Health professions education: A bridge to quality.* Washington, DC: National Academies Press.

Knopper, M. (2008). The clinician is in, but how good is the service? *Clinician Reviews, 18*(3), 18.

National League for Nursing. (2005). *Position statement transforming nursing education.* Retrieved April 22, 2008, from www.nln.org//aboutnln/PositionStatements/ transforming 052005.pdf

Porter-O'Grady, T., & Malloch, K. (2007). *Quantum leadership. A resource for health care innovation.* Sudbury, MA: Jones and Bartlett.

Reed, P. G. (1995). A treatise on nursing knowledge development for the 21st century: Beyond postmodernism. *Advances in Nursing Science, 17,* 70–84.

Reed, P. G. (2006). Commentary on neomodernism and evidence-based nursing: Implications for the production of nursing knowledge. *Nursing Outlook, 54,* 36–38.

Roy, Sr. Callista (2000a) A theorist envisions the future and speaks to nursing administrators. *Nursing administration quarterly, 24*(2), 1–12.

Roy, Sr. Callista. (2000b). The visible and invisible fields that shape the future of the nursing care system. *Nursing Administration Quarterly, 25*(1), 119–131.

Shorten, A., Wallace, M., & Crookes, P. (2001). Developing information literacy: A key to evidence-based nursing. *International Nursing Review, 48,* 86–92.

U.S Department of Health and Human Services & Centers for Disease Control. (2008). Public Health Preparedness: Mobilizing State by State. A CDC Report on the Public Health Emergency Preparedness Cooperative Agreement. Retrieved August 27, 2008, from http://emergency.cdc.gov/publications/feb08phprep/pdf/feb08phprep.pdf

Whall, A., Sinclair, M., & Parahoo, K. (2005). A philosophic analysis of evidence based nursing: Recurrent themes, metanarratives, and exemplar cases. *Nursing Outlook, 54,* 30–35.

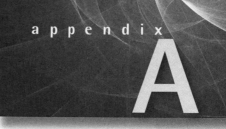

Code of Ethics for Nurses

Preface

Ethics is an integral part of the foundation of nursing. Nursing has a distinguished history of concern for the welfare of the sick, injured, and vulnerable and for social justice. This concern is embodied in the provision of nursing care to individuals and the community. Nursing encompasses the prevention of illness, the alleviation of suffering, and the protection, promotion, and restoration of health in the care of individuals, families, groups, and communities. Nurses act to change those aspects of social structures that detract from health and well-being. Individuals who become nurses are expected not only to adhere to the ideals and moral norms of the profession but also to embrace them as a part of what it means to be a nurse. The ethical tradition of nursing is self-reflective, enduring, and distinctive. A code of ethics makes explicit the primary goals, values, and obligations of the profession.

The Code of Ethics for Nurses serves the following purposes:

- It is a succinct statement of the ethical obligations and duties of every individual who enters the nursing profession.
- It is the profession's nonnegotiable ethical standard.
- It is an expression of nursing's own understanding of its commitment to society.

There are numerous approaches for addressing ethics; these include adopting or ascribing to ethical theories, including humanist, feminist, and social ethics, adhering to ethical principles, and cultivating virtues. The

Code of Ethics for Nurses reflects all of these approaches. The words "ethical" and "moral" are used throughout the Code of Ethics. "Ethical" is used to refer to reasons for decisions about how one ought to act, using the above-mentioned approaches. In general, the word "moral" overlaps with "ethical" but is more aligned with personal belief and cultural values. Statements that describe activities and attributes of nurses in this Code of Ethics are to be understood as normative or prescriptive statements expressing expectations of ethical behavior.

The Code of Ethics uses the term *patient* to refer to recipients of nursing care. The derivation of this word refers to "one who suffers," reflecting a universal aspect of human existence. Nevertheless, it is recognized that nurses also provide services to those seeking health as well as those responding to illness, to students and to staff, in healthcare facilities as well as in communities. Similarly, the term *practice* refers to the actions of the nurse in whatever role the nurse fulfills, including direct patient care provider, educator, administrator, researcher, policy developer, or other. Thus, the values and obligations expressed in this Code of Ethics apply to nurses in all roles and settings.

The Code of Ethics for Nurses is a dynamic document. As nursing and its social context change, changes to the Code of Ethics are also necessary. The Code of Ethics consists of two components: the provisions and the accompanying interpretive statements. There are nine provisions. The first three describe the most fundamental values and commitments of the nurse; the next three address boundaries of duty and loyalty, and the last three address aspects of duties beyond individual patient encounters. For each provision, there are interpretive statements that provide greater specificity for practice and are responsive to the contemporary context of nursing. Consequently, the interpetive statements are subject to more frequent revision than are the provisions. Additional ethical guidance and detail can be found in ANA or constituent member association position statements that address clinical, research, administrative, educational, or public policy issues.

Code of Ethics for Nurses with Interpretive Statements provides a framework for nurses to use in ethical analysis and decision making. The Code of Ethics establishes the ethical standard for the profession. It is not negotiable in any setting nor is it subject to revision or amendment except by formal process of the House of Delegates of the ANA. The Code of Ethics for Nurses is a reflection of the proud ethical heritage of nursing, a guide for nurses now and in the future.

Code of Ethics for Nurses

1   The nurse, in all professional relationships, practices with compassion and respect for the inherent dignity, worth, and uniqueness of every individual, unrestricted by considerations of social or economic status, personal attributes, or the nature of health problems.
    1.1 Respect for human dignity
    1.2 Relationships to patients
    1.3 The nature of health problems
    1.4 The right to self-determination
    1.5 Relationships with colleagues and others

2   The nurse's primary commitment is to the patient, whether an individual, family, group, or community.
    2.1 Primacy of the patient's interests
    2.2 Conflict of interest for nurses
    2.3 Collaboration
    2.4 Professional boundaries

3   The nurse promotes, advocates for, and strives to protect the health, safety, and rights of the patient.
    3.1 Privacy
    3.2 Confidentiality
    3.3 Protection of participants in research
    3.4 Standards and review mechanisms
    3.5 Acting on questionable practice
    3.6 Addressing impaired practice

4   The nurse is responsible and accountable for individual nursing practice and determines the appropriate delegation of tasks consistent with the nurse's obligation to provide optimum patient care.
    4.1 Acceptance of accountability and responsibility
    4.2 Accountability for nursing judgment and action
    4.3 Responsibility for nursing judgment and action
    4.4 Delegation of nursing activities

5   The nurse owes the same duties to self as to others, including the responsibility to preserve integrity and safety, to maintain competence, and to continue personal and professional growth.
5.1 Moral self-respect
5.2 Professional growth and maintenance of competence
5.3 Wholeness of character
5.4 Preservation of integrity

6   The nurse participates in establishing, maintaining and improving health care environments and conditions of employment conducive to the provision of quality health care and consistent with the values of the profession through individual and collective action.
6.1 Influence of the environment on moral virtues and values
6.2 Influence of the environment on ethical obligations
6.3 Responsibility for the health care environment

7   The nurse participates in the advancement of the profession through contributions to practice, education, administration, and knowledge development.
7.1 Advancing the profession through active involvement in nursing and in health care policy
7.2 Advancing the profession by developing, maintaining, and implementing professional standards in clinical, administrative, and educational practice
7.3 Advancing the profession through knowledge development, dissemination, and application to practice

8   The nurse collaborates with other health professionals and the public in promoting community, national, and international efforts to meet health needs.
8.1 Health needs and concerns
8.2 Responsibilities to the public

9   The profession of nursing, as represented by associations and their members, is responsible for articulating nursing values, for maintaining the integrity of the profession and its practice, and for shaping social policy.
9.1 Assertion of values
9.2 The profession carries out its collective responsibility through professional associations
9.3 Intraprofessional integrity
9.4 Social reform

American Nurses Association Constituent Member Associations

Links to all state agencies can be found at http://www.ncsbn.org

Alabama State Nurses' Association (ASNA)
360 North Hull Street
Montgomery, Alabama 36104-3658
(334) 262-8321
Fax (334) 262-8578
E-mail: edasna@bellsouth.net
www.alabamanurses.org/
*Office Hours: 8:00am–4:00pm
Central

Alaska Nurses Association (AaNA)
3701 East Tudor Road, Suite 208
Anchorage, Alaska 99507-1069
(907) 274-0827
Fax (907) 272-0292
E-mail: tom@aknurse.org
www.aknurse.org/
*Office Hours: 8:00am–4:30pm
Alaska Time

Arizona Nurses Association (AzNA)
1850 E. Southern Ave, Suite #1
Tempe, Arizona 85282
(480) 831-0404
Fax (480) 839-4780
E-mail: info@aznurse.org
www.aznurse.org/
*Office Hours: 8:30am–4:30pm
Mountain

Arkansas Nurses Association (ArNA)
1123 S. University Avenue, #1015
Little Rock, Arkansas 72204
(501) 244-2363
Fax (501) 244-9903
E-mail: arna@arna.org
www.arna.org/
*Office Hours: 8:00am–4:30pm Central

ANA\California (ANA\C)
Louise Timmer, EdD, RN, President
(04/09)
Tricia Hunter, RN, Executive Administrator
1121 L Street, Suite 409
Sacramento, California 95814
(916) 447-0225
Fax (916) 442-4394
E-mail: ANAC@anacalifornia.org
www.anacalifornia.org/
*Office Hours: 9:00am–5:00pm Pacific

Colorado Nurses Association (CNA)
1221 South Clarkson Street, Suite 205
Denver, Colorado 80210
(303) 757-7483
Fax (303) 757-8833
E-mail: cna@nurses-co.org or
pstearnsrn@aol.com
www.nurses-co.org/
*Office Hours: 8:30am–4:30pm Mountain

Connecticut Nurses Association (CNA)
Meritech Business Park
377 Research Parkway, Suite 2D
Meriden, Connecticut 06450
(203) 238-1207
Fax (203) 238-3437
E-mail: polly@ctnurses.org
www.ctnurses.org/
*Office Hours: 9:00am–5:00pm Eastern

Delaware Nurses Association (DNA)
2644 Capitol Trail, Suite 330
Newark, Delaware 19711
(302) 368-2333 or (800) 381-0939
Fax (302) 366-1775
E-mail: sarah@denurses.org
www.denurses.org/
*Office Hours: 9:00am–4:00pm Eastern

**District of Columbia Nurses
Association, Inc. (DCNA)**
5100 Wisconsin Ave, NW Suite 306
Washington, DC 20016
(202) 244-2705
Fax (202) 362-8285
www.dcna.org/
*Office Hours: 9:00am–5:00pm Eastern

Federal Nurses Association (FedNA)
8515 Georgia Avenue, Suite 400
Silver Spring, MD 20910
(301) 628-5019
Fax (301) 628-5006
E-mail: FedNA@ana.org
www.nursingworld.org/FedNA
*Office Hours: 9:00am–4:30pm Eastern

Florida Nurses Association (FNA)
P.O. Box 536985
Orlando, Florida 32853-6985
(407) 896-3261
Fax (407) 896-9042
E-mail: info@floridanurse.org
www.floridanurse.org/
*Office Hours: 8:30am–4:30pm Eastern

Georgia Nurses Association (GNA)
3032 Briarcliff Road, NE
Atlanta, Georgia 30329-2655
(404) 325-5536
Fax (404) 325-0407
E-mail: ceo@georgianurses.org
www.georgianurses.org/
*Office Hours: 8:00am–4:30pm Eastern

Guam Nurses Association (GNA)
P.O. Box CG
Hagatna, Guam 96932
Tel/Fax (671) 477-6877
E-mail: guamnurs@ite.net
*Office Hours: 11:00am–1:00pm Pacific

Hawaii Nurses Association (HNA)
677 Ala Moana Boulevard
Suite 301
Honolulu, Hawaii 96813
(808) 531-1628
Fax (808) 524-2760
E-mail: info@hawaiinurses.org
www.hawaiinurses.org/
*Office Hours: 8:00am–4:30pm Aleutian Time

Idaho Nurses Association (INA)
2417 Bank Drive, Suite 111
Boise, Idaho 83705
(208) 345-0500
Fax (208) 345-1163
www.nursingworld.org/snas/id/index.htm
*Office Hours: 9:00am–5:30pm Mountain

Illinois Nurses Association (INA)
105 West Adams Street, Suite 2101
Chicago, Illinois 60603
(312) 419-2900 ext. 229
Fax (312) 419-2920
www.illinoisnurses.com/
*Office Hours: 9:00am–5:00pm Central

Indiana State Nurses Association (ISNA)
2915 North High School Road
Indianapolis, Indiana 46224
(317) 299-4575
Fax (317) 297-3525
ISNA@indiananurses.org
www.indiananurses.org/

Iowa Nurses Association (INA)
1501 42nd Street, Suite 471
West Des Moines, Iowa 50266
(515) 225-0495
Fax (515) 225-2201
E-mail: Info@iowanurses.org
www.iowanurses.org/
*Office Hours: 8:30am–4:00pm Central

Kansas State Nurses Association (KSNA)
1109 SW Topeka Blvd
Topeka, Kansas 66612
(785) 233-8638
Fax (785) 233-5222
www.nursingworld.org/snas/ks/index.htm
*Office Hours: 8:00am–4:30pm Central

Kentucky Nurses Association (KNA)
1400 South First Street
P.O. Box 2616
Louisville, Kentucky 40201-2616
(502) 637-2546
Fax (502) 637-8236
E-mail: executivedirector@kentuckynurses.org
www.kentucky-nurses.org/
*Office Hours: 8:00am–4:30pm Eastern

Louisiana State Nurses Association (LSNA)
5713 Superior Drive, Suite A-6
Baton Rouge, Louisiana 70816
(225) 201-0993
(800) 457-6378
Fax (225) 201-0971
E-mail: lsna@lsna.org
www.lsna.org/
*Office Hours: 9:00am–4:00pm Central

ANA-Maine (ANA-ME)
P.O. Box 3000, PMB #280
York, Maine 03909
(207) 667-0260
E-mail: info@anamaine.org
www.anamaine.org/

Maryland Nurses Association (MNA)
21 Governor's Court
Suite 195
Baltimore, Maryland 21244
(410) 944-5800
Fax (410) 944-5802
E-mail: info@marylandrn.org
www.marylandrn.org/
*Office Hours: 8:30am–4:30pm Eastern

**Massachusetts Association of
Registered Nurses (MARN)**
P.O. Box 285
Milton, Massachusetts 02186
(617) 990-2856
E-mail: info@marnonline.org
www.marnonline.org/

Michigan Nurses Association (MNA)
2310 Jolly Oak Road
Okemos, Michigan 48864-4599
(517) 349-5640 ext. 14
Fax (517) 349-5818
www.minurses.org/
*Office Hours: 9:00am–5:00pm Eastern

Minnesota Nurses Association (MNA)
1625 Energy Park Drive
St. Paul, Minnesota 55108
(651) 646-4807 ext. 152
or (800) 536-4662
Fax (651) 647-5301
www.mnnurses.org/
*Office Hours: 8:15am–4:30pm Central

Mississippi Nurses Association (MNA)
31 Woodgreen Place
Madison, Mississippi 39110
(601) 898-0670
Fax (601) 898-0190
www.msnurses.org/
*Office Hours: 8:00am–4:30pm Central

Missouri Nurses Association (MONA)
1904 Bubba Lane, P.O. Box 105228
Jefferson City, Missouri 65110-5228
(888) 662-MONA (toll-free)
(573) 636-4623
Fax (573) 636-9576
E-mail: info@missourinurses.org
www.missourinurses.org/
*Office Hours: 8:30am–4:30pm Central

Montana Nurses Association (MNA)
120 Old Montana State Highway
Clancy, Montana 59634
(406) 442-6710
Fax (406) 442-1841
E-mail: info@mtnurses.org
www.mtnurses.org/
*Office Hours: 8:30am–4:30pm
Mountain

Nebraska Nurses Association (NNA)
P.O. Box 82086
Lincoln, Nebraska 68501-2086
(402) 475-3859
Fax (402) 475-3961
E-mail: execnna@alltel.net
www.nebraskanurses.org/
*Office Hours: 8:00am–4:30pm Central

Nevada Nurses Association (NNA)
P.O. Box 34660
Reno, Nevada 89533
(775) 747-2333
Fax (775) 329-3334
E-mail: NNA@NVNurses.org
www.nvnurses.org/
*Office Hours: 8:30am to 4:30pm Pacific

New Hampshire Nurses Association (NHNA)
210 N. State St., Suite 1-A
Concord, New Hampshire 03301
(603) 225-3783
Fax (603) 228-6672
www.nhnurses.org/
*Office Hours: 9:00am–5:00pm Eastern

New Jersey State Nurses Association (NJSNA)
1479 Pennington Road
Trenton, New Jersey 08618-2661
(609) 883-5335 ext. 10
Fax (609) 883-5343
E-mail: njsna@njsna.org
www.njsna.org/
*Office Hours: 8:30am–4:30pm Eastern

New Mexico Nurses Association (NMNA)
P.O. Box 29658
Santa Fe, New Mexico 87592-9658
(505) 471-3324
Fax (877) 350-7499
www.nmna.org/
*Office Hours: 8:00am–5:00pm
Mountain

New York State Nurses Association (NYSNA)
11 Cornell Road
Latham, New York 12110
(518) 782-9400 ext. 279
Fax (518) 782-9530
www.nysna.org/
*Office Hours: 8:30am–5:00pm Eastern

North Carolina Nurses Association (NCNA)
103 Enterprise Street
Box 12025
Raleigh, North Carolina 27605
(919) 821-4250
Fax (919) 829-5807
www.ncnurses.org/
*Office Hours: 8:30am–4:30pm Eastern

North Dakota Nurses Association (NDNA)
531 Airport Road, Suite D
Bismarck, North Dakota 58504-6107
(701) 223-1385
Fax (701) 223-0575
E-mail: ndna@prodigy.net
www.ndna.org/
*Office Hours: 8:30am–4:30pm Central

Ohio Nurses Association (ONA)
4000 East Main Street
Columbus, Ohio 43213-2983
(614) 237-5414 ext. 1020
Fax (614) 237-6081
www.ohnurses.org/
*Office Hours: M–Th. 8:30am–4:00pm;
Fri. 8:30 am–2:00pm Eastern

Oklahoma Nurses Association (ONA)
6414 North Santa Fe, Suite A
Oklahoma City, Oklahoma 73116
(405) 840-3476
Fax (405) 840-3013
E-mail: ona.ed@oklahomanurses.org
www.oklahomanurses.org/
*Office Hours: 8:30am–5:00pm Central

Oregon Nurses Association (ONA)
18765 SW Boones Ferry Road
Tualatin, Oregon 97062
(503) 293-0011
Fax (503) 293-0013
E-mail: ona@oregonrn.org
www.oregonrn.org/
*Office Hours: 8:30am–5:00pm Pacific

Pennsylvania State Nurses Association (PSNA)
2578 Interstate Drive, Suite 101
Harrisburg, Pennsylvania 17110-9601
(717) 657-1222 x200 or (888) 707-7762
Fax (717) 657-3796
www.panurses.org/
*Office Hours: 8:30am–4:30pm Eastern

Rhode Island State Nurses Association (RISNA)
67 Park Place
Pawtucket, Rhode Island 02860
(401) 305-3330
Fax (401) 305-3332
E-mail: risna@prodigy.net
www.risnarn.org/
*Office Hours: Monday–Thursday
10:00am–3:30pm Eastern

South Carolina Nurses Association (SCNA)
1821 Gadsden Street
Columbia, South Carolina 29201
(803) 252-4781
Fax (803) 779-3870
www.scnurses.org/
*Office Hours: 8:30am–4:30pm Eastern

South Dakota Nurses Association (SDNA)
P.O. Box 1015
116 N. Euclid
Pierre, South Dakota 57501-1015
(605) 945-4265
Fax (605) 945-4265
E-mail: sdnurse@midco.net
www.sdnursesassociation.org/
*Office Hours: 8:00am–5:00pm Central

Tennessee Nurses Association (TNA)
545 Mainstream Drive, Suite 405
Nashville, Tennessee 37228-1296
(615) 254-0350
Fax (615) 254-0303
www.tnaonline.org/
*Office Hours: 8:30am–4:30pm Central

Texas Nurses Association (TNA)
7600 Burnet Road Suite 440
Austin, Texas 78757-1292
(512) 452-0645
Fax (512) 452-0648
E-mail: memberinfo@texasnurses.org
www.texasnurses.org/
*Office Hours: 8:00am–5:00pm Central

Utah Nurses Association (UNA)
Donna Eliason, RN, President (01/08)
Executive Director (vacant)
4505 South Wasatch Blvd. #290
Salt Lake City, Utah 84124
(801) 272-4510
Fax (801) 293-8458
E-mail: una@xmission.com
www.utahnurses.org/
*Office Hours: Monday–Thursday
7:30am-3:30pm Mountain

Vermont State Nurses Association (VSNA)
100 Dorset Street, Suite 13
South Burlington, Vermont 05403-6241
(802) 651-8886
Fax (802) 651-8998
E-mail: vtnurse@prodigy.net
www.vsna-inc.org/
*Office Hours: Monday–Thursday
9:00am–3:00pm Eastern

Virgin Islands State Nurses Association (VISNA)
PO Box 3617
Christiansted, U.S. Virgin Islands 00822
(340) 713-0293

Virginia Nurses Association (VNA)
7113 Three Chopt Road, Suite 204
Richmond, Virginia 23226
(804) 282-1808/2373
Fax (804) 282-4916
E-mail: VNA@virginianurses.com
www.virginianurses.com/
*Office Hours: 8:30am–5:00pm Eastern

Washington State Nurses Association (WSNA)
575 Andover Park West, Suite 101
Seattle, Washington 98188-3321
(206) 575-7979
Fax (206) 575-1908
E-mail:wsna@wsna.org
www.wsna.org/
*Office Hours: 8:30am–4:30pm Pacific

West Virginia Nurses Association (WVNA)
405 Capitol Street, Suite 600
P.O. Box 1946
Charleston, West Virginia 25301
(304) 342-1169 or (800) 400-1226
Fax (304) 414-3369
www.wvnurses.org/
*Office Hours: 8:30am–4:30pm Eastern

Wisconsin Nurses Association (WNA)
6117 Monona Drive, Suite 1
Madison, Wisconsin 53716
(608) 221-0383
Fax (608) 221-2788
www.wisconsinnurses.org/
*Office Hours: 7:30am–4:00pm Central

Wyoming Nurses Association (WNA)
PMB 101; 501 S Douglas Hwy, Ste A
Gillette, Wyoming 82717
(800) 795-6381
Fax (307) 266-2010
www.wyonurse.org/
*Office Hours: Monday–Friday 8:00am–5:00pm Mountain

*All office hours listed are local times.

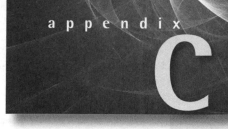

C

State Boards of Nursing

Alabama Board of Nursing
770 Washington Avenue
RSA Plaza, Ste 250
Montgomery, Alabama 36130-3900
Phone: 334.242.4060
Fax: 334.242.4360
Online: http://www.abn.state.al.us/

Alaska Board of Nursing
550 West Seventh Avenue Suite 1500
Anchorage, Alaska 99501-3567
Phone: 907.269.8161
Fax: 907.269.8196
Online: http://www.dced.state.ak.us/
   occ/pnur.htm

American Samoa Health Services
Regulatory Board
LBJ Tropical Medical Center
Pago Pago, American Samoa 96799
Phone: 684.633.1222
Fax: 684.633.1869
Online: N/A

Arizona State Board of Nursing
4747 North 7th Street, Suite 200
Phoenix, Arizona 85014-3653
Phone: 602.889.5150
Fax: 602.889.5155
Online: http://www.azbn.gov/

Arkansas State Board of Nursing
University Tower Building
1123 S. University, Suite 800
Little Rock, Arkansas 72204-1619
Phone: 501.686.2700
Fax: 501.686.2714
Online: http://www.arsbn.org/

California Board of Registered
   Nursing
1625 North Market Boulevard, Suite
   N-217
Sacramento, California 95834-1924
Phone: 916.322.3350
Fax: 916.574.8637
Online: http://www.rn.ca.gov/

California Board of Vocational Nurse and Psychiatric Technicians
2535 Capitol Oaks Drive, Suite 205
Sacramento, California 95833
Phone: 916.263.7800
Fax: 916.263.7859
Online: http://www.bvnpt.ca.gov/

Colorado Board of Nursing
1560 Broadway, Suite 1370
Denver, Colorado 80202
Phone: 303.894.2430
Fax: 303.894.2821
Online: http://www.dora.state.co.us/nursing/

Connecticut Board of Examiners for Nursing
Dept. of Public Health
410 Capitol Avenue, MS# 13PHO
P.O. Box 340308
Hartford, Connecticut 06134-0328
Phone: 860.509.7624
Fax: 860.509.7553
Online: http://www.state.ct.us/dph/

Delaware Board of Nursing
861 Silver Lake Blvd.
Cannon Building, Suite 203
Dover, Delaware 19904
Phone: 302.739.4500
Fax: 302.739.2711
Online: http://dpr.delaware.gov/boards/nursing/

District of Columbia Board of Nursing
Department of Health
Health Professional Licensing Administration
District of Columbia Board of Nursing
717 14th Street, NW
Suite 600
Washington, DC 20005
Phone: 877.672.2174
Fax: 202.727.8471
Online: http://hpla.doh.dc.gov/hpla/cwp/view,
    A,1195,Q,488526,hplaNav,|30661|,.asp

Florida Board of Nursing
Mailing Address:
4052 Bald Cypress Way, BIN C02
Tallahassee, Florida 32399-3252
Physical Address:
4042 Bald Cypress Way
Room 120
Tallahassee, FL 32399
Phone: 850.245.4125
Fax: 850.245.4172
Online: http://www.doh.state.fl.us/mqa/

Georgia Board of Nursing
237 Coliseum Drive
Macon, Georgia 31217-3858
Phone: 478.207.2440
Fax: 478.207.1354
Online: http://www.sos.state.ga.us/plb/rn

Georgia State Board of Licensed Practical Nurses
237 Coliseum Drive
Macon, Georgia 31217-3858
Phone: 478.207.2440
Fax: 478.207.1354
Online: http://www.sos.state.ga.us/plb/lpn

Guam Board of Nurse Examiners
Bldg. #123 Chalan Kareta
Vietnam Veteran's Highway
Mangilao, Guam 96923
Phone: 671.735.7406
Fax: 671.735.7413
Online: N/A

Hawaii Board of Nursing
Mailing Address:
PVLD/DCCA
Attn: Board of Nursing
P.O. Box 3469
Honolulu, Hawaii 96801

Physical Address:
King Kalakaua Building
335 Merchant Street, 3rd Floor
Honolulu, Hawaii 96813
Phone: 808.586.3000
Fax: 808.586.2689
Online: www.hawaii.gov/dcca/areas/pvl/
boards/nursing

Idaho Board of Nursing
280 N. 8th Street, Suite 210
P.O. Box 83720
Boise, Idaho 83720
Phone: 208.334.3110
Fax: 208.334.3262
Online: http://www2.state.id.us/ibn

Illinois Board of Nursing
James R. Thompson Center
100 West Randolph Street
Suite 9-300
Chicago, Illinois 60601
Phone: 312.814.2715
Fax: 312.814.3145
Online: http://www.idfpr.com/dpr/WHO/nurs.asp

Indiana State Board of Nursing
Professional Licensing Agency
402 W. Washington Street, Room W072
Indianapolis, Indiana 46204
Phone: 317.234.2043
Fax: 317.233.4236
Online: http://www.in.gov/pla/

Iowa Board of Nursing
RiverPoint Business Park
400 S.W. 8th Street
Suite B
Des Moines, Iowa 50309-4685
Phone: 515.281.3255
Fax: 515.281.4825
Online: http://www.iowa.gov/nursing

Kansas State Board of Nursing
Landon State Office Building
900 S.W. Jackson, Suite 1051
Topeka, Kansas 66612
Phone: 785.296.4929
Fax: 785.296.3929
Online: http://www.ksbn.org/

Kentucky Board of Nursing
312 Whittington Parkway, Suite 300
Louisville, Kentucky 40222
Phone: 502.429.3300
Fax: 502.429.3311
Online: http://www.kbn.ky.gov/

Louisiana State Board of Nursing
5207 Essen Lane, Suite 6
Baton Rouge, Louisiana 70809
Phone: 225.763.3570
225.763.3577
Fax: 225.763.3580
Online: http://www.lsbn.state.la.us/

Louisiana State Board of Practical Nurse
Examiners
3421 N. Causeway Boulevard, Suite 505
Metairie, Louisiana 70002
Phone: 504.838.5791
Fax: 504.838.5279
Online: http://www.lsbpne.com/

Maine State Board of Nursing
Regular mailing address:
158 State House Station
Augusta, Maine 04333
Street address (for FedEx & UPS):
161 Capitol Street
Augusta, Maine 04333
Phone: 207.287.1133
Fax: 207.287.1149
Online: http://www.maine.gov/boardofnursing/

Maryland Board of Nursing
4140 Patterson Avenue
Baltimore, Maryland 21215
Phone: 410.585.1900
Fax: 410.358.3530
Online: http://www.mbon.org/

Massachusetts Board of Registration in Nursing
Commonwealth of Massachusetts
239 Causeway Street, Second Floor
Boston, Maine 02114
Phone: 617.973.0800
800.414.0168
Fax: 617.973.0984
Online: http://www.mass.gov/dpl/boards/rn/

Michigan/DCH/Bureau of Health Professions
Ottawa Towers North
611 W. Ottawa, 1st Floor
Lansing, Michigan 48933
Phone: 517.335.0918
Fax: 517.373.2179
Online: http://www.michigan.gov/healthlicense

Minnesota Board of Nursing
2829 University Avenue SE
Minneapolis, Minnesota 55414
Phone: 612.617.2270
Fax: 612.617.2190
Online: http://www.nursingboard.state.mn.us/

Mississippi Board of Nursing
1935 Lakeland Drive, Suite B
Jackson, Mississippi 39216-5014
Phone: 601.987.4188
Fax: 601.364.2352
Online: http://www.msbn.state.ms.us/

Missouri State Board of Nursing
3605 Missouri Blvd.
P.O. Box 656
Jefferson City, Missouri 65102-0656
Phone: 573.751.0681
Fax: 573.751.0075
Online: http://pr.mo.gov/nursing.asp

Montana State Board of Nursing
301 South Park
P.O. Box 200513
Helena, Montana 59620-0513
Phone: 406.841.2345
Fax: 406.841.2305
Online: http://www.nurse.mt.gov

Nebraska Board of Nursing
301 Centennial Mall South
Lincoln, Nebraska 68509-4986
Phone: 402.471.4376
Fax: 402.471.1066
Online: http://www.hhs.state.ne.us/crl/nursing/nursingindex.htm

Nevada State Board of Nursing
5011 Meadowood Mall Way, Suite 300
Reno, Nevada 89502
Phone: 775.688.2620
Fax: 775.688.2628
Online: http://www.nursingboard.state.nv.us/

New Hampshire Board of Nursing
21 South Fruit Street
Suite 16
Concord, New Hampshire 03301-2341
Phone: 603.271.2323
Fax: 603.271.6605
Online: http://www.state.nh.us/nursing/

New Jersey Board of Nursing
P.O. Box 45010
124 Halsey Street, 6th Floor
Newark, New Jersey 07101
Phone: 973.504.6430
Fax: 973.648.3481
Online: http://www.state.nj.us/lps/ca/medical/
nursing.htm

New Mexico Board of Nursing
6301 Indian School Road, NE
Suite 710
Albuquerque, New Mexico 87110
Phone: 505.841.8340
Fax: 505.841.8347
Online: http://www.bon.state.nm.us/index.
html

New York State Board of Nursing
Education Bldg.
89 Washington Avenue
2nd Floor West Wing
Albany, New York 12234
Phone: 518.474.3817, Ext. 280
Fax: 518.474.3706
Online: http://www.nysed.gov/prof/nurse.htm

North Carolina Board of Nursing
3724 National Drive, Suite 201
Raleigh, North Carolina 27602
Phone: 919.782.3211
Fax: 919.781.9461
Online: http://www.ncbon.com/

North Dakota Board of Nursing
919 South 7th Street, Suite 504
Bismarck, North Dakota 58504
Phone: 701.328.9777
Fax: 701.328.9785
Online: http://www.ndbon.org/

**Northern Mariana Islands Commonwealth
  Board of Nurse Examiners**
Regular Mailing Address
P.O. Box 501458
Saipan, MP 96950
Street Address (for FedEx and UPS)
#1336 Ascencion Drive
Capitol Hill
Saipan, MP 96950
Phone: 670.664.4812
Fax: 670.664.4813
Online: N/A

Ohio Board of Nursing
17 South High Street, Suite 400
Columbus, Ohio 43215-3413
Phone: 614.466.3947
Fax: 614.466.0388
Online: http://www.nursing.ohio.gov/

Oklahoma Board of Nursing
2915 N. Classen Boulevard, Suite 524
Oklahoma City, Oklahoma 73106
Phone: 405.962.1800
Fax: 405.962.1821
Online: http://www.youroklahoma.com/nursing

Oregon State Board of Nursing
17938 SW Upper Boones Ferry Rd
Portland, Oregon 97224
Phone: 971.673.0685
Fax: 971.673.0684
Online: http://www.osbn.state.or.us/

Pennsylvania State Board of Nursing
P.O. Box 2649
Harrisburg, Pennsylvania 17105-2649
Phone: 717.783.7142
Fax: 717.783.0822
Online: http://www.dos.state.pa.us/bpoa/cwp/
view.asp?a=1104&q=432869

Rhode Island Board of Nurse Registration and Nursing Education
105 Cannon Building
Three Capitol Hill
Providence, Rhode Island 02908
Phone: 401.222.5700
Fax: 401.222.3352
Online: http://www.health.ri.gov/

South Carolina State Board of Nursing
Mailing Address:
P.O. Box 12367
Columbia, South Carolina 29211
Physical Address:
Synergy Business Park, Kingstree Building
110 Centerview Drive, Suite 202
Columbia, South Carolina 29210
Phone: 803.896.4550
Fax: 803.896.4525
Online: http://www.llr.state.sc.us/pol/nursing

South Dakota Board of Nursing
4305 South Louise Ave., Suite 201
Sioux Falls, South Dakota 57106-3115
Phone: 605.362.2760
Fax: 605.362.2768
Online: http://www.state.sd.us/doh/nursing/

Tennessee State Board of Nursing
227 French Landing, Suite 300
Heritage Place MetroCenter
Nashville, Tennessee 37243
Phone: 615.532.5166
Fax: 615.741.7899
Online: http://health.state.tn.us/Boards/
Nursing/index.htm

Texas Board of Nursing
333 Guadalupe, Suite 3-460
Austin, Texas 78701
Phone: 512.305.7400
Fax: 512.305.7401
Online: http://www.bon.state.tx.us

Utah State Board of Nursing
Heber M. Wells Bldg., 4th Floor
160 East 300 South
Salt Lake City, Utah 84111
Phone: 801.530.6628
Fax: 801.530.6511
Online: http://www.dopl.utah.gov/licensing/
nursing.html

Vermont State Board of Nursing
Office of Professional Regulation
National Life Building North F1.2
Montpelier, Vermont 05620-3402
Phone: 802.828.2396
Fax: 802.828.2484
Online: http://www.vtprofessionals.org/opr1/
nurses/

Virgin Islands Board of Nurse Licensure
P.O. Box 304247, Veterans Drive Station
St. Thomas, Virgin Islands 00803
Phone: 340.776.7131
Fax: 340.777.4003
Online: http://www.vibnl.org/

Virginia Board of Nursing
Department of Health Professions
Perimeter Center
9960 Mayland Drive, Suite 300
Richmond, Virginia 23233
Phone: 804.367.4515
Fax: 804.527.4455
Online: http://www.dhp.virginia.gov/nursing/

Washington State Nursing Care Quality Assurance Commission
Department of Health
HPQA #6
310 Israel Rd. SE
Tumwater, Washington 98501-7864
Phone: 360.236.4700
Fax: 360.236.4738
Online: https://fortress.wa.gov/doh/hpqa1/
hps6/Nursing/default.htm

West Virginia Board of Examiners for Registered Professional Nurses
101 Dee Drive
Charleston, West Virginia 25311
Phone: 304.558.3596
Fax: 304.558.3666
Online: http://www.wvrnboard.com/

West Virginia State Board of Examiners for Licensed Practical Nurses
101 Dee Drive
Charleston, West Virginia 25311
Phone: 304.558.3572
Fax: 304.558.4367
Online: http://www.lpnboard.state.wv.us/

Wisconsin Department of Regulation and Licensing
1400 E. Washington Avenue, RM 173
Madison, Wisconsin 53708
Phone: 608.266.0145
Fax: 608.261.7083
Online: http://www.drl.state.wi.us/

Wyoming State Board of Nursing
1810 Pioneer Avenue
Cheyenne, Wyoming 82001
Phone: 307.777.7601
Fax: 307.777.3519
Online: http://nursing.state.wy.us/

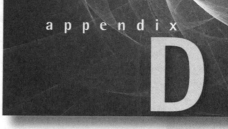

Professional Nursing Organizations

Academy of Medical Surgical Nurses
www.medsurgnurse.org

Academy of Neonatal Nursing
www.academyonline.org

Air & Surface Transport Nurses
Association
www.astna.org

American Academy of Ambulatory
Care Nursing
www.aaacn.org

American Academy of Nurse
Practitioners
www.aanp.org

American Academy of Nursing
www.aannet.org

American Assembly for Men in
Nursing
www.aamn.org

American Association for the History
of Nursing
www.aahn.org

American Association of Colleges of
Nursing
www.aacn.nche.edu

American Association of Critical-
Care Nurses
www.aacn.org

American Association of Diabetes
Educators
www.aadenet.org

American Association of Legal Nurse
Consultants
www.aalc.org

American Association of Managed
Care Nurses
www.aamcn.org

American Association of
Neuroscience Nurses
www.aann.org

American Association of Nurse
Anesthetists
www.aana.com

American Association of Nurse Attorneys
www.taana.org

American Association of Occupational Health Nurses
www.aaohn.org

American Association of Spinal Cord Injury Nurses
www.aascin.org

American Association on Intellectual and Development Disabilities
www.aamr.org

American College of Nurse Midwives
www.midwife.org

American College of Nurse Practitioners
www.acnpweb.org

American Holistic Nurses Association
www.ahna.org

American Medical Informatics Association
www.amia.org

American Nephrology Nurses' Association
www.annanurse.org

American Nurses Association
www.nursingworld.org

American Nursing Informatics Association
www.ania.org

American Organization of Nurse Executives
www.aone.org

American Psychiatric Nurses Association
www.apna.org

American Public Health Association
www.apha.org

American Radiological Nurses Association
www.arna.net

American Society of Ophthalmic-Registered Nurses, Inc.
www.asorn.org

American Society of Pain Management Nurses
www.aspmn.org

American Society of Perianesthesia Nurses
www.aspan.org

American Society of Plastic/Surgical Nurses
www.aspsn.org

Association for Professionals in Infection Control and Epidemiology
www.apic.org

Association of Pediatric Hematology/ Oncology Nurses
www.aphon.org

Association of periOperative Registered Nurses (AORN)
www.aorn.org

Association in AIDS Care (ANAC)
www.anacnet.org

Association of Camp Nurses
www.campnurse.org

Association of Community Health Nursing Educators
www.achne.org

Association of Nurses in AIDS Care
www.anacnet.org

Association of Pediatric Oncology Nurses
www.apon.org

Association of Rehabilitation Nurses
www.rehabnurse.org

Association of Women's Health, Obstetric and Neonatal Nurses
www.awhonn.org

Center for American Nurses
www.centerforamericannurses.org

Commission on Graduates of Foreign Nursing Schools
www.cgfns.org

Dermatology Nurses' Association
www.dna.inurse.com

Developmental Disabilities Nurses Association
www.ddna.org

Emergency Nurses Association
www.ena.org

Endocrine Nurses Association
www.endo-nurses.org

Hospice and Palliative Nurses Association
www.hpna.org

Infusion Nurses Society
www.ins1.org

International Council of Nurses
www.icn.ch

International Nurses Society on Addictions
www.intnsa.org

International Organization of Multiple Sclerosis Nurses
www.iomsn.org

International Society of Nurses in Genetics
www.isong.org

International Society of Psychiatric-Mental Health Nurses
www.ispn-psych.org

National Association for Associate Degree Nursing
www.noadn.org

National Association for Home Care and Hospice
www.nahc.org

National Association of Clinical Nurse Specialists
www.nacns.org

National Association of Directors of Nursing Administration Long Term Care
www.nadona.org

National Association of Hispanic Nurses
www.thehispanicnurses.org

National Association of Neonatal Nurses
www.nann.org

National Association of Nurse Massage Therapists
www.nanmt.org

National Association of Nurse Practitioners in Women's Health
www.npwh.org

National Association of Orthopedic Nurses
www.orthonurse.org

National Association of Pediatric Nurse Associates & Practitioners
www.napnap.org

National Association of School Nurses
www.nasn.org

National Black Nurses Association
www.nbna.org

National Conference of Gerontological Nurse Practitioners
www.ncgnp.org

National Gerontological Nurses Association
www.ngna.org

National League for Nursing
www.nln.org

National Nurses in Business Association, Inc.
www.nnba.net

National Nursing Staff Development Organization
www.nnsdo.org

National Organization of Nurse Practitioner Faculties
www.nonpf.com

National Student Nurses' Association
www.nsna.org

North American Nursing Diagnosis Association International
www.nanda.org

Nurses Christian Fellowship
www.intervarsity.org/ncf

Oncology Nursing Society
www.ons.org

Pediatric Endocrinology Nursing Society
www.pens.org

Preventive Cardiovascular Nurses Association
www.pcna.net

Respiratory Nursing Society
www.respiratorynursingsociety.org

Society for Vascular Nursing
www.svnnet.org

Society of Gastroenterology Nurses & Associates
www.sgna.org

Society of Otorhinolaryngology and Head-Neck Nurses
www.sohnnurse.com

Society of Pediatric Nurses
www.pedsnurses.org

Society of Trauma Nurses
www.traumanursesoc.org

Society of Urologic Nurses and Associates
www.suna.org

Space Nursing Society
www.spacenursingsociety

Transcultural Nursing Society
www.tcns.org

Wound, Ostomy and Continence Nurses Society
www.wocn.org

Index

Italicized page locators indicate a figure; tables are noted with a *t*